Cell and Tissue Based Molecular Pathology

Other books in this series:

Prayson: Neuropathology

Iacobuzio-Donahue & Montgomery: Gastrointestinal and Liver Pathology

Thompson: Head and Neck Pathology

O'Malley & Pinder: Breast Pathology

Thompson: Endocrine Pathology

Zhou & Magi-Galluzzi: Genitourinary Pathology

Hsi: Hematopathology

Sidawy & Ali: Fine Needle Aspiration Cytology

Nucci: Gynecologic Pathology

Zander & Farver: Pulmonary Pathology

Coming soon in this series:

Busam: Dermatopathology

Folpe & Inwards: Bone and Soft Tissue Pathology

Procop: Pathology of Infectious Disease

MOLECULAR PRINCIPLES

1 Molecular Biology Basics for the Pathologist

Ilka Warshawsky

INTRODUCTION

The completion of the Human Genome Project and research in molecular medicine are making genomic medicine an important area to enhance the quality of medical care, with genetics playing an increasingly significant role in the diagnosis, monitoring, and treatment of diseases. Genomic medicine is standard practice for diseases in which a single gene plays a prominent role; the role of genetic testing in complex disease traits in which multiple genes and nongenetic factors are implicated is less established.

Molecular pathology can be broadly defined as the testing of nucleic acids within a clinical context. The applications of molecular diagnostics span a range of human disorders, including hereditary, neoplastic, and infectious diseases. Molecular-based assays are used for specific purposes, including the following:

- Establishing the basis of an existing disorder (diagnostic testing)
- Determining the presence of a genetic condition when there are no obvious symptoms (predictive testing)
- Carrier testing
- Assessing a fetus for abnormalities (prenatal testing)
- Detecting cancer-causing gene mutations
- Selecting pharmacotherapy

Technologic advances such as automation for sequencing and genotyping, as well as the use of array technologies to screen for genetic alterations, to classify diseases, and to provide prognostic information, are allowing the translation of scientific knowledge into medical applications, both diagnostic and therapeutic.

The chapters that make up this book discuss molecular tools and techniques used in diagnostic molecular pathology laboratories, describe specific testing applications, and highlight quality assurance and regulatory aspects of molecular pathology.

THE HUMAN GENOME

All normal nucleated human cells other than sperm or ova contain 46 chromosomes arrayed in 23 pairs, with 1 chromosome in each pair maternally inherited and the other paternally inherited. Each chromosome is a highly ordered structure of double-stranded DNA that is compacted many times with the aid of structural DNA-binding proteins, including histone and nonhistone proteins.

It is estimated that the haploid genome contains approximately 3×10^9 base pairs of DNA, which are distributed among 22 autosomes, 2 sex chromosomes (X and Y), and mitochondria. Approximately 30,000 genes are encoded by this DNA, and these genes are distributed unevenly both across the human genome and within each chromosome; chromosome 1 has the most genes, and the Y chromosome has the fewest. It is estimated that more than 100,000 proteins are derived from the approximately 30,000 genes through the mechanism of alternative splicing.

Less than 10% of the human genome sequence encodes proteins; the remaining noncoding DNA consists of repetitive DNA and other sequences whose importance is not completely understood. Repetitive DNA may be repeats just a few nucleotides long, like CACACA, or the repeats can be up to a few hundred nucleotides long. Examples of the latter include short interspersed nuclear elements and long interspersed nuclear elements. In shorter repeats like di- and trinucleotide repeats, the number of repeating units can occasionally change during evolution and descent. Thus, they are useful markers for familial relationships and have been used in paternity testing and forensics. In pathology, they have been used to determine donor hematopoietic engraftment after allogeneic bone marrow transplantation, resolve specimen mix-ups, determine whether tissue fragments suspected of being contaminants in tissue blocks are "floaters," and identify maternal contamination in cultured amniocytes or chorionic villus samples.

GENE STRUCTURE AND FUNCTION

In its simplest form, a gene can be thought of as a segment of DNA containing the code for the amino acid sequence of a polypeptide chain and the regulatory sequences necessary for expression. Few genes, however, exist as continuous coding sequences; instead, most are interrupted by one or more noncoding regions or intervening sequences (introns). Introns alternate with coding sequences (exons), which ultimately encode the amino acid sequence of a protein. Introns are not present in the final messenger RNA (mRNA) but instead are removed during RNA splicing. Other important regions in genes include "start" and "stop" sequences for mRNA production, a 5' promoter region that includes sequences responsible for the proper initiation of transcription, and additional regulatory elements, including enhancers, silencers, and locus control regions that interact with cellular machinery to determine when, where, and to what level transcription (gene expression) occurs. At the 3' end of the gene is an untranslated region that contains a signal for the addition of adenosine residues (polyA tail), which aids in the stability of the RNA transcript (Figure 1-1).

DNA AND DNA REPLICATION

Each DNA molecule contains two polynucleotide strands that form an antiparallel double helix. Nucleotides, the building blocks of DNA, are composed of a nitrogenous base, a five-sided sugar molecule (deoxyribose), and a phosphate group. Successive nucleotides are joined together by phosphodiester bonds, and the two polynucleotide strands of DNA are held together by specific complementary pairs of bases. Adenine base-pairs with thymine using two hydrogen bonds; guanine base-pairs with cytosine using three hydrogen bonds. During DNA replication, a process mediated by several different proteins (including DNA polymerases), each existing DNA strand acts as a template for the production of a complementary strand. The base-pairing requirements ensure that each newly synthesized DNA strand has the correct nucleotide sequence (Figure 1-2).

TRANSCRIPTION AND TRANSLATION

The central dogma of molecular biology is that genes are composed of DNA, which is transcribed into RNA and then translated into proteins that make up living organisms (Figures 1-3 and 1-4).

RNA polymerase II mediates transcription and generates a single-stranded mRNA identical in sequence to the sense (coding) strand of DNA and complementary to the antisense (noncoding) strand except that RNA possesses uracil instead of thymine. Precursor mRNA for each gene is processed extensively in the nucleus, during which time a highly sophisticated ribonucleoprotein assembly, known as the *spliceosome,* catalyzes intron removal and exon ligation and, with the help of other regulatory proteins such as exonic and intronic splicing enhancers and silencers, orchestrates alternative splicing that allows the production of different pre-mRNA isoforms. mRNA crosses the nuclear membrane and enters the cytoplasm, where it serves as a template for protein synthesis.

Translation is the process whereby the mRNA sequence directs the amino acid sequence during protein synthesis. Translation occurs on ribosomes, complexes of ribosomal RNA (rRNA) and proteins. During protein synthesis, codons (a three-nucleotide sequence) are read by transfer RNA (tRNA), short RNA molecules that have a sequence complementary to an amino acid codon (anticodon) and bind to the amino acid molecule specified by the codon (Figure 1-5). Because there are 64 possible codons, most of the 21 amino acids are specified by more than one codon (Table 1-1). The ribosome moves along the mRNA until a stop codon is reached and synthesis is complete. The ribosome and protein product dissociate from the mRNA.

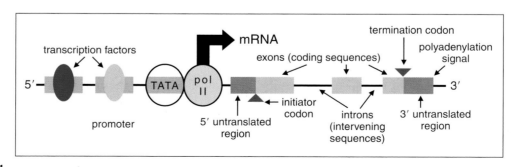

FIGURE 1-1

Structure of a typical human gene. Mammalian genes are transcribed from promoter sequences located 5' to the beginning of the coding sequence. Genes contain 5' and 3' untranslated regions, as well as exons that code for proteins and introns that are removed during splicing.

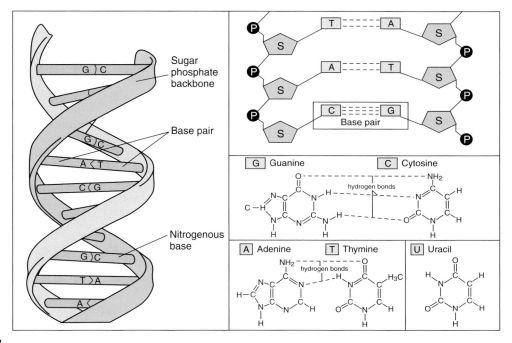

FIGURE 1-2

The structure of DNA. Schematic drawing *(left)* of the DNA double helix showing the sugar–phosphate backbone and bases arranged toward the middle. Expanded view *(right)* of the four nucleotides showing adenine (A) always pairing with thymine (T) using two hydrogen bonds and cytosine (C) always pairing with guanine (G) using three hydrogen bonds. Structure of the bases, including uracil (U), which is found in RNA, is shown.

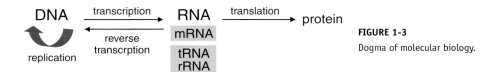

FIGURE 1-3

Dogma of molecular biology.

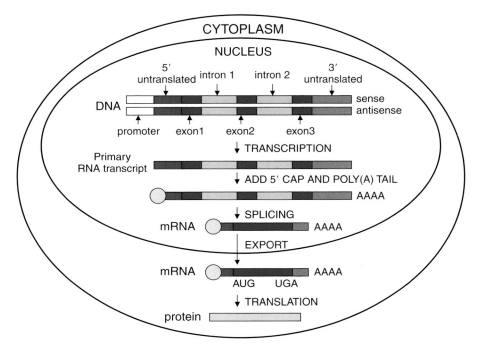

FIGURE 1-4

Transcription and translation. Transcription yields a primary RNA transcript that gets a cap added to the 5′ end and undergoes polyadenylation and splicing to produce messenger RNA (mRNA). Following transport of mRNA to the cytoplasm, mRNA is translated in the cytosol to protein molecules.

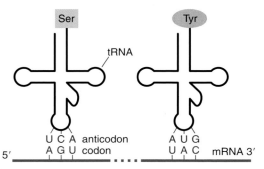

FIGURE 1-5

Transfer RNA (tRNA). A, adenine; C, cytosine; G, guanine; mRNA, messenger RNA; Ser, serine; Tyr, tyrosine; U, uracil.

GENE EXPRESSION

The control of gene expression is complex, and several diverse and highly specific processes exist that either activate or repress gene expression. Such regulation occurs at transcriptional and post-transcriptional levels and allows specific genes to be "turned on" (expressed) or "turned off" in specific tissues and at specific times. "Housekeeping genes" are involved in basic functions needed for the sustenance of cells and are typically constitutively expressed (they are always turned on). Examples of some common housekeeping genes are actin and glyceraldehyde 3-phosphate dehydrogenase.

Eukaryotic transcription control is mediated by proteins collectively called transcription factors, which bind directly to DNA sequences (named boxes, response elements, initiator elements) that usually lie upstream of the transcription start site in the promoter region. Subsequently RNA polymerase II binds to a transcription complex to initiate transcription. Some transcription factors increase the rate of transcription by binding to enhancer sequences, which may be located hundreds or thousands of base pairs from the transcription start site. Conversely, silencer elements exist, which are DNA sequences to which transcription factors bind to repress transcription. Mutations that occur in promoters or other regulatory elements

TABLE 1-1			
Genetic Code			
Amino Acid	Three-Letter Designation	Single-Letter Designation	Codon(s)
Alanine	Ala	A	GCA, GCC, GCG, GCT
Cysteine	Cys	C	TGC, TGT
Aspartic acid	Asp	D	GAC, GAT
Glutamic acid	Glu	E	GAA, GAG
Phenylalanine	Phe	F	TTC, TTT
Glycine	Gly	G	GGA, GGC, GGG, GGT
Histidine	His	H	CAC, CAT
Isoleucine	Ile	I	ATA, ATC, ATT
Lysine	Lys	K	TTT, TTG
Leucine	Leu	L	TTA, TTG, CTA, CTC, CTG, CTT
Methionine	Met	M	ATG (start codon)
Asparagine	Asn	N	AAC, AAT
Proline	Pro	P	CCA, CCC, CCG, CCT
Glutamine	Gln	Q	CAA, CAG
Arginine	Arg	R	AGA, AGG, CGA, CGC, CGG, CGT
Serine	Ser	S	AGC, AGT, TCA, TCC, TCG, TGT
Threonine	Thr	T	ACA, ACC, ACG, ACT
Valine	Val	V	GTA, GTC, GTG, GTT
Tryptophan	Trp	W	TGG
Tyrosine	Tyr	Y	TAC, TAT
Stop codons			TAA, TAG, *TGA

* TGA can code for either a stop codon or selenocysteine.
A, adenine; C, cytosine; G, guanine; T, thymine.

and at exon–intron boundaries can interfere with the normal expression of a gene and cause disease.

Regulation of gene expression also occurs at a post-transcriptional level. Examples of components regulated post-transcriptionally include the export of mRNA from the nucleus to the cytoplasm, alternative splicing, mRNA stabilization, and mRNA degradation. Over the past decade, small RNAs—microRNAs (miRNAs) and short interfering RNAs (siRNAs)—have emerged as important regulators of knocking down gene expression. The regulatory pathways mediated by these small RNAs are collectively referred to as *RNA interference* or *RNA silencing.* miRNAs and siRNAs are approximately 21 to 26 nucleotides long and function to inactivate specific mRNAs in sequence-specific manners: small RNAs, together with a RNA-induced silencing complex (RISC) protein complex, bind to target mRNA sequences. When RISC is coupled with siRNAs, target mRNA is cleaved and degraded; when RISC is coupled with miRNAs, the miRNAs base-pair (even though they are not completely complementary) with the 3′ untranslated region of target mRNAs and translation and subsequent protein expression are inhibited.

Gene expression can also be altered by "epigenetic" phenomena. *Epigenetics* refers to processes that alter gene function by mechanisms other than those caused by changes in DNA sequence. Two well-known examples of epigenetic changes that function to silence expression are DNA methylation and histone modification.

MODES OF INHERITANCE

Modes of inheritance have been established for numerous genetic disorders caused by mutations in single genes (monogenic inheritance), and an online database known as Online Mendelian Inheritance in Man (OMIM) catalogs these. Most single-gene conditions, some of which occur with increased frequency in specific ethnic groups, are relatively uncommon and typically follow one of three patterns of inheritance: autosomal dominant (disease is transmitted on a non-sex chromosome and is expressed when only a single copy of the mutant gene is present), autosomal recessive (disease is transmitted on a nonsex chromosome and is only expressed when both copies of a gene are mutant), or X-linked (disease is transmitted on the X chromosome). An additional pattern of inheritance is mitochondrial: several dozen genes involved in energy metabolism do not reside on nuclear chromosomes but instead are on the mitochondrial chromosome; because ova are rich in mitochondria but sperm are not, mitochondrial DNA and disease caused by mutations on mitochondrial DNA are maternally inherited.

Genetic transmission may also be affected by anticipation (progressively earlier onset and increased severity of a certain disease in successive generations of a family because of expansion of the number of triple repeats within or associated with the gene responsible for the disease), mosaicism (at least two cell lines differing in genotype or karyotype derived from a single zygote), genomic imprinting (different expression of alleles depending on parent origin), and uniparental disomy (both copies of a specific chromosome inherited from one parent).

Common chronic diseases such as hypertension, heart disease, and diabetes are known to run in families, indicating a genetic contribution to etiology. Such multifactorial conditions are not inherited according to Mendel's patterns but result from the interplay of environmental factors (such as diet, exercise, smoking, and exposure to pollutants) with susceptibility genes and involve the additive effect of many genes interacting with one another and with the environment.

MUTATIONS AND POLYMORPHISMS

Mutation refers to a change in the DNA sequence. The term can also imply that the change causes disease. *Polymorphism* has been used to indicate a non-disease-causing change or a change found at a frequency of 1% or greater in the population. Because confusion between the terms *mutation* and *polymorphism* may occur, neutral terms such as *sequence variant, alteration,* or *allelic variant* have been proposed. Recommendations for the description of sequence variants are summarized by the Human Genome Variation Society.

Deleterious sequence variants can cause disease by a variety of means. Most often, they cause loss of function, whereby there is a reduction or complete loss of one or more of the normal functions of a protein. Some alterations, however, cause disease through a gain of function, whereby the protein acquires some new toxic function. Such gain-of-function alterations are often dominantly inherited.

There are many types of sequence variants, including missense, nonsense, and splice site alterations. Other alterations include deletions, insertions, frameshifts, duplications, amplifications, and trinucleotide repeat expansions.

There are two main types of databases storing sequence variation information: comprehensive and locus specific (e.g., cystic fibrosis). The Human Gene Mutation Database (HGMD) collates known (published) sequence variants within the coding regions of human nuclear genes responsible for inherited disease and provides links to many locus-specific databases. Somatic alterations and alterations in the mitochondrial genome are not included in the HGMD, but the HGMD provides links to the latter (Mitomap) and to other useful databases. Because of the data generated from the Human Genome Project, new disease-associated genes are being discovered almost every week; in 2006, the HGMD cataloged more than 50,000 alterations in approximately 2000 genes, with approximately 50% of these changes being missense or nonsense sequence variants (Figure 1-6).

GeneTests is an online yellow pages that gives information on more than 250 genetic diseases and provides testing and contact information for laboratories offering testing for a particular disease. The Coriell Institute's Human Genetic Cell Repository supplies scientists with materials for genetic research and contains highly characterized cell cultures and derived DNA samples for a large number of genetic disorders. The Centers for Disease Control and Prevention also has validated quality control materials for several genetic disorders.

SINGLE NUCLEOTIDE POLYMORPHISMS AND HAPLOTYPES

Single nucleotide polymorphisms (SNPs) are single base differences in the DNA of individuals. For example, some people may have a chromosome with an adenine on one allele and a cytosine on the other allele (Figure 1-7). There are approximately 10 million SNPs in the human genome, including approximately 1000 deletion variants with deletion lengths ranging from 500 base pairs to 10.5 kilobases.

One use for SNP genotyping has been in the field of pharmacogenetics, where genetic differences in the cytochrome P450 (CYP) enzymes CYP2C9, CYP2C19, and CYP2D6 determine differences in the metabolism (poor, intermediate, extensive, or ultrarapid metabolizer) of approximately 25% of prescription drugs. By correlating SNP genotype with outcome, one can use SNP genotype to aid in selecting medications and doses. Several methods that rely on hybridization (e.g., molecular beacons), primer extension, oligonucleotide ligation, or nuclease cleavage (e.g., TaqMan™) and use various detection platforms are available for rapid SNP or allelic discrimination genotyping assays.

Alleles of SNPs that are close together tend to be inherited together. A set of associated SNP alleles in a region of a chromosome is called a *haplotype* (Figure 1-7). The International HapMap Project is

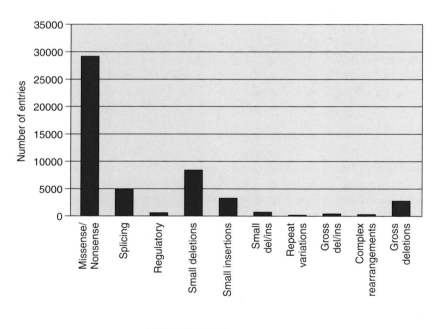

FIGURE 1-6

Numbers of mutations and mutation types in the Human Gene Mutation Database.

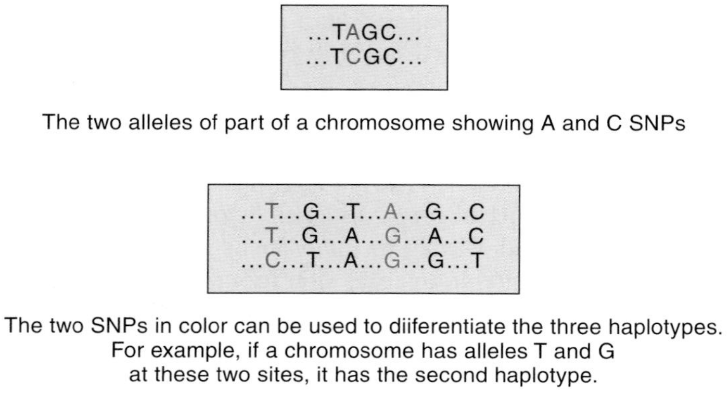

The two alleles of part of a chromosome showing A and C SNPs

The two SNPs in color can be used to differentiate the three haplotypes. For example, if a chromosome has alleles T and G at these two sites, it has the second haplotype.

FIGURE 1-7

Single nucleotide polymorphisms (SNPs) and haplotypes. SNPs are single base differences in the DNA of individuals and have a frequency of more than 1%. Haplotypes are sets of associated SNPs that tend to be inherited together. A, adenine; C, cytosine; G, guanine; T, thymine.

an ongoing project to establish the common patterns of human DNA sequence variation and is expected to be a key resource for researchers to find genes associated with common diseases such as heart disease, stroke, diabetes, and depression, as well as drug response.

GENOMIC REPOSITORIES

Online public molecular databases (Table 1-2) that collect, manage, store, and distribute data are an invaluable resource for researchers and molecular pathologists. Molecular databases exist for chromosome abnormalities, gene expression, gene structure, mutations, gene sequences, genetic disorders, protein motifs, and protein structure; details on many databases are available at the Oxford Journals website.

The United States, Europe, and Japan have their own comprehensive DNA and protein sequence databases of the human genome and genomes from other species, which are available at websites for the National Center for Biotechnology Information (NCBI), EMBL Nucleotide Sequence Database, and DNA Data Bank of Japan, respectively. The NCBI provides extensive cross-linking among its resources, such as finding disease description (OMIM), sequence variations (dbSNP), and tissue expression (UniGene). Several annotated databases also exist, such as Ensembl, a joint project of the European Bioinformatics Institute, the Wellcome Trust Sanger Institute, and Swiss-Prot.

TABLE 1-2
Public Molecular Databases

URL	Description
http://www.ncbi.nlm.nih.gov	Nucleotide sequence database (American)
http://www.ebi.ac.uk/embl	Nucleotide sequence database (European)
http://www.ddbj.nig.ac.jp	Nucleotide sequence database (Japanese)
http://www.ensembl.org	Annotated information on eukaryotic genomes
http://www.ncbi.nlm.nih.gov/projects /SNP	Single nucleotide polymorphisms
http://www.genetests.org	Medical genetics information
http://www.hgmd.org	Links to locus-specific mutation databases
http://www.mitomap.org	Human mitochondrial genome
http://www.ncbi.nlm.nih.gov/sites/entrez?db=omim	Catalog of human genes and genetic disorders
http://locus.umdnj.edu/ccr	Repository of cell cultures and DNA from human diseases
http://www.hapmap.org	Haplotype mapping project
http://www.hgvs.org	Guidelines for mutation nomenclature

SUGGESTED READINGS

Beaudet AL, Scriver CR, Sly WS, Valle D: Genetics, biochemistry, and molecular basis of variant human phenotypes. In Scriver CR, Beaudet AL, Sly WS, Valle D (eds): The Metabolic and Molecular Bases of Inherited Disease, vol 4. New York, McGraw-Hill, 2001, pp 3–45.

Burke W: Genetic testing. N Engl J Med 2002;347:1867–1875.

Burtis CA, Ashwood ER, Bruns DE (eds): Tietz Textbook of Clinical Chemistry and Molecular Diagnostics, 4th ed. St Louis, Elsevier Saunders, 2006, chapters 36–43.

Cardiff University Institute of Medical Genetics: Human Gene Mutation Database. Available at http://www.hgmd.org.

Centers for Disease Control and Prevention: RM Materials: Material Availability. Available at http://wwwn.cdc.gov/dls/genetics/rmmaterials/materialsavailability.aspx.

Collins FS, Green ED, Guttmacher AE, Guyer MS: A vision for the future of genomics research. Nature 2003;422:835–847.

Coriell Institute for Medical Research: NIGMS Human Genetic Cell Repository. Available at http://locus.umdnj.edu/nigms.

DNA data bank of Japan: DDBJ. Available at http://www.ddbj.nig.ac.jp.

European Bioinformatics Institute: EMBL Nucleotide Sequence Database. Available at http://www.ebi.ac.uk/embl.

European Bioinformatics Institute, the Wellcome Trust Sanger Institute, and Swiss-Prot: Ensembl. Available at http://www.ensembl.org.

Guttmacher AE, Collins FS: Genomic medicine: A primer. N Engl J Med 2002;347:1512–1520.

Human Genome Variation Society: HGV. Available at http://www.hgvs.org.

International HapMap Project: Home. Available at http://www.hapmap.org.

National Center for Biotechnology Information: dbSNP: Single Nucleotide Polymorphism. Available at http://www.ncbi.nlm.nih.gov/projects/SNP.

National Center for Biotechnology Information: UniGene: An Organized View of the Transcriptome. Available at http://www.ncbi.nlm.nih.gov/sites/entrez?db=unigene.

National Center for Biotechnology Information: What Does NCBI Do? Available at http://www.ncbi.nlm.nih.gov.

National Center for Biotechnology Information, Johns Hopkins University: Online Mendelian Inheritance in Man. Available at http://www.ncbi.nlm.nih.gov/sites/entrez?db=omim.

National Institutes of Health: GeneTests. Available at http://www.genetests.org.

Oxford Journals: Nucleic Acids Research. Available at http://nar.oxfordjournals.org.

Swiss-Prot: UniProtKB/Swiss-Prot. Available at http://www.ebi.ac.uk/swissprot.

2 Quality Assurance of Molecular Assays

Wayne W. Grody

INTRODUCTION

Molecular assays are by nature highly complex and usually quite sophisticated and esoteric. They more often resemble the assays performed in basic research laboratories than those that occur in routine clinical laboratories. This is not surprising when one considers that virtually all applications in molecular pathology have derived from research discoveries, many of them quite recent. Thus, there is a continual flow of test translation from the research to the clinical laboratory, which for the purposes of this book is the surgical pathology laboratory. This is an essential part of the evolution of molecular pathology and, indeed, the thing that makes it so exciting. Yet it causes problems for the practice of molecular pathology, especially in the area of quality assurance. It is a basic tenet of laboratory medicine that clinical and research activities are not to be mixed or performed concurrently on the same specimens or in the same space. This is because the needs and goals of research and clinical laboratories are vastly different. Research must be creative, flexible, ever-changing, and always open to new ideas and directions. It is performed by a diverse team of principal investigators, graduate students, postdoctoral fellows, and technicians, all of different backgrounds and levels of experience. Clinical laboratory practice, in contrast, must be consistent, unalteringly adherent to written protocols, and performed by licensed laboratorians who have completed mandatory training content and passed state and professional board examinations. The laboratories in which they work must be inspected regularly to ensure that these conditions are being met.

Still, this dichotomy inevitably breaks down to some degree in molecular pathology. More than almost any other area of laboratory medicine, the successful practice of molecular pathology requires and encourages close collaboration with research laboratories. Given the ever-increasing pace of advances in molecular biology and the Human Genome Project, the time interval between gene discovery and clinical test translation becomes ever shorter, sometimes even a matter of days. How can we ensure that such tests have received sufficient scientific scrutiny before they are put into practice? Importantly, has the test had adequate clinical validation and had its predictive value defined? Can it be performed accurately by technologists who may have had only limited or no training in the new molecular technique? To address these and other critical quality issues, it was appreciated early in the evolution of molecular pathology that new and dedicated quality assurance standards were critically needed, because those existing in pathology and laboratory medicine were neither applicable nor sufficiently specific for such a highly specialized field. These standards have been developed and continue to be modified in parallel with practice through a constellation of governmental, professional, and private organizations.

DEVELOPMENT OF QUALITY ASSURANCE STANDARDS

For most of the history of pathology, and of clinical medicine in general, there were no codified standards of practice, and test development, validation, performance, and interpretation were left solely to the discretion of the pathologist or laboratory director. Then, in the 1970s and 1980s, a series of widely publicized quality lapses in pathology laboratories led to increased governmental scrutiny of these operations. What resulted was the Clinical Laboratory Improvement Amendments (CLIA) of 1988, a series of federal regulations overseen by an agency within the U.S. Department of Health and Human Services now called the Centers for Medicare and Medicaid Services. Yet despite the regulations' tremendous effects on some aspects of pathology practice, such as cytology, other areas of laboratory medicine are not covered specifically in these guidelines or are absent. For the guidelines to apply to a specific laboratory activity, that subspecialty must be defined as such in the regulations. At present, there is no named laboratory activity in the CLIA regulations corresponding to anything in molecular pathology and only one that is relevant to genetics (cytogenetics). Thus, molecular diagnostic testing essentially does not exist in the eyes of the U.S. government; therefore, it is not specifically regulated. Of course, all laboratories doing clinical work, with results reported to physicians for use in medical management, must be licensed under the CLIA. To do this, they must undergo CLIA inspections and be shown to adhere to the standards contained therein. But in the absence of standards specific and relevant to the performance of molecular assays, CLIA inspection defaults to a rather cursory (or picky, depending on one's point of view) focus on water-bath temperatures, equipment maintenance records, and the like. It was not long after the birth of molecular pathology in the mid-1980s that its practitioners recognized a need for more specific, meaningful, and stringent standards that all laboratories could adhere to. It was felt that this would not only improve overall laboratory quality but also introduce a needed uniformity to a field that was highly fragmented because its test migration originated independently from many research laboratories.

The entity that took the lead in this effort is the one already inspecting and accrediting pathology laboratories in all other subspecialties around the country, the College of American Pathologists (CAP). In addition to its educational and lobbying efforts, the CAP has had a long-standing program of laboratory inspections and nationwide proficiency testing. In fact, it has "deemed" status from the government such that its inspections can be used in lieu of CLIA inspections for laboratory accreditation. The CAP programs are highly specialized, with inspection checklists (the compilation of guidelines that the inspector must examine) and proficiency testing challenges targeted to each section of the laboratory. What was lacking was a program for molecular pathology, and this was launched in 1989. The CAP's checklists and proficiency programs are developed by resource committees composed of experts in the field (drawn mostly from academic institutions, along with some commercial reference laboratories) who meet face to face at least three times a year. In 1989, the Molecular Pathology Resource Committee was established, and its members immediately began work writing a Molecular Pathology Checklist and developing proficiency tests in the area (the first being directed at gene rearrangements for clonality in lymphoma and leukemia). The checklist now contains hundreds of items covering all aspects of the molecular pathology laboratory, from specimen accessioning, to procedures, to personnel, to physical facilities and equipment. In the absence of anything relevant in the CLIA regulations, this document, which is constantly being revised and updated to reflect the advent of new techniques, has established

the de facto standards for the field. Its concepts have been borrowed or adapted by other agencies, both public and private; conversely, some of its items have been adapted from those of other entities, such as the American College of Medical Genetics (ACMG), which publishes its own standards and guidelines for molecular testing of genetic diseases, and the Clinical and Laboratory Standards Institute (CLSI, formerly the National Committee for Clinical Laboratory Standards), which develops voluntary consensus standards for laboratory testing in close partnership with in vitro diagnostics manufacturers.

As presently envisioned, any laboratory that wishes to become CAP accredited must be inspected using the Molecular Pathology Checklist if it performs any nucleic acid–based tests, with the exception of certain self-contained kits approved by the Food and Drug Administration (FDA) of the type that exist in molecular microbiology; if a laboratory is doing that sort of testing exclusively, it can be inspected using the Microbiology Checklist only (because it contains items that address these particular molecular assays). For its part, CAP has made an effort in the last few years to ensure that the individual doing the inspection is a true peer experienced in molecular pathology, because the oversight and educational value of the inspection is determined primarily from this factor. Having an unqualified inspector who is not familiar by personal experience with the concepts in the checklist results in a superficial effort that is of no real benefit. Because inspections of large clinical laboratories and pathology departments cover many different sections and are conducted by a large team of inspectors, it is the responsibility of the team leader to select a qualified individual to inspect the molecular pathology laboratory. There is a mechanism in place for feedback to CAP if the laboratory is not satisfied with the inspection experience.

In parallel with its writing of the checklist, the CAP Molecular Pathology Resource Committee embarked on the challenging effort to develop proficiency testing programs in all areas of molecular diagnostics. Although many of these had their origin in this committee, they have since been farmed out to other resource committees, such as those for microbiology, molecular genetics, and forensics. At present, there are proficiency challenges available for all applications described in this book, if not necessarily for every target analyte. There are challenges for in situ hybridization, immunoglobulin gene rearrangements, microsatellite instability, chromosome translocation analysis, etc. For a laboratory to be CAP accredited, it must enroll in an available proficiency testing program for every analyte it tests for. If a formal program is not available from the CAP (e.g., for certain rare analytes), the laboratory is obligated to set up an acceptable alternative, such as sample exchange with another laboratory, blinded retesting of its own samples, or retesting in-house by a different method (Table 2-1).

At the time of this writing, the CAP guidelines are considered the "gold standard" in the field, and laboratories that adhere to them are deemed to have met the highest applicable standards of practice. In other areas of molecular diagnostics, stringent guidelines have been developed by other agencies (e.g., ACMG and the American Society for Histocompatibility and Immunogenetics), but for tissue-based applications the CAP guidelines remain paramount. Supplemental guidance can be obtained from the CLSI documents, as well as several publications emanating from the Association for Molecular Pathology. However, only the CAP has the regulatory "teeth" for enforcement.

In parallel with accreditation of laboratories, there have been efforts to certify the qualification of laboratory personnel, at both the director and the staff levels. Depending on individual state law, a clinical laboratory may be directed by a physician, a doctoral-level scientist, or a board-certified pathologist. But there has been a general feeling that, just as molecular pathology laboratories required their own quality assurance guidelines, so should the personnel performing and interpreting these tests have special training and experience beyond that of general clinical laboratorians. Hence, we have seen the growth of fellowships in molecular diagnostics and examinations to ensure a minimal knowledge base in the area. The first recognized board certification in molecular diagnostics was the examination in Clinical Molecular Genetics offered by the American Board of Medical Genetics (ABMG) as one of its subspecialties. Eligibility for this exam requires a doctoral degree, a 2-year fellowship in an accredited medical genetics training program, and accrual of a "logbook" of 150 molecular genetics cases in which the fellow

has participated in various capacities. The ABMG examination focuses almost exclusively on molecular testing for inherited diseases, which is just one facet of molecular diagnostics. Because most pathologists are interested in the other areas as well or instead, such as testing for cancer markers and infectious disease, the ABMG track did not really satisfy their needs. In 2001, after years of negotiation, a new examination was introduced, jointly sponsored by the ABMG and the American Board of Pathology (ABP), called Molecular Genetic Pathology. It covers all areas of molecular diagnostics and requires 1 year of fellowship training in a molecular pathology laboratory. It is open only to physicians with primary certification in either pathology or medical genetics.

Other board certifications are open to doctoral scientists who specialize in other areas or are not eligible for the ABMG or ABP examinations. These are offered by the American Board of Clinical Chemistry, the American Board of Medical Microbiology, the American Board of Bioanalysis, etc., but they are not recognized officially by the American Board of Medical Specialties. For technical staff, examinations in clinical molecular biology are offered by the National Credentialing Agency and the American Society for Clinical Pathology (ASCP). Eligibility is usually at least 1 year of experience in a clinical molecular diagnostic laboratory (CLIA) or a combination of appropriate education and experience (ASCP).

All of these fellowships and certifying examinations are aimed at ensuring appropriate experience and knowledge of the individuals working in molecular diagnostic laboratories. Although in and of themselves they do not carry any regulatory imprimatur, they may be required under certain state laws, and at the time of this writing there are proposals to introduce them as requirements in the CLIA regulations.

TABLE 2-1

Acceptable Routes for Proficiency Testing

Formal CAP program—if available for analyte of interest

Alternative proficiency testing provider program

Splitting of samples with another laboratory

Testing of samples against another in-house method

"Chart review" or other clinical correlation with test results

CAP, College of American Pathologists.

EXAMPLES OF SPECIFIC QUALITY ASSURANCE GUIDELINES FOR TISSUE-BASED MOLECULAR ASSAYS

There is not space in this chapter to go over in detail all aspects of quality assurance in the anatomic molecular pathology setting; for this the reader is referred to the CAP Molecular Pathology Checklist and the other resources listed in the previous section and in the Suggested Readings section. This section only highlights several quality assurance issues that are unique or particularly relevant to molecular assays conducted on cells and tissues in the anatomic pathology laboratory.

TEST VALIDATION

For most of the molecular assays performed in anatomic pathology, there are no FDA-approved kits available. Therefore, most of the tests in use are developed in-house and designated in the vernacular as "home brews." It is the responsibility of the laboratory director to ensure that each assay is robust and clinically useful before putting it into practice. Test validation consists of two arms: analytic validation and clinical validation. Of these, the first is the more straightforward and easier to accomplish. It is done to ensure that the technical results are accurate: i.e., the assay in the laboratory's hands is capable of detecting the DNA or RNA target (mutation, translocation, microbial gene) when it is there and not detecting it when it is absent. The measures of these parameters are analytic sensitivity and analytic specificity, and they are determined by running a series of known positive and negative samples or by doing blinded comparisons with another laboratory experienced with the same test. There are no set minimum numbers specified in the regulations for performing test validation; it depends on the nature of the assay, the complexity of the technique, and the relative rarity of the nucleic acid target. The laboratory must decide on the acceptable minimum level of sensitivity and specificity, considering the nature of the assay, the nature of the disease, and the clinical implications of false-negative and false-positive results. The CAP Molecular Pathology Checklist has recently been beefed up in the area of test validation, and inspectors will demand to see records that proper validation was conducted and achieved for each newly introduced test.

Clinical validation is more problematic and often will be beyond the means of the individual laboratory to prove or document. Does detection of human papillomavirus (HPV) DNA in a cervical sample necessarily correlate with dysplasia or risk of dysplasia? Does detection of microsatellite instability in a colon tumor necessarily prove that it is genetic in origin? Only through the study and correlation of large numbers of patients can such questions be answered. Recognizing this, it is considered acceptable for the laboratory to refer to peer-reviewed medical literature as evidence of clinical validation for certain assays. However, well-performed clinical trials, statistically powered to answer the questions of clinical validation, are increasingly recognized as being necessary for the establishment of medical validity. Given the critical management decisions that often depend on these results, proof of clinical validation is rapidly becoming necessary before a test can be implemented or expected to be reimbursed.

PROBES AND PRIMERS

DNA and RNA probes and polymerase chain reaction (PCR) primers lie at the heart of virtually every molecular assay. Therefore, it is critical that their properties be well known, tested, and understood. The laboratory's procedure manuals must contain sufficient documentation of probe–primer sequence and hybridization behavior to ensure robust performance and appropriate interpretation of test results. The records must contain information about the sequence, genomic location, source, polymorphisms, restriction enzyme recognition sites, and any other applicable features for each probe and primer in use.

CONTROLS

Second in importance only to the probes and primers are the controls, both positive and negative, used in the assay. These must be selected with care and used religiously, with test results discounted if one or more control samples register out of range. Probes directed at particular mutations or infectious targets must be tested against a positive control known to contain the target sequence of interest and a negative control known not to contain it. Suboptimal hybridization to the positive control, or appearance of a hybridization signal in the negative control, invalidates that run of the assay. Unfortunately, positive controls in molecular pathology are not always easy to come by, especially for rare mutations. In such cases, an artificial or synthetic control may need to be used, such as a plasmid carrying the gene region or mutation of interest. Several procedures for constructing such controls have been published, and several commercial firms sell prepackaged artificial controls. Unfortunately, manufacturers of test reagents are not allowed to include controls if the products are marketed as analyte-specific reagents (ASRs) and have not gone through formal FDA review.

For all PCR assays, a "no DNA" or "no template" control is essential. This control contains all ingredients of the PCR assay except for the target template. If any signal is seen, it indicates a contamination problem in the assay that must be investigated. Quantitative tests, such as real-time PCR, require positive controls at low, medium, and high levels so that a standard curve can be constructed for the assay and the patient results can be quantified accurately. Even qualitative assays may require some degree of quantitation, if only to ensure that a minimum expected level of sensitivity is in force. Thus, for clonal gene rearrangement studies in lymphoid lesions, a "sensitivity control" should be run, consisting of a positive clonal sample diluted into a negative one down to the level of sensitivity claimed for the assay (e.g., 5%). Any PCR test in which a blank result (no amplification) is indicative of a negative result must be controlled by the simultaneous amplification of a second target sequence in the sample (different from the target in question) to ensure that the blank result was not caused by PCR failure or endogenous inhibitors of amplification.

Southern blot assays must be controlled at multiple levels. A sample showing expected target sizes must be run, e.g., human placental DNA to show the position of germline bands in gene rearrangement studies. This control also monitors adequate performance of the restriction endonuclease digestion. Sensitivity controls of the type described earlier are also essential.

CLIA stipulates that a positive control must be included for every analyte in every run of an assay. This rule was formulated long ago when assays typically measured a single analyte. In molecular pathology, an increasing number of assays involve multiplex detection of many possible targets at once. At the extreme of this trend are high-density microarrays that interrogate hundreds or thousands of mutations or gene expression messenger RNA species simultaneously. It soon became obvious that the old requirement for positive controls would not be practicable in this setting. The CAP checklist item on this subject has been revised to permit the rotation of controls (one or two at a time) for multiplex assays run in an array format. In addition, it is felt that assays using DNA sequencing (described later) do not require a positive control, because the visualized sequence itself serves as an internal control; it would be impossible to select controls for every potential nucleotide change in any case. It is prudent, however, to run a negative control so that the wild-type sequence can be visualized in comparison to the test sample.

POLYMERASE CHAIN REACTION CONTAINMENT

PCR and other powerful amplification technologies present a serious risk of false-positive results because of product carryover or contamination, simply because the mass of target sequence is so large after amplification. Therefore, quality assurance guidelines require adequate physical separation of pre- and postamplification samples and procedures. Ideally, these should be in separate rooms with one-way sample flow. Other helpful precautions include use of dedicated pipettes, meticulous liquid transfer procedures, frequent glove changes, and use of closed-sample reactions. Despite much press about this artifact in the early days of PCR, it should be fairly easy to avoid if these guidelines are followed.

TYPES OF CONTROLS USED IN MOLECULAR PATHOLOGY—FACT SHEET

Positive Mutation Controls
▶ For allele-specific assays
▶ Not needed for DNA sequencing

Negative Mutation Control

No-Template Control for PCR

Sensitivity Control
▶ For gene rearrangement Southern blots

Endogenous Nontarget Control
▶ For PCR assays that give a blank result for negative
▶ For in situ hybridization

Germline Control
▶ For gene rearrangement Southern blots

Restriction Digestion Control
▶ For Southern blots and amplified fragment length polymorphism assays

Quantitation Controls
▶ For quantitative PCR and other quantitative assays
▶ Range of low, medium, and high controls

IN SITU HYBRIDIZATION

In situ hybridization technique is in a sense the most wedded of all molecular procedures to the practice of anatomic pathology because it is performed on intact tissues and cells. Therefore, it is accepted that additional personnel requirements are needed beyond those listed earlier for general molecular pathology. It almost goes without saying that meaningful interpretation of an in situ hybridization result on a tissue section requires assessment not only of the probe signal but also of its location within particular tissue regions, cell types, and pathologic processes. Thus, the interpreter not only should have expertise in molecular biology but also must be skilled in the morphologic assessment of histopathology and cytology specimens; in other words, this technique should be under the supervision of a pathologist who can include these morphologic findings in the test report. Although this is the only area of molecular pathology for which an anatomic pathology background is explicitly recommended in the guidelines, it is certainly helpful in many other areas. For example, one may be called upon to examine a skin or lymph node biopsy to make sure the lesion was appropriately sampled to be able to observe a T cell receptor gene rearrangement by Southern blot or PCR, given the lower limit of sensitivity of the assay.

As in certain PCR assays, a blank result (no probe signal) is a possibility in some in situ hybridization assays, such as those targeting viruses like HPV. As for the analogous situation in PCR, it is recommended that an endogenous positive control be used—in this case, a probe known to hybridize to some other target in the tissue section to ensure that the submitted tissue is adequately preserved so that its nucleic acid targets are intact and accessible.

DNA SEQUENCING

As molecular pathology analytes become more specific, even down to the individual patient level, DNA sequencing becomes increasingly central as a technique. It is the best way to detect any of numerous possible mutations in a gene or gene region and to detect subtle differences in the genotype of patients, tumors, or infectious organisms. But because it queries much more data (hundreds or thousands of individual nucleotides) than probe-specific assays, it demands special quality assurance and interpretive considerations. First, no gene can be addressed at this level until its normal (wild type) sequence is known; otherwise, it will not be clear which nucleotide variants represent clinically significant results. Furthermore, recurring mutations and common polymorphisms (clinically benign or silent missense changes) should be known to the extent possible. Even with this foreknowledge, it is inevitable that new or novel missense variants will be detected when sequencing oncogenes in tumors, tumor suppressor genes in blood cells, etc. In such cases, it is the responsibility of the laboratory director to assess the likely clinical significance of the result and include this information in the report. Although there are no rules for doing so that will be 100% predictive, some hints can be gleaned from the location of the nucleotide substitution in the gene, the nature of the resulting amino acid substitution in the protein product, the degree of evolutionary conservation at that codon position, or the concordance of the variant with clinical phenotype in other family members (if they can be tested as well).

One must also be comfortable enough with the technology used to feel confident that sequence anomalies observed are real. Although most laboratories have now switched from manual radioactive sequencing and autoradiography to automated sequencing on DNA analyzers using fluorescent labels, the latter are in some sense more prone to interpretation problems, both overcalls and undercalls. When the expected result is a heterozygous nucleotide substitution, it is prudent to run the sequencing in both forward and reverse directions (i.e., sequencing both strands of the gene) to check whether the change is clearly observed both times; if not, it may be an artifact. Also, one must always keep in mind that large deletions may be invisible by standard sequencing methods, because only the remaining normal allele will be replicated and sequenced. This is exactly what happens to produce the phenomenon of loss of heterozygosity in tumors.

REQUISITIONS AND REPORTS

Paper requisitions and reports (or their electronic counterparts) are essential for the appropriate ordering and reporting of tests throughout the clinical laboratory. However, there may be certain features of them that differ in the molecular pathology setting. For example, in addition to the standard patient demographic data, some tests require precise racial and ethnicity information to determine which mutations to target, because these may be ethnic specific. Some tests may require informed consent, especially those with implications for other family members. For example, there is much discussion about whether microsatellite instability testing in colon tumors should be considered a genetic test (because it has genetic implications) and, if so, whether informed consent should be required (because it is in many other molecular tests for heritable cancer syndromes). The CAP checklist skirts this issue by requiring informed consent to be documented on the requisition form "when appropriate"; presumably it is left to the laboratory director to make the determination of appropriateness for each test or clinical situation.

Much discussion has also ensued in recent years about which and how much information should be included in the molecular pathology test report. All laboratorians are cognizant of the inherent conflict between including sufficient information so that the clinician can properly understand the result and including so much that none of it is read. Because molecular assays are not familiar to many practicing physicians, it is important that the meaning and limitations of the test be spelled out understandably in the report. The sensitivity of the assay, its ability to detect some proportion of possible mutations less than 100%, and the clinical predictive value of a positive result should all be included. If a missense variant is detected, the report must make some attempt to address its likely clinical significance, as detailed earlier in the section on sequencing. Tests based on in situ hybridization should include a correlation of the probe findings within the histologic context. It is probably not necessary to list every probe and restriction enzyme used for most tests; these will be meaningless to the clinician anyway. But sufficient information should be provided so that, if the patient is subsequently seen in another center, it will be understood what test was performed to prevent needless duplication and to appreciate how comprehensive the assay was. Test reports with genetic implications, such as microsatellite instability, may need to contain a recommendation for genetic counseling. Lastly, any test that uses ASR products must contain a disclaimer stating that the assay has not been reviewed by the FDA but has been individually validated by the laboratory.

LABORATORY SAFETY

Safety is an essential part of all clinical laboratory practice—in fact, the most important aspect for those working in the laboratory—and for the most part the guidelines are generic and well covered in general laboratory manuals. However, some unique and particularly noxious materials are sometimes used in molecular pathology laboratories that deserve special attention. Although used less than in earlier years because of the advent of colorimetric, fluorescent, and chemiluminescent signaling methods, radioactive materials are still employed and have special storage, shielding, and disposal requirements that are specific for each isotope. Other hazards that require protection are ethidium bromide used to stain DNA in agarose gels, ultraviolet light sources used to photograph those gels, various other chemicals and biologics, and the clinical specimens themselves, which may contain obvious or occult infectious organisms. Containment of recombinant DNA materials (plasmids, etc.) is not the issue it was in the early days of the field, and most are now considered of negligible hazard, requiring no more than standard laboratory decontamination procedures.

CONCLUSION

Like the scientific discipline itself, quality assurance in molecular pathology is a constantly changing landscape. It is almost impossible to codify guidelines in stone, because the advent of new and more powerful techniques always demands new approaches. Therefore, most professional and private (if not governmental) entities that have tried to tackle these challenges have deliberately left many of the guidelines somewhat flexible or discretionary to give qualified laboratory directors and pathologists the most latitude in setting up whatever procedures and safeguards work best for their particular laboratory and clinical application. Those in the field consider such decisions to be part of the practice of medicine, and board-certified laboratory directors should be trusted to make them in the patients' best interest. As long as this trust is not violated and the quality assurance landscape for molecular pathology is always recognized as fluid, we should continue to offer the highest-quality molecular assays, no matter what unexpected advances occur in the future.

SUGGESTED READINGS

American College of Medical Genetics: ACMG Standards and Guidelines for Genetic Laboratories. Available at http://www.acmg.net.

American College of Medical Genetics Laboratory Practice Standards Committee Working Group: Recommendations for standards for interpretation of sequence variations. Genet Med 2000;2: 302–303.

Association for Molecular Pathology: Recommendations for in-house development and operation of molecular diagnostic tests. Am J Clin Pathol 1999;111:449–463.

Centers for Medicare and Medicaid Services: Clinical Laboratory Improvement Amendments. Available at http://www.cms.hhs.gov/clia.

College of American Pathologists: Checklist 12: Molecular Pathology. Available at http://www.cap.org.

Grody WW: Quest for controls in molecular genetics. J Mol Diagn 2003;5:209–211.

Killeen AA, Leung WC, Payne D, et al: Certification in molecular pathology in the United States. J Mol Diagn 2002;4:181–184.

National Committee for Clinical Laboratory Standards: Nucleic Acid Amplification Assays for Molecular Hematopathology: Approved Guideline. NCCLS document MM5-A, vol 23, no 17. Wayne, PA, NCCLS, 2003.

Seabrook JM, Hubbard RA: Achieving quality reproducible results and maintaining compliance in molecular diagnostic testing of human papillomavirus. Arch Pathol Lab Med 2003;127:978–983.

Tatum T, Hendrix E: Training technologists for the genomic age. Clin Lab Sci 2006;19:148–152.

available from several vendors; and adaptable to high-throughput robotic manipulation; it is therefore a popular choice for clinical molecular laboratories.

Anion-exchange chromatography columns are made of a unique anion-exchange resin that selectively binds nucleic acids, allowing rapid separation of DNA. Crude lysate is applied to the column under conditions that favor binding. Binding is facilitated by a series of buffers of differing salt concentrations and pH. These conditions allow the phosphates in the backbone of the molecule, which are negatively charged, to bind with positive residues contained in the resin. Contaminants are removed using a moderate salt buffer, and the DNA is eluted off the column with a high salt buffer. The result is highly purified nucleic acid.

The use of magnetic particles for rapid nucleic acid isolation is an easy and fast method that has been adapted for use in many automated systems. With this technology, the nucleic acid is captured onto magnetic particles, typically using a biotinylated probe that binds streptavidin-coated paramagnetic particles. A magnet pulls the paramagnetic particles to the side of the tube, and cellular debris is removed using a series of wash steps. The nucleic acid is eluted from the probe in pure form.

RNA versus DNA Isolation

RNases are ubiquitous, highly stable, and active in virtually any aqueous environment, and they can regain their activity after denaturation. RNA is therefore subject to rapid degradation by RNases, and scrupulous care must be taken in the laboratory setting to overcome the lability of RNA. RNA isolation requires steps to inhibit or degrade cellular RNases and prevents their reintroduction into the isolated RNA; it must be performed promptly. If RNA isolation is delayed, samples should be stored at $-86°$ C (erythrocytes should be eliminated as discussed earlier) or less or temporarily in buffer with RNase inhibitors. Addition of GITC or β-mercaptoethanol to the RNA isolation reagents inhibits or denatures RNase. Purified RNA is rehydrated in nuclease-free water and stored at $-86°$ C to further inhibit any remaining RNase activity.

Nucleic Acid Measurement of Quantity and Quality

Nucleic acid quantification may be optional for many protocols; however, some methods require accurate measurement of nucleic acid concentration. Typically, this is done by measuring the absorbance of a nucleic acid solution at several wavelengths of ultraviolet light in a spectrophotometer. Maximal absorbance is 260 nm (A_{260}) for nucleotides and 280 nm (A_{280}) for proteins. The quantity of nucleic acids is determined by the A_{260} measurement, and an A_{260}-to-A_{280} ratio provides an estimate of the purity of the sample. Pure DNA has an A_{260} of 1.0 at 50 μg/mL and an A_{260}-to-A_{280} ratio of 1.8; pure RNA has an A_{260} of 1.0 at 40 μg/mL and an A_{260}-to-A_{280} ratio of 2.0. Lower ratios indicate protein contamination. Additional contaminants can be detected by absorbance at other wavelengths.

Electrophoresis and Visualization of DNA

Electrophoresis separates charged molecules in an electric field because of their differential mobilities in a sieving matrix, whether liquid or solid (gel). Agarose and acrylamide are the matrices most commonly used to separate DNA molecules of differing molecular weights. For both gel types, samples, controls, and sizing standards are loaded into the matrix, along with a dye allowing visualization of the samples. Electrodes are attached to the buffer chambers and connected to a power supply that generates an electric field. DNA, negatively charged, migrates toward the anode (+) in the electric field.

The differential mobility is determined by the size of the molecule and its conformation, the net charge of the molecule (as modified by pH), temperature, and the pore size of the matrix. The mobility of a molecule through the matrix is inversely proportional to the log of its size. Therefore, smaller molecules travel through the gel more quickly than larger molecules. The size of DNA can be modified by restriction endonuclease (RE) digestion (see below), rendering it small enough to be mobile in the matrix.

Intercalating agents such as ethidium bromide (EtBr) cause DNA to fluoresce upon illumination with ultraviolet light, thereby enabling visualization of DNA. By staining sample DNA with EtBr in an electrophoretic gel and comparing to mass standards in adjacent lanes, DNA size can be estimated. As importantly, the image of the EtBr-stained DNA sample in a gel can be used to assess quality. High-quality, substantially intact DNA forms a tight band close to the origin of electrophoresis. A smear of EtBr-stained DNA extending downward from the well, on the other hand, is indicative of DNA degradation. SYBR® Green is an alternative dye for these purposes.

Polyacrylamide forms small pores useful for high resolution of DNA fragments of tens to hundreds of base pairs. Single base-pair resolution can be achieved, making polyacrylamide gels ideal for sequencing under denaturing conditions (described later). Agarose gels with a concentration of 1% are used to separate DNA fragments of 1 to 20 kilobases, and higher concentration gels are useful to separate smaller DNA fragments. Agarose is safer than acrylamide (in the unpolymerized state, a lung irritant and neurotoxin) but still must be handled and disposed of properly if stained with EtBr.

Capillary electrophoresis is a widely used separation technology in analysis of macromolecules, including DNA. In the molecular diagnostics laboratory, DNA sequencing and fragment analysis are the most common applications employing capillary electrophoresis. With this technology, electrophoretic separation takes place in a capillary tube ranging from 25 to 100 cm in length and approximately 50 to 75 μm in diameter. Most capillary tubes are made of glass, and the internal walls are usually covered with a coating containing acid silanol groups that impart a negative charge. An acrylamide-based polymer acts as the electrolyte solution and sieving matrix in the capillary. DNA fragments, in typical electrophoretic nature, separate by size in the capillary and are detected through a window at the far end of the capillary. Several vendors manufacture excellent capillary electrophoresis and DNA sequencing instruments, which are highly automated and an important part of the 21st-century molecular pathology laboratory.

RESTRICTION FRAGMENT LENGTH POLYMORPHISM

REs are proteins that occur naturally in bacteria and cleave DNA into small fragments. REs recognize highly specific stretches of bases, recognition sites (commonly four to eight base pairs long), and cleave foreign DNA (a bacterial defensive "immune system" to protect against phage activity) at or near the recognition site. Unique DNA restriction fragment families are generated by digestion with an RE, creating a range of DNA fragments differing in molecular weight. If a single nucleotide polymorphism or mutation is present that modifies a restriction site, incubating DNA with the RE and visualizing the "restricted" fragments using electrophoresis can identify the creation or removal of that site. RE digestion is commonly used as a component in several molecular techniques.

Polymorphisms, or differences in DNA sequence among individuals in a population, are heritable. *Polymorphism* is not synonymous with *mutation*. Mutations are variations found less frequently in a population than polymorphisms, and they occur as nongermline (somatic cell) changes, usually in a tumor cell, or as inherited (and transmissible) alterations of a "wild type" DNA sequence. Restriction fragment length polymorphisms are differences in DNA that manifest as removal or creation of an RE site; removal results in a larger restriction fragment in individuals containing the polymorphism, while creation of an RE site results in two smaller fragments relative to the unaffected individual. In either case, the polymorphism is detectable through routine molecular pathology laboratory methods

and can be detected by observing the restriction fragment pattern, i.e., a restriction fragment *length* polymorphism.

SPECIFIC METHODOLOGIES

DNA SEQUENCING

Molecular pathology owes its existence to the ability to sequence DNA. Specific sequence information is a prerequisite for designing the primers and probes used in diagnostic tests. The DNA sequencing method originally developed by Sanger, Nicklen, and Coulson is the basis for most DNA sequencing performed in clinical laboratories. It was also the backbone technology that enabled the sequencing of the human genome.

The original Sanger sequencing reaction uses a single primer and DNA polymerase. Components include (1) electrophoresis with single base-pair resolution, (2) sequence-specific complementary primers, and (3) small proportions of dideoxyribonucleotide triphosphates (ddNTPs), in addition to the conventional deoxyribonucleotide triphosphates (dNTPs). ddNTPs lack the oxygen attached to the 3′ carbon, thus preventing elongation. This results in a set of newly synthesized DNA chains complementary to the template DNA but varying in length, with the length determined by the point of incorporation of the ddNTP into the growing chain.

Today, sequencing is similar to the original method developed 30 years ago except that radioactive labeling has largely been replaced by fluorescent labeling. Two categories of fluorescent labeling exist; one exploits fluorescently labeled primers, and the second uses ddNTPs individually labeled with different fluorophores, enabling the reactions to be performed in a single tube. Dye-primer labeling may be used in fragment analysis for detection of, e.g., microsatellite instability, loss of heterozygosity, forensic investigation, or allogeneic bone marrow transplantation monitoring using short tandem repeat polymorphisms. Dye-terminator labeling is used where entire sequences must be analyzed, e.g., human immunodeficiency virus resistance testing. Automated sequencers have been developed using both types of fluorescent technology, as well as adaptations of these technologies. The various instruments' detection software generates an electropherogram of the DNA sequence, correlating each dye's fluorescence intensity to a specific ddNTP migration time. The introduction of capillary electrophoresis facilitated widespread incorporation of sequencing and fragment analysis into the clinical laboratory.

is characterized by gradual increase or decrease in fluorescence without amplification of product. All software packages included with the instruments available commercially for clinical laboratory use are loaded with tools to assist in the preceding calculation and analyses.

In the plateau phase of amplification, critical reaction components become rate limiting and amplicon accumulation slows or stops; therefore, increase in fluorescent signal slows or stops. In turn, as rate of accumulation of product slows or stops in the plateau phase, the curve levels. In conventional PCR, the end point for analysis is in this plateau phase. Real-time PCR, on the other hand, uses built-in software packages that quantify product during the log-linear phase, making it more amenable to quantification. In quantitative real-time PCR, the standard curve generated from known standards is used to determine the concentration of unknown samples based on the C_t value. Real-time instrumentation software packages are powerful and versatile; in choosing a system, ensure full training by the vendor for all users.

Melting curve analysis of the final amplified product may be performed in real-time PCR. In real-time PCR, dsDNA that undergoes melting curve analysis is the amplicon to which a fluorescently labeled probe is bound. The melting point is the temperature at which 50% of the strands are single-stranded DNA and the other 50% are dsDNA. The nucleotide sequence of the hybrid dictates the T_m. Thus, guanosine–cytosine–rich sequences are more resistant to denaturation, i.e., have a higher T_m, because of the three hydrogen bonds holding guanosine and cytosine together; only two hydrogen bonds bind an adenine–thymidine dyad. Real-time instruments capable of melting curve analysis slowly increase the temperature after the final extension and monitor the denaturation of hybrids through measurement of fluorescence. In this way, single base changes, whether mutations or clinically significant polymorphisms, can be identified, because different sequences will melt at different T_m. Software makes these differences obvious to the human eye.

METHYLATION-SPECIFIC POLYMERASE CHAIN REACTION

Cells regulate gene expression in several ways, including DNA methylation, an enzyme-mediated modification that adds a methyl ($-CH_3$) group at selected sites in genes. Of relevance to diagnostics, methylation occurs only at a specific motif known as CpG dinucleotides: cytosine followed by a guanosine. CpG dinucleotides suffer spontaneous mutations and are selectively depleted from the genome. Some regions of DNA, however, retain CpG dinucleotides; these are known as *CpG islands* and are usually found in the 5′ region of expressed genes, often in association with promoters. Gene expression is silenced when the promoter–CpG island is methylated; transcription is inhibited.

Important clinical questions may be addressed by assessing methylation using methylation-specific PCR (MSP). In MSP, DNA is first treated with sodium bisulfite, which converts unmethylated cytosine to uracil, thereby differentiating methylated cytosine, which is left unaffected. Primer pairs that specifically identify either methylated or unmethylated DNA are employed, followed by gel electrophoresis used to detect the presence or absence of the amplicon in each of the two reactions. In this way, the presence of unmethylated alleles, methylated alleles, or both is assessed. Clinically, MSP may be used to study imprinted genes, presence of clonality (based upon X chromosome inactivation through methylation), and presence of abnormally methylated CpG islands present in neoplasia. In quantitative MSP, real-time PCR is employed to distinguish high-level CpG methylation, which is common to neoplasia, from low-level methylation, which is more common in aging or in non-neoplastic conditions, e.g., metaplasia.

IN SITU POLYMERASE CHAIN REACTION

In situ PCR can be performed directly on cellular material that is contained in solution or adhered to glass slides. Experimental protocols for in situ PCR include steps that take into account specimen type, fixative, and processing methods used. Paraffin-embedded specimens have been adapted to in situ PCR and involve removal of the paraffin and rehydration of the tissue (see nucleic acid isolation, described earlier) before the reaction. If the specimen is in solution, the reaction components are added directly to the tube. For specimens on a glass slides, the components are added to the specimen, covered with a coverslip, and sealed to prevent evaporation. Conventional thermal cyclers or specially designed thermal cycling ovens are used for amplification. Detection of the amplicons is usually accomplished indirectly with hybridization to specific probes or directly with the use of labeled nucleotides that have been incorporated into PCR. The practical effectiveness of in situ PCR is limited by amplicon diffusion and suboptimized target localization.

PROTEIN TRUNCATION TEST

The protein truncation test (PTT), as the name implies, is employed to identify mutations, at the protein level, that result from premature termination of protein translation. The test has been used for detecting the large deletions in the dystrophin gene and the resulting protein responsible for Duchenne muscular dystrophy. PTT is also used to detect protein-truncating mutations associated with multiple types of hereditary cancer syndromes, particularly breast, ovarian, and colon cancers. In PTT, following amplification of the sequence of interest, amplicons are used for in vitro transcription and translation and the generated proteins are separated using sodium dodecyl sulfate polyacrylamide gel electrophoresis. Truncated protein migrates more quickly in the gel than the wild-type protein.

IN VITRO NUCLEIC ACID AMPLIFICATION ALTERNATIVES TO POLYMERASE CHAIN REACTION

The exclusive use of PCR in the research laboratories of the 1980s, as well as its early commercialization in the 1990s, caused PCR to be the only amplification process in use for many years. Because it was clear that amplification is the key to molecular diagnostics, companies other than Roche (the historical patent holder for PCR) worked to develop alternatives to PCR for the clinical laboratory. Three are described here: transcription-mediated amplification (TMA), strand displacement amplification (SDA); and nucleic acid sequence–based amplification (NASBA). Each is performed on dedicated equipment using analyte-specific kits for various analytes that may be obtained from Gen-Probe, Becton Dickinson, and bioMerieux, respectively. For a time, ligase chain reaction was popular in the molecular diagnostics laboratory, but it has been withdrawn from the marketplace and so will not be covered here.

TRANSCRIPTION-MEDIATED AMPLIFICATION

RNA is the template for amplification in TMA and includes, as components of the reaction template, two primers, reverse transcriptase, and RNA polymerase. One primer contains a promoter sequence for subsequent binding of RNA polymerase. Initially, the primer containing the promoter sequence hybridizes to the target RNA and reverse transcriptase synthesizes a copy with the promoter sequence incorporated into the cDNA (Figure 3-3). This generates an RNA:DNA hybrid, and the RNase H nuclease activity inherent in reverse transcriptase digests the RNA component of the hybrid in the next step of the reaction. The second primer then hybridizes to the cDNA and a dsDNA molecule is synthesized. RNA polymerase, also present, initi-

ates transcription by binding the promoter sequence in the DNA template. Each of the newly synthesized RNA amplicons also enters the TMA cycle, serving as templates for subsequent rounds of amplification. Eight to nine orders of magnitude of amplification can be achieved quickly in an autocatalytic, isothermal process. Proprietary labeled DNA probes are employed to initiate chemiluminescent detection and quantification.

STRAND DISPLACEMENT AMPLIFICATION

In SDA, a proprietary isothermal, in vitro, nucleic acid amplification technique, hemimodified DNA is polymerized using three conventional dNTPs and one containing a 5′-[a-thio]triphosphate. The primer or primers are designed with an RE recognition site in the 5′ overhang end. RE included in the reaction mixture nicks the unmodified DNA strand at a double-stranded hemiphosphorothioate recognition site, which occurs when the 5′-[a-thio]triphosphate nucleotide is incorporated. Linear amplification occurs when a single primer is used. Exponential amplification is achieved by using two primers, both containing RE recognition. This complicated biochemistry occurs in a reaction transparent to the user in proprietary instrumentation in common use in the molecular microbiology laboratory. SDA has also been adapted to microarray formats and may find future applications.

NUCLEIC ACID SEQUENCE–BASED AMPLIFICATION

NASBA, marketed in a line of products under the NucleSens™ brand name by bioMerieux, is an isothermal amplification method for single-stranded nucleic acids using two sequence-specific primers (Figure 3-4) and three enzymes: avian myeloblastosis virus–reverse transcriptase (AMV-RT), RNase H, and T7 RNA polymerase. One primer contains a T7 RNA polymerase recognition sequence at its 5′ end and facilitates transcription of a target fed by AMV-RT to cDNA. The RNA strand is then destroyed by RNase H, and dsDNA is synthesized off the second primer by AMV-RT. T7 RNA polymerase synthesizes multiple antisense RNA transcripts, and the cycle is repeated. Generally, amplification is approximately 10^{12}-fold in 1 to 2 hours at a constant 41° C. Because RNA is single stranded at this temperature, it is preferentially amplified, permitting RNA detection in a genomic DNA background without generation of false-positive results. Specific DNA amplification may be done by introducing a denaturation step before amplification. End-point and real-time NASBA assays are commercially available for several infectious disease tests.

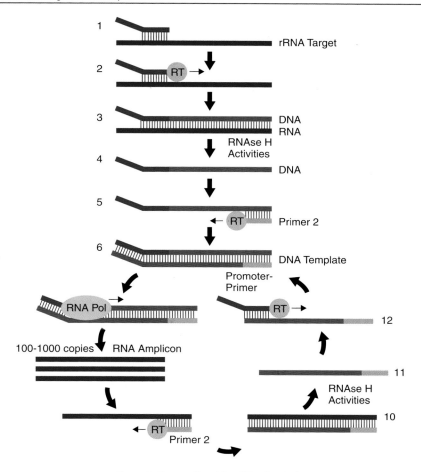

FIGURE 3-3

Transcription-mediated Amplification Cycle

Step 1: Promoter primer binds to rRNA target
Step 2: Reverse transcriptase creates DNA copy of rRNA target
Step 3: RNA:DNA duplex
Step 4: RNAse H activities of reverse transcriptase degrade rRNA
Step 5: Primer 2 binds to DNA, and reverse transcriptase creates new DNA copy
Step 6: dsDNA template with promoter sequence
Step 7: RNA polymerase (RNA Pol) initiates transcription of RNA from DNA template
Step 8: 100–1000 copies of RNA amplicon are produced
Step 9: Primer 2 binds to each RNA amplicon, and reverse transcriptase creates DNA copy
Step 10: RNA:DNA duplex
Step 11: RNAse H activities of reverse transcriptase degrades rRNA
Step 12: Promoter primer binds to newly synthesized DNA; reverse transcriptase creates dsDNA, and autocatalytic cycle repeats, resulting in a billionfold amplification Reprinted with permission from Gen-Probe.

SIGNAL AMPLIFICATION TECHNOLOGIES

BRANCHED DNA TECHNOLOGY

Branched DNA technology, proprietary to Siemens and automated in commercially available systems for viral analytes (kits plus automated analyzers), employs multiple capture extenders (oligonucleotides) that hybridize to complementary regions of the target nucleic acid of interest. Capture probes, attached to the surface of a microtiter plate, bind the capture extenders anchoring the target to the plate. Target probes are then added that hybridize to different, conserved sequences on the target nucleic acid. The target probes contain key sequences that bind the following reaction components in sequential order, which in turn, precipitates signal amplification: preamplifier (complementary to a region of the target probes), amplifier (complementary to a region of the preamplifier molecule), and alkaline phosphatase–modified label probes (complementary to portions of the amplifier molecule). The series of probes results in formation of large hybridization complexes on the target RNA or DNA, which can contain more than 10,000 alkaline phosphatase molecules. Addition of dioxetane substrate for the alkaline phosphatase results in chemiluminescence proportional to the amount of target RNA or DNA present in the sample.

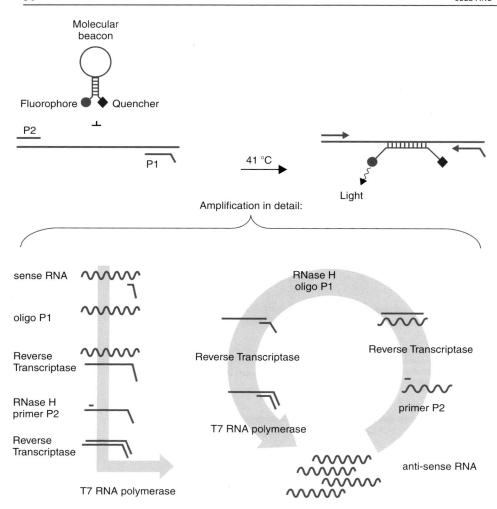

FIGURE 3-4

The nucleic acid sequence–based amplification reaction. The P1 antisense primer contains a T7 RNA polymerase promoter sequence for in vitro transcription and a second, Ps, sense primer. Detection is through a probe containing a fluorophore and a quencher molecule, which are dissociated upon binding, resulting in fluorescence.

HYBRID CAPTURE

Hybrid capture is the generic term for proprietary technology marketed by Qiagen for the detection of various pathogens in the molecular diagnostics laboratory environment. Hybrid capture is a signal amplification system based on antibody binding to RNA:DNA hybrids. In the assay, denatured target DNA hybridizes to unlabeled RNA probes, creating RNA:DNA hybrids. The hybrids are captured by an anti-RNA:DNA antibody bound to the surface of individual wells of a microtiter plate. A second anti-RNA:DNA monoclonal antibody conjugated to alkaline phosphatase is used to initiate the detection phase. Addition of a dioxetane-based substrate, cleaved by the alkaline phosphatase, generates a chemiluminescent signal that is proportional to the amount of starting material.

FLUORESCENCE IN SITU HYBRIDIZATION

Fluorescence in situ hybridization (FISH) is something of a hybrid between cytogenetics and molecular diagnostics. FISH-based assays are marketed by several companies, and Abbott Molecular boasts several FDA-approved applications. In FISH, fluorescently tagged DNA or RNA probes are used to identify genomic sequences of interest. FISH may be used to identify sequences of interest in FFPE tissue sections, an advantage that permits correlation of probe hybridization with tissue morphology. When coupled to conventional cytogenetics, FISH provides high resolution for identification of specific abnormalities, e.g., gene amplification, deletions, and translocations.

Akin to Southern blot, FISH requires denaturation, hybridization with a probe, and washing. First, a probe specific for the target of interest is applied to the slide, along with a nuclear counterstain and reagents that enhance denaturation of target DNA and reduce background. The slides are sealed and incubated in a humid environment under conditions that denature the DNA, allowing hybridization to occur between the probe and its cDNA sequence. The unbound probe is then removed by washing, and patterns of fluorescence are interpreted by fluorescence microscopy.

In dual-color FISH (dFISH), two probes with different fluorescence wavelengths are used to identify structural chromosomal rearrangements. Although each probe generates a characteristic color individually, a distinct third color is formed when the two probes are juxtaposed (fusion signal). For example, two probes can bind to a region of chromosomal rearrangement, generate a fusion signal, and thereby identify mutations that involve two partner genes.

In spectral karyotyping and multiplex FISH, multiple fluorochromes, specialized optics, and image analysis identify all chromosomes in a specimen. In a variation of FISH called comparative genomic hybridization (CGH), relative gains or losses in the genome may be assessed for clinical investigation. In CGH, the ratio of patient specimen DNA, labeled with one fluorochrome, and that of normal DNA, labeled with a different fluorochrome, are compared. CGH is a powerful research and discovery tool and has applications in translational research for potential clinical application. In another variation on the FISH theme, bright field in situ hybridization employs colorimetric probes, which provide a relatively stable signal that also does not require fluorescence microscopy.

DNA ARRAYS AND CHIPS

In the context of molecular diagnostics, the term *array* may be considered jargon for a collection of molecules orderly arranged on solid supports, e.g., nylon membranes, printed circuit board, glass slides, and silicon surfaces. Macroscopic arrays include the example of reverse line blots on nylon membranes, and microarrays include DNA chips. Many synonyms for *microarray* exist: *GeneChip®, DNA chip, genome chip, biochip, gene array, DNA array,* and *DNA microarray.* Liquid phase arrays also exist, e.g., Luminex.

Line probe assays are the simplest type of array. Generally, reverse hybridization is employed. Using this method, DNA is amplified using biotinylated primers, denatured, and hybridized to probes bound to a nylon or nitrocellulose strip in a parallel line format. The probes are specific for mutations or polymorphisms of interest. After hybridization, alkaline phosphatase–labeled streptavidin is added, which binds to the biotin in the amplicons. Colorimetric detection with a specific chromogen generates a purple-brown precipitate, which is interpreted as positive result.

DNA chips may be thought of as miniaturized platforms for allele-specific oligonucleotide hybridization, some with thousands of unique sequences. In general, DNA is fluorescently labeled, denatured, and hybridized to the oligonucleotide probes on the chip akin to many hybridization style assays described in this chapter. Upon completion of the assay, the chip is scanned and the fluorescence patterns are measured and examined to detect the presence of mutant or wild-type sequences and/or gene expression changes that might be indicative of disease or part of a pattern specific for a disease, known as a *disease profile* or *genetic signature.*

Although clinical laboratory diagnostic applications for DNA chips were limited at the time of this writing, it seems clear that the complex nature of disease at the molecular level will yield to our knowledge, at which time multiple analytes (genes or specific genes' expression) will need to be assessed simultaneously. Once this occurs, DNA chips will serve as the natural platform choice for such investigation and clinical testing. Assays using chips for applications in pharmacogenomics, sepsis, leukemia genotyping, and identifying solid and hematologic tumors are in use or in development. In the second half of this decade, it is likely that the major commercial supplier of such assays will be Roche, in partnership with the original developer of these chips, Affymetrix. To be fair, other companies are working on similar and other applications. Currently, technology is relatively expensive, applications are limited, and experience in the clinical arena is limited (as opposed to the extensive experience in the research arena), so readers interested in this technology are advised to use the Internet and discussion groups to learn more. (An excellent resource for this sort of investigation is available to members of the Association of Molecular Pathology through its listserv, CHAMP, which is an acronym for CHat AMP.)

Informatics software used to analyze data generated by DNA chips requires simplification and modification for clinical laboratory application. Useful algorithms for data analysis must be developed to assist in disease diagnosis and prognosis. The great potential that this "marriage" of Silicon Valley to molecular diagnostics possesses promises to advance laboratory medicine to a new level before much more time passes.

SUGGESTED READINGS

Baltimore D: Viral RNA-dependent DNA polymerase. Nature 1970;226:1209–1211.

Bernard PS, Wittwer CT: Real-time PCR technology for cancer diagnostics. Clin Chem 2002;48:1178–1185.

Bustin SA: Absolute quantification of mRNA using real-time reverse transcription–polymerase chain reaction assays. J Mol Endocrinol 2000;25:169–193.

DiDomenico N, Link H, Knobel R, et al: Cobas Amplicor™: Fully automated RNA and DNA amplification and detection system for routine diagnostic PCR. Clin Chem 1996;42:1915–1923.

du Manoir S, Speicher MR, Joos S, et al: Detection of complete and partial chromosome gains and losses by comparative genomic in situ hybridization. Hum Genet 1993;90:590–610.

Dyanov HM, Dzitoeva SG: Method for attachment of microscopic preparations on glass for in situ hybridization, PRINS, and in situ PCR studies. BioTechniques 1995;18:823–826.

Esch RK: Basic nucleic acid procedures. In Coleman WB, Tsongalis GJ (eds): Molecular Diagnostics for the Clinical Laboratorian. Totowa, NJ, Humana Press, 1997, pp 55–58.

Farkas DH: Specimen procurement, processing, tracking, and testing by the Southern blot. In Farkas DH (ed): Molecular Biology and Pathology: A Guidebook for Quality Control. San Diego, Academic Press, 1993, pp 51–75.

Farkas DH: Thermal cyclers. In Laboratory Instrument Evaluation Verification and Maintenance Manual. Northfield, IL, College of American Pathologists, 1998, pp 130–133.

Guan XY, Zhang H, Bittner M, et al: Chromosome arm painting probes. Nat Genet 1996;12:10–11.

Lay MJ, Wittwer CT: Real-time fluorescence genotyping of factor V Leiden during rapid-cycle PCR. Clin Chem 1997;43:2262–2267.

Lo Y, Wong I, Zhang J, et al: Quantitative analysis of aberrant p16 methylation using real-time quantitative methylation-specific polymerase chain reaction. Cancer Res 1999;59:3899–3903.

Loeffelholz MJ, Lewinski CA, Silver SR, et al: Detection of *Chlamydia trachomatis* in endocervical specimens by polymerase chain reaction. J Clin Microbiol 1992;30:2847–2851.

Mullis K, Faloona F, Schart S, et al: Specific enzymatic amplification of DNA in vitro: The polymerase chain reaction. CSH Symp Quant Biol 1986;51:263–273.

Olek A, Oswald J, Walter JAA: A modified and improved method of bisulfite based cytosine methylation analysis. Nucleic Acids Res 1996;24:5064–5066.

Roest PA, Roberts RG, Sugino S, et al: Protein truncation test (PTT) for rapid detection of translation-terminating mutations. Hum Mol Genet 1993;2:1719–1721.

Ronaghi M, Karamohamed S, Pettersson B, et al: Real-time DNA sequencing using detection of pyrophosphate release. Anal Biochem 1996;242:84–89.

Sanger F, Nicklen S, Coulson AR: DNA sequencing with chain-terminating inhibitors. Proc Natl Acad Sci USA 1977;74:5463–5467.

Schmaizing D, Koutny L, Salas-Solano O, et al: Recent developments in DNA sequencing by capillary and microdevice electrophoresis [review]. Electrophoresis 1999;20:3066–3077.

Schrock E, du Manoir S, Veldman T, et al: Multicolor spectral karyotyping of human chromosomes. Science 1996;273:494–497.

Sooknanan R, van Gemen B, Malek LT: Nucleic acid sequence-based amplification. In Wiedbrauk DL, Farkas DH (eds): Molecular Methods for Virus Detection. San Diego, Academic Press, 1995, pp 261–285.

Walker GT, Little MC, Nadeau JG, Shank DD: Isothermal in vitro amplification of DNA by a restriction enzyme/DNA polymerase system. Proc Natl Acad Sci USA 1992;89:392–396.

Westin L, Xu X, Miller C, et al: Anchored multiplex amplification on a microelectronic chip array. Nat Biotechnol 2000;18:199–204.

4

Conventional and Real-Time Polymerase Chain Reaction

Aaron Bossler • Vivianna Van Deerlin

INTRODUCTION

The polymerase chain reaction (PCR), first conceived by Kary B. Mullis in 1983, revolutionized the ability to perform biologic research and has become a technologic foundation in the molecular diagnostic laboratory. With its high sensitivity for detecting and copying a target region from even a single DNA molecule, PCR amplification has many applications in research and in the clinical laboratory for testing in genetics, oncology, infectious diseases, pharmacogenetics, and identity testing. Myriad commercial products and reagent kits are available, some with predesigned protocols that simplify the validation and implementation process for many assays, as well as manual and automated instrument platforms. Most molecular diagnostic tests incorporate target amplification by PCR, and although variations and new technologies are being introduced at a rapid pace, PCR will undoubtedly continue to play a major role in diagnostic applications. This chapter delves into the principles of PCR, variations and applications of PCR, and the necessary controls that can help ensure its appropriate use and interpretation in clinical testing.

PRINCIPLES OF POLYMERASE CHAIN REACTION

PCR mimics the natural process of DNA replication and, like DNA replication, requires the presence of a DNA template, a DNA polymerase, and four deoxyribonucleotide triphosphates (dNTPs): adenine (dATP), guanine (dGTP), thymidine (dTTP), and cytosine (dCTP). PCR amplification also requires a reaction buffer optimal for the activity of the polymerase and two primers (a forward and a reverse primer) designed to flank a target region. Primers are chemically synthesized, single-stranded oligonucleotides that are complementary to the flanking ends of the target region of the template DNA sequence to be amplified. The complementary strands of the input DNA provide the sequence template for synthesis of the DNA copies. By convention, the DNA sequence is written in the 5′ to 3′ orientation, which is determined by the chemical structure of the phosphate–sugar backbone of the DNA chain (Figure 4-1A). DNA polymerase catalyzes the unidirectional addition of the appropriate dNTP to the 3′ end of the growing DNA chain. In this way, the primers in the reaction each provide an anchoring hydroxyl group (−OH) at the 3′ carbon position of the sugar moiety to which a phosphodiester bond with the 5′ phosphate group of an incoming dNTP can be formed (Figure 4-1).

The essential element for the success of PCR is thermal cycling. The PCR amplification process is based on repeated cycles of three steps: denaturation (usually 95° C), annealing (usually 45° C to 60° C), and extension (usually 72° C). These thermal cycles are performed in a programmable instrument, or thermal cycler, which can generally hold 24, 48, 96, or 384 tubes, or multiwell plates, and adjusts the temperature of the wells for each of the PCR steps for the number of indicated cycles. In the first step or denaturation phase, the reaction is heated to 95° C for a brief period (15 to 30 seconds) to break the hydrogen bonds between the two strands of the double-stranded DNA (Figure 4-2A) and allow them to separate, thus forming single-stranded DNA, which will anneal to oligonucleotide primers in the next step. This annealing step occurs when the temperature is lowered to between 45° C and 60° C; the forward and reverse primers bind to their complementary sequences on the template DNA. The DNA polymerase recognizes and binds to the double-stranded primer–target molecule hybrid and proceeds along the template, adding dNTPs that are complementary to the target to the 3′ end of the primer strand. This extension phase is carried out at a temperature optimal for the function of the DNA polymerase. Thermostable DNA polymerases work most efficiently at 68° C to 75° C; thus, the temperature is typically raised to 72° C for a period sufficient to complete the extension, which depends

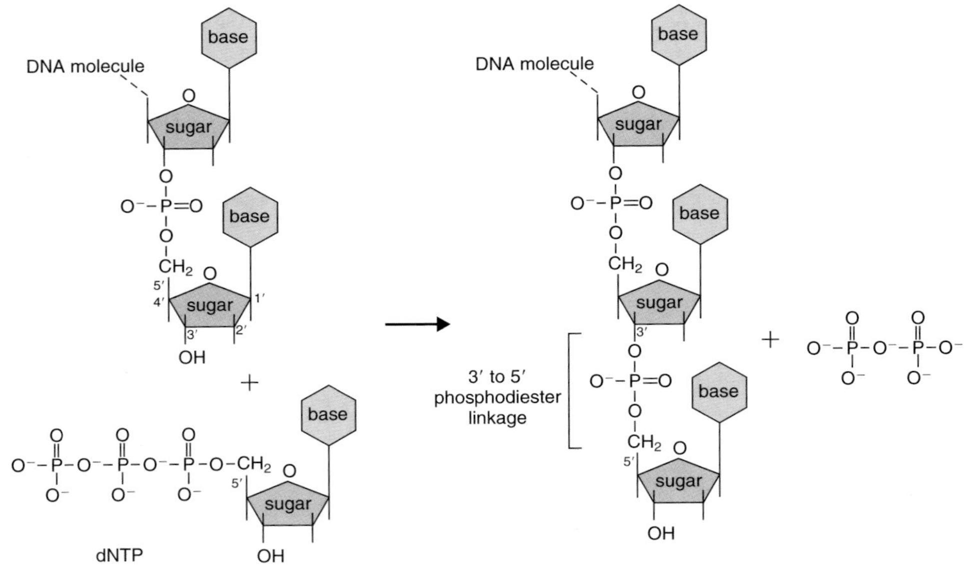

FIGURE 4-1

Phosphodiester bond formation. The carbon atoms of the sugar ring (in pink) are numbered 1′ through 5′. The primer DNA molecule has a hydroxyl group (−OH) at the 3′ carbon, which initiates the nucleophilic attach of the alpha phosphate group at the 5′ carbon atom of the incoming nucleotide, resulting in elongation of the DNA chain by one nucleotide.

on the length of the target. At the end of this first cycle of amplification, two daughter strands, one from each original template strand, are produced and can serve as templates in the next cycle, which is repeated following the same steps (Figure 4-2B). A PCR amplification usually consists of 30 to 50 cycles.

The resulting product represents an exponential amplification of the starting target in the sample. The amplicon yield can be estimated using the following formula:

$$X_n = X_0 \times (1 + E)^n$$

where X_n is the amount of amplicon made in n PCR cycles, X_0 is the amount of starting template, and E is the efficiency of the reaction, which varies from zero to one. Theoretically, the number of amplicons doubles with each cycle (Table 4-1). In reality, the efficiency of the reaction decreases over the course of PCR amplification (Figure 4-3). At first, the PCR efficiency is close to 1.0 and the growth is exponential, but as the cycles progress, the amplification efficiency plateaus with no further increase in amplicon production. This plateau effect is thought to occur either because one of the reagents becomes limiting (such as primers or dNTPs) or because of instability of the DNA polymerase with repeated heating cycles. It may also be caused by end product inhibition, competition by nonspecific products, and incomplete denaturation of strands at higher product concentration or reannealing of product at higher concentrations, which prevents the extension process.

DNA Polymerase

Heat stability of the DNA polymerase is an essential characteristic required for thermal cycling. Incubation at 95° C denatures and inactivates most proteins. The identification and isolation of thermostable DNA polymerases from organisms that survive in extreme environments like hot springs or thermal vents was instrumental in the development of automated PCR. Three commonly used DNA polymerases are *Taq* polymerase (originally isolated from the microorganism *Thermus aquaticus*), Pfu *(Pyrococcus furiosus)*, and Vent or Tli *(Thermococcus litoralis)*. *Taq* DNA polymerase was the first heat-stable polymerase to be applied for use in the PCR in 1987, and it remains one of the most commonly used polymerases. Although these enzymes are most active at 70° C, they synthesize DNA at a broad range of temperatures as long as a primer–template hybrid is present. At low temperatures, where specificity of primer binding is lower (i.e., primers may hybridize to template DNA despite one or more mismatches), the DNA polymerase may begin to extend a nonspecific product, which can cause high background and low specific product yield. To overcome this problem, hot-start PCR was developed in which one essential reagent is withheld from the mixture until the system has reached a favorable temperature for specific primer annealing, usually the polymerase. Hot-start processes include use of heat-labile physical barriers like wax to separate the polymerase from the reaction and polymerase-inactivating antibodies that block the polymerase until the antibody is denatured in the

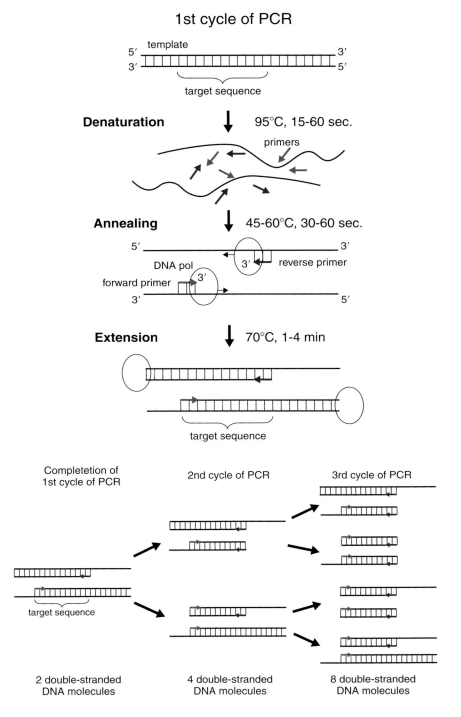

1st cycle of PCR

FIGURE 4-2

Thermal cycling steps in a polymerase chain reaction (PCR) reaction. **A,** A target sequence is selected. The template denatures at 95° C. Forward primers (red arrows) and reverse primers (blue arrows), which are present in the reaction in excess, anneal to the complementary sequence of the target during the annealing step. The polymerase (black oval) extends the PCR product during the extension phase. **B,** The first three cycles of PCR and the resulting products. Note that only at the end of the third cycle are the first correctly sized amplicons representing the target sequence produced.

95° C step. Another approach has been to modify the polymerase either through the selection of thermally activated polymerase mutants or by the design of heat-sensitive specialty molecules that block the polymerase. Several types of hot-start polymerases are commercially available.

PRIMERS

Two PCR primers, one forward and one reverse, are necessary for exponential PCR amplification to occur. The forward primer is complementary to the reverse template strand at the beginning of the target

TABLE 4-1
Exponential Amplicon Production

Number of Cycles	Number of Copies
1	$2^1 = 2$
2	$2^2 = 4$
3	$2^3 = 8$
4	$2^4 = 16$
10	$2^{10} = 1024$
20	$2^{20} = 1,048,576$
30	$2^{30} = 1,073,741,824$

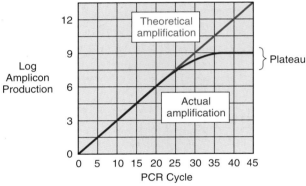

FIGURE 4-3

Plateau effect in polymerase chain reaction (PCR). Theoretically, the product should double with each cycle, as depicted by the straight line on the graph. In reality, with increasing PCR cycle numbers, the reagents become limiting and the amplification slows to a stop, depicted as the plateau of the curve. Thus, between cycles 35 and 45 in this example, if one were to measure the amount of product formed at each cycle end point, the amount of product produced would be the same.

temperatures, and may decrease the final yield of product. The optimal annealing temperature for any given PCR reaction is primarily a function of the melting or dissociation temperature (T_m) of the oligonucleotide primers, i.e., the temperature at which 50% of the oligonucleotide primers are bound to their complementary sequence and the other 50% are separated into single-stranded molecules. The T_m of the primers depends on both its length and its nucleotide sequence composition, i.e., the ratio of the number of guanines and cytosines to the number of adenines and thymidines. The T_m of the primers can serve as a rough guide to determine the optimal annealing temperature to favor specific primer template binding over nonspecific DNA interactions that could lead to misextension. In practice, however, this is ultimately determined by trial and error. Of note, in some cases a mismatched nucleotide is intentionally designed in a primer sequence in combination with a lower annealing temperature in the PCR, for example, to introduce a restriction enzyme cleavage site to the final product. Additional factors to consider in designing primers are the presence of intra- and intersequence complementarity. A primer that anneals to its own complementary sequence, its paired primer, or other primers in a multiplex reaction may result in spurious product formation referred to as *primer-dimers*. Any of these intra- or inter-primer interactions could unfavorably influence the PCR reaction, decreasing the yield of the specific product. Software applications for selecting optimal primer sequences are available commercially, as well as freely on the Internet. Several websites listed in Suggested Readings have tools for designing primers.

In multiplex PCR, where more than one pair of primers is used for simultaneous amplification of multiple targets in a single reaction, the primers can be selected to vary the length of the amplicons, allowing the products to be differentiated. Primers can also be designed to carry additional molecules or labels that become incorporated into the amplicons. These can include radioactive labels, fluorescent dyes, protein adducts, or other molecules that can be used to help detect the amplicon. For example, the primer can be labeled with radioactive phosphorus-32 or numerous fluorescent dyes, such as 6-carboxyfluoroscein or tetrachloro-6-carboxyfluorescein. Primers labeled with a protein adduct such as biotin use the high-avidity binding of streptavidin for detection by linking enzymes such as horseradish peroxidase to the streptavidin molecule. The biotin-labeled amplicons are incubated first with the streptavidin horseradish peroxidase, washed, and then incubated with an oxidizable chromogenic substrate such as tetramethylbenzidine and hydrogen peroxide to produce a color change.

sequence, and the reverse primer is complementary to the forward strand at the end of the target sequence (Figure 4-2A). For the PCR amplification to be successful, the primers must bind to opposite strands of the DNA template so that both strands of the target are copied with each cycle. They are added to the reaction in molar excess (usually at a final concentration of 200 to 900 nM) because with each cycle they become incorporated into the daughter strands, thus decreasing their concentration in the reaction.

There are several attributes of a good primer that determine its performance. One is that the primer sequence must be unique in the sequence of the DNA of the targeted specimen. Primers that match (or partially match) regions of DNA other than the target may lead to the generation of nonspecific PCR products, particularly at lower annealing

THE TEMPLATE

DNA

The template is the DNA molecule to which the primers and polymerase bind and whose target sequence is copied. Sources of DNA are numerous and may be genomic, mitochondrial, recombinant, or microbial. For clinical testing, DNA is usually isolated from the nuclei or mitochondria of fresh, frozen, or formalin-fixed paraffin-embedded tissue specimens; peripheral blood, bone marrow, body fluids, genital tract, or fine needle biopsy specimens; buccal cells; or microorganisms that may be present in any of these types of specimens. Leukocytes in blood are a common source of DNA for molecular testing. Formalin-fixed specimens are generally suitable for PCR; however, the DNA is partially fragmented because of protein cross-linking to DNA, which can be problematic for some assays. Therefore, it is generally advisable to design the amplicon target lengths to be short (usually less than 300 base pairs) to make it more likely that the sequence of interest will be detected from a pool of smaller fragmented pieces of DNA. DNA may also be extracellular from the breakdown of cells releasing free nucleic acid into blood, urine, or cerebrospinal fluid. There is a developing interest in obtaining "free" nucleic acid as a means to detect or monitor neoplastic disease. Finally, DNA that has been excised from a host genome and cloned into vector DNA molecules such as plasmids or cosmids is often used as positive control material in PCR amplification.

RNA

To detect or quantify RNA transcripts or the RNA genomes of some viruses, RNA must be converted into DNA so that it can serve as a template in a PCR amplification. This process is called *reverse transcription* (RT) and harnesses enzymes from retroviruses that are used to integrate their RNA genomes into host genomic DNA. In the laboratory, these reverse transcriptases convert RNA (total RNA or messenger RNA [mRNA]) templates into complementary DNA. Two commonly used reverse transcriptase enzymes are derived from the avian myeloblastosis virus and the Moloney murine leukemia virus. The initiating step in RT is similar to PCR in that oligonucleotide primers anneal to the template, but the reaction is different in that it is performed isothermally, i.e., at a single temperature, rather than with thermal cycling. Three types of primers are commonly used to initiate RT: oligo-dT, a string of thymidines that anneals to the polyadenylated tract present at the end of most mRNA molecules; random hexamer primers, which anneal randomly throughout the sequence; or target-specific primers, which are designed to bind selectively to the RNA molecule of interest and can be used as primers in the subsequent PCR amplification.

RT is usually combined with subsequent PCR amplification (known as RT-PCR) in either the same reaction tube (one step) or as a separate reaction (two step). In a one-step RT-PCR reaction, all the reagents needed for the RT and for the PCR amplification, including the target-specific primers, are added at the start. One-step reactions can use either reverse transcriptase with a DNA polymerase or a DNA polymerase that also has reverse transcriptase activity, such as *rTth,* derived from the organism *Thermus thermophilus,* which in the presence of manganese ions exhibits high reverse transcriptase activity and replaces the use of a separate RT enzyme. The advantage of a one-step RT reaction is that contamination risk is reduced because the tube does not need to be opened, and because the entire reaction is used for a template, the analytic sensitivity for low copy number transcripts may be increased. A disadvantage of one-step RT-PCR is that several targets cannot be tested for in the same sample unless several reactions are set up independently or multiplex PCR, which can be difficult to optimize, is used. One might want to evaluate several targets and a control gene in the same sample, e.g., several breakpoints for a chromosomal translocation that results in a novel chimeric transcript (e.g., *BCR/ABL1* arising from t(9;22) (q34; q11)) and a "housekeeping" control gene. Two-step RT-PCR is ideal in these situations because aliquots of the RT reaction are used as the template in one or more PCR reactions, which are set up like a standard PCR reaction.

RNA templates are found in almost all the same sources as DNA. However, RNA is more labile than DNA and is prone to degradation mostly because ribonucleases, enzymes that degrade RNA, are present almost everywhere. Special care must be taken to preserve RNA in the specimen when it is collected. When quantification of RNA species is important, stabilizing agents, which are commercially available, can be used. For tissue, flash freezing in liquid nitrogen is ideal soon after collection. Alternatively, special RNA stabilization liquid can be used for RNA preservation without fixation. Formalin-fixed paraffin-embedded specimens can be used for evaluation of RNA; however, like DNA but even more so, the RNA is susceptible to degradation and fragmentation.

OPTIMIZING THE REACTION

The DNA polymerase, primers, dNTPs, and template are combined in a buffered solution of Tris hydrochloride (pH, 8.0) containing potassium chloride and magnesium chloride. A reaction buffer for each enzyme is generally provided by the manufacturer for each specific polymerase as a 10X concentrated solution with or without magnesium. Magnesium ions are bound by DNA and the polymerase and are important for the reaction because they affect the T_m of the template, primers, and PCR products; the specificity of PCR product formation; and the activity and fidelity of the DNA polymerase. The optimal concentration for magnesium in each reaction must be determined case by case, but it generally ranges from 0.5 to 5.0 MM. In addition, the concentrations of the primers and the ratio of primers to template can be altered empirically to maximize the yield of the specific product.

Additives may also be required in some cases to improve the specificity of the PCR amplification, the yield of PCR products, or both. Several organic additives that have been described include dimethylsulfoxide (DMSO, 1% to 10% v/v), 1-carboxy, *N-N-N*-trimethylmethanammonium inner salt (betaine, ~1M), tetramethylammonium chloride (TMAC, up to 100mM), polyethylene glycol (5% to 15% w/v), glycerol (2% to 8% v/v), spermidine (0.5 to 3mM), and formamide (1.25% to 10%). The mechanism of action for each of these additives may be multifactorial and may include effects on primer T_m, the catalytic activity of the enzyme, or nonspecific structures that may form within and between the different DNA molecules once they become single stranded. For DMSO, betaine, and formamide, the effect likely is to lower the T_m so that specific interactions are

favored and nonspecific secondary structures are less likely to form at the annealing temperature of the reaction. Nonionic detergents such as Tween 20 and Triton-X-100 have also been used. Bovine serum albumin is another additive that may work to help bind protein inhibitors of the PCR amplification. Titration of the concentration of these additives in the reaction is usually required to determine the optimal concentration.

ANALYSIS OF POLYMERASE CHAIN REACTION PRODUCTS

Electrophoresis

Following PCR amplification, the amplicon products can be detected using several methods (Figure 4-4). An inexpensive and easy way of identifying PCR products has traditionally been to separate them using agarose gel electrophoresis and to visualize the products with ethidium bromide dye under ultraviolet light (Figure 4-5). Because of their inherent negative charge at mildly alkaline pH, the DNA molecules migrate through the sieve-like agarose gel using an electric current. Separation occurs based on size, with small fragments migrating more rapidly toward the anode than larger fragments. The concentration of agarose can be varied (commonly from 0.5% to 4%) to modify the separation properties of the gel. Polyacrylamide gels can also be used to separate DNA when the fragments are smaller. Ethidium bromide can be added to the gel

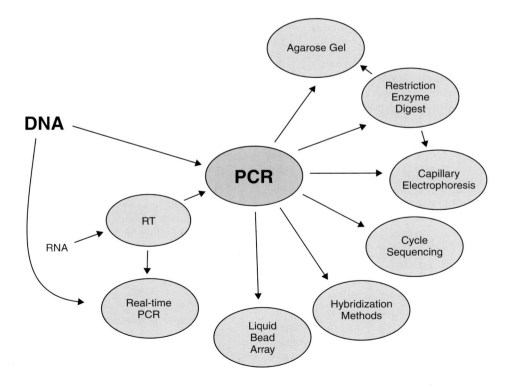

FIGURE 4-4

Detection methods for analyzing polymerase chain reaction (PCR) products. DNA or RNA after initial reverse transcription can be amplified using PCR and detected using several methods. DNA or RNA can also be amplified and detected using real-time PCR.

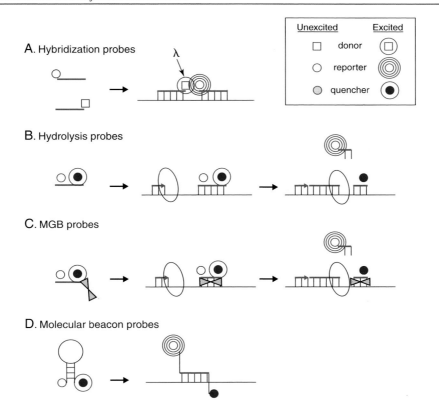

FIGURE 4-8

Real-time polymerase chain reaction (PCR) probe variations. **A,** Hybridization probes. Two separate, single-labeled oligonucleotides anneal to the target, bringing the donor fluorophore into proximity of the reporter fluorophore. After the donor fluorophore is excited by a certain wavelength of light energy (λ) its emission is absorbed by the reporter fluorophore, which then emits a different wavelength of light. Open square, donor dye; Open circle, reporter dye. **B,** Dual-labeled hydrolysis probe. When the reporter and quencher fluorophores are in proximity on the probe, the quencher absorbs the light emission from the exited reporter fluorophore. After the 5′ nuclease activity of the DNA polymerase hydrolyzes the end nucleotides from the probe, releasing the reporter fluorophore from the probe, the reporter fluorophore is excited and its light emission is not quenched. Open circle, reporter dye; closed circle, quencher dye. **C,** Minor groove binding (MGB) probes. Fluorescence is generated in the same manner as the hydrolysis probes. The MGB molecule covalently attached to the dual-labeled probe binds to the minor groove of the resulting double-stranded molecule when the probe anneals to the target, helping stabilize the binding of shorter probes. **D,** Molecular beacon probes. Note the stem–loop structure in the unbound target conformation. Annealing to the target after denaturation allows the reporter fluorophore to escape the quenching effect of the quencher fluorophore.

such molecule is dihydrocyclopyrroloindole tripeptide, which is typically attached to the 3′ end of the probe and folds into the minor groove of the duplex probe–target molecule through Van der Waals forces. This effectively raises the T_m of the probe and allows the use of shorter probes. This is an advantage in situations in which the conserved target sequence is short.

Molecular Beacons

Molecular beacons are single oligonucleotide sequences with reporter and quencher dyes at opposite ends, similar to hydrolysis probes but different in that the terminal sequences of the probe are complementary to each other (Figure 4-8D). In the unbound state, this allows the probe to fold back and anneal to itself, forming a double-stranded stem and single-stranded loop structure. This places the quencher dye adjacent to the reporter dye and prevents the reporter signal from being detected. The loop sequence is designed to be complementary to the target sequence. In amplification, the stem is melted during the denaturation step, allowing the intervening loop sequence to bind to the target sequence during the annealing step. When bound to the target sequence, the quencher is separated from the reporter, allowing its fluorescence to be detected. Unlike hydrolysis probes, the molecular beacon is displaced by the *Taq* polymerase but not hydrolyzed, leaving it intact to reform its original stem–loop structure in preparation for the next amplification cycle.

ADVANTAGES OF POLYMERASE CHAIN REACTION

The sensitivity, specificity, speed, and versatility of PCR have made it an indispensable tool for much of the testing done in molecular diagnostics. PCR instruments are affordable, some reagents are relatively inexpensive and standardized, and assays can be readily optimized. PCR set-up, amplification, and analysis can be performed quickly and easily, with results available in hours (not including specimen extraction and post-PCR analysis); in comparison, its predecessor, Southern blot hybridization, is time and labor intensive, taking days to yield results, and is less sensitive. PCR has been simplified and increasingly automated with the advent of real-time PCR for simultaneous detection and amplification of many samples in a closed system. This eliminates the need for postamplification manipulation, reducing the analysis time and decreasing the risk of contaminating subsequent PCR amplifications in the laboratory. In addition, Q-PCR has made quantification of a target over a range of seven logs or more relatively straightforward to perform for both DNA and RNA templates.

PCR does not require intact DNA, so almost any type of biologic specimen can be used to obtain nucleic acid—in contrast to Southern blot hybridization, which requires fresh tissue with full-length DNA. This feature makes analysis of tissues or cells that have been formalin-fixed and paraffin-embedded for histologic analysis feasible for PCR. DNA from formalin-fixed tissues is fragmented, making it unusable in most Southern blot applications, but PCR primers can be designed to accommodate the fragmentation of the DNA by limiting the size of the target.

In theory, a target can be amplified exponentially from even a single molecule or cell, which exemplifies the exquisite analytic sensitivity of PCR-based methods, although in practice attaining this level of sensitivity requires special assay design. Nevertheless, other methods such as Southern or northern blot hybridizations or fluorescence in situ hybridization (FISH) do not match the sensitivity of PCR because they lack an amplification step. The ability to achieve high analytic sensitivity with PCR-based applications has made it possible to monitor for residual disease after therapy in some neoplastic conditions using disease-specific markers.

DISADVANTAGES OF POLYMERASE CHAIN REACTION

Despite all the attributes of PCR, there are some limitations to its use and diagnostic utility. Several factors may influence the suitability of a particular DNA target. First, the target sequence needs to be known so that primer sequences can be designed. Second, the primer-annealing sequence in the target DNA needs to be conserved among individuals; otherwise, the primers may not work reliably. Polymorphisms in the primer region of the target may disrupt the ability of the primer to anneal, leading to failed amplification and possibly a false-negative result. Third, the primer sequence needs to be unique to reduce the possibility of the primer annealing to an unrelated DNA sequence. Comparison of the target sequence with a sequence of related genes or organisms is necessary to

determine how specific the primer pair is for the desired target.

Another limitation of PCR is the maximum length of the PCR product that can be synthesized. Characteristics of the DNA polymerase, including the processivity (length of product extension) and fidelity (whether incorrect nucleotides are inserted during the synthesis), vary with different polymerases, but most work well for generating products from a few hundred to a few thousand base pairs in length. Amplification of longer stretches of DNA requires special DNA polymerases or it may not work. Diseases that may be problematic for testing by PCR include trinucleotide repeat expansion diseases like Huntington's disease, fragile X, or myotonic dystrophy, which can be detected by PCR amplification if the trinucleotide repeat expansions are small. However, if the expansions are several hundreds or thousands of repeats long, Southern blot hybridization is necessary to identify the expanded alleles reliably.

Testing for other chromosomal alterations like translocations, inversions, or large additions or deletions can hamper the use of PCR if the primer-binding sites are disrupted by the genetic alteration. Methods such as traditional cytogenetics or FISH are more effective in these situations. FISH is useful for detecting chromosomal abnormalities because the probes are not negatively affected by small changes in the DNA, as is the case with PCR primers. Using PCR alone in these cases may result in false-negative results.

Exponential amplification is an essential component of PCR; however, it is also a weakness: it can potentially lead to contamination of subsequent PCR amplifications, which may result in false-positive results. Negative controls containing all reagents except the template DNA are required for correct interpretation of results. Good clinical laboratory practices to avoid contamination include physical separation of pre-PCR handling steps from the amplification and postamplification analysis areas, use of aerosol barrier pipette tips, and frequent changing of gloves and laboratory coats. Another means of control is the use of heat-labile uracil N-glycosylase (UNG) in PCR reactions substituting deoxyuridine (dUTP) for dTTP. The UNG enzyme hydrolyses the N-glycosidic bond between the deoxyribose sugar and the uracil base. Amplicons containing uridines are susceptible to hydrolytic cleavage by the enzyme at 50° C. The enzyme is included in the PCR reaction, and a pre-PCR incubation at 50° C cleaves any contaminating amplicons that were previously synthesized containing uridines. The enzyme is inactivated at high temperature, which occurs during the denaturation step of the PCR cycle, thus preventing it from degrading any new amplicons.

APPLICATIONS

Innumerable variations in the PCR method have been designed to detect disease. Its versatility has made it an unparalleled success in the research and clinical laboratories. PCR amplification of nucleic acids can be used to detect and query human and nonhuman genomes, as well as to detect or quantify gene expression. Application to the clinical molecular diagnostic laboratory involves selecting methods from a "molecular toolbox" and joining them to obtain the desired answer. Generally, the methods involve obtaining the nucleic acid, either DNA or RNA, from the sample; selecting primers specific for the task; amplifying the nucleic acid; and then detecting it with myriad options. Target amplification, whether by conventional PCR or real-time methods, is the most commonly applied method in the molecular toolbox, although many new variations, including methods based on signal amplification, are being developed. Applications for detecting the amplified product are numerous and have utility in several areas, including forensic or identity testing, detecting specific polymorphic or pathogenic genetic variations, and detecting the presence of specific new targets, such as chromosomal rearrangements or microorganisms. The use of target amplification in clinical medicine and pathology is so pervasive that it is difficult to describe all applications of PCR. However, a few examples will be used here to illustrate basic categories of applications that combine target amplification with different detection methods to answer a variety of questions.

USING POLYMERASE CHAIN REACTION TO DETECT KNOWN MUTATIONS

PCR methodology is particularly effective for mutation and polymorphism detection of small sequence alterations, including one or a few nucleotide substitutions, and small insertions or deletions. Such alterations account for most genetic diseases and are associated with many oncologic diseases. Identification of these alterations not only aids in diagnosis but also may identify carriers of a genetic disease, carry prognostic information, guide selection of therapy, or be used to monitor for disease recurrence. Many variations in PCR-based methods are used to detect mutations, and some of them are described here.

Numerous design modifications can be incorporated at the primer level for mutation detection. One example, referred to as allele-specific amplification or amplification refractory mutation testing, is used to detect SNPs by designing one of the primers so that the 3' end of the primer includes the mutated or polymorphic nucleotide. Both normal and mutant primer sets are separately amplified under conditions (i.e., relatively high annealing temperature) that favor only extension of the matched 3' end. In this way, both of the alleles can be detected, if present. This method can be applied to conventional or real-time PCR, and these assays can be multiplexed so that more than one alteration can be detected simultaneously.

Another design example uses a restriction enzyme site for detection of sequence alterations, referred to as restriction fragment length polymorphism (RFLP) analysis. Restriction enzymes have the ability to cleave DNA at or near specific recognition sequences. Mutations may disrupt a site or create a new restriction site. The normal sequence can be differentiated from the mutation by the pattern of fragments following the restriction enzyme digestion. The primers are designed to flank the mutation, along with the restriction site. Following PCR amplification, the amplicons are digested with the specific restriction enzyme or enzymes and separated by size with electrophoresis to differentiate the presence of normal or mutant sequences. The primer design can also be used to introduce new restriction enzyme sites, using primers altered to contain sequence to create the restriction site. One example of RFLP discrimination is in the detection of the mutated FMS-like tyrosine kinase 3 *(FLT3)* gene, where characteristic sequence changes are associated with prognosis in acute myeloid leukemia (Figure 4-9). The codon for the aspartic acid at position 835 (Asp835) is often mutated, with either substitution mutations, resulting in a different amino acid at that position, or in-frame deletion of the codon, removing the aspartic acid from the sequence. These alterations are believed to constitutively activate the tyrosine kinase function of the protein. In either case, the alterations at Asp835 in the *FLT3* gene eliminate an *Eco*RV restriction enzyme site (sequence 5'-_GAT_/ATC-3' underlined sequence is the aspartic acid codon). Primers are designed to flank Asp835 and a second *Eco*RV site within the target sequence. Thus, the resulting amplification product is cut twice if the sequence is normal but cut only once if the *FLT3* Asp835 mutation is present. The presence of a second restriction site, which occurs in all samples, is considered ideal in the design of RFLP assays because it serves as an internal control for the activity of the restriction enzyme.

USING POLYMERASE CHAIN REACTION TO DETECT CHROMOSOMAL REARRANGEMENTS

Diseases that involve chromosomal rearrangements such as translocations, inversions, deletions, or insertions are amenable to PCR detection when

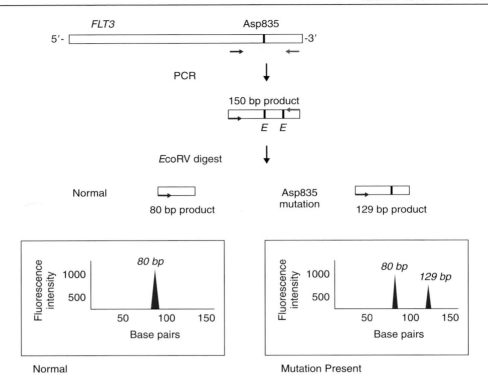

FIGURE 4-9

FLT3 mutation testing using polymerase chain reaction (PCR) amplification and restriction fragment length polymorphism detection. The location of the codon for the aspartic acid at position 835 (Asp835) mutated in the *FLT3* gene is depicted at the top, along with the primers that flank it. The forward primer only is fluorescently-labeled with 6-carboxyfluoroscein for capillary electrophoresis detection (blue arrow). The mutations at this codon disrupt the restriction site for the restriction enzyme *Eco*RV (5'-GAT/ATC-3'). Following amplification, the PCR products are digested with *Eco*RV and separated by capillary electrophoresis. As a control for the *Eco*RV digestion, the amplicon contains a second *Eco*RV restriction site that is unaffected by the mutation. The products of the PCR amplification and *Eco*RV digestion containing the fluorescent label from the forward primer are detected using capillary electrophoresis, and the size of the products indicates whether the codon is mutated. The absence of a mutation results in a detectable 80-base-pair fragment only, and the presence of a somatic mutation will be represented by detection of both the 80-base-pair and the 129-base-pair fragments.

the breakpoints of the two segments of adjoining DNA are known and conserved. PCR primers are designed to amplify across the breakpoints in the two genes; thus, an amplification product is generated if the rearrangement is present. One well-characterized translocation is the chromosome 14 and chromosome 18 translocation [t(14;18)(q32;q21)] of the *BCL2* gene on 18q with the immunoglobulin heavy chain locus *(IGH)* gene enhancer on 14q commonly associated with follicular center-cell lymphomas. Translocation of the *BCL2* gene does not disrupt its coding sequence but rather approximates the *BCL2* gene to the *IGH* enhancer, resulting in increased Bcl2 protein expression (Figure 4-10). The *IGH* gene enhancer breakpoint is relatively constant, and the *BCL2* gene breakpoint occurs primarily in two regions such that two separate amplification reactions can be used to detect most rearrangements.

Chromosomal rearrangements that result in chimeric transcripts can be detected at the mRNA level. This approach is preferred, rather than trying to amplify the DNA across the breakpoints, because the chromosomal breakpoints can occur anywhere within the introns spanning several hundreds or thousands of base pairs, which makes primer design difficult, if not impossible, to detect a small-enough target for successful amplification. In contrast, the introns are spliced out in the mRNA and the exons are constant, making the novel transcript an ideal target for detection. Therefore, these rearrangements are detected by RT-PCR of mRNA using fusion gene specific primers in a conventional or real-time PCR amplification. Examples of translocations detected in this way include the *BCR/ABL1*, t(9;22)(q34;q11), in chronic myeloid leukemia and acute lymphoblastic leukemia; *PML/RARA*, t(15;17)(q22;q12), in acute promyelocytic leukemia; *PAX3/FKHR* or *PAX7/FKHR*, t(2;13)(q35;q14) or t(1;13)(p36;q14), in alveolar rhabdomyosarcoma; and *EWS/FLI1*, t(11;22)(q24;q12), in Ewing's sarcoma.

AMPLIFICATION OF MICROSATELLITES

Microsatellites consist of 1 to 9 base-pair sequences repeated several times, and they are found throughout the human genome. Their repetitive nature makes them prone to adding or deleting repeats during replication, which introduces mismatches that can be corrected by the DNA mismatch repair system. Defects in mismatch repair genes are seen in hereditary nonpolyposis colon cancer (HNPCC) and

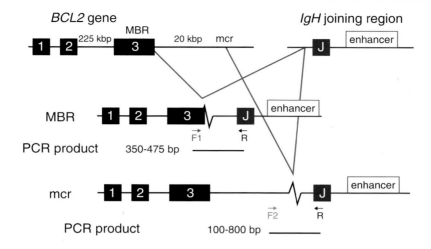

FIGURE 4-10

Polymerase chain reaction (PCR) amplification of the *BCL2* translocation with the immunoglobulin heavy chain *(IGH)* enhancer. The *BCL2* and *IGH* joining region loci are depicted, along with the two most common breakpoints in the *BCL2* locus (MBR and mcr). Exons are represented by boxes and introns by connecting lines. Two different forward primers and one common reverse primer are used in two separate PCR amplifications to detect the translocation at the DNA level.

in up to 15 % of sporadic colorectal cancer, and they lead to microsatellite instability (MSI) or variations in the number of repeats at some microsatellite loci because they fail to be repaired. Several genes are involved in the DNA mismatch repair system, including MutS homologue 2 *(MSH2)* and MutS homologue 6, MutL homologue 1 *(MLH1),* and *PMS2.* Germline mutations in *MSH2* and *MLH1* reduce their expression and account for 80% to 90% of HNPCC cases. Loss of expression due to epigenetic silencing, primarily methylation of the *MLH1* promoter, contributes to MSI in sporadic colorectal cancer. These genetic defects can be uncovered by performing immunohistochemistry on tumor sections, looking for reduced expression, or performing sequencing to identify the mutations. However, PCR amplification is an effective means to test for MSI as a marker for possible DNA mismatch repair gene mutations and to identify individuals with HNPCC.

The microsatellite sequence is amplified from DNA from tumor and from normal tissue using primers to the unique regions upstream and downstream of each microsatellite. In cases in which tumor and normal tissue are both present in the tissue section, some form of microdissection is used to separate the two before extracting the DNA. Amplification products are separated by capillary electrophoresis, and a normal specimen will demonstrate either two predominant peaks (one for each allele) or one predominant peak (if both alleles are the same repeat size) and accompanying *stutter peaks* (Figure 4-11). These artifactual peaks, or "stutters," result from slippage of the DNA polymerase during amplification. Stutter peaks are more pronounced when the microsatellite repeat unit is small; e.g., mono- and dinucleotide repeats have more stutter than tri- or

tetranucleotide repeats. Thus, for the mononucleotide examples shown in Figure 4-11, a Gaussian distribution of peaks is produced around the center main allele peak. The presence of MSI is determined by comparing the amplification pattern at each locus in the tumor to the normal tissue, looking for additional peaks or a change in the overall peak pattern.

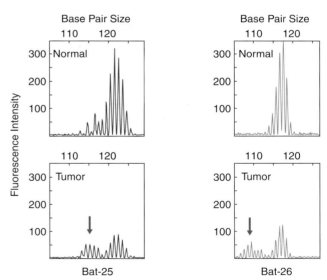

FIGURE 4-11

Capillary electropherograms of amplification products of the BAT-25 and BAT-26 microsatellites. Both normal and tumor tissue are amplified using fluorescently-labeled primers that flank the mononucleotide repeat microsatellites BAT-25 and BAT-26. For the normal tissue (top panels), a single homozygous allele is detected, but it appears as a Gaussian distribution of peaks because of polymerase slippage, known as stutter, as it amplifies the repeated target sequence. Compared to the normal tissue, the tumor tissue (lower panels) has additional peaks (highlighted by red arrows). These peaks represent microsatellite instability in the tumor DNA from failure to correct the DNA during replication and indicate that mutations may be present in the DNA mismatch repair genes.

The 1997 Bethesda guidelines recommend a panel of five microsatellite markers: two mononucleotide (BAT-25 and BAT-26) and three dinucleotide (D5S346, D2S123, and D17S250) repeats. The results are interpreted as positive for MSI if two or more of the five microsatellites demonstrate additional peaks. Using PCR to screen for mutations in mismatch repair genes is highly sensitive and specific, is relatively quick and easy to perform on formalin-fixed paraffin-embedded tissue biopsies, and helps identify individuals who need further testing with immunohistochemistry or sequencing to identify mutations in the DNA mismatch repair genes.

USING POLYMERASE CHAIN REACTION TO DETECT RESIDUAL DISEASE IN CANCER

PCR is an ideal methodology for testing for residual cancer cells because of its high analytic sensitivity. Identification of a specific mutation, translocation, or rearrangement in the cancer specimen at diagnosis provides a disease-specific marker that can then be used to monitor the patient during and after therapy. Cancer treatments are numerous, including traditional chemotherapy, monoclonal antibody therapy, small molecule inhibitors, and bone marrow and peripheral stem cell transplantation. The goal is to achieve disease remission, which can be assessed using PCR to detect a specific marker of the disease, if one is available. Many of the examples of mutation and translocation testing presented earlier can be used as disease markers. One scenario that has been shown to be particularly useful for guiding therapy is the quantitative monitoring of the *BCR/ABL1* transcript in chronic myeloid leukemia. The fusion gene product is a constitutively active tyrosine kinase. Therapy with imatinib mesylate (Gleevec™), which inhibits the *BCR/ABL1* kinase activity, has been highly successful with relatively few side effects, unlike peripheral stem cell or bone marrow transplants. RT Q-PCR can be used not only to detect the disease-associated transcript but also to quantify it to follow the response to Gleevec therapy. Patients who exhibit a drop in *BCR/ABL1* transcript levels greater than 3 logs by 12 months following therapy have a better probability of disease-free survival than those who do not. In addition, detection of relapse by RT-PCR may precede detection of cytogenetic relapse by up to 6 months.

CONCLUSION

Molecular diagnostic testing has been fundamentally based on PCR methodology because it was the first easily performed nucleic acid amplification method, it

is relatively straightforward to translate PCR-based research testing to the clinical diagnostic laboratory, and PCR technology is readily accessible. The required assay validation, quality control, and potentially difficult interpretations require laboratories using this technology—or, for that matter, any molecular technology—to have experienced and well-trained technical laboratory professionals. Board certification for laboratory directors in the subspecialty of molecular genetic pathology is available, along with credentialing for laboratory professionals. For any laboratory, entry into the molecular diagnostics arena should be carefully considered because of its high complexity (regardless of how easy a kit's instructions seem to be) and required expertise. In-house testing for a specific molecular abnormality may be extremely useful to clinicians in determining the correct modality of treatment in an appropriate time frame for certain patients.

For laboratory-developed or "home brew" assays, PCR methods will likely continue to be essential for the near future. However, competition with commercially available diagnostic methods based on target or signal amplification will continue to grow. Some advantages of these methods are simplified protocols, isothermal reactions not requiring a thermal cycler, less risk of contamination (signal amplification methods), and greater reproducibility in some cases. Assays must be evaluated case by case to select the most appropriate method.

Performance improvements will continue to advance the use of PCR technology, and these will probably come in the form of automation and miniaturization of the technology, along with simplification of the test protocols. Automation that includes specimen processing, PCR amplification, and detection in an "all in one" instrument, with few manual steps other than placing the patient's specimen into the reaction chamber or cartridge and reading the results, is slowly becoming a reality. Importantly, having instruments that interface with the laboratory information system will simplify the process of molecular testing as well. Another improvement to PCR will come in the form of miniaturization. This has the potential to make PCR faster and able to use fewer reagents and patient specimens. PCR is quite amenable for microscale integrated biochemical analysis, referred to as *microPCR* or colloquially as "lab on a chip" design, because all steps, including nucleic acid extraction, PCR reaction preparation, PCR amplification, and detection, can be performed in a liquid environment. Advances in the technical design and manufacturing capacity are beginning to make this a reality. Research advances in silicon technology, micromachining, and biologic microelectromechanical systems continue.

Another revolution in biotechnology that will have a significant impact on molecular diagnostics is occurring at the nanometer scale and is referred to as *nanotechnology*. This is the science of manufacturing structures, devices, and systems with a length scale of approximately 1 to 100 nM. These structures have the capacity to act as platforms for analysis or as detectors of specific molecules using structures with names like *quantum dots, nanopores,* and *cantilevers,* as well as many other *nano-*named particles and devices. The use of metallic atoms, single organic molecules, and inorganic molecules has been described. Electric, optical, magnetic, chemical, or nanomechanical properties can all be applied for measuring these molecules, and the potential applications for these technologies seem almost limitless. Nanotechnologies are desirable because the level of sensitivity is at the single molecule level and because the ability to process and detect many more specimens at once is orders of magnitude higher than current technologies. As these systems develop, become cost efficient in their production, and are validated for clinical testing, they have the potential to replace traditional PCR and real-time PCR, thereby changing the approach to clinical molecular diagnostic testing that we use today.

SUGGESTED READINGS

Principles of Polymerase Chain Reaction

Bielefeld University: Bioinformatics Server. Available at bibiserv.techfak.uni-bielefeld.de/genefisher.

Csako G: Present and future of rapid and/or high-throughput methods for nucleic acid testing. Clin Chim Acta 2006;363:6–31.

Gibbs R: DNA amplification by the polymerase chain reaction. Anal Chem 1990;62:1202–1214.

Helmholtz Center: ExonPrimer. Available at ihg.gsf.de/ihg/ExonPrimer.html.

Kermekchiev MB, Tzekov A, et al: Cold-sensitive mutants of *Taq* DNA polymerase provide a hot start for PCR. Nucleic Acids Res 2003;31:6139–6147.

Killeen AA: Principles of Molecular Pathology. Totowa, NJ, Humana Press, 2004.

Leonard DGB: Diagnostic Molecular Pathology. Philadelphia, Elsevier Saunders, 2004.

Leonard DGB, Bagg A, Caliendo A, et al: Molecular Pathology in Clinical Practice. New York, Springer, 2006.

Pavlov AR, Pavlova NV, et al: Recent developments in the optimization of thermostable DNA polymerases for efficient applications. Trends Biotechnol 2004;22:253–260.

SourceForge: Primer3. Available at frodo.wi.mit.edu/cgi-bin/primer3/primer3_www.cgi.

Coleman WB, Tsongalis GJ: Molecular Diagnostics for the Clinical Laboratian. Totowa, NJ, Humana Press, 2005.

Real-Time Polymerase Chain Reaction

Bustin SA: Real-time, fluorescence-based quantitative PCR: A snapshot of current procedures and preferences. Expert Rev Mol Diagn 2005;5:493–498.

Bustin SA, Mueller R: Real-time reverse transcription PCR (qRT-PCR) and its potential use in clinical diagnosis. Clin Sci (Lond) 2005;109:365–379.

Holland PM, Abramson RD, et al: Detection of specific polymerase chain reaction product by utilizing the 5′→3′ exonuclease activity of *Thermus aquaticus* DNA polymerase. Proc Natl Acad Sci USA 1991;88:7276–7280.

Jochen W, Pingoud A: Real-time polymerase chain reaction. ChemBioChem 2003;4:1120–1128.

Marras SAE, Tyagi S, et al: Real-time assays with molecular beacons and other fluorescent nucleic acid hybridization probes. Clin Chim Acta 2006;363:48–60.

Peters IR, Helps CR, et al: Real-time RT-PCR: Considerations for efficient and sensitive assay design. J Immunol Methods 2004;286:203–217.

Applications

Abu-Duhier FM, Goodeve AC, et al: Identification of novel FLT-3 Asp835 mutations in adult acute myeloid leukaemia. Br J Haematol 2001;113:983–988.

Armstrong SA, Mabon ME, et al: FLT3 mutations in childhood acute lymphoblastic leukemia. Blood 2004;103:3544–3546.

Bagg A: Chronic myeloid leukemia: A minimalistic view of post-therapeutic monitoring. J Mol Diagn 2002;4:1–10.

Giles FJ: FLT3 inhibitor KRN383 on xenografted human leukemic cells harboring FLT3-activating mutations: FLT3 in AML: Much more to learn about biology and optimal targeting. Leuk Res 2006;30: 1469–1470.

Hochhaus A: Minimal residual disease in chronic myeloid leukaemia patients. Best Pract Res Clin Haematol 2002;15:159–178.

Söreide K: Microsatellite instability in colorectal cancer. Br J Surg 2006;93:395–406.

Murphy KM, Levis M, et al: Detection of FLT3 internal tandem duplication and D835 mutations by a multiplex polymerase chain reaction and capillary electrophoresis assay. J Mol Diagn 2003;5:96–102.

Ryuzo O: Treatment of chronic myeloid leukemia with imatinib mesylate. Int J Clin Oncol 2006;V11:176–183.

Yamamoto Y, Kiyoi H, et al: Activating mutation of D835 within the activation loop of FLT3 in human hematologic malignancies. Blood 2001;97:2434–2439.

Zheng R, Small D: Mutant FLT3 signaling contributes to a block in myeloid differentiation. Leuk Lymphoma 2005;46:1679–1687.

Perspectives

Auroux, PA, Koc Y, et al: Miniaturised nucleic acid analysis. Lab Chip 2004;4:534–546.

Cheng MMC, Cuda G, et al: Nanotechnologies for biomolecular detection and medical diagnostics. Curr Opin Chem Biol 2006;10:11–19.

Jain KK: Nanotechnology in clinical laboratory diagnostics. Clin Chim Acta 2005;358:37–54.

Lee SJ, Lee SY: Micro total analysis system (µ-TAS) in biotechnology. Appl Microbiol Biotechnol 2004;V64:289–299.

McNeil SE: Nanotechnology for the biologist. J Leukocyte Biol 2005;78:585–594.

Pammer P: Nanopatterning of biomolecules with microscale beads. ChemPhysChem 2005;6:900–903.

Rosi NL, Mirkin CA: Nanostructures in biodiagnostics. Chem Rev 2005;105:1547–1562.

Thaxton CS, Georganopoulou DG, et al: Gold nanoparticle probes for the detection of nucleic acid targets. Clin Chim Acta 2006;363: 120–126.

Yu-Ting Li, H: Gold nanoparticles for microfluidics-based biosensing of PCR products by hybridization-induced fluorescence quenching. Electrophoresis 2005;26:4743–4750.

Zheng G, Patolsky F, et al: Multiplexed electrical detection of cancer markers with nanowire sensor arrays. Nat Biotechnol 2005;23: 1294–1301.

5

Loss of Heterozygosity

Jennifer L. Hunt

PRINCIPLES OF LOSS OF HETEROZYGOSITY

TUMOR SUPPRESSOR GENES

Tumorigenesis through the inactivation of tumor suppressor genes was first described by Alfred G. Knudson in the early 1970s. Knudson elegantly showed that hereditary retinoblastoma and sporadic tumors had similar molecular mutations involving the retinoblastoma gene. His theory, which is now known as *Knudson's hypothesis,* predicted that both copies of the retinoblastoma gene had to harbor mutations for tumorigenesis to occur. This type of gene is now known as a *tumor suppressor gene* (*TSG*).

In the sporadic, nonhereditary situation, normal cells have two functional copies of a wild-type (non-mutated) TSG, one inherited from each parent. In the process of tumorigenesis, one copy of the TSG develops an inactivating mutation. This first mutation is often a point mutation or small deletion mutation, and this is termed the first genetic *hit.* This first hit can also be inherited in cancer syndromes that make patients susceptible to tumors. Alone, the first mutation is not tumorigenic and may have no ramifications for cell function, because the second copy of the TSG is still functioning. TSGs are referred to as *recessive genes*—they require both copies to be mutated for loss of function to occur. The second genetic hit alters the second copy of the TSG; this hit commonly occurs from larger deletion mutations. It is uncommon for cells to have two large deletion mutations (biallelic deletion). The cells that harbor two mutated copies of the TSG have a loss of function of the TSG activity, and this contributes to carcinogenesis.

One of the most famous illustrations of Knudson's hypothesis is the Vogelstein model of familial colon cancer progression. In this classic model, germline mutations in the familial adenomatous polyposis gene (*APC*, on chromosome 5q21) are inherited as the first hit, and somatic mutations (usually deletions) in the second copy of the *APC* gene represent the second hit. With both copies of the gene functionally lost, colon carcinogenesis is initiated. The colonic adenoma–to–carcinoma pathway is probably one of the best-studied examples of tumorigenesis using a tumor suppressor pathway.

Some of the most common TSGs are listed in Table 5-1. TSG mutations and losses are common in dysplastic and neoplastic conditions. In fact, TSGs have been implicated as being a part of tumorigenesis in nearly every type of sporadic tumor.

Point mutations are more difficult to measure in tumors than are deletions. Many studies have used the deletion of a TSG as a surrogate marker for inactivation of the TSG. Deletions of TSGs can be assessed in several assays. One of the most common is the loss of heterozygosity (LOH) assay, which is discussed in detail here.

DNA POLYMORPHISMS

Before discussing LOH, it is important to gain an understanding of DNA polymorphisms. A huge percentage of the genetic code is redundant, with up to 99.9% homology among individuals. Each human still has a unique DNA genetic code, which accounts for major phenotypic differences, and the differences in the genetic code are predominantly the result of variable regions, called *polymorphisms.*

The types of variable areas within the genetic code include short tandem repeats (STRs), single nucleotide polymorphisms (SNPs), and longer repeat polymorphisms. STRs are short nucleotide sequences (2 to 7 base pairs in length) that are repeated for a variable number of times. The most common types of STR are dinucleotide repeat (2 base pairs long), trinucleotide repeat (3 base pairs long), and tetranucleotide repeat (4 base pairs long). Figures 5-1 and 5-2 demonstrate sequences from a typical SNP and a typical STR. Figure 5-3 demonstrates the typical peak and stutter patterns seen for various types of STRs, using a capillary electrophoresis analysis.

When an individual has inherited two copies of a polymorphism that are different from each other (have different numbers of repeats on each copy), they are said to have an "informative genotype" at

TABLE 5-1

Common Tumor Suppressor Genes and Their Chromosomal Location, Function, and Any Associated Inherited Syndromes

Tumor Suppressor Gene	Chromosomal Location	Function	Inherited Syndromes
VHL	3p26-p25	Regulation of transcription elongation	Von Hippel-Lindau syndrome
APC	5q21	Signaling through adhesion molecules	Familial adenomatosis polyposis
PTEN	10q23	Regulated cell survival	Cowden syndrome
WT1	11p13	Transcriptional regulation	Wilms' tumor
BRCA2	13q12.3	Repair double-stranded breaks	Familial breast cancer
RB1	13q13	Cell cycle regulation	Retinoblastoma
P53	17p13	Cell cycle regulation, apoptosis	Li-Fraumeni syndrome
NF1	17q11.2	Catalysis of Ras inactivation	Neurofibromatosis type 1
BRCA1	17q21	Repair double-stranded breaks	Familial breast cancer
DCC	18q21.3	Transmembrane receptor	Colon cancer
NF2	22q12.2	Linkage of cell membrane to cytoskeleton	Neurofibromatosis type 2

First copy: a-allele   Second copy: t-allele

ttgatttgagattaatctactta   ttgatttgagattattctactta

FIGURE 5-1

A single nucleotide polymorphism with two different allele possibilities.

that locus. An informative genotype means the person is heterozygous for the polymorphism. Informative loci are essential diagnostically because the two copies can be discriminated from each other by simple polymerase chain reaction (PCR)–based assays, which discriminate on the basis of size. If an individual is homozygous for the polymorphism, the locus is noninformative and the PCR products will be identical whether both are present or one allele is deleted.

LOSS OF HETEROZYGOSITY ANALYSIS

LOH is a technique used to identify loss of genetic material. It is most often used to identify TSG loss. But one fundamental requirement for the assay is that one has to be able to discriminate between the two copies of a particular gene. Because the coding regions of genes contain few intragenic sequence polymorphisms, the maternal allele and the paternal allele usually have an identical sequence. Therefore, LOH analysis uses polymorphisms that occur near TSGs as surrogate markers for the gene itself.

In LOH analysis, PCR primers are designed to flank a known polymorphism that is in proximity to a gene of interest. In an informative locus, the PCR amplicons will have different lengths because the two copies have different numbers of repeated units. In

---

First copy: 11 repeats

61   ttgattgagattaatctacttaaccgtaactgggtggaagtctttctagttaaaatctg

121 ttta**gatagatagatagatagatagatagatagatagatagatagatagata**acaactttatat

Second copy: 15 repeats

61   ttgattgagattaatctacttaaccgtaactgggtggaagtctttctagttaaaatctg

121 ttta**gatagatagatagatagatagatagatagatagatagatagatagatagatagatagat**

181 **agata**acaactttatat

FIGURE 5-2

A tetranucleotide repeat unit that is heterozygous or informative. The repeat sequence is GATA, and it repeats for 11 and 15 units on the two different alleles. The polymerase chain reaction (PCR) products, assuming that the entire sequence shown is amplified, would be 181 and 197 base pairs. The difference in the sizes of the two PCR products is caused by the different number of repeated GATA in the short tandem repeat.

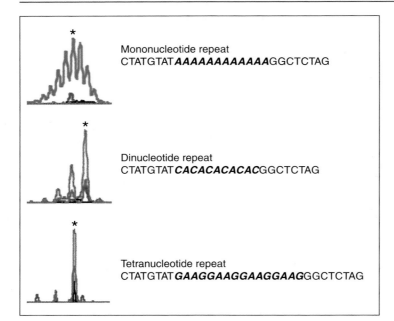

Mononucleotide repeat
CTATGTAT***AAAAAAAAAAAA***GGCTCTAG

Dinucleotide repeat
CTATGTAT***CACACACACAC***GGCTCTAG

Tetranucleotide repeat
CTATGTAT***GAAGGAAGGAAGGAAG***GGCTCTAG

FIGURE 5-3

The appearance of mononucleotide, dinucleotide, and tetra-nucleotide short tandem repeats (STRs). The STRs illustrated are homozygous (only one allele present). By convention, the highest peak is considered to be the length of the allele (*), and the rest of the peaks are stutter peaks.

the example in Figure 5-4, the PCR product from the first copy will be have 181 base pairs (with 11 repeat units of a tetranucleotide repeat) and the second copy will have a 197-base-pair product (with 16 repeat units of a tetranucleotide repeat).

PCR products of different sizes will migrate separately, either in traditional gel electrophoresis or in capillary electrophoresis analysis; the longer fragments migrate more slowly than shorter ones. In normal cells, the amount of each PCR product will be approximately equal, because the amount of DNA template from diploid cells should have equal copies of each allele. In tumor cells that harbor deletions, the quantity of PCR product from the two different alleles will not be equal. When one copy of the STR is completely lost, only one PCR product will be visualized. This loss makes the genotype of the tumor cell homozygous at the locus, which is where the term *loss of heterozygosity* is derived from.

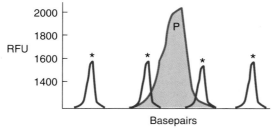

FIGURE 5-4

The typical appearance of a single polymerase chain reaction (PCR) product (P) analyzed by capillary electrophoresis. The x-axis shows the number of base pairs, which is calculated by the machine through comparison to the number of base pairs in the known size standards (each peak with a * is a size standard peak). The relative fluorescence of the PCR product is given along the y-axis.

In analyzing for the presence of LOH in a traditional gel, the bands are visualized for their intensity. By convention, when one band is less than 50% of the intensity of the other, this is considered to be evidence of LOH. In capillary electrophoresis, the ratio of the amount of PCR product for the two alleles is derived from the relative peak heights. To determine whether LOH has occurred, a ratio of the peak heights in the normal tissue is compared to that obtained from the tumor tissue. Comparing the ratio of peak heights in tumor cells to that from normal cells is a standardization that helps account for variability in PCR efficiency. The Figure 5-5 diagram illustrates the typical findings in both a gel analysis and a capillary electrophoresis analysis for LOH. Figure 5-6 shows a true electropherogram printout from an LOH analysis in which an allele ratio is calculated from peak heights in capillary electrophoresis.

Advantages of Loss of Heterozygosity Analysis

With adequately sensitive methods, cells can also be individually examined for deletion mutations using in situ hybridization assays. Although these assays are important in molecular pathology, they may lack sensitivity. The advantages of using the PCR-based LOH assays include the ability to detect small deletions and the ability to enrich for tumor cells through microdissection.

Enrichment of tumor cells through microdissection is especially helpful in working with paraffin-embedded samples. Microdissection can be done by hand using simple laboratory equipment or using laser capture microdissection instruments. It is important to remember that even with microdissection the DNA from thousands of cells will be assessed together. Minor changes in small populations of cells

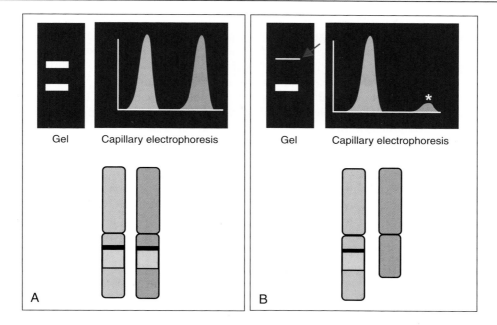

FIGURE 5-5

What would be seen in a loss of heterozygosity analysis of normal cells **(A)** and tumor cells that have lost the locus of interest **(B)**. The gel electrophoresis is shown on the left, and the capillary electropherograms are shown on the right. The lost larger allele is seen in panel B by the much-lighter-intensity top band in the gel (→) and a much shorter second peak in the electropherograms (*).

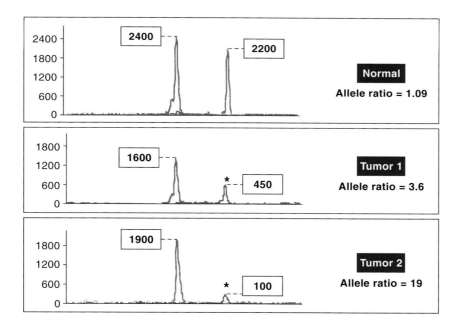

FIGURE 5-6

Electropherograms from a normal sample from a patient with an oligodendroglioma. Two different areas of tumor were microdissected, and polymerase chain reaction was performed for a marker on 1p. The two tumor samples show loss of the larger allele (*). The ratio of the peak heights is measured in relative fluorescent units and given in the box next to each peak. The ratio of the allele heights in the tumor is compared to that in the normal sample to assess for loss of heterozygosity.

will not usually be identified by most PCR-based assays. Therefore, PCR-based LOH assays are best used to detect clonal DNA damage.

Disadvantages of Loss of Heterozygosity Analysis

There are several pitfalls that can affect the reliability and sensitivity of an LOH analysis. As with any molecular test, it is critical to understand good

controls and potential problems before using the assay.

CONTAMINATED TUMOR SAMPLES. Histologic sections of tumors usually contain a mixture of tumor cells, inflammatory cells, stromal cells, and other cellular contaminants. This tissue heterogeneity can cause problems in molecular analyses of all types but especially in amplification-based procedures. For example,

LOH can be masked by heavy contamination by normal DNA. The best technique to minimize the level of contamination is to microdissect tumor cells from the contaminating tissues in a tissue section. There are many methods to perform microdissection, including manual methods and automated methods. Usually, a manual microdissection will be sufficient to eliminate the gross contamination that is problematic in LOH analysis.

POOR MARKERS. It is critical to realize that polymorphic repeat units present near TSGs are only surrogate markers for the gene itself. The distance between the TSG and the polymorphism will affect how tightly the polymorphism is linked to the TSG. If a polymorphism is far from the TSG of interest, it will not represent an accurate measurement of the TSG. Online databases can be used to judge the distance between the polymorphisms and the TSGs.

LOW DNA CONCENTRATIONS. Another major problem in LOH analysis can arise if there is inadequate DNA. When the DNA concentration is very low, one allele may be preferentially amplified over the other. When one allele has insufficient amplification, this is termed *allelic dropout*. The extreme of this situation can be seen in assays that use whole genome amplification for single cells, such as in single-cell analysis for preimplantation genetic analysis. When allelic dropout occurs, the PCR product allele ratio no longer reflects the original amount of starting DNA of each allele. Allelic dropout can yield false-positive results for LOH. Determining whether allelic dropout has occurred is difficult. One of the most reliable ways to detect false-positive results from allelic dropout is to run samples in duplicate. When DNA concentrations are low, allele ratios will be inconsistent between duplicates.

LACK OF A NORMAL COMPARISON SAMPLE. Sometimes in tumor pathology, a concordant normal sample from the patient may not be available. It is always preferable to use normal controls that have undergone identical tissue-processing procedures. But, when paraffin-embedded normal tissue is not available, other normal tissues from the patient can be requested, such as blood or a buccal swab.

Applications of Loss of Heterozygosity Analysis

Currently, there are several situations in which an LOH analysis is commonly used in the clinical assessment of tumors.

Loss of 1p and 19q are characteristic findings in oligodendrogliomas. Concurrent loss of 1p and 19q is thought to be prognostic, as well as predictive of the response to chemotherapy. In contrast, LOH of p53 and p16 may be associated with poor survival or with tumor progression. PCR-based testing for multiple markers on both 1p and 19q spanning the

minimal deletion areas has become a standard clinical assay in neuropathology (Figure 5-6). Loss of 1p and 19q can also be assessed using fluorescence in situ hybridization (FISH) or through combined FISH and LOH testing.

Another application of the LOH assay occurs when a patient has two tumors in different sites and the question arises of whether the second tumor is a metastasis or a second primary. Differentiating between these scenarios can be difficult, especially when the histology is similar. And the clinical implications can be important, because a second primary tumor can be treated with the intention to cure but a recurrence or distant metastasis equates to a high stage with limited treatment options.

Because carcinogenesis is accompanied by an accumulation of mutations over time, TSG deletion patterns can be used as a clonality assessment. Any tumor will have a relatively unique set of genetic losses that is conserved despite progression. By assessing a panel of multiple TSGs for LOH, the relationship between these two tumors can be predicted. These are just a few examples. Other clinical applications of LOH testing are emerging, both for diagnostic and for prognostic use.

CONCLUSION

LOH analysis can be a powerful tool for solid tumor analysis. At this point, however, there are few validated, established LOH assays that have clinical applications. As our understanding of tumor genetics and of important prognostic and diagnostic markers increases, assessment of tumors with an LOH analysis is likely to become more important. Many laboratories already have the equipment in place to implement LOH assays. Because many of these assays will be improved by microdissection, collaboration between morphologists and molecular pathologists will be essential in designing high-quality assays.

SUGGESTED READINGS

Fearon ER., Hamilton SR, Vogelstein B: Clonal analysis of human colorectal tumors. Science 1987;238(4824):193–197.

Findlay I, Quirke P, Hall J, Rutherford A: Fluorescent PCR: A new technique for PGD of sex and single-gene defects. J Assist Reprod Genet 1996;13(2):96–103.

Fujiyama A, Watanabe H, Toyoda A, Taylor TD, et al: Construction and analysis of a human–chimpanzee comparative clone map. Science 2002;295(5552):131–134.

Hunt JL, Finkelstein SD: Microdissection techniques for molecular testing in surgical pathology. Arch Pathol Lab Med 2004;128(12):1372–1378.

Iwasa Y, Michor F, Komarova NL, Nowak MA: Population genetics of tumor suppressor genes. J Theor Biol 2005;233(1):15–23.

Kelley TW, Tubbs RR, Prayson RA: Molecular diagnostic techniques for the clinical evaluation of gliomas. Diagn Mol Pathol 2005;14(1):1–8.

Knudson AG Jr: Genetics and the etiology of childhood cancer. Pediatr Res 1976;10(5):513–517.

Knudson AG Jr, Strong LC: Mutation and cancer: A model for Wilms' tumor of the kidney. J Natl Cancer Inst 1972;48(2):313–324.

Payne SR, Kemp CJ: Tumor suppressor genetics. Carcinogenesis 2005;26(12):2031–2045.

Ronchetti D, Arisi E, Neri A, et al: Microsatellite analyses of recurrence or second primary tumor in head and neck cancer. Anticancer Res 2005;25(4):2771–2775.

Sieben NL, ter Haar NT, Cornelisse CJ, et al: PCR artifacts in LOH and MS analysis of microdissected tumor cells [comment]. Hum Pathol 2000;31(11):1414–1419.

Slebos RJ, Umbach DM, Sommer CA, et al: Analytical and statistical methods to evaluate microsatellite allelic imbalance in small amounts of DNA. Lab Invest 2004;84(5):649–657.

Thiagalingam S, Foy RL, Cheng KH, et al: Loss of heterozygosity as a predictor to map tumor suppressor genes in cancer: Molecular basis of its occurrence. Curr Opin Oncol 2002;14(1):65–72.

Vogelstein B, Fearon ER, Hamilton SR, et al: Genetic alterations during colorectal-tumor development. N Engl J Med 1988;319(9):525–532.

6

Direct Genome Sequencing in Diagnostic Pathology

Gurunathan Murugesan • Gary W. Procop

INTRODUCTION

Molecular diagnostics identify or confirm genetic variants associated with diseases or that can serve as surrogate markers of disease. DNA is the primary target for molecular diagnostics because of its simplicity, relative stability, and wide applicability. DNA variants associated with diagnostic or prognostic value can include simple abnormalities such as point mutations, single nucleotide polymorphisms (SNPs), small additions and deletions, repeat sequences of varying length, translocations, and gross chromosomal abnormalities. Molecular methodologic approaches routinely used for diagnostics include polymerase chain reaction (PCR) coupled with multiple detection systems, real-time PCR, fluorescence in situ hybridization, restriction fragment length polymorphism analysis (RFLP), denaturing gradient gel electrophoresis, single-stranded conformation polymorphism (for insertions and deletions), hybrid capture, and the hybridization protection assay. However, only direct genome sequencing using the template DNA generated from genome by PCR will be sufficiently robust for some applications.

BASIS OF DIRECT DNA SEQUENCING FOR MOLECULAR DIAGNOSTICS

Although most genetic variations attributed to altered DNA sequence can be identified by PCR-based assays and detection systems, direct sequencing of DNA is still the "golden" reference standard and in some instances is essential for the identification of certain DNA variations that cannot be confirmed by PCR-based assays. Examples include diseases or clinical conditions associated with multiple mutations in tandem or within the same gene and identification of certain disease-causing and drug-resistance pathogens. In addition, assays that yield limited information can only be resolved by sequencing the target DNA. For instance, RFLP can demonstrate that a particular restriction site (4- to 6-base-pair region) has a mutation but cannot identify the exact mutated base. Similarly, assays identifying SNPs can only identify the specific nucleotide being interrogated, not the nucleotides in proximity. Any atypical pattern can only be resolved by sequencing. Not too long ago, sequencing was a labor-intensive, time-consuming, and expensive proposition. However, the Human Genome Project has tremendously advanced DNA sequencing technologies, leading to cost-effective diagnostics based on direct sequencing of DNA. This chapter presents the basics of DNA sequencing, various sequencing methods, and illustrative examples used in molecular diagnostics.

BASICS OF DNA SEQUENCING

CONCEPT

Resolution of the double-helix structure of DNA by James D. Watson and Francis Crick in 1953 was the landmark discovery in the field of DNA research. This discovery established that the DNA molecule, composed of four deoxyribonucleotide triphosphates (dNTPs: deoxyadenylate, dATP; deoxyguanylate, dGTP; deoxycytidylate, dCTP; and deoxythymidylate, dTTP), has two strands that are complementary to each other and are held together by noncovalent weak hydrogen bonds between base pairs on the opposing strands (dATP and dTTP, dCTP and dGTP). Two strands of the DNA can be separated from each other into single strands under denaturing conditions (high temperature, low salt, and extremes of $p^H - <3$ or >10). Each of the DNA strands can then serve as a template for replication or synthesis of its complementary strand. This concept is central to DNA sequencing as currently practiced.

PRINCIPLE AND METHODS

DNA sequencing is the process of determining the exact order of the four bases (adenine, A; thymine, T; cytosine, C; guanine, G) in a given DNA

TABLE 6-2

Applications of Pyrosequencing: Select Examples

Areas of Application	Specific Uses	Comments
Bacteriology	Identifies *Bordetella pertussis, Neisseria* spp., *Helicobacter pylori,* and *Streptococcus* spp.	Targets sequences in the 16S rRNA gene or similar genes; identifies genetic determinants of resistance
Mycobacteria	Identifies or categorizes mycobacteria to the species level or to clinically relevant groups (e.g., *Mycobacterium tuberculosis* complex)	Targets hypervariable region A of the 16S rRNA gene; identifies genetic determinants of resistance
Mycology	Identifies clinically important fungi, including *Aspergillus, Fusarium,* and *Candida* spp.	Targets the internal transcribed spacer region
Virology	Identifies herpes simplex virus, influenza, and human papillomavirus	Targets virus-specific DNA or RNA sequences
Human genetics	Cytochrome 450 analysis	Analyzes single nucleotide polymorphisms
Oncology	Genetic analysis and methylation	Determines variety of cancer

determination of certain subtypes of hepatitis C virus (HCV) that are more likely to respond to therapy than other types; this can be determined by sequencing the 5′ untranslated region of the HCV. Resistance of cytomegalovirus to antiviral agents such as ganciclovir and foscarnet can also be established by DNA sequencing.

APPLICATIONS IN CLINICAL GENETICS

Identification of polymorphisms related to multiple disorders, methylation analysis, and pharmacogenomics presents opportunities for diagnostics based on pyrosequencing. Select examples where pyrosequencing can be used in a clinical setting are summarized in Table 6-2. A pyrogram depicting the identification of a pathogenic mycobacterium causing a granulomatous pulmonary nodule is illustrated in Figure 6-4.

CONCLUSION

The Sanger method of DNA sequencing and, more recently, pyrosequencing are becoming incorporated as routine assays in many modern molecular pathology laboratories. These techniques are commonly used to identify wide-ranging genetic variations in human DNA and to identify bacteria, mycobacteria, and fungi, particularly infectious agents that are difficult to identify using phenotypic methods or that are slow growing. Direct sequencing of DNA has the advantage of identifying the genetic variation in the context of flanking sequences, which offers the most reliable confirmation. When PCR-based assays are not available or inconclusive and need confirmation, DNA sequencing is often necessary. One major caveat of sequencing is that the methods require sequence alignment and visual

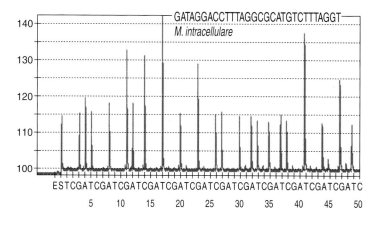

FIGURE 6-4

Pyrogram showing the "signature" sequence of *Mycobacterium intracellulare.* A target DNA template generated by polymerase chain reaction was subjected to pyrosequencing to establish the identity of the bacterium in a patient with a pulmonary granuloma. The order of nucleotides incorporated revealed the sequence unique for *M. intracellulare,* which was the causative agent of the nodule, as subsequently confirmed by culture. Note that the peak height or signal strength as shown in the y-axis is proportional to the number of nucleotides incorporated.

matching, consuming substantial personnel and instrument time. Therefore, PCR-based diagnostics will continue to dominate molecular pathology assays based on detection of specific DNA sequence alterations until a system capable of performing automated sequence alignment to score the variant DNA species is developed and implemented. Such an automated system will make direct sequencing of DNA even more attractive as a routine molecular pathology assay.

SUGGESTED READINGS

Chan EY: Advances in sequencing technology. Mutat Res 2005;573: 13–40.

Graham CA, Hill AJM: Introduction to DNA sequencing. In Graham CA, Hill AJM (eds): DNA Sequencing Protocols, 2nd ed. Methods in Molecular Biology, vol 167. Totowa, NJ, Humana Press, 2001, chapter 1, pp 1–12.

Hall N: Advanced sequencing technologies and their wider impact in microbiology. J Exp Biol; 2007;209:1518-1525.

Heller C: Principles of DNA separation with capillary electrophoresis. Electrophoresis 2001;22:629–643.

Highsmith WE Jr: Electrophoretic methods for mutation detection and DNA sequencing. In Coleman WB, Tsongalis GJ (eds): Molecular Diagnostics for the Clinical Laboratorian, 2nd ed. Totowa, NJ, Humana Press, 2006, chapter 9, pp 85–109.

Kan CW, Fredlake CP, Doherty EAS, Barron AE: DNA sequencing and genotyping in miniaturized electrophoresis systems. Electrophoresis 2004;25:3564–3588.

Metzker ML: Emerging technologies in DNA sequencing. Genome Res 2005;15:1767–1776.

Nunnally BK: Introduction to DNA sequencing. In Nunnally BK (ed): Analytical Techniques in DNA Sequencing. Boca Raton, FL, Taylor & Francis, 2005, chapter 1, pp 1–12.

Ronaghi M: Pyrosequencing sheds light on DNA sequencing. Genome Res 2001;11:3–11.

Sanchez-Vega B: Introduction to capillary electrophoresis of DNA. In Walker JM, Rapley R (eds): Medical Biomethods Handbook. Totowa, NJ, Humana Press, 2005, chapter 10, pp 95–116.

Schuster SC: Next-generation sequencing transforms today's biology. Nat Methods 2008;5:16–18.

Shendure JA, Porreca GJ, Church GM: Overview of DNA sequencing strategies. Curr Protoc Mol Biol 2008; Chapter 7, Unit 7.1.1-7.1.11.

Strom CM: Mutation detection, interpretation, and applications in the clinical laboratory setting. Mutat Res 2005;573:160–167.

7

Array-based Comparative Genomic Hybridization in the Analysis of Genomic Alterations in Human Disease

Marek Skacel • Ana Ambu Siva • Raymond R. Tubbs

INTRODUCTION

Besides their utilization in gene expression studies, the concept of using microarrays has been explored in the study of other molecular genetic aspects of human disease. This includes the use of arrays for the detection of gains and losses of genomic DNA. Fluctuations in DNA sequence copy number with concomitant microscopic or cryptic chromosomal aberrations are becoming increasingly correlated with phenotypic abnormalities. Characteristic isolated DNA copy abnormalities occur in a variety of inherited syndromes, and genomic DNA amplification, deletion, or both is a common alteration occurring in cancer cells. The development of many human neoplasms follows a defined series of histopathologic stages, a process that involves multiple genetic changes such as translocations, deletions, duplications, and alterations in chromosomal copy number changes. Importantly, such abnormalities often involve areas of DNA harboring oncogenes and tumor suppression genes that play an important role in the cell cycle control, and their alteration affects cancer growth.

It is now possible to screen tumors for genomic changes, as an alternative to the examination of the transcriptional activity of the tumor cells. Compared to messenger RNA expression, the genomic changes are less variable and less likely to be subject to transient changes in the tissue environment. This reduced complexity greatly simplifies the identification of potentially causal genetic changes in individual tumors. Also, the dynamic range of the genomic changes is more manageable (the locus-to-locus variation of DNA is small, including either allele loss or locus amplification), and messenger RNA levels present in cells typically vary over several orders of magnitude. The knowledge of genetic changes common to specific tumor types may facilitate the development of markers for early detection, diagnosis, and monitoring during clinical intervention. Furthermore, the identification of these genomic alterations may define causal molecular changes that may lead to more targeted therapeutic approaches to disease. The best illustration of the power of this approach is the identification of the amplification of the *ERBB2 (HER2)* gene in breast carcinoma, which has not only served as a prognostic parameter but also led to the development of individualized, targeted therapy.

CLASSICAL CYTOGENETICS AND METAPHASE-BASED COMPARATIVE GENOMIC HYBRIDIZATION

Classical cytogenetics has been used for decades to karyotype cells, but its use is limited by the need to culture cells to produce metaphase chromosomes. It also requires specialized expertise in interpreting the chromosomal spreads. In addition, cytogenetics only provides a crude analysis of the chromosome number and has limited sensitivity in identifying deletions and amplifications. The introduction of comparative genomic hybridization (CGH) to metaphase chromosomes (M-CGH) revolutionized clinical cytogenetics by permitting a genomewide analysis of cancer specimens with chromosomal aberrations that were either too many or too complex to be fully characterized by routine cytogenetics. Moreover, because CGH requires only genomic DNA from the sample, it permits the analysis of specimens from which chromosomal preparations cannot be obtained because of poor cell growth.

Using this technique, the genomic DNA from the tumor is labeled with a fluorescent dye in one color while a normal reference DNA sample is labeled in a different color. The labeled samples are then cohybridized to normal metaphase chromosome spreads. Chromosomal imbalances across the genome in the tumor DNA are then quantified and positionally defined by analyzing the ratio of fluorescence of the two colors along the target metaphase chromosomes.

However, the resolution of CGH applied to the metaphase spreads is limited by cytogenetic resolution of approximately 5 megabases (Mb), and considerable cytogenetics expertise is required to accomplish such analysis. Therefore, M-CGH has never become a widely used technique and has remained limited to specialized research applications, verification of probe specificity, and clarification of complex genetic rearrangements preliminarily identified by classical banded cytogenetics. The inherently low resolution associated with metaphase chromosomes banding, along with the labor intensiveness of this procedure, make M-CGH largely incapable of accomplishing genomewide screens for chromosomal aberrations less than 5 Mb, a limitation which makes this approach unsuitable for a high-throughput study of human neoplasms.

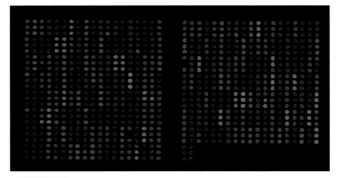

FIGURE 7-1

The spectrum of genomic amplifications (green) and losses (red) in a tumor sample as detected by array-based CGH (GenoSensor™ 300 from Abbott Molecular). A relatively high number of loci with color change is seen in this colonic adenocarcinoma sample. Each target clone is arrayed in triplicate, and a high concordance can be seen among each of the replicate spots in this particular array.

BACTERIAL ARTIFICIAL CHROMOSOME ARRAYS AND OTHER ALTERNATIVES

Recently, the advent of bacterial artificial chromosome (BAC) array technology has refocused attention upon the applicability of CGH to the study of genomic alterations in human disease. BACs are large-insert DNA clones that have been cytogenetically and physically mapped to the human genome. Currently, more than 8800 such clones are known, with at least 1 clone on average per megabase available on each chromosome. This resource affords the opportunity to generate an ordered array of DNA segments at a high genomic resolution and replace the metaphase spreads as the hybridization template. Such array-based CGH (A-CGH) circumvents the considerable limitations associated with the use of chromosome spreads. A high-resolution fluorescent scanner is used to capture the fluorescence intensity of each spot in the array and converts them into an intensity ratio. The fluorescence ratio of the two colors can be compared among different spots representing different genomic regions. (An example of one of the commercially available platforms is shown in Figure 7-1.) This provides a genomewide molecular profile of the sample with respect to regions of the genome that are deleted or amplified. The resolution of this approach depends on a combination of the number, size, and map positions of the DNA elements within the array. BAC arrays provide an opportunity to perform high-resolution genomic scans in a rapid and highly reproducible fashion.

The strength of signals provided by BACs has enabled exploration of human neoplasms in numerous studies since their original description by Pinkel et al.

(1998). Most recently, these arrays were used to identify important genomic copy number alterations in a variety of neoplasms, including breast cancer, gastric cancer, glioblastoma multiforme, neuroblastoma, rhabdomyosarcoma, nasopharyngeal carcinoma, osteosarcoma, adrenocortical tumors, and ovarian, bladder, and prostate cancers. Selected references are included at the end of this chapter as suggested readings.

A-CGH resolution has improved substantially over the past decade. Abbott Molecular has produced an array containing 300 BACs, providing fairly low resolution but offering a more standardized approach to data classification using a proprietary scanner and software package. Spectral Genomics has produced a 2500-clone BAC array capable of approximately 1-Mb resolution, which has been used successfully to assess DNA copy number alterations in a variety of studies. Roswell Park Cancer Institute and Fred Hutchinson Cancer Research Center have constructed 6000 and 20,000 BAC arrays with resolutions of 500 kilobases (kb) and about 200 kb, respectively, shown to identify characteristic losses of chromosome 1p and 19q material in oligodendrogliomas. A 32,000-clone BAC array achieving a 45-kb resolution has been shown to identify single copy number alterations in oral squamous cell carcinoma.

BACs are not the sole platform used for the construction of CGH arrays. Similar to their use for gene expression studies, complementary DNA (cDNA) arrays can also serve as a template for comparative genomic hybridization. cDNA arrayed in the form of individual sequences typically longer than 100 nucleotides provides the advantage of being more readily available for construction of such arrays by the spotting of polymerase chain reaction (PCR) products. Based on the experience with these arrays in the literature, they may enable study of small deletions and amplifications (high resolution) and eliminate some representational bias. However, cDNA arrays may be limited by their inability to effectively measure deletions because of the background noise encountered when using single probes. cDNA arrays have recently been used in studies of bilateral breast carcinomas and pediatric osteosarcoma, as well as to detect DNA copy number alterations, in addition to methylation abnormalities.

Oligonucleotide arrays are similar to cDNA arrays except that their hybridization templates are short, typically composed of less than 25 nucleotides. The advantage of oligonucleotide arrays is that an almost infinite amount of oligonucleotides can be rapidly synthesized for a specific region of interest, whereas the resolution of BACs is limited by their size. The oligonucleotide design may provide improved specificity and sensitivity even when using longer oligonucleotides as probes. Apart from their potential for achieving a higher density of probes on the array slide, there is the flexibility of choice and layout of probes, which can be customized. Published studies using oligonucleotide-based A-CGH include those studying breast carcinoma and cancer cell lines.

Oligonucleotides not only are able to detect copy number alterations but also are used to detect single nucleotide polymorphisms (SNPs), thus expanding their future utility tremendously. SNP arrays have been previously used to detect 14 mutations in the exon 11 of the BRCA1 gene or to study loss of heterozygosity in prostate carcinoma. A 1500-probe SNP oligonucleotide array compared favorably to conventional microsatellite PCR in a transitional cell carcinoma study focused on detection of loss of heterozygosity of 9p and 9q. In addition, the array-based approach was shown to offer distinct advantages over traditional microsatellite analysis in this study. The high-density mapping array was quicker, more accurate, and readily adaptable. The array data was generated in about 6 weeks, while completion of conventional PCR studies required 8 times as much time. A commercially available two-array Gene Chip® Mapping 100K array set (Affymetrix) can be used to genotype more than 100,000 SNPs—10 times more than its predecessor—and the complexity of well-characterized SNP arrays will continue to expand. A plethora of studies have emerged using this and related products (Affymetrix, Agilent).

CHALLENGES AND LIMITATIONS OF ARRAY-BASED COMPARATIVE GENOMIC HYBRIDIZATION

An array can produce thousands of data variables, corresponding to the number of individual probes used. The high cost of these arrays often makes it difficult to ensure reproducibility of the data by repetitive assessment of identical samples, but that does not diminish the importance of such observations. Ensuring data validity becomes especially important when comparing findings from fresh and fixed tissues or when comparing the data from various investigators.

When choosing an array, other important considerations should be taken into account. The resolution—determined by the number of BACs, cDNA sequences, or oligonucleotides on the array—is of utmost importance. However, the greater the array resolution, the greater the noise level and the complexity of the data generated. Although denser or higher-resolution arrays can detect smaller deletions and amplifications, the bioinformatics aspect of data analysis becomes more challenging—especially when analyzing a series of relatively small sample sizes or DNA samples of less-than-superior quality. Various statistical approaches have been used in data analysis; their complexity goes beyond the scope of this chapter.

In addition to resolution, signal quality is a key parameter because it affects the accuracy of each of the respective platforms. Types of fluorescent dyes selected can also influence the results recorded by the excitation lasers and detection systems, as can the location of the spots on the chip, unevenness, or dust on the array slides. The quality of separation of fluorescent signals of differing wavelengths is critical, in addition to accurate quantitative measurements of fluorescence intensities. Reliable scoring of ratio differences may be difficult in practice because of nonhomogenous genomic balances within the cells populations, background fluorescence, and background DNA within the probe solution. The presence of background "noise" can affect the microarray experiments at all stages, from the preparation of tissue samples and DNA purification, to the hybridization and washing processes themselves, and finally to the extraction of data and bioinformatic analysis. A-CGH requires at least 35% "target" tumor cells in the sample, which may require microdissection or flow sorting for enrichment. Currently, although several publications have reported successful A-CGH analysis using PCR–amplified samples, there are still no standardized protocols available that will guarantee uniform nonpreferential amplification of selected genomic regions in such samples. Another limitation of A-CGH is that most tissue samples available in pathology archives have been formalin fixed and paraffin embedded and therefore are unable to provide superior-quality, high molecular weight DNA. Therefore, frozen tissue or fresh cells are preferred where possible.

A-CGH can only detect nonbalanced alterations such as gains and losses of chromosomal DNA, not balanced translocations. In addition, it only provides an overall estimate of the net genomic imbalance within a tumor. Therefore, genomic changes affecting minor clones of cells within the sample or masked by concurrent changes of a reciprocal translocation may not be detected by this powerful technique.

NONONCOLOGIC APPLICATIONS OF ARRAY-BASED COMPARATIVE GENOMIC HYBRIDIZATION

Besides its clear role in oncologic research, A-CGH is of value in prenatal analysis of amniotic fluid cells or chorionic villous sampling in cases of suspected chromosome abnormality syndromes. A-CGH could also be used for genetic counseling of patients with cancer predisposition syndromes. In addition, fluctuation in DNA sequence copy number associated with chromosomal aberrations or microdeletion syndromes is increasingly correlated with postnatal phenotypic abnormalities, such as unexplained mental retardation.

Microdeletion syndromes such as Angelman/Prader-Willi (15q deletion) syndromes and DiGeorge (22q deletion) syndrome may be quickly and efficiently identified using A-CGH. The contribution of submicroscopic, subtelomeric chromosome rearrangements to mental retardation has been studied using a 3569-clone BAC array to detect novel deletions and duplications as small as 1 Mb and as large as 8.6 Mb present in 7 of 20 mental retardation patients of unknown etiology. It has been shown by A-CGH that submicroscopic chromosomal anomalies represent a major cause of mental retardation. Interstitial microdeletions or microduplications detected with DNA arrays are comparable or may even exceed the 5% submicroscopic, subtelomeric rearrangements currently reported among individuals with mental retardation. References to this work are included in the Suggested Readings section at the end of this chapter. This testing is currently offered for clinical diagnosis through Signature Genomic Laboratories.

Specific deletions have been shown to predispose 10% of patients with retinoblastoma to mental retardation and dysmorphic features. Using a 6000-clone BAC array with 750-Mb resolution, investigators from the Roswell Park Cancer Center Institute identified 32- to 64-Mb deletions in the esterase D *(ESD)* gene in patients with retinoblastoma. The *ESD* gene normally lies 650 kb centromeric to the *RB1* gene. The size of deletion and genotype (homozygosity) was associated with reduction of ESD enzyme activity and severity of phenotypical features. Similarly, sporadic cases of aniridia show a 50% increase of Wilms' tumor of the kidney in pediatric patients.

Patients at risk of this malignancy have deletions of both 11p13 regions containing both the *WT1* and the *PAX6* genes. Patients with mutations of the *PAX6* gene alone represent the hereditary form of the disease, which is not at increased risk of the disease. cDNA arrays for molecular cytogenetic analysis were shown to rapidly identify these differences.

The potential for A-CGH implementation as a practical and effective tool in genetic screening is compelling. Three possible applications of this technology in future genetic assessment can be envisioned. First, array-based copy number screening may partially replace karyotyping in the previously discussed patient groups. Second, this technology could be instrumental in detection of genes involved in physical and mental development. Third, systematic analysis of genomic polymorphisms in human population may provide more insight into the variability of the human genome as a whole.

FLUORESCENCE IN SITU HYBRIDIZATION IN VALIDATION OF ARRAY-BASED COMPARATIVE GENOMIC HYBRIDIZATION DISCOVERIES

Following array-based genomic profiling, the discovered alternations can be validated by several other molecular genetic approaches in various types of specimens. Quantitative PCR and fluorescence in situ hybridization (FISH) are two methods often used for achieving this goal. FISH is a straightforward technology and can be performed in most molecular genetic pathology or cytogenetics laboratories. One of the greatest challenges for FISH validation is the availability (or lack thereof) of good-quality probes for regions of interest to be used for validation FISH experiments. Commercial sources such as Abbott Molecular provide basic directly labeled, ready-to-use probes, but this armamentarium of probes is limited to centromeres or chromosome arms or well-known disease-related loci. Therefore, frustration is often caused by lack of specific probes for significant alterations detected in A-CGH experiments. One of the solutions for investigators is to label their own probes using readily available resources.

To accomplish a successful validation, the correct BAC clone needs to be obtained and DNA must be extracted from this clone. The A-CGH result is defined by a genomic alteration (amplification or deletion) seen at a given BAC. Human genome browsers provide a rapid and reliable display of any requested portion of the human genome at a desired scale. They also reveal dozens of annotated tracks containing information on known or predicted genes, expressed sequence tags, messenger

been developed, but conventional techniques are still regarded as best for most applications. Chloroform–phenol extractions are incredibly efficient but are not well suited to automation, which is an important goal for in vitro diagnostics. RNA stabilizing preservatives have also been sought as an alternative to cryogenic processing, the best characterized of which is RNALater® (Qiagen). This is an aqueous fixative that rapidly permeates thin tissue segments and appears to have favorable properties for RNA and specimen preservation. Drawbacks include expense and some changes in antigenicity and morphology.

IN VITRO LABELING

The next step is to convert the isolated RNA to labeled targets, which may be prepared as cDNA or cRNA depending on the protocol. For direct labeling and generation of fluorescent cDNA targets, at least 20 mg of total RNA are required, corresponding to approximately 2 million cells. The small fraction of polyadenylated mRNA is specifically labeled using reverse transcriptase with oligo-dT primers, and a variety of labeled nucleotides can be incorporated into newly synthesized cDNA. Biotin- or digoxigenin-modified nucleotides can be used and coupled to fluorescent reporters in subsequent steps; otherwise, the high-performance Cy3 (green fluorescing) and Cy5 (red fluorescing) dyes are commonly used. Labeling with Cy3 is less efficient than with Cy5, so the former is often used for labeling reference RNA rather than precious sample RNA. More recently, dye bias has been avoided using aminoallyl-labeled nucleotides, which may be subsequently conjugated to either of the cyanine dyes.

For smaller samples (e.g., aspirates, core biopsies, and laser-microdissected sections), it may be necessary to incorporate an amplification step; indeed, in Affymetrix protocols, amplification is inherent in the design of the assay. These protocols are based on the Eberwine method, shown in Figure 8-3. As in direct labeling methods, a reverse transcription reaction using oligo-dT primers is used—however, the primer sequence is extended to include the promoter element for bacteriophage T7 RNA polymerase. Second-strand cDNA synthesis is performed using *Escherichia coli* DNA polymerase I, and the resulting template is then repeatedly transcribed using T7 RNA polymerase. This method produces labeled cRNA targets with linear amplification, from as little as 200 ng starting total RNA (~20,000 cells). Some specimens may require a further round of amplification, which can be performed by repeating the reverse transcription reaction on newly amplified RNA. Amplification reactions are efficient, but in general some loss of fidelity should be

expected compared to direct labeling. In particular, amplification may introduce inaccuracies in the amplification of rare mRNA species, where small degrees of technical variability in template quality and yield may become greatly magnified.

HYBRIDIZATION

Labeled targets are then hybridized to the array of immobilized probes. For oligonucleotide arrays, target preparations are usually sheared by chemical means to produce uniformly small fragments. Depending on the platform and strategy, competitive hybridization between a specimen and an external reference RNA may be used, producing a relative measure of transcript abundance. External RNA references are constructed from pooled cell lines, providing representation of a broad spectrum of transcripts.

An absolute measure of RNA abundance may also be obtained using single-channel measurements, and manufacturers typically claim enhanced ability to detect extremely rare transcripts with this approach. This appears reasonable because at minimum the experimental noise is halved by elimination of the second channel.

Hybridization protocols are straightforward, involving the application of labeled target molecules to the DNA-modified surface of the array. Control probes for hybridization may be numerous, including probes for "housekeeping" genes, with high expression in most tissues. The same probe may be distributed in multiple locations across the array and may be used to monitor spatial variations in hybridization. Miniaturization has been an important goal because modern applications require higher probe density and because small volumes can be hybridized and circulated more efficiently over smaller areas. Hybridizations are lengthy (~16 hours) and require the use of a hybridization chamber, with methods to ensure circulation of the labeled target.

IMAGE CAPTURE

After hybridization, the microarray is washed, stained with secondary reagents if required, and submitted to imaging to record probe intensity. Typical microarray reader hardware employs laser-scanning confocal microscopy, and a digital image of fluorescence intensity is obtained representing the amount of hybridized target within the image spot. The scanned microarray images are matched to the map of probe elements, reviewed for gross errors (e.g., spot defects or physical scratches), and processed in a semiautomated or automated manner.

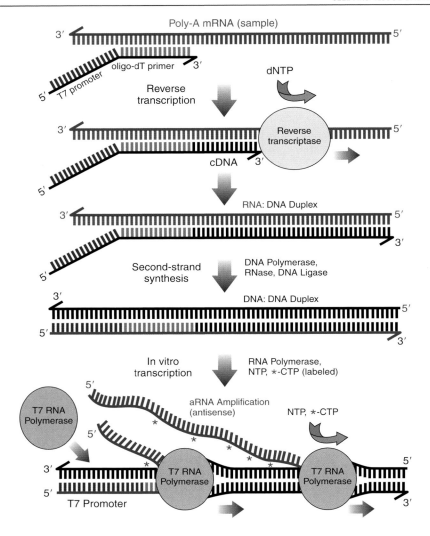

FIGURE 8-3

In vitro labeling of messenger RNA (mRNA). The Eberwine protocol for linear amplification of input mRNA produces targets from as few as 20,000 cells. cDNA, complementary DNA; CTP, cytidine triphosphate; dNTP, deoxyribonucleotide triphosphate; oligo-dT, oligo-deoxythymidine; poly-A, polyadenine; RNase, ribonuclease.

DATA PROCESSING

TWO-CHANNEL MEASUREMENTS

To compare measurements between arrays, it is necessary to ensure that they are on the same scale (normalized); it may also be important to apply various corrections for systematic error. In two-channel applications (cDNA arrays, Agilent arrays), normalization is fairly straightforward, because all measurements are relative to a common reference standard and many probe effects are canceled between channels in ratio intensity measurements. Figure 8-4A is a plot of the Cy5 intensity (tumor) versus Cy3 intensity (reference) for a representative cDNA array. In most cases, as in tumor tissue, it is apparent that a large fraction of genes show no differential expression, and ratio measurements are usually scaled to a median of 1.0 to reflect this effect. Data are usually log transformed, which is a standard method for convenient analysis of ratio measurements. Thus, to divide by the median intensity ratio, one subtracts the median log ratio and the data are said to be *median centered*.

Many two-color arrays show a dependence of ratio measurements on the measured intensity, which may be seen most clearly in "M versus A" plots (Figure 8-4B). Here, M refers to the log ratio measurement, and A refers to the average log intensities of both channels. The value of A represents an estimate of the total log intensity in both channels. In the figure, a smooth curve has been fitted to the data for each print tip in the arrayer, showing different performance for different tips. Figure 8-4C shows the effect of removing these dependencies, although in practice this method is rarely used because of instabilities in the fit at the intensity extremes (with fewer data points).

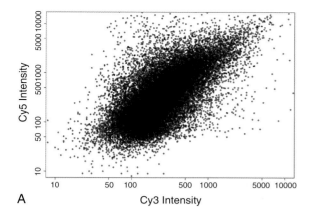

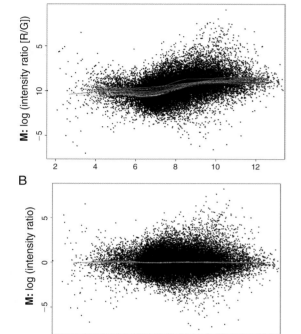

FIGURE 8-4

Raw data from microarray measurements. **(A)** Plot of fluorescence signal intensity in specimen and control channels. **(B)** Diagnostic "M versus A" plot with smooth curves fitted to the data from each of 48 print tips in the arrayer. M refers to the log ratio measurement, and A refers to the average log intensities of both channels. **(C)** Pin dependencies removed by subtracting the fitted curves from intensity data. Plots were generated using the marray package from the academic freeware BioConductor, in the R-statistical software environment.

Two-channel measurements are always relative to the reference standard, and for a given set of experiments, a data matrix is constructed, with columns representing individual arrays and each row representing a given gene. Expression measurements are centered about the mean (or median) for each gene, reflecting the relative degree of expression across the experiment set. Expression measurements are also centered about the mean (or median, as often preferred) for each array, reflecting the usual situation in which the expression of most genes is unchanged between reference and test

samples. Trends in the data are often removed by performing an iterative centering strategy, whereby genes and arrays are consecutively centered, and this is repeated until no further change is observed.

SINGLE-CHANNEL MEASUREMENTS

Preprocessing and normalization of single-channel measurements has proved more problematic, in particular for the 25-mer probes of Affymetrix. The commonly used Affymetrix algorithm, MicroArray Suite 5.0 (MAS 5.0), involves subtraction of the mismatch (MM) intensity from the perfect match (PM) intensity. MAS 5.0 determines a confidence level for each probe set and provides a present, absent, or marginal call for each transcript.

A remarkable (and worrisome) observation is that the MM intensities can be higher than the PM intensities, especially in the lower intensity regions (e.g., for up to 30% of probes). Moreover, MM intensities are reported to show significantly high correlations with PM intensities for many probes. This has been referred to as the "riddle of the bright mismatch" and has been most recently explained in terms of the lower stringencies used for the shorter probes and unexpected hybridization kinetics for RNA:DNA mismatches under these conditions.

The MAS 5.0 algorithm performs accurately for controlled spike-in experiments but is associated with high variance and low precision and does not treat the MM intensity problem. Several alternatives exist that outperform MAS in benchmark comparisons, including the recent Affymetrix release Probe Logarithmic Intensity Error (PLIER). Different algorithms may supply corrections for probe affinity, may supply different normalizations, and may use physical or statistical models for nonspecific hybridization.

Competing algorithms involve fundamentally different data transformations and are known to generate divergent results. Many software utilities provide a suite of normalization methods, with facilities for comparison of results. The use of MAS 5.0 has been standard practice, and expression levels using this algorithm are incorporated in many public repositories. In more recent articles, newer algorithms are often preferred.

UNSUPERVISED ANALYSIS

After preprocessing, large volumes of microarray data are typically filtered to select genes with reliable changes in expression across comparison groups. First, measurements of spot intensity are associated with several quality parameters, and spots may be discarded if they have low signal-to-noise, irregular morphology or if they have been otherwise flagged as unreliable. Any criterion or statistic may be used to select genes: e.g., a second filter is often applied that selects only genes expressed at high levels across a specified number of arrays.

The most commonly used unsupervised strategy is cluster analysis, which is used to group genes that show common patterns of variation across microarray experiments and which has been extensively employed to infer relationships among genes. A variety of methods are used, most commonly hierarchic agglomerative clustering as implemented in the popular Eisen algorithm: Cluster. The standard Pearson correlation coefficient is most often used as a measure of similarity, and gene clusters are iteratively merged with the cluster they most closely resemble.

The content of each cluster is a group of genes whose expression levels are correlated across cases, and the algorithm has proved useful in delineating programs of transcription activity. Numerous disease processes have been identified by hypothesis-driven inspection of correlated genes: (1) upregulated transcription factors often cluster with their targets, (2) clustered genes may be present in the same amplicon, (3) genes reflect cell lineage or differentiation antigens (including normal cell components in tumor tissue samples), (4) genes present in a breakpoint region activated by translocation, and (5) specific biologic pathways are activated by coordinated upregulation of their components.

It is also informative to cluster cases in the same fashion, based on global similarities in their expression profiles. This represents a direct and powerful method for distinguishing homogeneous groupings within a set of heterogeneous lesions, a process that has been termed *class discovery.* A biclustered graph can be constructed by separately clustering both cases and genes; in this manner, it may be possible to visualize distinct clusters of genes that characterize clustered specimen groupings. In Figure 8-5, cases from several classes of soft-tissue tumors are clustered and show distinct homogeneous groupings that largely reflect diagnostic categories. Thus, the gene expression profiles alone categorize tumors in much the same way as does histopathologic diagnosis (although interestingly, leiomyosarcomas are not well distinguished from malignant fibrous histiocytoma or undifferentiated sarcoma). Numerous distinct clusters of genes are also apparent in the figure, including a cluster related to the Wnt pathway, which is shown in the zoomed image. The canonic Wnt pathway is known to be classically upregulated in desmoid-type fibromatosis (DTF), and this pattern shows a degree of overlap with synovial sarcoma, where specific Wnt pathway components are also upregulated.

Other features of the soft-tissue tumor expression profile can be examined by projecting gene lists onto the clustered tumors. In Figure 8-6A, confining the analysis to transcription factors, it can be noted that translocation-associated sarcomas again show distinctive and sharply defined clusters, intriguingly defined by some of the major morphogenetic regulators in mesenchymal tissues (e.g., homeobox genes, runt-related transcription factor, and lymphoid enhancer-binding factor 1). Collagens and metalloproteinases are highly expressed in DTF, as evident in Figure 8-6B,C, consistent with the matrix remodeling and fibrosis characteristic of these tumors. Genes involved in cell motility can also been highlighted (Figure 8-6D), consistent with the infiltrative behavior of DTF.

Unsupervised techniques have been used with extraordinary success. The work of Alizadeh, Eisen, Davis, et al. (2000) in lymphoma is a celebrated example of the use of clustering to delineate heterogeneous disease groups. The authors constructed an array that is widely known as the "LymphoChip," an array of 17,856 clones (12,069 from a germinal-center B-cell cDNA library, and other clones from cDNA libraries of various B-cell malignancies). A dominant feature of the diagnostic category of *diffuse large B-cell lymphoma* was revealed, i.e., on the basis of gene expression profile, tumors with this diagnosis can be sharply divided into germinal-center-like cases with good prognosis and activated B cell–like cases with poor prognosis. This new distinction was dramatically evident and represented fundamental differences in disease processes, and the new disease entities so defined have been rapidly adopted.

SUPERVISED ANALYSIS

Supervised analyses use external clinical information to test specific hypotheses, such as association of expression with survival or differences among defined groupings of cases. For example, the familiar t-test is commonly used to test genes for differential regulation among comparison groups. As with any statistic, the t-test suffers from the problem of false positives because of multiple testing: when testing N independent genes at significance level alpha, we may expect $N \times \alpha$ false positives because of chance fluctuations alone (e.g., for 10,000 genes at significance level $p = 0.05$, 500 false positives are expected). There are several methods for controlling the false-positive error rate, and the available without charge Excel add-in, significance analysis of microarrays (SAM), is most often referenced in this context. Alternatives exist, and commercial systems usually offer methods to deal with this problem.

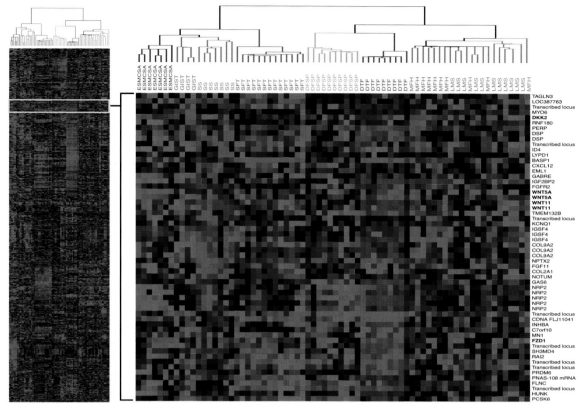

FIGURE 8-5

Cluster diagram of gene expression profiles from soft-tissue tumors; the right hand image represents an expanded view of the highlighted sector at left. Here, 1941 genes were selected, which were differentially expressed in more than four cases. Duplicated gene names represent clones for different regions of the same transcript, provided as hybridization controls. Data were downloaded and processed from the public login of the Stanford Microarray Database; clusters were generated using the Eisen software Cluster. DFSP, dermatofibrosarcoma protuberans; DTF, desmoid-type fibromatosis; ESMCSA, extraskeletal myxoid chondrosarcoma; GIST, gastrointestinal stromal tumor; LMS, leiomyosarcoma; MFH, malignant fibrous histiocytoma; SFT, solitary fibrous tumor; SS, synovial sarcoma.

Comparison studies of this sort are extremely powerful and may be strategically designed to identify differential expression in a variety of situations: chemosensitivity (response versus no response), disease progression, normal versus disease, drug response (before versus after), disease subtypes, and others. SAM is widely used because it provides multiplicity corrections for t-tests, paired sample tests, and nonparametric tests, as well as for time course and survival analyses.

Continuous variables may also be evaluated for correlation of expression measurements with survival, or dose response, and multiple stratifications of the sample may be required. The output of each of these analyses is a list of genes significantly regulated in association with a biologic process, together with quantitative estimates of expression levels and significance. In practice, the first step is to directly examine such lists and to identify known biologic markers, or activation of known biologic systems. Microarray experiments are always designed and interpreted in light of an enormous wealth of prior knowledge, and a thorough analysis of agreement with previous molecular findings is the best starting point.

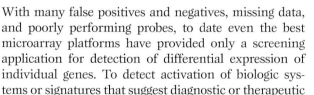

EXPRESSION SIGNATURES

With many false positives and negatives, missing data, and poorly performing probes, to date even the best microarray platforms have provided only a screening application for detection of differential expression of individual genes. To detect activation of biologic systems or signatures that suggest diagnostic or therapeutic strategies, a good start is to show enrichment for coordinately regulated genes from a known biologic system.

This process may be cast into a formal statistical framework using a method known as *enrichment analysis.* A gene list may be projected onto any of several gene classifications, and enrichment analysis is used to test for significant overrepresentation of common genes between two lists. Several websites provide facilities for such analyses, and many are dedicated to ontologies from the Gene Ontology (GO) Consortium. The GO Consortium provides three separate hierarchic classification schemes for each gene: molecular function, biologic process, and cellular compartment. It is common practice

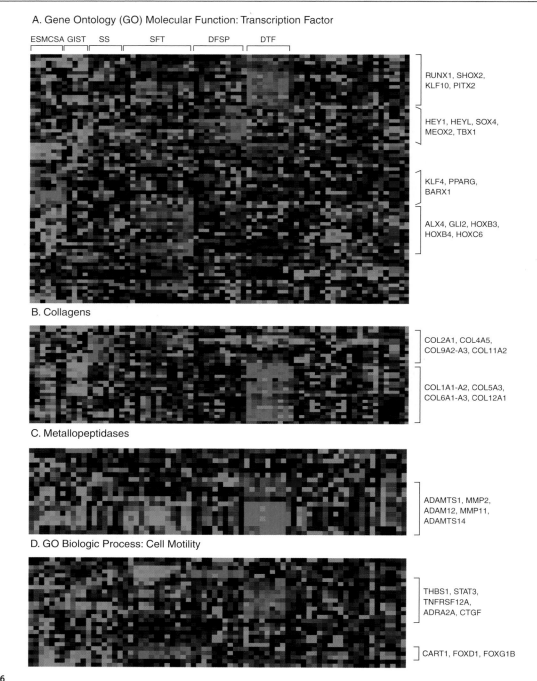

A. Gene Ontology (GO) Molecular Function: Transcription Factor

ESMCSA GIST   SS   SFT   DFSP   DTF

RUNX1, SHOX2, KLF10, PITX2

HEY1, HEYL, SOX4, MEOX2, TBX1

KLF4, PPARG, BARX1

ALX4, GLI2, HOXB3, HOXB4, HOXC6

B. Collagens

COL2A1, COL4A5, COL9A2-A3, COL11A2

COL1A1-A2, COL5A3, COL6A1-A3, COL12A1

C. Metallopeptidases

ADAMTS1, MMP2, ADAM12, MMP11, ADAMTS14

D. GO Biologic Process: Cell Motility

THBS1, STAT3, TNFRSF12A, ADRA2A, CTGF

CART1, FOXD1, FOXG1B

FIGURE 8-6

Analysis of expression signatures in the soft-tissue tumors from Figure 8-5. Subclusters from various gene classification schema reveal distinctive biologic themes for translocation-associated and nonpleomorphic tumors. DFSP, dermatofibrosarcoma protuberans; DTF, desmoid-type fibromatosis; ESMCSA, extraskeletal myxoid chondrosarcoma; GIST, gastrointestinal stromal tumor; SFT, solitary fibrous tumor; SS, synovial sarcoma.

to project gene lists onto different levels of GO categories.

There are, of course, many gene classification schemes that can be considered, and gene expression data may be projected onto any number of categories, such as proliferation, drug response, cell lineage commitments, and cell type–specific expression. Common transcription factor–binding sites can be identified in the regulatory regions of coordinately regulated genes, and lists of known targets for a transcription factor

may be examined for enrichment in the same way. *Pathway signatures* can also be evaluated, and there are Web-based facilities for projection of microarray results onto common pathway diagrams.

GENE EXPRESSION PROFILING OF BREAST CANCER

An example of the insights gained from the use of microarrays is given for breast cancer, where one of the most pressing clinical needs is to identify good-prognosis patients who may safely avoid adjuvant chemotherapy. Current prognostic indices refer up to 90% of node-negative breast cancers for chemotherapy, although this treatment is not required for many of these patients. A plethora of molecular studies in breast cancer have identified individual markers or panels of markers, elucidating different functional aspects of breast cancer biology. Microarrays have unique capacity to examine relationships among differentially regulated genes and have illuminated distinct patterns of expression that more clearly delineate breast cancer heterogeneity.

Seminal work in this area relates to an important series of cDNA array measurements known as the *Norway/Stanford set*. This data is also referred to as the *molecular portraits set,* from the title of the original article by Perou, Sorlie, Eisen, et al. (2000), referenced in the Suggested Readings section. The study included 65 specimens from 42 individuals, and measurements were related to profiles from a panel of 17 cell lines. Using cDNA arrays with probes representing 8102 genes, the investigators identified distinct clusters of cases that were postulated to form intrinsic subtypes of breast cancer. Expression signatures that could be discerned from cluster diagrams suggested fundamentally different tumor phenotypes and included (1) the Luminal/ER+ cluster, the most dominant feature of the cluster diagram (further subdivided into good- and poor-prognosis subsets), represented by the estrogen receptor (ER) and coregulated genes, including known ER targets; (2) the proliferation cluster, a broad swath of genes whose expression varies with the cell cycle; (3) signatures characteristic of nonepithelial components, including adipocytes, macrophages, B and T lymphocytes, and stromal and endothelial cells; (4) the basal-like cluster, which is ER− and with high expression of genes associated with basal differentiation; (5) genes associated with the HER2 amplicon and defining the HER2+/ER− group; and (6) a cluster defining similarity to normal breast samples, including signatures from adipose and other nonepithelial cell types, and expressing basal markers.

In their original study, these investigators defined a set of 496 "breast cancer–intrinsic" genes, which showed large differences among subtypes but also showed reliably uniform expression between paired samples from the same tumor (e.g., before and after doxorubicin treatment). The subtypes defined in these initial studies appear to reflect a pervasive and robust pattern of gene expression, which has since been confirmed on multiple platforms and in independent series. Subtype distinctions have since been refined, and intrinsic gene lists have been elaborated with greater genome coverage and in larger series.

Other published expression profiles of breast cancer with potential clinical utility include the Amsterdam (van't Veer, et al) and Rotterdam (Wang, et al)

signatures, also referenced in the Suggested Readings section. The 70-gene Amsterdam signature is a prognostic signature developed at the Dutch National Cancer Institute on the Agilent platform. The signature was derived from studies of sporadic cases from 97 young women (<55 years), with node-negative breast cancer measuring less than 5 cm (stage I and II). Also evaluated were 18 carriers of BRCA1 germline mutations and 2 BRCA2 carriers. The studies used the Agilent Hu25K array, including probes for multiple transcripts. The 70-gene Amsterdam signature was derived from supervised analysis linking to patient outcomes and has been further evaluated on an unselected cohort of 295 cases. The signature includes a spectrum of genes related to diverse malignant processes: in the poor-prognosis group, high expression is detected for genes involved in proliferation, invasion and metastasis, angiogenesis, and receptor signaling pathways. Interestingly, many established markers of breast cancer prognosis were not included in the signature, including ER, cyclin D1, and HER2, indicating more significant effects from other reporters in this system. The authors also concluded that many of the features prognostic for distant metastases are present early in the primary tumor cells, before apparent lymph node involvement, and that these modes of spreading are independent events.

This Amsterdam signature is under evaluation in a large international study known as the Microarrays in Node-negative Disease May Avoid Chemotherapy (MINDACT) trial. The MINDACT trial is designed to randomize adjuvant treatment for patients with discordant prognostic indices between standard clinical or pathologic criteria and the Amsterdam signature, with additional goals related to alternative hormonal and chemotherapeutic regimens. The trial is a prospective study of 6000 patients; accrual began in September 2005, and end points are designed at 3 to 6 years follow-up.

Another published prognostic signature, known as the 76-gene Rotterdam signature, was developed at Erasmus Medical Center from studies of 286 lymph node–negative cases, primarily of stages I and II. Measurements were performed with the Affymetrix Hu133 chip, and survival analysis with training and validation sets were used. Comparisons with the Amsterdam signature are favorable, and numerous common pathways are identified between the two measurement series.

VALIDATION

Expression profile studies are prone to false positives, as well as apparently discordant results. This is because of their nature as discovery-based tools, measuring thousands of genes over a more limited number of specimens. With evolving nonstandardized methods of data processing and analysis, validation of important findings is therefore especially important. Current algorithms for validation require a test and training set, although these are often too small for statistical validity.

RNA-level validation may be obtained by applying real-time quantitative PCR (Q-PCR), to aliquots of total RNA reserved from samples submitted for microarray analysis. A more scientifically convincing validation of key genes comes through the use of independent specimens, which are most readily available as formalin-fixed, paraffin-embedded archival tissue blocks. With appropriate primer design, Q-PCR can often be made to work on samples from archival blocks. Tissue microarrays are also useful as a high-throughput method for validation on large numbers of independent clinical specimens, using immunohistochemistry or nucleic acid in situ hybridization. Thus, an entire study cohort can be arrayed within single or multiple blocks and assayed for protein, RNA, and DNA content with the added advantage of retaining morphologic context. These techniques are discussed in other chapters in this volume.

A lack of comparability among results from different platforms has been previously identified, and this problem has even been apparent using different versions of Affymetrix chips. In recent studies, problems with discordance among platforms largely have been addressed; e.g., although there are only five genes in common between the Amsterdam and the Rotterdam signatures, further analysis indicated that the signatures show activation of numerous common pathways. This suggests that different array platforms provide probes sets with complementary coverage of the genome and that the quality of probe response may be quite different between systems.

A major difficulty with cross-platform comparisons involves mapping common genes among platforms, which until recently has been done using Unigene clusters. Previous studies of cross-platform validation sacrificed resolution and clarity, because the first step was to discard large numbers of probes that were apparently not common among platforms. However, Unigene clusters represent predicted genes based on clustering of expressed sequence tags and are not necessarily accurate. For example, probe sequences for the Affymetrix U133A chip were based on Unigene build 133 (April 2001), but there have been more than 60 modifications to the Unigene build since that time. Improved correspondence has been realized with verified and updated probe annotations, and several reports have outlined the need for direct sequence verification in cross-platform comparisons. Improved agreement among platforms is consistently achieved with these methods, and newer annotations and array designs should largely eliminate these problems.

The U.S. Food and Drug Administration has moved to define standards in the microarray arena in cooperation with many academic and industrial groups, including the National Institutes of Health, National Cancer Institute, National Institute of Standards and Technology, and External RNA Control Consortium. Data acquisition has recently been completed for the Microarray Quality Control (MAQC) study, comparing six different high-density commercial platforms, as well as alternate expression profiling techniques, including Q-PCR systems. The same commercial RNA specimens were used in all assays, and three sites were selected by each manufacturer to run five replicate specimens. Platforms differed in genome coverage, with roughly 65% of 24,000 defined genes common to all platforms.

This study provided estimates of quantitative precision of expression measurements within each platform, with coefficients of variation between 5% and 15% for replicate measurements within a single laboratory and between 10% and 20% for combined measurements from three laboratories. The concordance of overexpression calls was determined to be between 80% and 95% for replicate measures from a single laboratory and between 70% and 85% when measures from three laboratories were combined. Interplatform comparisons were more limited in initial reports because of differences in data analysis and threshold calls among platforms. Different sites concurred on lists of overexpressed genes by as little as 60%, although good agreement on the rank (highest to lowest) of expression values was seen (the median correlation coefficient among sites, including all platforms, was 0.87). Thus, the MAQC study defined reference specimens and performance metrics that may provide the basis for proficiency testing and provided one of the more rigorous protocols for comparisons among microarray platforms.

CONCLUSION

Gene expression profiling using DNA microarrays is a powerful and revolutionary technique for the measurement of patterns of gene expression on a genomic scale, which has been used to characterize a variety of biologic processes in health and disease. As a discovery-based technology, DNA microarrays have incredible power for examining relationships among overexpressed genes and for resolving transcriptional programs related to disease processes. As has already been seen in lymphomas and breast cancer, these findings may suggest new disease classifications and new methods for stratifying treatment, although their clinical utility critically depends on formal validation studies with unselected cohorts.

Expression profiling also presents the exciting opportunity to identify new therapeutic targets and specific disease signatures and may have its major clinical impact in this area through functional dissection of cancer genomes. With new therapeutics targeting specific pathways, expression arrays are expected to play a larger role in support of investigational drug studies.

Microarray measurements are technically demanding and involve extensive precautions to avoid degradation of sample RNA, which may be impractical in a routine clinical context. Despite these demanding issues in the United States, some referral laboratories may currently offer microarray analyses as an ancillary diagnostic test and must be certified for high-complexity clinical testing.

Translation to clinical practice is likely to come from evaluation of more limited panels of markers, which can serve as surrogate markers for the full expression profile. These could be evaluated using smaller standardized microarrays with focused content or by Q-PCR employing a defined set of primer pairs. Immunochemical or other protein-based assays may provide a more readily applicable and cost-effective platform for routine evaluation and await the development of validated panels of surrogate markers, the composition of which will be derived from the output of array analyses.

SUGGESTED READINGS

Alizadeh AA, Eisen MB, Davis RE, et al: Distinct types of diffuse large B-cell lymphoma identified by gene expression profiling. Nature 2000;403(6769):503–511.

Blue Cross Blue Shield: GENE EXPRESSION PROFILING for Managing Breast Cancer Treatment. Blue Cross Blue Shield Technology Evaluation Center Assessment Program, vol 20, no 3, May 2005. Available at http://www.bcbs.com/tec/vol20/20_03.html.

The Chipping Forecast I: Nat Genet 1999;21(Suppl).

The Chipping Forecast II: Nat Genet 2002;32(Suppl).

The Chipping Forecast III: Nat Genet 2005;37(6s).

Dunphy, CH: Gene expression profiling data in lymphoma and leukemia: Review of the literature and extrapolation of pertinent clinical applications. Arch Pathol Lab Med 2006;130:483–520.

Eisen MB, Spellman PT, Brown PO, Botstein D: Cluster analysis and display of genome-wide expression patterns. Proc Natl Acad Sci USA 1998;95(25):14863–14868.

Eisen Lab: Cluster. Available at http://rana.lbl.gov/EisenSoftware.htm.

National Center for Biotechnology Information: What Does NCBI Do? Available at http://www.ncbi.nlm.nih.gov/.

Perou CM, Sorlie T, Eisen MB, et al: Molecular portraits of human breast tumours. Nature 2000;406(6797):747–752.

Stanford University: Stanford Microarray Database. Available at http://genome-www5.stanford.edu/.

Staudt LM, Sandeep D: The biology of human lymphoid malignancies revealed by gene expression profiling. Adv Immunol 2005;87:163–208.

U.S. Food and Drug Administration Center for Toxicogenomics: Microarray Quality Control Project. Available at http://www.fda.gov/nctr/science/centers/toxicoinformatics/maqc/.

University of California, Santa Cruz: UCSC Genome Browser. Available at http://genome.ucsc.edu/cgi-bin/hgGateway.

van't Veer LJ, Dai H, van de Vijver MJ, et al: Gene expression profiling predicts clinical outcome of breast cancer. Nature 2002;415(6871):530–536.

Wang Y, Klijn JG, Zhang Y, et al: Gene-expression profiles to predict distant metastasis of lymph-node-negative primary breast cancer. Lancet 2005;365(9460):671–679.

9 Epigenetics: DNA Hypermethylation in Cancer

Bin Yang

INTRODUCTION

According to Alfred G. Knudson's two-hit theory of tumorigenesis, disruption of the function of a tumor suppressor gene requires a complete loss of function of both copies of the involved gene. Many tumor suppressor genes have been identified by chromosomal analysis that has lost one allele referred to as *loss of heterozygosity*. However, the mode of inactivation of the second allele was not always understood. Traditionally, it is believed that the second hit can be carried out genetically by point mutations, either germline mutation in familial cancers or somatic mutation in noninherited tumors. It has been debated for decades whether the initiation and progression of cancer can also be caused by epigenetic changes, such as DNA methylation, that are not caused by alterations in the primary DNA sequence. Recent molecular studies have demonstrated that, indeed, gene inactivation can occur by aberrant DNA methylation. It is now established not only that epigenetic changes are as common as genetic changes in cancers but also that both genetic and epigenetic processes are also intricately related in tumorigenesis.

EPIGENETIC CONTROL OF GENE EXPRESSION IN NORMAL CELLS

Epigenetics is defined as a heritable change in gene expression without an alteration in the DNA sequence. Among epigenetic changes, DNA methylation is the major alteration that takes place during aging, embryogenesis, and carcinogenesis. All cells in the body are descendants of a fertilized egg and in almost all cases contain the same set of genes. But there is great diversity in normal cell types that carry out a variety of specific functions. These specific properties mostly are determined by activating expression or repression of sets of genes by epigenetic controls. Such epigenetic events reprogram the

genome in normal development into different types of differentiated somatic cells. Therefore, cell differentiation requires cell type–specific silencing of some genes and activation of others. It has been shown that the major change that leads to gene silencing during embryogenesis and development is methylation of DNA at CpG sites, cytosine (C) base followed by a guanosine (G). This form of methylation prevents the binding of transcription factors to CpG dinucleotides in gene promoter regions. In mammals, patterns of DNA methylation are species and tissue specific. Prohibition of DNA methylation stops development (embryogenesis), switches on apoptosis, and is usually lethal. Aberrant patterns of DNA methylations can result in malignant transformation of cells. One of the best examples of the tight control of gene expression through epigenetic mechanisms involving methylation silencing of genes is the inactivation of the X chromosome in females. Recent studies further indicate that DNA methylation is a primary mechanism for silencing primordial germ cell genes in both germ cell and somatic cell lineages. In all, epigenetic changes are responsible for chromatin structure stability, genome integrity, modulation of tissue-specific gene expression, embryonic development, genomic imprinting, and X chromosome inactivation in females.

The epigenetic methylation of DNA has other functions. One of the major functions appears to be to permanently silence the large proportion of "junk" DNA, repetitive sequences, etc., that has entered our genomes throughout the course of evolution, mostly by viral transfection. It has been estimated that 45% of the human genome consists of viral transposons, endogenous retroviruses, and repeat sequences capable of moving around the genome and causing instability and inappropriate expression of local genes if not kept in check by strong silencing mechanisms. Epigenetic changes play critical roles in controlling host–viral interactions in several DNA virus infections. It has been found that latency or episomal expression of Epstein-Barr virus infection, a virus linked to several human neoplasms, is tightly controlled through host cell DNA methylation, whereas

TABLE 9-1

Epigenetics

DEFINITION

Heritable change in gene expression without an alteration in the DNA sequence

INVOLVEMENT OF EPIGENETIC CONTROL IN NORMAL CELLS

Embryonic development and cell differentiation

Genomic imprinting

Inactivation of the X chromosome in females

Silencing of intragenomic parasitic DNA elements, such as transposons

DNA METHYLATION, HISTONE DEACETYLATION, AND CHROMATIN STRUCTURE

Euchromatin state (gene activated) that associates with the DNA promoter hypomethylation and the histone acetylation

Heterochromatin state (gene silenced) that associates with the DNA promoter hypermethylation and histone deacetylation

DIFFERENCE BETWEEN EPIGENETICS AND GENETICS

Genetic alterations: point mutation and deletion

Epigenetic alterations: DNA methylation, histone deacetylation, and histone methylation

Both genetic and epigenetic changes are inheritable

Epigenetic change is usually *reversible,* and most genetic alterations are *irreversible*

latency of herpes simplex virus type 1 infection is linked to histone modifications. Methylation in regulatory and L1 open reading frame regions in human papillomavirus (HPV) type 16 and HPV-18 is implicated in promoting the switch from an episomal to an integrated state of HPV DNA in infected cervical epithelial cells. Thus, many strategies have evolved for viral–host interaction that involves epigenetic regulation (Table 9-1).

PROTEINS THAT REGULATE DNA METHYLATION

The DNA methyltransferases (DNMTs) are the enzymes responsible for the generation of genomic methylation patterns leading to gene silencing. However, the underlying mechanisms by which DNMTs repress transcription and how they are targeted to preferred DNA sequences is still largely unknown. Emerging evidence points to an intricate web of interactions between DNMTs and the chromatin

environment in which they function. There are three known biologically active DNMTs in mammalian cells: DNMT1, DNMT3a, and DNMT3b. Although much remains to be determined about how each participates in establishing normal DNA-methylation patterns and the aberrant patterns in cancer, it is certain that each of these proteins is vital for embryonic development because disabling any of these three genes in mice causes embryonic or early postnatal death.

DNMT1 is responsible for maintaining DNA methylation patterns in adult cells. The substrate for this DNA methylase is hemimethylated DNA. Methylation occurs immediately after DNA replication with the enzyme's primary function to ensure that the methylation pattern of the parental cells is identically reproduced in each daughter cell.

There is considerable evidence indicating an upregulation of DNMT1 in cancer. Experimental evidence indicates that forced overexpression of the murine *Dnmt1* gene in NIH3T3 cells results in cellular transformation. In human fibroblasts, sustained overexpression of DNMT1 leads to the processive time-dependent hypermethylation of several CpG islands. Conversely, reduction of DNMT1 levels appears to have protective effects. Reduction of DNMT1 through an antisense approach can block tumorigenesis. Therefore, inhibition of DNMT function may be a promising target for future pharmacogenomics therapy.

DNMT3a and DNMT3b are the enzymes responsible for establishing de novo methylation. These enzymes use unmethylated DNA as their template and play an important role in embryonic development. Although DNMT1 seems to be responsible for most of the DNA-methylating capacity in cancer cells and has long been suspected to be the main factor in maintaining abnormal promoter methylation in neoplasia, recent studies suggest that an interaction between DNMT1 and DNMT3b may be vital for this function. Recent work has also revealed that these DNMTs may contribute to the transcriptional repression of chromatin by mechanisms other than just DNA methylation. Such chromatin consists of DNA that forms complexes in promoter regions with groups of proteins that act to prevent the transcription of genes. Thus, each of the DNMTs interacts directly with histone deacetylases and can recruit them to sites of gene promoters. DNMTs also bind to other proteins with the potential to repress gene transcription and thus may coordinate transcriptional repression. For example, in leukemic cells, abnormal transcription factors arising from translocated genes may recruit complexes of DNMTs with other proteins to gene promoters. This is a good example of how DNMTs, in addition to mediating DNA methylation, may act as platforms to help coordinate other chromatin-mediated aspects of gene silencing (Table 9-1).

DNA METHYLATION, CHROMATIN STRUCTURE, AND GENE EXPRESSION

It has been known for many years that DNA methylation, chromatin structure, and gene silencing are closely interconnected processes. For example, early studies revealed that high levels of CpG methylation coincide with heterochromatic regions and hypomethylation or demethylation is associated with euchromatin formation. In human cells, histones undergo many post-translational modifications, such as methylation, phosphorylation, ubiquitination, and ribosylation. Among the histone modifications implicated in gene silencing, the best characterized to date are histone deacetylation and methylation of histone H3 at lysine 9. Aberrant epigenetic silencing of tumor suppressor genes by promoter DNA hypermethylation and histone deacetylation plays an important role in the pathogenesis of some cancers. It is increasingly clear that histone deacetylation and methylation of histone H3 at lysine 9 work hand in hand with DNA methylation to repress transcription. It has been observed that DNA hypermethylation is often coupled with histone deacetylation and unmethylated CpG-island chromatin is enriched in hyperacetylated histones. Chromatin modification provides the other major epigenetic mechanism of gene silencing by rendering methylated promoter regions inaccessible for transcription. The potential reversibility of epigenetic abnormalities has promoted the development of pharmacologic inhibitors of DNA methylation and histone deacetylation as possible anticancer therapeutics. Recent preclinical studies of DNMT and histone deacetylase inhibitors have yielded encouraging results, especially against hematologic malignancies (Table 9-1).

DNA METHYLATION IN CANCER

TWO MAJOR METHYLATION CHANGES IN CANCER CELLS

Although the underlying mechanisms are still largely unknown, recent studies have shown that two major changes in methylation status occur during carcinogenesis: regional promoter hypermethylation and genomewide hypomethylation. The most studied alteration of DNA methylation in cancer is the aberrant hypermethylation of CpG islands surrounding promoter regions. These methylation changes are critically associated with transcriptional silencing of the involved genes. DNA methylation of genes tends to occur primarily in promoter regions that contain CpG islands, defined as a 1.0-kilobase stretch of DNA

that contains this sequence at a higher frequency than the rest of the genome. Methylation of CpG islands in the promoter region silences gene expression and is a normal event that occurs in cells to regulate gene expression, particularly during embryogenesis. However, when aberrant DNA methylation of tumor suppressor genes occurs in tumors, it is implicated in neoplastic transformation.

Although hypermethylation of promoter regions of tumor suppressor genes is one of the hallmarks of cancer cells, relative genomewide hypomethylation was recognized many years ago in tumors using methylation-sensitive restriction digestion and Southern blot analysis. Malignant cells may have 20% to 40% reduced methylation at CpG islands genomewide relative to their normal counterparts. This form of hypomethylation mainly occurs at the coding region and introns of genes. The mechanism and significance of genomewide hypomethylation is still unknown. It is also not clear whether global hypomethylation and promoter CpG-island hypermethylation are mechanistically linked during tumorigenesis. It has been postulated, however, that global hypomethylation may contribute to carcinogenesis through three mechanisms: chromosome instability, reactivation of transposons, and loss of imprinting (Table 9-2).

MULTIPLE GENE METHYLATION IS THE HALLMARK IN CANCER CELLS

Genomic screening of 98 primary human tumors has revealed that each tumor contains on average about 600 aberrantly methylated CpG islands out of approximately 45,000 CpG islands in the genome. Genes often altered genetically in cancers, such as p15, p16, and adenomatous *Polyposis coli,* can be silenced through promoter methylation as well, although many of these methylated CpG islands are present in genomic regions containing genes that have not yet been identified yet may play an important role in tumorigenesis. To date, most studies have focused on aberrant CpG-island methylation status of less than 50 relatively well-characterized candidate tumor suppressor genes in the most common human cancers, such as cancer of the colon, lung, breast, and prostate. These tumor suppressor genes have been found to be the key elements involved in major signaling pathways, including p53, Wnt/β-catenin, pRb, AKT/PKB, JAK/STAT, and Ras/BRAF/MAPK pathways. Aberrant methylation is also involved in regulating many cellular and biologic functions, such as cell cycle control, genome stability, DNA repair, apoptosis, angiogenesis, invasion, and metastasis. Therefore, DNA promoter hypermethylation not only silences the expression of the specific target genes but, more importantly, also disrupts the fundamental pathways thought

---

TABLE 9-2

Epigenetic Alterations in Cancer and Other Human Disorders

EPIGENETIC CHANGES IN CANCER CELLS

Hypermethylation of DNA promoter regions of a set of genes, mostly candidate tumor suppressor genes, is the major alteration during tumorigenesis

Genomewide hypomethylation, mainly at the coding sequences and repetitive introns

Histone deacetylation and methylation, which are closely linked to chromatin structure and DNA methylation

EPIGENETIC ABNORMALITY IN OTHER HUMAN DISORDERS

Inactivation of the silent allele at imprinted loci: Beckwith-Wiedemann syndrome, Prader-Willi syndrome, and Angelman syndrome

Methylation machinery abnormality:

1. Rett syndrome, an X-linked neuropsychiatric disorder, with mutation of the gene encoding methyl-CpG-binding protein MeCP2

2. Immunodeficiency–centromeric instability– facial anomalies syndrome, a rare disorder characterized by immunodeficiency, facial anomalies, and hypomethylation of the satellite DNA of chromosomes 1 and 16, with mutation of the *Dnmt3b* gene

---

to lead to cancer (Figure 9-1). The evidence suggests that concurrent methylation of multiple CpG islands is the hallmark in almost all human cancers. This epigenetic hallmark in cancer cells can be used as a potential molecular biomarker for the accurate detection of cancer cells in pathologic specimens.

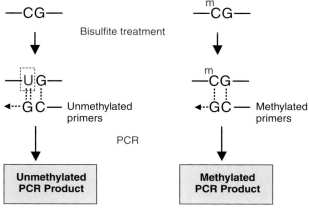

FIGURE 9-1

Detection of DNA promoter hypermethylation by methylation-specific polymerase chain reaction (PCR). Genomic DNA was first treated with bisulfite, which converts unmethylated cytosine (C) to uridine. By designing PCR primers specific to methylated and unmethylated alleles, both methylated and unmethylated alleles of any specific gene can be detected.

METHYLATION IN CANCER IS TISSUE AND STAGE SPECIFIC

Aberrant DNA methylation has been demonstrated in almost all kinds of tumors, from epithelial carcinomas to mesenchymal sarcomas and from melanoma to hematopoietic malignancies. The aberrant methylation of genes that suppress tumorigenesis appears to occur early in tumor development and increases progressively, eventually contributing to the malignant phenotype. Based on published DNA methylation profiles in different tumors, it seems that similar patterns of CpG-island methylation are shared within tumor types. However, methylation of CpG islands can be quantitatively different in individual tumors within a tumor type and may be nonrandom and tumor type and stage specific. Clearly, studies have shown that late-stage cancers tend to harbor more aberrant methylation of CpG islands and candidate tumor suppressor genes than early precursors. Consistent with the concept of multistep tumorigenesis, accumulation of multiple epigenetic alterations is present in most human neoplasms.

DNA METHYLATION AS A MOLECULAR BIOMARKER IN CANCER DETECTION

As stated earlier, methylation of multiple candidate tumor suppressor genes is a hallmark in cancer cells in comparison to their normal counterparts. Thus, molecular changes associated with epigenetic gene silencing may serve as potential markers for risk assessment, early diagnosis, and prediction of prognosis. Molecular signatures of cancer cells can be used to improve cancer detection and assessment of cancer risk. Hypermethylation of the promoter region of cancer-related genes provides some of the most promising markers for cancer diagnosis. DNA-based markers have advantages because of the inherent stability of DNA compared with RNA and some proteins. Also, the constant patterns of abnormal CpG-island methylation at the promoter region in genes of interest allow a simpler detection strategy than is possible for many common mutations in cancer. Such mutations, even for the same tumor type, may differ widely from patient to patient in their position within the gene. In contrast, for any given gene, a single assay for the detection of promoter-methylation abnormalities will work in virtually all patients and all types of cancers. Another possible advantage to hypermethylation as a marker for cancer diagnosis is the evidence from recent studies indicating that specific methylation profiles exist in different types of cancer. Using specific methylation profiles will be helpful in differentiating one cancer type from another, particularly in certain clinical settings, such as the differential diagnosis of whether a liver nodule is a primary tumor versus metastasis. Finally, although methylation of individual tumor suppressor genes occasionally can be seen in benign processes, methylation of multiple tumor suppressor genes is a relatively unique observation to malignancy. Therefore, concurrent methylation of several tumor suppressor genes can be applied as a surrogate marker in detection of malignancy in clinical samples.

Aberrant CpG-island methylation has been used as a molecular tool for detection of cancer cells in a variety of tissue and cytologic samples. Liquid-based cytology samples, such as body fluids and fine-needle aspiration, provide excellent materials for polymerase chain reaction (PCR)–based methylation assays because of the absence of formalin fixation. A recent study demonstrated that methylation-specific PCR (MSP) detected aberrant promoter methylation in sputum of patients with lung cancer up to 3 years before clinicopathologic detection of tumors in individuals who smoke. Similar approaches have been applied to breast ductal lavage, bronchial lavage, cervical smears, urine, peritoneal washing, and fine-needle aspiration biopsies. In some patients, dying tumor cells can release fragments of genomic DNA, which can be used as biomarkers for the diagnosis of cancer. Using MSP, it is possible to detect methylated genes released from tumors in the serum of patients. In some studies, there has been a good correlation between the detection of the methylated gene in serum and the methylation of the identical gene in the primary tumor. This approach has the potential to be used for early diagnosis of cancer and to monitor the response to chemotherapy.

THE EPIGENOME AS A TARGET FOR CANCER CHEMOPREVENTION AND TREATMENT

The fundamental difference between genetic alterations and epigenetic changes is that the former are irreversible and the latter are potentially reversible. The potential reversibility of epigenetic changes in neoplasia presents new opportunities for the clinical treatment of cancer. This has drawn great attention from clinicians and pharmaceutical professionals searching for agents that can reverse abnormal DNA methylation and inhibit DNA hypermethylation as potential tumor therapies. The potent and specific inhibitor of DNA methylation 5-aza-deoxycytidine has been demonstrated to reactivate most silenced genes in human tumor cells. This provides the rationale for further investigations into the potential of this demethylating agent as a cancer therapeutic. Because it is unlikely

that a single agent has the potential to cure malignant disease because of the rapid development of drug resistance to single-drug therapy, the interaction of 5-aza-deoxycytodine with other agents that enhance its antineoplastic activity is also being investigated. The discovery of the "cross-talk" between DNA methylation and chromatin remodeling pathways has also provided a novel opportunity for therapeutic intervention. Gene silencing by aberrant methylation and histone deacetylation can be reversed by a combination of an inhibitor of DNA methylation with an inhibitor of histone acetylation. An alternative approach would be to inhibit DNA methylation by targeting DNMT. It has been shown that inhibition of the function of DNMT1 and DNMT3b using small interfering RNAs dramatically enhances the chemosensitivity of ovarian cancer cells to cisplatin-based chemotherapy. From the preceding information, it seems certain that ongoing analyses of epigenetic changes in cancers will play an important role not only in early detection of cancer but also in refining therapeutic strategies and in monitoring chemotherapeutic responses.

DNA METHYLATION AS A PROGNOSTIC OR PREDICTIVE BIOMARKER FOR CANCER

Another potential application of the assessment of CpG-island hypermethylation involves using the function of the silenced genes to gauge prognosis. Glioblastoma is the most common brain tumor and is notoriously chemoresistant. Recent epigenetic studies have identified a DNA methylation marker that seems to strongly predict a patient's tumor chemosensitivity. Alkylating agents such as temozolomide are the primary form of glioblastoma chemotherapy and injure DNA, culminating in apoptotic cell death. (O^6-methylguanine-DNA methyltransferase, or MGMT, is an enzyme that can repair the DNA damage caused by this agent). Methylation of the promoter of *MGMT* turns off transcription of the gene, reducing the intracellular level of MGMT and thereby inhibiting the repair mechanism. In principle, therefore, interference with MGMT should accentuate the antitumor effect of the alkylating agent. Investigators have found that the prognosis is better for patients who have tumors in which there is methylation of the *MGMT* promoter than for patients who have tumors without methylation at this locus. Furthermore, almost all benefit of adding temozolomide to radiotherapy occurs within subgroups of patients who have this promoter methylated. Therefore, detection of MGMT promoter methylation in biopsy samples from glioblastoma patients may be a useful epigenetic tool in predicting a patient's sensitivity to alkylating agents such as temozolomide. Similar studies have been done in lymphoma and male germ cell tumors. DNA promoter hypermethylation of RASSF1A and HIC1 genes associates with chemoresistance, and the transcriptional inactivation of MGMT by epigenetic alterations confers exquisite sensitivity to cisplatin. Another example with prognostic importance is the gene for death-associated protein kinase (DAPK), an antiapoptotic factor. Patients with lung tumors containing a hypermethylated DAPK gene have a shorter survival after diagnosis than those with tumors that do not. Larger studies must be performed to determine the clinical applicability of such findings, but the results suggest that the relatively easy and rapid detection of hypermethylated CpG islands of specific genes may prove clinically valuable.

DNA METHYLATION ANALYSIS TECHNIQUES AND CLINICAL APPLICATIONS

The central role of DNA methylation in maintaining cellular function and the recognition that aberrant DNA methylation patterns may be one of the driving forces in tumorigenesis have created a strong need for techniques to reliably detect and measure methylation in DNA from clinical samples. DNA hypermethylation can be detected by several methods, which are grouped into two major categories for the purpose of simplification: global or genomewide CpG-island methylation analysis and focused regional CpG-island methylation analysis. The global or genomewide CpG-island methylation analyses involve complete enzymatic hydrolysis of genomic DNA, followed by high-resolution separation to obtain the total base composition of the genome. The assays include methylation-sensitive restriction endonuclease Southern blot (MSRE-Southern), restriction landmark genomic scanning, differential methylation hybridization, methylation CpG-island amplification–representational difference analysis, high-performance liquid chromatography, high-performance capillary electrophoresis, and methylation-sensitive arbitrarily primed PCR. An exception to these DNA-based methods is immunohistochemical analysis of genomewide methylation using monoclonal antibodies raised against 5-methylcytosine or DNMT. The focused regional CpG-island methylation analyses available mostly involve chemical treatment of genomic DNA with bisulfite followed by PCR-based analysis. The assays include MSP, Cobra, MethyLight, methylation-sensitive single nucleotide primer extension, methylation-specific microarray, and direct bisulfite genomic sequencing (Table 9-3). Sequence analysis of PCR products generated from bisulfite treated DNA is

considered the gold standard for gene-specific methylation analysis, because it provides information about the methylation status of every cytosine residue within the target sequence. Most methods mentioned earlier are nonquantitative assays. Recently, several quantitative or semiquantitative methods have been developed for the detection of the percentage of methylation of a single CpG island or overall methylation of a group of CpG islands. These include pyrosequencing, Methy-Light, and Sequenom's MassArray for Methylation (Table 9-3). No doubt these quantitative methylation assays will facilitate the process of translating epigenetic research assay into clinical practice for the early and accurate detection of cancer cells.

MSP is currently the most widely used technique to investigate the methylation status of specific CpG sites in CpG islands. The basic principle of this method is PCR-based discrimination between methylated and unmethylated DNA in bisulfite-converted DNA. Briefly, bisulfite treatment of DNA results in a deamination of unmethylated cytosines to form uracil; 5-methyl-cytosine is resistant to this chemical treatment. In a standard PCR, all uracil and thymine residues will be amplified as thymine and only 5-methylcytosine residues will be amplified as cytosine. Because of the differences in the DNA sequence of methylated and unmethylated CpGs after bisulfite treatment, it is possible to design specific primers for methylated and unmethylated alleles and differentially detect both methylated and unmethylated alleles simultaneously by MSP. There are several notable advantages of using MSP in clinical settings. First, MSP is a rapid and sensitive method for the detection of promoter methylation. Methylated target molecules can be detected down to a level of 0.1% to 0.01% of the total population. Therefore, only small quantities of starting DNA template are required for MSP analysis. Second, because MSP can differentially and simultaneously detect methylated (present mostly in cancer cells) and unmethylated (present mostly in normal cells) alleles of any genes of interest, it is unnecessary to isolate or enrich cancer cells from a background of reactive cells, inflammatory cells, or stromal cells. This is particularly useful for cytology samples, such as pleural effusion or urine, where microdissection is not possible. It may also be possible to make a semiquantitative assessment of allele types in an isolated homogenous population by comparing methylated with unmethylated signals. Finally, the methylation status of several tumor suppressor genes can be analyzed in a single MSP reaction using a nested approach. Therefore, a panel of candidate tumor suppressor genes, involved in different signaling pathways, can be analyzed simultaneously. In general, the information obtained by MSP should be considered only qualitative, and the semiquantitative estimates should be further validated using a more

TABLE 9-3

DNA Methylation Analysis Techniques

Global/Genome-wide Methylation	MSRE-southern blot HPLC or HPCE Immunochemical stain
Regional CpG island Methylation (chemically converting genome with bisulfite treatment)	MSP MethyLight Cobra Pyrosequencing Direct bisulfite genomic sequencing
Methylation Microarray	MassArray by Sequenom Methylscope by Orion Methylation Oligoarray
Quantitative Methylation Assays	Pyrosequencing MethyLight
Methylation Sequencing	Bisulfite sequencing Pyrosequencing (less than 250 bp)

HPCE, high-performance capillary electrophoresis; HPLC, high-performance liquid chromatography; MSP, methylation-specific polymerase chain reaction; MSRE-Southern, methylation sensitive restriction endonuclease Southern blot.

quantitative method, such as pyrosequencing. Limitations of MSP are that usually only a limited number of CpG sites are reliably probed and that CpG sites outside CpG islands are not amenable to analysis.

CONCLUSION

Epigenetic changes occur often during tumor development. The major change is aberrant DNA methylation, which in turn silences the expression of genes that suppress tumorigenesis. Aberrant DNA methylation profiling is a promising ancillary molecular tool in the early and accurate detection of cancer cells in clinical samples. In addition, aberrant DNA methylation profiling may be a useful molecular biomarker in prediction of chemoresponsiveness or prognosis of patients with cancer. Finally, epigenetic changes are potential targets for therapeutic intervention using inhibitors of DNA methylation and histone deacetylation.

SUGGESTED READINGS

Baylin SB, Herman JG: DNA hypermethylation in tumorigenesis: Epigenetics joins genetics. Trends Genet 2000;16:168–174.

Costello JF, Fruhwald MC, Smiraglia DJ, et al: Aberrant CpG-island methylation has non-random and tumour-type-specific patterns. Nat Genet 2000;24:132–138.

Esteller M, Sanchez-Cespedes M, Rosell R, et al: Detection of aberrant promoter hypermethylation of tumor suppressor genes in serum DNA from non-small cell lung cancer patients. Cancer Res 1999;59:67–70.

Evron E, Dooley WC, Umbricht CB, et al: Detection of breast cancer cells in ductal lavage fluid by methylation-specific PCR. Lancet 2001;357:1335–1336.

Feinberg AP, Vogelstein B: Hypomethylation distinguishes genes of some human cancers from their normal counterparts. Nature 1983;301:89–92.

Herman JG, Graff JR, Myohanen S, et al: Methylation-specific PCR: A novel PCR assay for methylation status of CpG islands. Proc Natl Acad Sci USA 1996;93:9821–9826.

Jones PA, Baylin SB: The fundamental role of epigenetic events in cancer. Nat Rev Genet 2002;3:415–428.

Knudson AG Jr: The genetic predisposition to cancer. Birth Defects Orig Artic 1989;25:15–27.

Yang B, Guo M, Herman JG, Clark DP: Aberrant promoter methylation profiles of tumor suppressor genes in hepatocellular carcinoma. Am J Pathol 2003;163:1101–1107.

10

Tissue Microarrays
Ziad Peerwani

INTRODUCTION

The tissue microarray (TMA) represents a high-throughput intermediary step between tissue blocks and various tissue-based assays. This technique produces a paraffin block embedded with numerous tissue cores of small diameter. The cores are preconfigured, allowing identification and manipulation of hundreds of specimens simultaneously. Initially, an area of interest is identified within a tissue paraffin block, also referred to as the *donor block*. Next, a thin-walled needle is used to obtain a core of the designated tissue. This step is repeated multiple times using the same or different blocks to obtain multiple cores. The cores are consecutively inserted into a blank preconfigured paraffin block, or *recipient block,* containing multiple preformed holes. When the completed TMA is sectioned, the slide contains many tissue sections laid out in a grid. The area of tissue contained within the tissue disc depends upon the needle diameter used to collect the tissue cores, usually 0.6 to 3 mm. Even the larger cores available for TMA construction sample a small but representable area of the original tissue. Depending upon the length of the initial tissue cores, which determines the depth of the suitable recipient block, approximately 100 to 200 consecutive 5-μm sections can be obtained from each TMA block. The advent of TMA technology has allowed efficient examination of many tissue samples under identical staining conditions on a single slide.

PRINCIPLES OF THE TECHNIQUE

INTRODUCTION TO THE TISSUE MICROARRAY METHOD

Various layouts, techniques, and analytic approaches are available for construction and analysis of TMAs. Experience in performing TMA construction improves both the quality and the efficiency of

TMA preparation. The purpose of the study and the type of tissues involved will dictate which combination of configuration and analysis to use. The investigator's familiarity with the various methods and instruments in the construction and analysis of TMAs is essential to successfully conduct a TMA study. Careful consideration of these choices before construction yields a powerful and efficient tool in the analysis of tissue specimens. This flexibility allows investigators to tailor this powerful technique to their specific clinical and research needs.

Core Size and Its Acquisition

The core diameter chosen for the TMA construction is critical. This decision is a key variable in determining the total number of specimens included within a TMA. Cores of various diameters are differentially susceptible to artifacts or complications of TMA construction. Consideration must be given to the integrity of the donor block, the study design and questions, and complications that may arise because of core size. These considerations should guide the investigator's selection of tissue core diameter.

The first step in the physical construction of a TMA is the identification of areas within a tissue block to include in the microarray. Most TMA protocols use paraffin-embedded blocks (Figure 10-1) as the tissue source. The literature does describe some experience using frozen section blocks for TMA construction, but its use is not as well established as paraffin block–based TMA construction. Using microscopy, the investigator identifies areas of interest within a representative slide of the block. This area is punched out (Figure 10-2) using a stylet. The area chosen depends upon the study objectives and tissue architecture. Although a preponderance of current research and validation studies involves neoplastic lesions, any tissue can be included within a TMA.

Because specimens can heterogeneously express markers, a recurrent concern within the literature is whether tissue cores adequately represent the disease process in the original specimen. Core stylets, used in the TMA construction, sample a small area. When comparing the area considered representative and

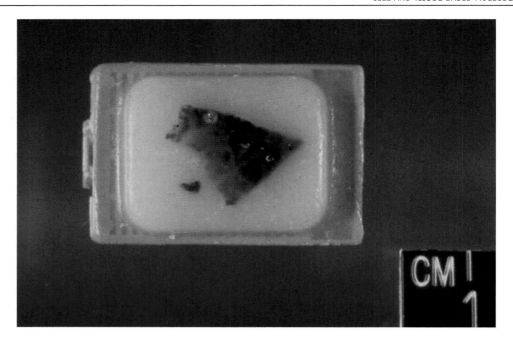

FIGURE 10-1

Donor block. The tissue is embedded within a paraffin block. Using microscopy, the area of interest is identified and mapped to this donor block. Multiple holes are seen here, reflecting previous core removal. The core removal minimally affected the block's integrity.

sufficient for clinical diagnosis, the TMA samples approximately 0.3% of the minimum area recommended for whole section diagnosis. Surprisingly, validation studies have demonstrated that TMAs adequately represent donor tissue in most instances. Including two to three cores per specimen in a TMA adequately compensates for specimen heterogeneity, resulting in concordance rates greater than 95% when compared to whole tissue sections. Larger-core TMAs and some specimen types yield satisfactory concordance rates using only two cores. A general recommendation for specimen core selection includes one core from the

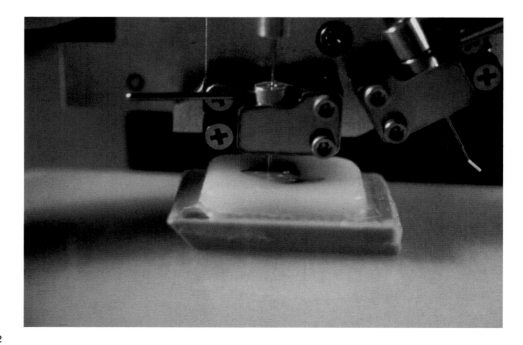

FIGURE 10-2

Coring the donor block. Once the areas of interest are mapped out, it is time to punch out the tissue cores. The stylet is inserted into the tissue block, creating the tissue core. The tissue core remains within the stylet as it is removed from the tissue block.

center of the lesion of interest, a second core from the periphery, and a random third core. This approach can be modified depending upon the study parameters. For instance, the collection of cores can be used to microdissect architectural patterns, such as various Gleason grades in prostatic adenocarcinoma.

TMA tissue discs contain a limited area of tissue. When selecting the area to core, focus should be directed toward identifying areas within the block that fulfill the study parameters and fit within the area of the recipient core position. Another consideration is the location of cells within tissue discs. Cells located on the periphery of the tissue disc are more susceptible to artifacts, such as nonspecific immunohistochemical staining of tissue edges, and can seriously confound the interpretation of the TMA study. Ideally, the cells of interest are located centrally within the tissue cores.

Stylets for procurement of various core sizes are available, although some options are instrument dependent. For most instruments and protocols, diameter options range between 0.6 and 2 mm. Beecher Instruments offers a 3-mm-diameter core needle for its automated arrayer (ATA-27). In general, smaller core diameters result in greater specimen number in each array block, resulting in higher throughput. The larger core diameters result in more tissue represented per specimen but fewer cases analyzed per slide. The decision of which diameter to use depends upon core-related artifact considerations, specimen number, and availability of donor tissue.

During sectioning of the array, individual cores can fold, completely disrupting the tissue disc. The larger core sizes result in greater tissue disc area per section. Therefore, folding or disruption of larger cores more often results in partial obstruction of the individual sample. However, there is usually sufficient intact tissue remaining to provide adequate analysis. With the larger core diameters, usually two cores are sufficient to provide acceptable concordance rates. This reflects the greater tissue area available with the larger cores and their decreased likelihood of complete loss during sectioning artifact.

On the other hand, the larger cores cause greater disruption of donor blocks. The larger needles are relatively more likely to crack and fragment the tissue block when punching cores. The fragmentation or disruption of the original block destroys its use for further studies. This is problematic if the tissue block is needed for further diagnostic or research purposes. In comparison, the smaller cores cause less disruption of the donor block and less artifact when the donor block is sectioned after core removal. Therefore, if the integrity of the original donor block is imperative, smaller core sizes should be considered.

Donor blocks have variable depths of residual tissue. These lengths depend upon the thickness of the original tissue when submitted for embedding, as well as the number of sections obtained from a block before TMA construction. The tissue within the block should be at least 1 mm thick to allow for adequate core length. Preferably, 3 to 4 mm of tissue thickness is recommended; which allows flexibility during TMA construction, flexibility while facing the block, and increased sections from each TMA block.

Different methods are available to compensate for thin donor blocks, particularly when it is imperative to include a specific donor. Multiple similar tissue cores can be placed on top of one another within a single recipient block hole. This creates a stack of tissue cores within the TMA. Alternatively, the donor block can be cored from the side. Lastly, the tissue can be melted and a lengthwise strip cut from the block. This strip of tissue is embedded within the recipient block as if it were a tissue core. These techniques compensate for thin donor blocks and help optimize the TMA thickness.

Placement of Tissue within the Array

The next consideration is the recipient block construction. The number of samples included per block depends upon the layout and spacing parameters. After the cores' locations are determined, careful attention to placing the cores in the recipient block is essential. Compensation for air pockets and cracks within the paraffin ensures proper sectioning of the TMA block.

There are a few factors to consider when deciding on the TMA configuration. Locating tissue on a slide is difficult when the microarray contains a high number of cores. Separating cores within the array into smaller dissymmetric matrices is recommended. This allows easier orientation while reviewing the slide and prevents misidentification of cores. The spacing of the submatrices results in a slight decrease in the total number of cores included in the microarray block. Nonetheless, correct identification of tissue cores is imperative to maintain the integrity of the derived data. Dissymmetry of the matrix allows superior orientation, and the submatrices facilitate manual review and orientation of the slide, preventing core misidentification and reducing errors in manual data acquisition. For digital scanning and computer review of the slides, the limitation placed by orientating large specimen numbers on a single slide is reduced. The computer programs can adequately orient and identify the tissues based upon user preset terms. Nonetheless, the volume of information and cores requires constant vigilance to ensure data integrity and analysis.

Placement of many cores close to one another distorts the TMA. Cores located within the center of the block will be higher than the cores in the periphery, making it difficult to face the block without losing significant amount of tissue. Therefore, the cores within the recipient block should be adequately spaced. Most protocols recommend a spacing of 0.7 to 0.8 mm between cores.

Once the layout is decided, the microarray recipient block is ready to be created. The recipient blocks usually begin as preformed blocks of paraffin. Standard techniques entail coring the block to create recipient holes (Figure 10-3) before obtaining the cores. The arrangement of the holes should reflect the predetermined layout. Creation of the recipient block requires a significant level of accuracy regarding hole placement. Manual techniques require more diligence by the operator to ensure the recipient block reflects the planned layout. The precision and accuracy limitations of the human hand should be considered during the creation of the TMA layout. By virtue of robotics, automated arrayers are more precise and accurate in creating the recipient block. Therefore, they are more adept at creating higher-density TMAs with smaller core diameters.

While creating the recipient holes within the microarray block, residual paraffin remains within the hole. As the donor cores are inserted into the recipient block, the residual paraffin is pushed into the hole. If the depth of the hole is insufficient, the compacted paraffin prevents proper insertion of the core with excessive tissue extrusion. This results in unnecessary tissue loss during block facing. Sufficiently deep holes allow space for residual paraffin to be compacted within the recipient block and prevent needless loss of the donor cores.

Although excessive extrusion of cores results in unnecessary loss of tissue, it is just as important to avoid insertion of the cores below the surface of the recipient block. Tissue length is inherently variable within the various cores. The length of tissue depends upon the thickness of tissue submitted for embedding, as well as the number of sections previously cut from the donor block. Therefore, many specimen cores will not span the entire depth of the TMA block. By inserting the cores below the surface of the block, multiple sections must be cut to face the block and ensure all tissue discs are represented. Depending upon how deeply the cores were inserted, significant amount of tissue can be lost while attempting to ensure complete representation of all cores. Therefore, it is advisable to leave the cores slightly protruding from the recipient paraffin block. The slight core protrusions can be corrected after completion of all core insertions.

Space remains between the inserted cores and the recipient holes. Miniscule cracks form within the tissue cores and the recipient block during their various manipulations. These air pockets and cracks disrupt tissue discs during sectioning. By heating the TMA after core insertion, the cores are merged with the surrounding paraffin, reducing the cracks and air

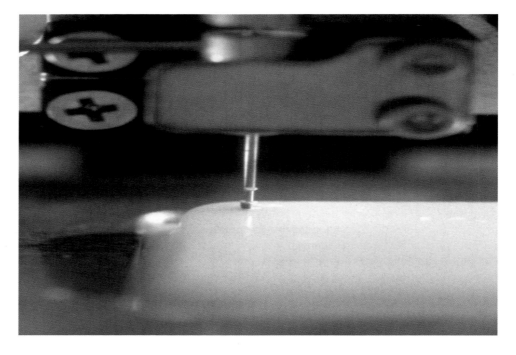

FIGURE 10-3

Deposition of the core. The recipient block is usually prepared before retrieval of the tissue cores. Once the layout of the tissue microarray is decided, a stylet is used to punch out holes. The recipient block is then ready to receive tissue cores. As seen here, the stylet contains the previously punched out tissue core. The core is deposited into its designated hole within the recipient block.

pockets. Ideally, complete melting of the paraffin allows appropriate merging of the cores with the recipient block. Unfortunately, completely melted paraffin does not support cores within the recipient block, which quickly lose their orientation in the heated liquid paraffin. Therefore, moderate heating to soften, but not melt, the TMA block is used to slowly merge the cores with the paraffin. Delicate pressure applied to the surface of the heated recipient block aids in the merging. This can be accomplished by applying gentle pressure with a glass slide to the surface of the block. This step evenly completes the insertion of the cores. Multiple cycles of heating and cooling are used to adequately merge the block with the tissue cores and complete the creation of a TMA block (Figure 10-4).

Various authors have suggested methods to address the merging of tissue cores with the TMA block. Chen et al. describe a method of TMA construction without prefabricating a recipient block. Instead, they suggest the creation of an adhesive platform that serves to maintain core orientation within an embedding mold. The cores are then heated slightly to soften them, followed by careful injection of heated paraffin. The use of melted paraffin allows adequate merging of cores with the paraffin. Their adhesive platform aligns the cores in a single plane and maintains core orientation within the melted paraffin milieu. Alternatively, Yan et al. (2006) have described a method of creating recipient paraffin blocks with an agarose matrix. Two percent agarose is cast within an embedding mold and the mold is allowed to solidify at room temperature. Multiple ethanol dehydration steps are applied to the agarose followed by clearing with xylene. The mold is then infiltrated with liquid paraffin and allowed to solidify at room temperature. Regarding TMA core insertion, the blank agarose paraffin recipient block is routinely handled. Preformed holes are punched out, and tissue cores are inserted. Once core insertion is complete, melting of the block allows adequate merging of the paraffin with the cores, and the agarose matrix maintains the integrity of the tissue core orientation. These are examples of alternate methods for TMA construction described within the literature. Although the authors of the protocols offer data validating their techniques, independent examination of these techniques within the literature is not generally available. The use of altered TMA techniques should be left to the discretion of individual investigators regarding their viability for use as TMA design alternatives.

Sectioning of the Block

The completed TMA block contains the valuable combination of specimen number and diversity in compact form (Figures 10-5 and 10-6). Maintaining the integrity of tissue discs during sectioning is a priority. Various problems may arise during sectioning, including disc folding or complete loss. Different

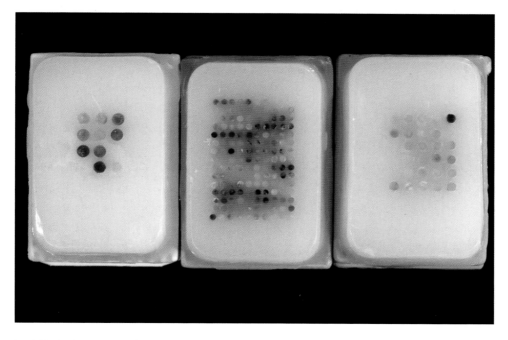

FIGURE 10-4
Tissue microarray (TMA) block. After insertion of the cores, the cores are merged with the recipient block through multiple cycles of heating to create the TMA block. As seen here, different core sizes result in different TMA densities. The block on the left contains 2-mm cores of various normal tissues. The middle block is a multitumor TMA created using 1-mm cores. The right block is a colon cancer TMA created using 1.5-mm cores.

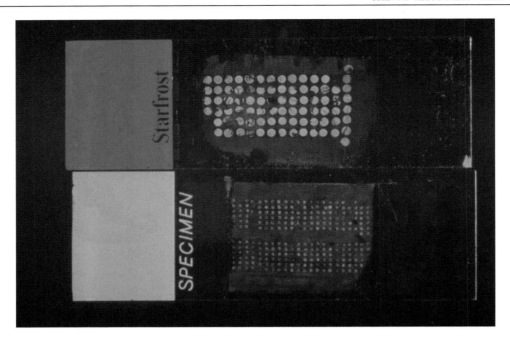

FIGURE 10-5

Unstained tissue microarray slide. Multiple tissue discs are arrayed on the unstained sectioned slide. Various assays that use paraffin sections, such as immunohistochemistry or fluorescence in situ hybridization, are applied to the unstained slides. Alternatively, sectioned slides can be saved for future projects or studies.

methods are available to maintain the integrity of tissue discs and assist in their transfer from the block to the slides during sectioning.

The original method of TMA construction used a paraffin sectioning aid system. The system from Instrumedics includes the use of adhesive-coated slides, adhesive tapes, and an ultraviolet lamp. Briefly, the adhesive tape is applied to the surface of the block before sectioning. The block is cut, with the resultant section adhered to the tape. The tape is applied to an adhesive-coated slide and incubated under ultraviolet light for a short time. Afterward, the slides are placed

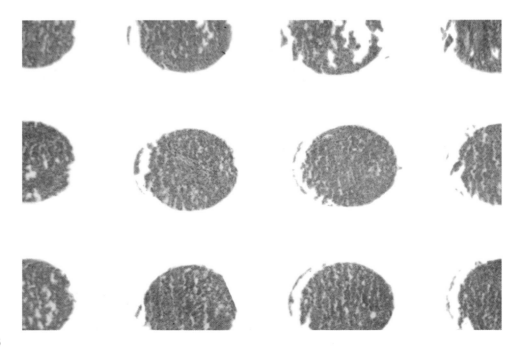

FIGURE 10-6

Multiple tissue discs. This hematoxylin and eosin–stained section illustrates the usefulness of the tissue microarray (TMA). The discs are efficiently organized to allow accurate study of the TMA section. The amount of tissue for each specimen is relatively small, allowing complete and focused examination of each specimen in minimal time. The investigator can easily study and compare sections with one another. Furthermore, this slide demonstrates the spacing of the tissue discs, which clearly delineates each specimen.

within a solvent bath and the tape is removed, leaving the cut section on the slide. This method aids in the transfer of sections to the slide and prevents folding and loss of tissue discs during transfer.

Skacel et al. (2002) reported less-than-optimal clarity of immunohistochemical and fluorescence in situ hybridization (FISH) results when using an adhesive tape section aid system. Particularly with FISH, their experience indicates disruption of the probe's penetration into the nuclei with consequential attenuation of signal when using the tape. These authors recommend using a water bath with electrostatically charged slides, a common procedure for routine immunohistochemistry. Their protocol included soaking of the blocks in a low-concentration detergent solution followed by cooling on ice before cutting. Retention of 90% to 95% of the tissue discs from small-diameter-core TMAs and usually 100% of discs from the larger-core TMAs was achieved. Although requiring more experience and skill than the adhesive tape systems, the authors reported clearer signals with both immunohistochemistry and FISH.

The number of sections obtained from a TMA depends upon the shortest tissue cores. As sections are cut from the block, the shorter tissue cores are cut through first. The utility of a given TMA rapidly diminishes as a number of cores are lost during sectioning. The average TMA generates between 100 and 200 consecutive 5-μm sections. Because tissue is lost during facing of the recipient block, the number of times one returns to the block to obtain a section decreases the total number of sections obtainable from the TMA.

Some protocols require cutting multiple sections at one time. This avoids facing the block when a section is needed and increases the yield of a TMA block. When sectioning and storing multiple paraffin sections, the question of antigen loss with time arises. Using a breast and mixed tumor microarrays, DiVito et al. (2004) showed significant preservation of estrogen receptor, Ki-67, and pancytokeratin antigenicity by dipping sectioned slides in paraffin followed by storage in a nitrogen environment when compared to storage under an ambient room environment. Alternatively, storage at 4° C or colder may be used to help preserve antigenicity. Nonetheless, the amount and significance of antigen loss is variable and depends upon local environment. The optimal storage method should be decided by individual investigation based upon local experience of antigen loss, storage times, and environmental considerations.

Instruments

Different options are available for the creation of TMAs. Multiple "home-brew" methods are found within the literature, offering alternative methods for TMA construction. Various companies offer both manual and automated arrayers for TMA construction.

The literature contains many examples of methods for TMAs construction using locally developed techniques. These options often reduce the cost of microarray construction by avoiding the purchase of a manual or automated workstation. Some methods attempt to address problems with microarray construction, such as alignment of the core faces within the recipient block for cutting or difficulty merging the donor cores with the recipient paraffin block. These techniques offer alternatives for microarray construction but necessitate further training and experience in a specific method that may not be found or used at other institutions.

Manual arrayers (Figure 10-7) offer a more standardized method of microarray construction. A platform is used to hold and stabilize the recipient and donor blocks, with a mounted, manually driven stylet for punching and depositing tissue cores. The area of interest is visually identified using either a magnifying glass or a stereomicroscope, often not sold with the manual arrayer. The Beecher Instruments' manual workstation product specification indicates a punch speed of 30 to 70 cores per hour using its equipment. The user must keep track manually of core placement and location. This equipment allows better control over the needle's angle during punching or deposition of cores, with less alteration or variability of the needle's angle during vertical, Z-axis, movement. Nonetheless, the needle may bend while coring relatively hard tissue, e.g., bone or bone marrow. Beecher currently offers two manual arrayers, MTA-I and MTA-II. The MTA-II has added features, such as enhanced control of the X- and Y-axis movement and localization during array construction. Furthermore, the MTA-II offers a convenient visual display of the X and Y position of the stylet. Nonetheless, the MTA-II currently costs approximately twice as much as the MTA-I.

Chemicon, now a part of Millipore, offers a manual tissue arrayer, the ATA-100, offering added features not found in other manual arrayers. This manual arrayer incorporates a stereomicroscope with a slide stage, where a representative microscopic slide of the block can be placed and viewed. The slide stage is indexed to its respective block, allowing precision coring of the block relative to the visual inspection of the slide. The second salient feature of this workstation is that the two needles are mounted in tandem. The first needle is used to obtain the tissue core from the donor block. The second needle is used to create the recipient hole for the tissue core. The second needle's Z-axis movement matches the movements and position of the first needle. Therefore, the recipient hole is created after the donor core is obtained, with its depth defined by the donor core

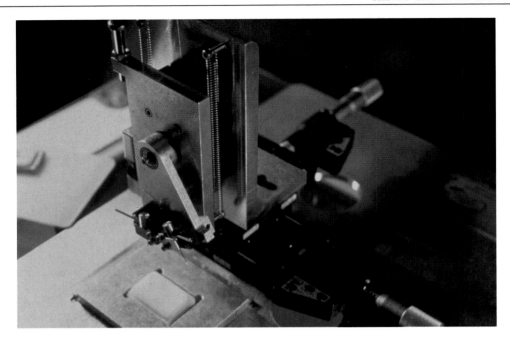

FIGURE 10-7

Manual workstation. This is an example of a manual arrayer. The block is secured during punching. Punching of both the donor block and the recipient block is performed at the manual workstation. The stylet is mounted to the machine, which restricts and defines its movement. The X-axis and Y-axis positions of the stylet is precisely controlled by knobs. These knobs are used to align the stylet to the predetermined areas of both the donor block and the recipient block. Once the stylet is correctly aligned, the user controls the Z-axis movement of the stylet to punch out the core.

length. This adjustable Z height allows delivery of cores to the same level within the recipient block, reducing tissue loss during facing of the block and sectioning. Currently, the ATA-100 costs approximately three times more than the Beecher MTA-II.

Automated tissue array workstations incorporate computer hardware and software, digital imaging, and robotics to automate the construction of the TMA. The donor block is digitally scanned, and the user designates areas to be incorporated in the TMA by digitally circling areas of interest on the computer display. The recipient block's layout is digitally mapped, and the location of tissue cores is assigned and tracked by the computer. The arrayer's robotic-driven stylet punches a core of tissue and deposits it within its designated hole within a recipient block. The automated arrayers can have multiple recipient blocks loaded into the machine, allowing simultaneous creation of multiple similar TMA blocks. Using the computer, multiple areas of interest can be selected for coring. The automated arrayer either can include multiple different cores of tissue from the same block within the same TMA or can create multiple similar TMAs by placing cores into different recipient blocks. The Beecher Automated Arrayer technical specifications include the creation of 26 replicate array blocks in a single run and a core transfer rate of 120 to 180 cores per hour. This equipment option is the most expensive, but it offers the most comprehensive set of tools and efficiency for TMA creation.

Tissue Microarray Analysis

The nature of TMA technology generates voluminous information. From the recipient block layout and the specimen features to the results from multiple assays and stains applied to different sections of the same TMA, the data can be staggering, complex, and overwhelming. Adequate organization, coupled with the appropriate analytic tools, is imperative for efficient and effective use of this technology. Although different approaches exist for organizing and analyzing the data, the choice of which methods to use depends upon the investigator and the demands of the tissue-based study.

Careful attention to specimen location during TMA construction, along with accurate recording of location, is imperative to ensure the integrity of the study results. Misidentified cores can skew data, as well as obfuscate the utility of the TMA. It is prudent to assign random identifiers to the specimens within the TMA and dissociate the data and results from patient identifiers. This allows accurate core orientation and identification while sharing and collaborating with TMA blocks and results. This dissociation preserves patient confidentiality while maintaining data integrity. Previously collected specimen information is useful to include within the TMA results database, such as patient age, diagnoses, therapy, and outcomes. This approach allows efficient analysis of experimental results by integrating various specimen and patient features with the TMA results.

Another consideration is whether a centralized institutional database containing TMA information and results may be appropriate. Because the TMA provides a medium in which various tissue-based assays are applied, the potential for diverse and different assays applied to the same TMA block is a distinct advantage for many institutions engaged in translational research and clinical method validation. The creation of a centralized database allows the addition of new results from different experiments by the same or different investigators upon their completion. This allows the integrated and comparative analysis of various immunohistochemical, FISH, protein expression profiling, and other assays with one another. Another consideration is whether image capture and digital storage of TMAs are used by an institution. Products are available, such as the LifeSpan Alias™, that allow automated image capture of multiple TMA slides. The images from a specimen core obtained by different assays applied to different sections of the same TMA block can be stored and linked within the TMA database. This allows individuals to revisit the images and reassess the interpretation of results from an experiment. By adding the results from different interpretations of the same data to a centralized database, studies of intraobserver and interobserver variability are also possible and relatively easily accomplished. The centralized database requires a significant technologic investment by an institution and requires diligent participation by all parties to maintain its usefulness, efficiency, and data integrity. Importantly, the centralized database further integrates the information obtained from various experiments on a single TMA block, increasing the productivity of the TMA.

For many projects, a simple spreadsheet suffices for the organization and compilation of data. The spreadsheet is less expensive than purchasing dedicated software but relies upon the user to create and organize the layout. By itself, the spreadsheet lacks the statistical and analytic tools to properly study the data produced from the TMA. Various statistical and analytic programs are available to assist with interpretation of a TMA study. Companies like Beecher offer analytic software that assist with identification of neoplasms and interpretation of various TMA projects. Some programs are available online without charge from various institutions, and others can be purchased from various companies. The combination of spreadsheets with statistical and analytic programs is sufficient for many TMA projects. Institutions with a higher volume of dense TMAs containing numerous data points and integrating multiple assays on the same block may benefit from an integrated image and data acquisition, database, and analytic software platform.

ADVANTAGES

The last decade has seen an exponential rise in the number of possible molecular markers of disease. The need to validate their usefulness in clinical settings and as diagnostic tools is imperative for the evolution of medicine. Concurrent with the increase in newly discovered markers, there are numerous examples of markers whose reported specificity within the literature declines after their initial description as the natural result of ongoing experimentation and verification. The decrease in usefulness and specificity reflects the broader experience and application of a given marker with time. The initial discrepancy likely arises from the inability of conventional tissue-based techniques to adequately sample the breadth of possible specimens seen within the clinical laboratory or reflects insufficient experimental design.

Conventional techniques entail the analysis of whole sections of tissue. Each specimen block included within the study design is represented by a tissue section. Every assay included within the study design must be applied to a section of tissue. The substantial economic, time, and labor savings of a study involving hundreds of specimens when using TMAs, rather than whole tissue sections, is apparent.

The greatest advantage of the TMA is the significant increase in throughput of tissue-based assays. This technique compacts hundreds of specimens into a single paraffin block. A tissue-based assay need only be applied to a single section of the block, instead of hundreds of separate slides, with huge savings in economic and labor resources. Although inconceivable with conventional techniques, literally thousands of specimens can be studied in a TMA-based study by including multiple sections from different TMA blocks.

The TMA offers superior standardization among specimens when compared to whole tissue section. Because the TMA contains multiple specimens on a single slide, identical staining and environmental parameters are simultaneously applied to all specimens within the slide. In comparison, conventional techniques are more susceptible to artifacts attributable to variations in technique, reagents, and environmental factors among individually stained whole sections.

TMAs sample a relatively small portion of a donor block. Excluding defects produced by tissue coring of donor cores, the original blocks are left essentially intact. The donor block is available for future clinical or research purposes. Whole section–based studies gradually cut through the block. Each time an assay is performed, less tissue is available for future clinical or research needs.

Once the TMA is created, it is an invaluable repository of tissue specimens and diversity. Construction of the TMA is the labor-intensive step. Once created, the TMA block provides numerous specimens neatly organized in a single paraffin section. Multiple different studies and assays can be performed at different times using the same TMA block. Coupled with its diverse tissues sampled, it streamlines and reduces cost for multiple projects. Finally, the TMA offers an archive of tissue to compare with or use when future needs dictate.

DISADVANTAGES

The imperfect concordance between TMAs and whole section studies prevents its usefulness as a diagnostic tool for individual lesions. The overall results of a TMA study are a strong reflection of the staining pattern across the numerous specimens contained within the microarray. For the individual patient or specimen, the question of whether the result is true or is one of the few discordant results prevents its usefulness as a diagnostic tool.

The tissue disc (Figure 10-8) contains a small sample of tissue offering limited architectural details. Although selective sampling of a specimen can allow microdissection and comparison of different

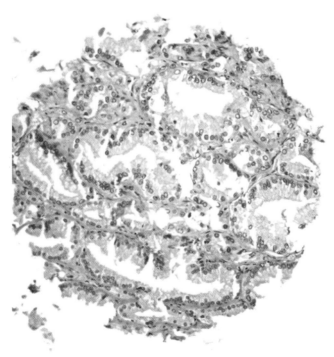

FIGURE 10-8

Tissue discs. This higher-power look at a prostate tissue microarray illustrates the information contained within the tissue disc. Numerous cells are included in each core, allowing adequate evaluation of the tissue. Furthermore, the tissue discs contain sufficient tissue to provide some architectural details.

architectural patterns within a lesion, the interaction and spatial relationship among architectural features within a specimen cannot be completely appreciated. Whole sections better correlate the assay's result to a specimen's architecture, including its interaction with surrounding structures.

The TMA is best suited as a screening tool of many specimens. The diversity of specimens included within the microarray allows it to gauge the specificity of different assays. Nonetheless, the investigator should consider confirming the results of a TMA study with whole sections when warranted. It is unnecessary to include the number and diversity of specimens within a confirmatory study. Rather, the follow-up study on whole sections allows the investigator to characterize the assay in relationship to the specimen's architecture. Furthermore, it allows a clearer understanding of the assay when applied to diagnostic specimens.

APPLICATIONS

The TMA interjects a new step between tissue blocks and various tissue-based assays. The creation of a TMA is not an end point but rather is an innovative intermediate tool altering current approaches to tissue-based validation and research studies. Various assays that use paraffin-embedded tissue as the specimen source are applied to the TMA sections. Therefore, the primary purpose of this technique is to significantly increase the throughput of other tissue-based diagnostic techniques.

Proteomics represents a current area of great research interest. The profiling and quantification of proteins is an important tool in advancing medical knowledge. Chung et al. (2006) recently described a method of paraffin-based quantification of protein expression using TMAs. The authors developed a method of transferring proteins from a formalin-fixed paraffin section to a stack of membranes. Antibodies against specific protein epitopes were applied to different membranes, and the complexes were detected using fluorescently labeled secondary antibodies. Total protein within each membrane was determined, allowing normalization for each antibody. By using a TMA section as the paraffin section source, the TMA essentially became a protein array, with the results easily correlated with tissue morphology.

Of all the assays applied to the TMA section, immunohistochemistry is the most common—and potentially the most powerful. The literature contains a multitude of validation studies confirming the utility and effectiveness of immunohistochemistry on TMA sections. Various studies within the literature have examined breast carcinoma and their immunohistochemical staining patterns by TMA. Camp et al. (2000) reported greater than 95% concordance with standard whole sections when staining for estrogen receptors, progesterone receptors, and *HER2* oncogene expression when using two or more cores. Skacel et al. (2002) provided validation of the TMA's ability to assess the estrogen receptor, progesterone receptor, and the HER2 amplification status when fewer than 100 cells are contained within the tissue disc. The TMA is a powerful tool in assessing the diagnostic utility of newly developed immunohistochemical markers in the diagnosis of disease.

FISH is another technique adaptable to the TMA (Figures 10-9 and 10-10). Diaz et al. (2004) investigated the validity of using TMA in FISH testing for HER2 gene amplification in breast cancer. The authors created two TMA blocks with paired cores from 41 breast cancer cases. FISH for the HER2 gene amplification status was performed in parallel at two separate institutions, one a reference center and the other a testing center, and showed strong concordance between the results from the two institutions. The reference center also compared TMA-based *HER2* FISH to *HER2* chromogenic in situ hybridization and HER2 immunohistochemistry, documenting a good concordance among the assays performed on TMA sections. Diaz et al. (2004) concluded that

FISH performed on TMA sections was relatively straightforward with no significant complications.

CONCLUSION

Although relatively straightforward, the TMA technique relies heavily upon operator skill. As the operator gains experience, the efficiency and quality of TMAs produced will improve significantly. Consideration for the inclusion of this technique within a laboratory or institution depends upon its projected use and the resources available for its implementation and maintenance. Nonetheless, this technique is useful in both basic and translational research and in clinical settings as a method validation tool.

The use of TMAs first found its solid footing within the research arena. Its ability to concurrently survey large numbers of specimens serves both basic and translational research studies. With the application of various techniques, like FISH and immunohistochemistry, the TMA block becomes quite versatile. Furthermore, the ability to apply a technique to

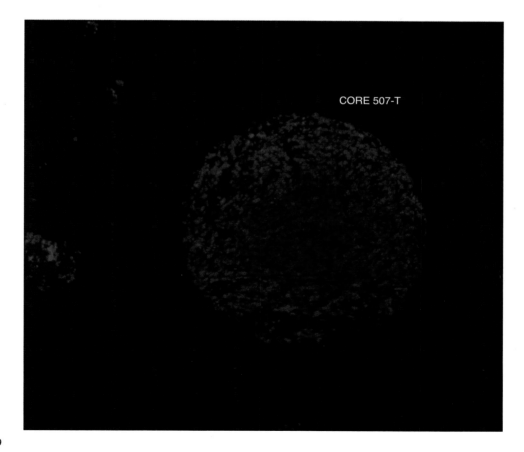

FIGURE 10-9

4'-6-Diamidino-2-phenylindole (DAPI) staining of a tissue disc. The tissue microarray (TMA) can be used with FISH. The picture illustrates DAPI staining of HER2 FISH performed on a breast adenocarcinoma TMA.

FIGURE 10-10

HER2 staining of a tissue disc. This high-power view illustrates HER2 FISH applied to a breast adenocarcinoma tissue microarray. The upper left corner is the edge of the tissue disc. Multiple cells are present that contain numerous HER2 signals (red dots).

multiple specimens in an identical environment decreases the variation among specimens while saving resources. If applied as a screening tool, the investigator should have little concern over the small sample area contained within the tissue disc. Although the concordance rate for TMAs is superb, a whole section of specimens remains the gold standard. The question of adequate representation must be assessed individually for specific specimens. Because the concordance rate is not perfect, a few tissue discs in a given TMA do not reflect the specimen's actual assay result. This explains why the technique is employed not as a diagnostic tool for specific specimens but rather to look at the assay results of numerous diverse specimens as a group.

Within the clinical setting, TMAs offer an efficient method for adjusting and validating tissue-based assays within clinical laboratories. This technique allows multiple positive and negative controls to be analyzed simultaneously. The specimens undergo assays simultaneously and are exposed to the same reagents and assay conditions, addressing the question of inter-assay variability. The inclusion of numerous samples under identical assay parameters and environments gives a clearer picture of a test's functionality. The TMA can gauge the staining and result parameters of a given assay in a diverse set of tissues, broadening the scope of the validation of new stains or reagents and

better gauging their specificity of an assay. Furthermore, the TMA offers laboratories the ability to compare and validate their tissue-based assay with one another using the same set of diverse tissues.

As discussed, different equipment options are available for TMA construction. High-end workstations increase the efficiency and ease of a TMA construction but at substantial additional cost. The automated arrayers are better suited for constructing high-density TMAs than are manual techniques. Consideration for their use includes a laboratory's or institution's projected volume of TMA construction and available capital resources. The investment of an automated arrayer may not be cost efficient if the volume of TMAs is not sufficiently high. For many institutions, a manual arrayer workstation offers suitable TMA construction capability at an affordable price. In comparison to the automated arrayers, the manual arrayer's primary drawback is its susceptibility to operator skill as the TMA is constructed. The various home-brew methods available within the literature offer alternatives to purchasing costly equipment and attempt to address various processing problems that arise when using standard techniques. As one would expect, operator familiarity and experience with a given laboratory-developed technique plays a critical role in the efficiency and quality of the TMA produced.

The exponential rise of tissue marker discovery creates a significant burden in identifying and confirming their clinical utility. The application of a new marker to a single section of a high-density TMA block offers simultaneous evaluation of hundreds of tissues. As emphasized in this chapter, TMAs offer a powerful supplemental tool in the analysis of tissues by combining conventional tissue-based techniques with high-throughput innovation. This technique creates a diverse compact tissue platform upon which a plethora of research and clinical assays can and have been applied. The result is an enormous increase in productivity and efficiency, along with decreasing labor and costs. This technology has provided a new paradigm for screening newly discovered markers and assisting investigators with management of the burden of evaluating the clinical utility of the numerous research advances.

SUGGESTED READINGS

Battifora H: The multitumor (sausage) tissue block: Novel method for immunohistochemical antibody testing. Lab Invest 1986;55: 244–248.

Braunschweig T, Chung JY, Hewitt SM: Tissue microarrays: Bridging the gap between research and the clinic. Expert Rev Proteomics 2005;2(3):325–336.

Camp RL, Charette LA, Rimm DL: Validation of tissue microarray technology in breast carcinoma. Lab Invest 2000;80(12):1943–1949.

Chen N, Zhou Q: Constructing tissue microarrays without prefabricating recipient blocks: a novel approach. Am J Clin Pathol 2005;124(1): 103–107.

Chung J, Braunschweig T, Baibakov, et al: Transfer and multiplex immunoblotting of a paraffin-embedded tissue. Proteomics 2006;6(3): 767–774.

Diaz LK, Gupta R, Kidwai N, et al: The use of TMA for interlaboratory validation of FISH testing for detection of HER2 gene amplification in breast cancer. J Histochem Cytochem 2004;52(4):501–507.

DiVito KA, Charette LA, Rimm DL, Campl RL: Long-term preservation of antigenicity on tissue microarrays. Lab Invest 2004;84(8): 1071–1078.

Frierson HF Jr, Moskaluk CA, Powell SM, et al: Large-scale molecular and tissue microarray analysis of mesothelin expression in common human carcinomas. Hum Pathol 2003;34(6):605–609.

Hicks DG, Longoria G, Pettay J, et al: In situ hybridization in the pathology laboratory: General principles, automation, and emerging research applications for tissue-based studies of gene expression. J Mol Histol 2004;35(6):595–601.

Kononen J, Bubendorf L, Kallioniemi A, et al: Tissue microarrays for high-throughput molecular profiling of tumor specimens. Nat Med 1998;4:844–847.

Liu CL, Prapong W, Natkunam Y, et al: Software tools for high-throughput analysis and archiving of immunohistochemistry staining data obtained with tissue microarrays. Am J Pathol 2002;161(5):1557–1565.

Makretsov RA, Huntsman DG, Nielsen TO, et al: Hierarchical clustering analysis of tissue microarray immunostaining data identifies prognostically significant groups of breast carcinoma. Clin Cancer Res 2004;10(18 Pt 1):6143–6151.

Schoenberg Fejzo M, Slamon DJ: Frozen tumor tissue microarray technology for analysis of tumor RNA, DNA, and proteins. Am J Pathol 2001;159(5):1645–1650.

Skacel M, Skilton B, Pettay JD, Tubbs RR: Tissue microarrays: A powerful tool for high-throughput analysis of clinical specimens: A review of the method with validation data. Appl Immunohistochem Mol Morphol 2002;10(1):1–6.

Yan P, Seelentag W, Bachmann A, Bosman FT: An agarose matrix facilitates sectioning of tissue microarrays blocks. J Histochem Cytochem 2007;55(1):2–4.

11 Fluorescence In Situ Hybridization

James R. Cook

PRINCIPLES OF TECHNIQUE

The first in situ hybridization (ISH) studies were reported more than three decades ago. These techniques originally employed radioactively labeled probes that were hybridized to cytologic preparations. Using autoradiography, these studies allowed, for the first time, the enumeration and spatial localization of specific DNA sequences within an intact nucleus. The subsequent development of fluorochromes that could be directly or indirectly linked to DNA probes led to the creation of fluorescence in situ hybridization (FISH). The use of fluorescently labeled probes was a major advance because it allowed laboratories to avoid the use of radioactive agents, provided a more rapid assay than autoradiography, and allowed the results to be visualized directly under a fluorescence microscope. Furthermore, the simultaneous use of two or more fluorochromes allows the analysis of multiple DNA sequences within the same hybridization (two-color or multicolor FISH). Today, a wide and ever-growing range of FISH probes and fluorochromes is commercially available for many constitutional and neoplasm-associated abnormalities, and FISH analysis has become a staple of modern molecular pathology and cytogenetic laboratories.

Fluorescence In Situ Hybridization Probes

Three basic types of DNA probes are generally employed: centromeric probes, whole chromosome probes, and locus-specific probes. *Centromeric probes,* also known as *chromosome enumeration probes* (CEPs), hybridize to highly repetitive 171-base-pair sequences of α satellite DNA present within the centromeres of each chromosome. The probes are carefully selected to target sequences unique to specific chromosomes, allowing the detection and enumeration of specific chromosomes in interphase nuclei or metaphase cytogenetic preparations. Because of the presence of highly homologous satellite sequences, not all chromosomes can be specifically

identified in this manner. In particular, the similarity between chromosomes 13 and 21 and between chromosomes 14 and 22 precludes the use of specific centromeric probes for these chromosomes. Locus-specific probes (described later in this chapter) must therefore be employed for detection and analysis of these chromosomes.

Whole chromosome probes (sometimes called *whole chromosome paints*) are a complex mixture of probes, all labeled with one fluorochrome, that hybridize to sequences distributed along the length of a given chromosome. Analysis of metaphase chromosomes with a whole chromosome paint therefore identifies the chromosome of interest, allows enumeration of the chromosome, and can identify regions of the chromosome of interest that may be located elsewhere because of structural karyotypic abnormalities (i.e., translocations). In an interphase nucleus, the DNA material from any given chromosome is widely spread throughout the nucleus. Whole chromosome paints therefore yield only diffuse staining in interphase cells, and this type of probe is suitable only for analysis of metaphase chromosome spreads.

Perhaps the type of FISH probe employed most often is the *locus-specific probe* (also known as the *locus-specific identifier,* or *LSI probe*). This probe hybridizes to specific genes of interest, allowing the assessment of copy number and location of particular chromosomal regions. By using the LSI probe in two-color or multicolor assays with other reference probes, one can assess for amplification of a target gene or design probes to detect translocations involving specific loci (these applications are discussed in detail later in this chapter). Locus-specific probes are generally in the range of 100 to 300 kilobases to produce an easily visible signal. Locus-specific probes may be prepared from a variety of sources, including bacterial artificial chromosomes (BACs), P1 artificial chromosomes, and yeast artificial chromosomes. Particularly useful are the recently available FISH-mapped BAC libraries, which allow rapid identification of BACs hybridizing to particular areas of interest that may be subsequently grown, purified, and labeled for "home-brew" applications. In addition, the number of commercially available locus-specific probes relevant to common inherited conditions and neoplasms continues to grow rapidly.

TYPES OF SPECIMENS ANALYZED

A variety of cytologic preparations and tissues are suitable for FISH analysis. For peripheral blood and bone marrow samples, direct smears or gravity preparations may be produced, which are subsequently fixed in Carnoy's solution or simply air dried. For body fluids of limited cellularity, such as urine samples, cytospin preparations similar to those used for cytopathology are employed. Whole cell preparations may be prepared from tissue biopsy samples in two ways. First, touch preparations can be prepared from fresh or frozen tissue samples and either air dried or fixed in Carnoy's. Alternatively, a portion of fresh tissue may be disaggregated and a cell suspension can be prepared, analogous to procedures used to perform flow cytometry on tissue biopsies. Lastly, fine-needle aspirate smears are also suitable for FISH studies. In each of the preceding situations, the goal is to produce, within at least focal areas of the slide, a monolayer of intact cells. Such preparations facilitate analysis through ease of scoring with a minimum amount of artifact because of nuclear overlap or disrupted nuclei.

Often in routine surgical pathology practice, the only available material for examination is formalin-fixed, paraffin-embedded (FFPE) tissue. Fortunately, FISH methods applicable to FFPE tissues have also been developed, creating the opportunity to bring this powerful analytic tool to retrospective analysis of archival samples. Two basic procedures have been developed, each with distinct advantages and disadvantages. In the first protocol, thick sections or needle core samples are taken from a paraffin block, and intact nuclei are purified from the paraffin sample. Gravity preparations of the intact nuclei may then be prepared, as with any other cellular suspension. Alternatively, thin paraffin sections (typically 5 μm) may be employed. Intact paraffin sections are pretreated to remove the paraffin wax, and proteinase treatment is employed to remove interfering proteins. FISH analysis may then be performed on the intact tissue. The primary advantage of the nuclear purification procedure is that the final result is a suspension of intact nuclei, without truncation artifacts that may be easily counted. However, the nuclear purification steps add time to the overall protocol, and it may be impossible to distinguish between malignant nuclei and contaminating admixed benign nuclei.

In the intact paraffin section technique, sectioning through some nuclei in a given plane produces truncation artifacts, such that some nuclei present will demonstrate only a partial signal pattern. For example,

analysis of a normal cell with a chromosome 3 centromere probe is expected to produce two signals in an intact nucleus. However, if a portion of the nucleus containing one chromosome 3 is not present because of plane of section artifact, the resulting truncated nucleus will display only one centromeric signal. Nuclear truncation artifacts, and methods employed to minimize their effects, are discussed further later in this chapter.

On the other hand, a powerful advantage of the intact paraffin section technique is the ability to correlate FISH results with tissue morphology. The image under a 4´-6-diamidino-2-phenylindole (DAPI) filter is quite similar to what a surgical pathologist might expect from a tissue section stained with hematoxylin. The pathologist can therefore easily identify particular regions of a section to be counted. For example, in whole section FISH analysis of a breast carcinoma, the pathologist may readily distinguish between areas of invasive carcinoma and those of in situ carcinoma, which generally could not be accomplished using isolated nuclear preparations.

When FISH analysis of intact paraffin sections is desired, it must be noted that the choice of fixative used is critical. Fixation using formalin or zinc formalin mixtures provides the most reliable results in most laboratories' experience. B5-fixed material is generally not suitable for FISH analysis. Alternative fixatives are becoming more widespread in many laboratories in an attempt to reduce the use of formalin. The use of alternative fixative agents, however, may yield suboptimal results with FISH analysis in some cases. Laboratories are encouraged to keep in mind the potential need for FISH or other molecular assays before implementing alternative fixative protocols and to ensure that the use of alternate fixatives does not compromise molecular analysis that may be required for optimal patient care.

BASIC METHOD

The basic steps in any FISH analysis are similar. DNA probes, usually but not always double stranded, are identified that are complementary to the target DNA sequence of interest. The cells to be analyzed are treated with protease to remove nuclear proteins that may interfere with hybridization. The target DNA is denatured (usually with heating and formamide), producing a single-stranded target DNA sequence. Double-stranded DNA probes must also be similarly denatured. Commonly, a probe is applied first, followed by codenaturation of the target and probe. The probe and target DNA are then allowed to hybridize. During hybridization, the specificity of target–probe interaction is strictly controlled by the stringency of the hybridization and wash buffers. The nuclei of the target cells are then counterstained with propidium iodide (PI) or, more commonly, DAPI. Using a fluorescence microscope with appropriate filters, the DAPI- or PI-stained nuclei will be readily localized, and the fluorescent probe signals will be visualized. The number of nuclei to be scored will vary with the particular application. When using intact paraffin sections and specifically targeting neoplastic cells, a relatively small number of cells may be sufficient. For example, scoring of 40 cells may be sufficient for analysis of *HER2* amplification in invasive breast carcinoma. To detect a small number of malignant cells in a background of benign elements, such as assays for residual or recurrent leukemias in bone marrow samples, analysis of 500 or more nuclei may be required.

CONTROLS AND ASSAY DEVELOPMENT

Because most commercially available FISH probes are currently marketed in the United States as analyte-specific reagents, a molecular pathology laboratory must perform internal validation studies before implementing new FISH assays. The initial development and validation of a FISH assay requires several phases. First, the probe of interest should be hybridized to normal control metaphases to ensure that the probe hybridizes to the expected chromosomal regions and does not exhibit cross-reactivity with other regions. Next, a reference range for abnormal nuclear signal patterns (false-positive nuclei) is determined by analysis of a series of normal control samples (usually at least 20 samples). For analysis of malignancy-associated abnormalities, it may be preferable to analyze malignant samples known to be negative for the abnormality of interest whenever possible, because malignant cells may produce slightly different reference ranges than benign negative control cells. Cutoffs for interpretation as a positive result are then established based upon the observed reference ranges. Criteria for establishing cutoffs have varied in the literature. Some have suggested direct binomial distribution analysis of the negative control samples, and others have set thresholds at more than 2 or more than 3 standard deviations above the mean of abnormal nuclei counted in the negative controls. Positive control samples, known to be positive for the abnormality of interest by other techniques, should similarly be analyzed. Correlation with results of a separate analysis performed on the same samples using another method, or with the same method performed by another laboratory, can also be used to validate the new probe assay. Tissue microarrays of cytogenetically characterized cell line xenograft preparations are also useful tools for validation studies.

ADVANTAGES

Many diagnostically and prognostically significant molecular abnormalities can be detected by multiple techniques, including classical cytogenetics, Southern blot studies, and polymerase chain reaction (PCR)–based or reverse transcriptase–PCR (RT-PCR)–based strategies, as well as FISH. FISH techniques offer several advantages over other techniques, at least within select circumstances. The primary advantage of FISH studies over classical cytogenetics is the ability to analyze nondividing (interphase) nuclei. FISH can therefore provide cytogenetic information from archived material (such as bone marrow aspirate smears or FFPE material) that could not be analyzed by classical cytogenetics. In addition, FISH analysis can identify abnormalities that are cryptic in normal cytogenetics, confirm or clarify suspected abnormalities with equivocal findings by G-banded karyotyping, and provide additional analysis when classical cytogenetic studies have been noninformative because of isolation of only normal metaphases or lack of metaphases for analysis. Some abnormalities (such as translocations involving the *BCL6* or *CCND1* genes) may be detected by Southern blot studies. FISH analysis, however, generally produces results with a faster turnaround time and offers the ability to identify the translocation partner genes using specific two-color, fusion probes. In many cases, FISH studies are also preferable to PCR- or RT-PCR-based approaches for detection of translocations at initial diagnosis. For example, the PCR primers commonly used to detect *IGH/BCL2* translocations (involving the so-called major breakpoint region and minor cluster region) do not detect a subset of translocations with variant breakpoints. Commercially available FISH probes, in contrast, span all known translocation breakpoints, resulting in the superior sensitivity of FISH analysis. Studies directly comparing FISH and PCR strategies for detection of lymphoma-associated translocations in FFPE material have also demonstrated better sensitivity using FISH.

DISADVANTAGES

Although FISH studies are a powerful tool for detection of molecular cytogenetic abnormalities, one must be aware of their intrinsic limitations. A major disadvantage of FISH analysis compared to classical cytogenetic studies is that FISH studies only provide information regarding the specific chromosomal regions targeted by the FISH probes. Classical cytogenetic studies, on the other hand, allow global screening of karyotypic abnormalities, including changes that were previously unsuspected by the pathologist. FISH analysis therefore can never serve as a complete substitute for classical cytogenetic studies. In the evaluation of hematopoietic neoplasms, or other tumors in which cytogenetic status will influence prognosis or classification, FISH studies are best performed as an adjunct to, and not a replacement for, classical cytogenetics.

FISH analysis may also be limited in the setting of minimal residual disease studies. Many FISH protocols will require 5% to 10% of the total cells present to be positive for the abnormality to distinguish a true positive case from background signals. In some settings, a lower cutoff may be employed. For example, protocols have been published for BCR/ABL detection in the bone marrow using dual fusion probes and scoring of at least 500 nuclei, yielding cutoffs of less than 1% of the total cells. Even these rigorous scoring methods, however, are much less sensitive than quantitative RT-PCR studies for BCR/ABL, which are reported to have a sensitivity of 1 in 1×10^5. When detection of a small percentage of abnormal cells is required, quantitative RT-PCR-based approaches are generally preferable to FISH studies.

FISH studies also do not provide allele-specific information that may be detected by other technologies. For example, loss of regions of chromosomes 1p and 19q in gliomas may be assessed by either FISH or PCR-based loss of heterozygosity (LOH) techniques. In some tumors, for example, one could see loss of a paternal allele but duplication of the other, maternal allele. LOH techniques would still detect this abnormality, but FISH studies, which do not discriminate between the maternal and the paternal alleles, would display a normal pattern. Furthermore, FISH studies generally cannot detect small changes, such as specific point mutations, which are better detected by PCR analysis or direct sequencing.

APPLICATIONS

In routine clinical practice, FISH techniques can be employed to identify several types of genetic abnormalities, including genomic gains at specific loci or entire chromosomes, gene amplification, loss of specific loci or entire chromosomes, and the presence of translocations (Table 11-1). Details of specific applications are discussed later in this text in organ system–specific chapters. Nevertheless, the following section describes examples of FISH probes used to detect each of these types of cytogenetic abnormalities and their utility in routine pathology practice.

TABLE 11-1

Examples of Commonly Employed FISH Techniques

GENOTYPING OF NEOPLASMS

Polysomy and other gains
  Trisomy 12 in B-cell chronic lymphocytic leukemia
Losses
  Deletions of chromosomes 1p and 19q in gliomas
Amplification
  HER2/neu amplification in invasive breast carcinoma
Translocations
  t(9;22)(q34;q11) BCR/ABL in chronic myeloid leukemia

CONSTITUTIONAL MOLECULAR CYTOGENETICS

Sex chromosome enumeration
  Gender determination with XY probes
Polysomy and other gains
  Trisomy 21 in Down syndrome
Losses of specific regions
  Del(22q11.2) in DiGeorge syndrome

FISH, fluorescence in situ hybridization.

GAINS: POLYPLOIDY

In some malignancies, the identification of gains of specific loci or entire chromosomes may be of diagnostic or prognostic significance. For example, in B-cell chronic lymphocytic leukemia, the presence of trisomy 12 is associated with atypical morphologic features and an intermediate prognosis (Figure 11-1). The evaluation of a sample for potential polysomy is most easily carried out using centromere-specific probes and intact, whole cell preparations such as peripheral blood smears or touch preparations of tissue biopsy specimens. The number of centromeric signals within each cell is readily discernible in intact cell preparations and, if clinically desired, one may separately score nuclei with three signals, four signals, etc., to accurately assess ploidy for the chromosome of interest. Gains of a particular chromosome may also be assessed in paraffin sections. However, because of the potential for nuclear truncation in paraffin sections, one cannot accurately distinguish trisomy from tetrasomy, etc., within any given nucleus. One can, however, score any nuclei showing three or more centromeric signals as a method to identify the presence of polysomy. When assessing intact paraffin sections for polysomy, one should ensure that sections are well cut without folded tissue, and areas with closely overlapping nuclei should be avoided whenever possible. Gains of specific chromosomal regions may also be assessed using locus-specific

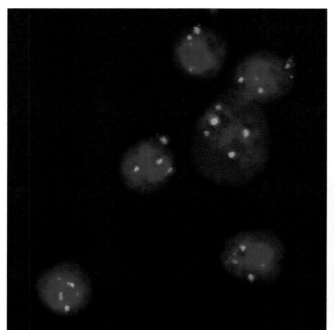

FIGURE 11-1

Trisomy 12 in B-cell chronic lymphocytic leukemia. Three copies of a chromosome 12 centromere probe (green signals) are visible, in addition to two copies of a 13q13 probe (red signal). Trisomy of chromosome 12 has been associated with an intermediate prognosis and atypical morphologic features in B-cell chronic lymphocytic leukemia.

probes. Analysis of specific loci may be most useful to detect abnormalities involving chromosomes for which centromere-specific probes are not available.

The enumeration of specific chromosomes may also be of value in some non-neoplastic conditions, such as prenatal assessment for chromosomal abnormalities. An example of this approach is a commercially available, U.S. Food and Drug Administration–approved kit including centromeric probes for chromosomes 18, X, and Y and locus-specific probes for chromosomes 13q and 21q. This probe cocktail allows detection of trisomy 13, 18, or 21; gender determination; and assessment for abnormalities of the sex chromosomes.

AMPLIFICATION

When identified by banded karyotyping, gene amplification may take one of two forms: repeated segments within one chromosome (known as *homogeneously staining regions*) or small extrachromosomal material (known as *double minutes*). Gene amplification is detected by FISH through the use of locus-specific probes, which will show many copies of a particular locus when amplified, as opposed to the expected two copies with a normal chromosome complement. The use of a differentially labeled reference probe, usually a centromeric probe for the same chromosome as the locus of interest, allows one to distinguish between polysomy and low-level amplification. Cases displaying

an increased ratio of locus-specific signal to centromeric signal are generally interpreted as evidence of amplification (precise cutoffs must be established for each application). In polysomy, one may find multiple (usually <5) copies of a locus-specific signal but with a ratio of locus-specific signal to centromeric signal of approximately 1.0. Examples of amplification detection that may be of diagnostic or prognostic utility include analysis of *HER2* in breast carcinoma (Figure 11-2),

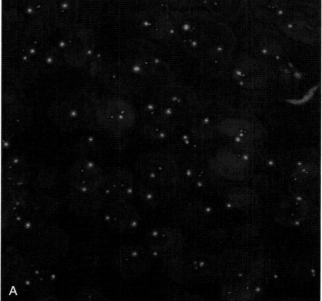

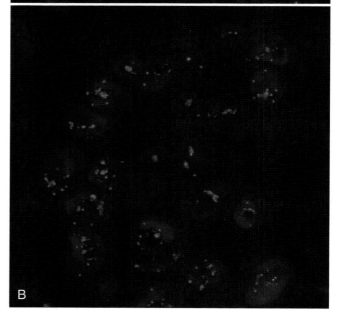

FIGURE 11-2

Amplification of *HER2* in breast carcinoma. FISH analysis of breast carcinomas in intact paraffin sections using probes to the *HER2* locus (red signal) and the chromosome 7 centromere (green signals). **A,** In the absence of *HER2* amplification most cells display two red and two green signals (*HER2*/CEP17 ratio < 1.8 per ASCO/CAP guidelines). **B,** In the presence of *HER2* amplification, numerous *HER2* signals are observed (*HER2*/CEP17 ratio > 2.2 per ASCO/CAP guidelines).

EGFR amplification in glioblastoma multiforme, or *MYCN (NMYC)* in neuroblastoma.

Amplification may be assessed through FISH using either intact cell preparations (cell suspensions or touch preparations from tissue biopsy samples) or in intact paraffin sections. The use of a reference centromeric probe and calculation of the ratio of locus signal to centromeric signal allows accurate assessment of amplification, even in the setting of nuclear truncation artifacts in paraffin sections. The use of FFPE material is particularly common in cases such as breast carcinoma, where FFPE tissue may be the only available specimen in routine practice. Analysis using intact sections in this setting also allows the pathologist to specifically target areas of invasive carcinoma for analysis, without scoring of nuclei from areas of benign epithelium, stromal cells, infiltrating lymphocytes, or in situ carcinoma.

DELETION

The loss of specific loci, chromosomal regions, or entire chromosomes may also be of diagnostic or prognostic interest in many neoplasms. For example, loss of the *TP53* locus at chromosome 17p13 or the *ATM* gene on chromosome 11q23 are each associated with an adverse prognosis in B-cell chronic lymphocytic leukemia. Similarly, losses of material on chromosomes 1p and 19q are often found in oligodendrogliomas (Figure 11-3) and are associated with a relatively favorable prognosis. Deletions of specific loci or loss of entire chromosomes is most easily identified using whole cell preparations (touch preparations, cell suspensions, etc.) for which the precise number of signals in each nucleus can be tabulated. However, deletion of specific loci (using loci-specific probes) or entire chromosomes (using centromeric probes) can also be detected using intact paraffin sections. When analyzing paraffin section material, it is particularly useful to include a separate, differentially labeled reference probe signal, either to the centromere of the chromosome of interest or to another region on the same chromosome. Calculating a ratio of locus-specific signal to reference signal assists in correcting for possible nuclear truncation artifacts. Although various scoring protocols have been described in the literature, a ratio of less than 0.7 (locus to reference) is generally considered to be consistent with loss of a specific locus. As noted earlier, care must be exercised to exclude apparent loss because of gain at the reference locus.

Several non-neoplastic, constitutional syndromes are also associated with loss of specific loci that may be assessed on prenatal samples. For example, commercially available LSI probes can be employed to identify cases of DiGeorge syndrome (associated with loss of material at 22q11.2) or Cri-du-chat syndrome (deletion of 5p15).

TRANSLOCATIONS

Many neoplasms, especially hematolymphoid malignancies and sarcomas, are associated with recurring, balanced translocations of diagnostic or prognostic significance. Assays for these translocations have therefore become one of the most commonly employed FISH procedures in routine clinical practice. Two general strategies have been employed in the design of FISH probes for detection of translocations: fusion probes and break-apart probes. Each of these types of probes has distinct advantages and disadvantages.

In the simplest type of fusion probe, a so-called single-fusion technique, differentially labeled probes hybridize to the two chromosomal loci involved in the translocation. Typically, one probe is labeled with a red and the other with a green fluorochrome. In a normal cell, two red and two green signals are expected. In the setting of a balanced translocation involving these two genes, the normal chromosomes yield separate red and green signals; one of the derivative chromosomes produces a yellow fusion signal, and the other derivative chromosome is no longer labeled (a one red, one green, one fusion, or 1R1G1F, pattern). Currently, most commercially available fusion probes are produced as *dual fusion* probes (Figure 11-4). In this approach, the differentially labeled probes to the two translocation partner genes are chosen so that the probes substantially overlap both sides of the known translocation breakpoints. In a dual fusion probe, the presence of a balanced translocation yields a one red, one green, two fusion (1R1G2F) pattern. Spurious fusion signals can be seen in occasional benign cells because of random overlap of the target loci being analyzed. Because it is unlikely that both sets of target loci would happen to overlap by chance alone, counting of cells with two fusion signals results in a much lower cutoff threshold with dual fusion probes than could be possible with a single fusion probe. Dual fusion probes are therefore particularly valuable when the number of malignant cells within a sample may be relatively low. It must be remembered, however, that unbalanced translocations will yield only one yellow fusion signal even with a dual fusion probe.

Alternatively, translocations involving a target gene may also be detected using break-apart probes (Figure 11-5). In a break-apart probe, differentially labeled probes are chosen to be located on each side of the translocation breakpoints. In a normal cell, two fusion signals are seen. In the presence of a translocation involving the target gene, one fusion

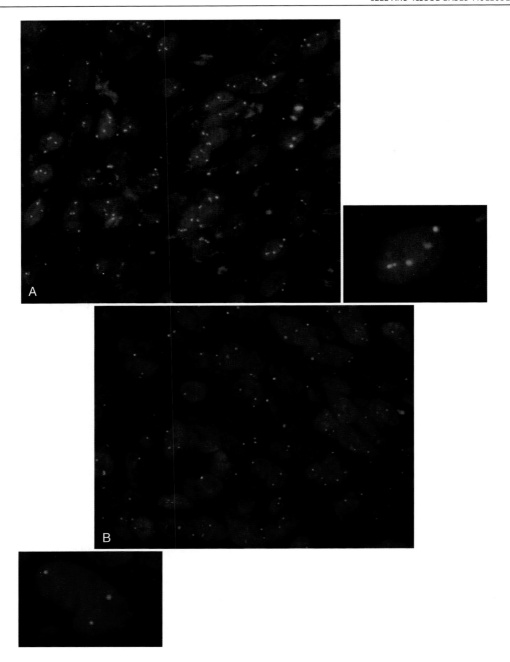

FIGURE 11-3

Del(19q) in gliomas. Using intact paraffin sections, gliomas are analyzed by FISH with probes hybridizing to 19q13 (red signal) and 19p13 (green signal).
A, In the absence of chromosome 19q deletion, most cells display two red and two green signals (inset). **B,** A decreased ratio of 19q13-to-19p13 signals indicates the presence of del(19q), with numerous cells displaying two green and one red signal (inset). The combined loss of chromosomes 19q and 1p has been associated with chemosensitivity and improved prognosis in oligodendrogliomas.

signal will be seen, corresponding to the normal chromosome, as will separate red and green signals, corresponding to the two derivative chromosomes. A positive break-apart or split-signal pattern identifies the presence of a translocation involving the target gene but provides no information regarding the translocation partner gene present. These probes are particularly valuable for genes known to have many translocation partners. For example,

more than 30 different genes have been described in translocations with the *MLL* gene at 11q23 in acute myeloid or acute lymphoid leukemias. Screening for such a range of abnormalities is obviously not practical with a fusion-based FISH approach. Using a break-apart strategy, however, one can screen for MLL translocations in a single assay. If clinically desired, follow-up analysis with fusion FISH probes or with PCR-based techniques and

Normal

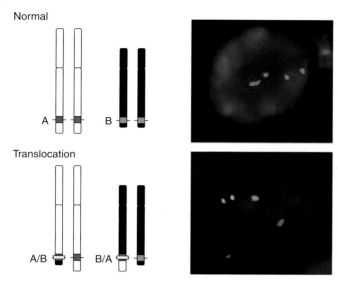

FIGURE 11-4

Dual fusion translocation probes. A dual fusion strategy employs separately labeled probes for gene *A* (red) and gene *B* (green). In a normal cell, two red and green signals are visualized. In the presence of an *A/B* translocation, two fusion signals are seen, in addition to one red and one green signal. (From Cook JR: Paraffin section interphase fluorescence in situ hybridization in the diagnosis and classification of non-Hodgkin lymphomas. Diagn Mol Pathol 2004;13(4):197–206 with permission.)

correlation with classical cytogenetics can assist in identification of the translocation partner gene involved. Break-apart probes are also of value in intact paraffin section FISH, because the break-apart probes generally yield a lower cutoff threshold than do fusion probes.

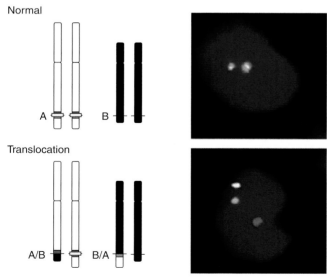

FIGURE 11-5

Break-apart translocation probes. Break-apart probes employ differentially labeled probes hybridizing to regions of gene *A* flanking the translocation breakpoints. In a normal cell, two intact fusion signals are detected. In the presence of an *A/B* translocation, one fusion pair is split, yielding a one yellow fusion, one red, one green pattern. (From Cook JR: Paraffin section interphase fluorescence in situ hybridization in the diagnosis and classification of non-Hodgkin lymphomas. Diagn Mol Pathol 2004;13(4):197–206.)

METAPHASE FLUORESCENCE IN SITU HYBRIDIZATION STUDIES: MARKER CHROMOSOME ANALYSIS, MULTIPLEX FLUORESCENCE IN SITU HYBRIDIZATION, AND SPECTRAL KARYOTYPING

The preceding discussion has focused primarily on interphase FISH analysis. FISH procedures performed on metaphase cytogenetic preparations can also be of clinical utility in many settings. For example, locus-specific probes can be used to detect submicroscopic deletions that would not be identified by G-banded karyotyping alone. Similarly, some translocations are not readily detected by standard metaphase cytogenetic studies. For example, some translocations involving the *MLL* locus at 11q23 can be misinterpreted as a del(11)(q23). FISH studies using a break-apart probe spanning the *MLL* locus on metaphase preparations not only can demonstrate the definitive presence of a translocation rather than a deletion but also can assist in identifying the translocation partner locus involved. Finally, FISH studies are useful for clarifying the nature of marker chromosomes, whose identities cannot be definitively established by karyotyping alone.

Two specialized protocols for metaphase FISH analysis have been developed in recent years: multiplex FISH (M-FISH) and spectral karyotyping (SKY). Both these techniques use whole chromosome paints labeled with various combinations of fluorochromes. Computer-assisted analysis of the combinatorial fluorescence allows identification of each chromosome as a unique false color in a single analysis. In M-FISH, a series of images is captured through multiple filter sets, each of which detects specific fluorochromes. Computer image analysis software then merges the data from each image and assigns a false color to each of the chromosomes based on the combinatorial fluorescence. In SKY analysis, a single, specially designed filter set and Fourier transformation analysis are employed to assign each chromosome a unique false color. The resulting multicolor image can clearly identify segments of each chromosome, including the origin of material in marker chromosomes or other abnormalities that may be missed by standard banded karyotyping (Figure 11-6). Although powerful, the complexity of M-FISH and SKY analysis and the associated costs have precluded routine clinical application of this type of technology in most laboratories at the current time.

FLUORESCENCE IN SITU HYBRIDIZATION WITH SIMULTANEOUS IMMUNOFLUORESCENCE

In 1992, Weber-Matthiesen et al. reported the development of a procedure using interphase FISH analysis with simultaneous immunofluorescence, a

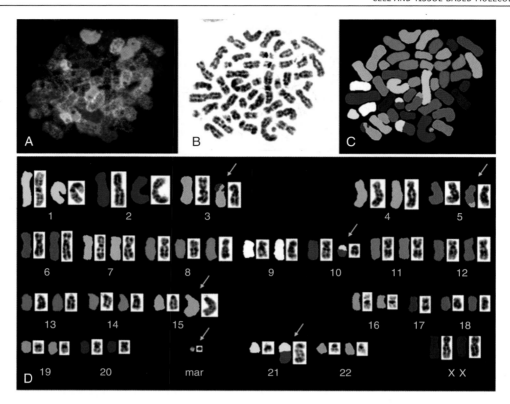

FIGURE 11-6

Complex karyotype detected in a patient with acute myeloid leukemia, analyzed using spectral karyotyping (SKY). **A,** Metaphase cell with chromosomes shown in SKY display colors. **B,** Inverted and contrast-enhanced 4'-6-diamidino-2-phenylindole (DAPI) image of the same metaphase cell. **C,** The same metaphase cell with chromosomes shown in spectra-based classification colors. **D,** Karyotype of the same cell with each chromosome represented twice, by SKY image shown in classification colors on the left and its inverted and contrast-enhanced DAPI-stained image on the right. Arrows denote structurally rearranged chromosomes. The karyotype interpretation is as follows:

47,XX,der(3)del(3)(p11.2p21)t(3;17)(p24~25;?),der(5)t(3;5)(p25;q31),+8,−10,
+der(10 or 21)(21q??21q?::10? ?10?::21q??21q?::10??10?), der(15)(15pter?15q26::15q??15q?::15q22?15q26::15q??15q?),−17,
der(21)(21pter?21q22::10??10?::21q22?21q22::10??10?::21q??21q?::10? ?10?),+mar
(Courtesy of Dr. Krzysztof Mrózek, Ohio State University, Columbus, OH.)

technique termed *fluorescence immunophenotyping and interphase cytogenetics as a tool for the investigation of neoplasms* (FICTION). Variations on FISH–immunofluorescence procedures have been applied to a range of sample types, including cytologic preparations, peripheral blood, and both frozen and paraffin section material. The use of an immunofluorescent marker allows evaluation of only cells of interest. Tyramide signal amplification may be used to maximize concurrent cell conditioning, nucleoprotein digestion, and target hybridization. For example, in diffuse large B-cell lymphoma, FISH results could be scored only on cells that were also CD20 positive. Properly chosen immunofluorescent markers allow the specific identification of tumor nuclei for analysis and the exclusion of non-neoplastic stromal or inflammatory cells, producing a more precise assessment of the tumor genotype. Although primarily a research tool, combined FISH–immunofluorescence procedures have been employed in some clinical laboratories, such as for analysis of plasma cell neoplasms (Figure 11-7).

CONCLUSION

The number of clinically relevant applications of FISH technology and the availability of commercially available, analyte-specific reagent FISH probes has increased dramatically in the last several years. In some areas of diagnostic pathology, especially in hematolymphoid neoplasms and sarcomas, FISH studies have become the technique of choice for genotypic evaluation. For example, FISH studies for t(9;22)(q34;q21) *BCR/ABL* or t(11;14)(q13;q32) *CCND1/IGH* are the current gold standards for initial diagnosis of chronic myeloid leukemia and mantle cell lymphoma, respectively. Similarly, FISH studies are generally considered to represent the gold standard for analysis of *HER2* amplification in breast carcinoma. FISH techniques, at least for these most widely employed applications, have therefore become an important part of routine clinical practice at most large

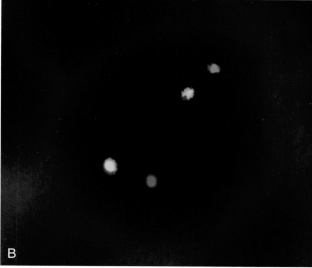

FIGURE 11-7

FISH analysis with simultaneous immunofluorescence. A case of plasma cell myeloma analyzed using a dual fusion probe for t(11;14)(q13;q32) *CCND1/IGH* with simultaneous immunofluorescence for CD138, a marker of plasma cells. **A,** Under a 4′-diamidino-2-phenylindole filter, plasma cells are identified by intense blue cytoplasmic staining in a bone marrow clot preparation. **B,** The plasma cells are positive for *CCND1/IGH,* as indicated by a two fusion, one red, one green signal pattern.

ratory capable of FISH analysis when circumstances make such studies clinically desirable.

As the number of recurring cytogenetic abnormalities associated with particular types of neoplasms and congenital disorders continues to grow every year, the demand for FISH studies will likely continue to expand through at least the short-term future. In the long term, it remains unclear to what extent FISH analysis might be replaced by array-based molecular techniques. Current array-based comparative genomic hybridization studies are capable of detecting numeric chromosomal abnormalities with high resolution. Similarly, gene expression profiling experiments in acute lymphoid leukemias have shown that expression profiles can be designed that allow the detection of recurring chromosomal translocations such as *BCR/ABL* or *TEL/AML1.* It remains to be seen whether array-based methodologies are ultimately able to be integrated into routine molecular pathology practice. It is likely that, even if array-based platforms or multiplexed PCR analysis becomes the technique of choice for initial screening for selected types of neoplasms, confirmation of the presence of particular chromosomal abnormalities by other techniques such as FISH will remain important. FISH analysis can therefore be expected to maintain an integral role in molecular pathology and cytogenetic laboratories for the foreseeable future.

SUGGESTED READINGS

Antonescu CR: The role of genetic testing in soft tissue sarcoma. Histopathology 2006;48:13–21.

Cook JR: Paraffin section interphase fluorescence in situ hybridization in the diagnosis and classification of non-Hodgkin lymphomas. Diagn Mol Pathol 2004;13:197–206.

Fuller CE, Perry A: Molecular diagnostics in central nervous system tumors. Adv Anat Pathol 2005;12:180–194.

Hicks DG, Tubbs RR: Assessment of the HER2 status in breast cancer by fluorescence in situ hybridization: A technical review with interpretive guidelines. Hum Pathol 2005;36:250–261.

Kelley TW, Tubbs RR, Prayson RA: Molecular diagnostic techniques for the clinical evaluation of gliomas. Diagn Mol Pathol 2005;14:1–8.

Landstrom AP, Tefferi A: Fluorescent in situ hybridization in the diagnosis, prognosis, and treatment monitoring of chronic myeloid leukemia. Leuk Lymphoma 2006;47:397–402.

National Center for Biotechnology Information: Human BAC Resource. Available at http://www.ncbi.nlm.nih.gov/genome/cyto/hbrc.shtml.

Tibiletti MG, Bernasconi B, Dionigi A, et al: The applications of FISH in tumor pathology. Adv Clin Path 1999;3:111–118.

University of California, Santa Cruz: UCSC Genome Bioinformatics. Available at http://genome.ucsc.edu/.

van Dongen JJ, van der Burg M, Langerak AW: Split-signal FISH for detection of chromosome aberrations. Hematology 2005;10(Suppl 1):66–72.

Ventura RA, Martin-Subero JI, Jones M, et al: FISH analysis for the detection of lymphoma-associated chromosomal abnormalities in routine paraffin-embedded tissue. J Mol Diagn 2006;8:141–151.

Weber-Matthiesen K., Winkemann M, Muller-Hermelink A, et al: Simultaneous fluorescence immunophenotyping and interphase cytogenetics: A contribution to the characterization of tumor cells. J Histochem Cytochem 1992;40:171–175.

Wolf AC, Hammond MD, Schwartz JN, et al: American Society of Clinical Oncology/College of American Pathologists guideline recommendations for human epidermal growth factor receptor 2 testing in breast cancer. J Clin Oncol 2007;25(1):118–45.

medical centers and reference laboratories. For smaller hospitals with lower volumes of such cases, the costs of implementing FISH techniques, including fluorescence microscopes, skilled technologists, and appropriate dark rooms for hybridization and counting of results, may be prohibitive. However, all pathologists should familiarize themselves with clinical scenarios in which submission of material to a reference laboratory for FISH analysis may be helpful in the diagnosis or classification of malignancy. In particular, pathologists routinely handling hematolymphoid malignancies, sarcomas, gliomas, and breast carcinomas should establish working relationships with a reference labo-

12 Bright-Field In Situ Hybridization

Ricardo V. Lloyd • Xiang Qian • Long Jin

INTRODUCTION

Bright-field in situ hybridization (ISH) is a widely used technique that allows visualization of specific gene products in cells and tissues under routine bright-field microscopy. A DNA or RNA probe is used to detect the presence of the complementary DNA (cDNA) or complementary RNA (cRNA) target sequences in cell specimens (smears, cytospins, or cell pellets) and tissue sections (frozen, paraffin, semithin, and ultrathin plastic sections) through colorimetric or metallographic techniques visualized with a light microscope.

The identification of gene expression patterns in tissues can provide information critical for understanding gene function. ISH also allows morphologic identification of viral, bacterial, and fungal organisms. The method involves a hybridization reaction between a labeled nucleotide probe and cRNA or cDNA target sequences. Those hybrids can be detected either by histochemical chromogen development for nonisotopically labeled probes, also called *chromogenic in situ hybridization* (CISH™), or by enzyme metallography, also called *silver in situ hybridization* (SISH™). Historically, autoradiographic emulsion for radioactively (isotopic) labeled probes have also been used (Figure 12-1).

Although isotopic methods (such as probes labeled with ^{3}H, ^{32}P, ^{35}S, or ^{125}I) have problems with long turnaround times, exposure risk, and waste disposal, they remain useful because of their greater sensitivity. Nonisotopic methods are considered better for application of ISH in diagnostic pathology. However, nonisotopic CISH often has lower sensitivity compared with an isotopic method. ISH detection limits on tissue sections are in the range of 40 kilobases of target DNA and 10 to 20 copies of messenger RNA (mRNA) or viral DNA per cell. The application of nucleic acid target and signal amplification techniques to ISH can allow detection of as few as one or two copies of specific DNA molecules in cell preparations and provide precise localization, yielding positive signals that are retained within the subcellular compartments. This chapter reviews the basic principles of bright-field approaches of ISH and its uses in diagnostic molecular pathology and research.

BASIC PRINCIPLES OF IN SITU HYBRIDIZATION

The basic requirements for a probe are specificity for the sequence of interest and labeling with a reporter to allow appropriate detection. The melting temperature (T_m) of hybrids is the point at which 50% of the double-stranded nucleic acid chains are separated. The optimal temperature for hybridization is 15° C to 25° C below the T_m. There are various formulas to calculate T_m, depending on probe length and type of hybrids. For DNA:DNA hybrids with probes longer than 22 base pairs, the following formula can be used:

$$T_m = 81.5 + 16.5 \log (Na) + 0.41 (\% GC) - 0.62 (\% \text{ formamide}) - 500 \text{ per length of base pairs of probe}$$

RNA:RNA hybrids are generally 10° C to 15° C more stable than DNA:DNA or DNA:RNA hybrids and therefore require more stringent conditions for hybridization and posthybridization washing. A variety of probes can be used for ISH (Table 12-1), and the appropriate type of probe is determined largely by the application.

TISSUE PREPARATIONS

ISH has been applied to cell specimens (smears, cytospins, and cell pallets) and tissue sections (frozen, paraffin, semithin, and ultrathin plastic sections). Tissue processing including storage and fixation should be optimized to detect intracellular nucleic acids. Both intact cells and frozen tissues (stored at −70° C) are ideal for ISH, because they contain better-preserved nucleotide sequences. Formalin-fixed archival tissues can be used for ISH after storage for several years; they are an almost limitless source of material for study

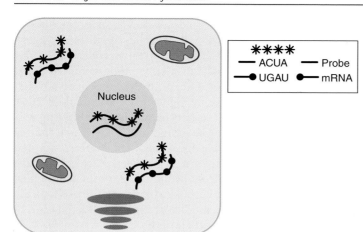

FIGURE 12-1

Schematic representation of an in situ hybridization reaction. A riboprobe or antisense RNA probe is labeled with a nonradioactive or radioactive reporter and then hybridized with the cells or tissues of interest. The hybridization product is usually present in the cytoplasm for RNA targets. Targets, such as many viral infections, are usually present in the nucleus of the cells.

using a variety of molecular techniques. Ideal fixation for ISH should preserve both RNA or DNA and tissue morphology. Cross-linking fixatives such as paraformaldehyde, formalin, and glutaraldehyde are most commonly used. Bouin's solution, which contains picric acid or other strong acids or heavy metals, preserves nucleic acids poorly. The nature of the fixation is a particularly important consideration when proteolytic digestion conditions are being optimized. Fixed frozen section or cytospin cells need relatively mild proteolytic digestion. Formalin-fixed archival tissues with better morphology require more rigorous proteolysis. The slides should be pretreated with a suitable coating solution, such as 3-aminopropyltrimethoxysilane or poly-L-lysine to ensure optimal adherence of tissue sections to the glass slides.

PRETREATMENT OF CELLS AND TISSUES

A series of pretreatment steps before hybridization can increase the efficiency of hybridization and reduce nonspecific background staining. Protease treatment

(e.g., proteinase K) is considered one of the most important steps to increase the accessibility of the target nucleic acid. The concentrations of proteinase K (1 to 50 μg/ml) and the length of treatment (5 to 30 min) depend on tissue type, fixative, and length of fixation. Prolonged incubation will lead to overdigested tissues, resulting in loss of signal and morphologic integrity. Underdigestion leads to suboptimal probe penetration. In both these situations, there is relative failure of the hybridization reaction because probe and target nucleic acids are not brought together under optimal conditions. Coupling of digestion to other unmasking techniques, such as treatment with sodium bisulfite, sodium thiocyanate, or hydrochloric acid, may increase the hybridization signal. Acetylation of sections using 0.25% acetic anhydride per 0.1-M triethanolamine can reduce charged probes binding to tissues. Acetic anhydride also reduces the nonspecific binding of unrelated digoxigenin-labeled probes to neuroendocrine cells. The presence of endogenous biotin or alkaline phosphatase (AP) should be anticipated in some

---

TABLE 12-1

Types of Probes

Probe Type	Probe Preparation	Probe Labeling
dsDNA, cDNA	DNA: Fragment isolation (optional)	dsDNA: Random primed DNA labeling, nick translation, PCR
ssRNA, oligonucleotide ssDNA	cDNA: Cloning	RNA: In vitro transcription, RT-PCR
	RNA: Cloning in transcription vectors	Oligonucleotides: End labeling or tailing
	Oligonucleotides: Chemical synthesis	

cDNA, complementary DNA; dsDNA, double-stranded DNA; PCR, polymerase chain reaction; RT-PCR, reverse transcriptase–polymerase chain reaction; ssDNA, single-stranded DNA.

tissues when using nonisotopic probes. Inhibition or elimination of endogenous horseradish peroxidase (HRP) enzyme activities (e.g., in erythrocytes, neutrophils, and macrophages) can be accomplished by treatment with hydrogen peroxide. Endogenous AP can be inhibited by treatment of sections with 0.2N HCl and levamisole and endogenous biotin by biotin-blocking agents. Microwave pretreatment can be used for formalin-fixed archival tissues to improve staining sensitivity. The mechanisms by which these steps improve nucleic acid unmasking are not clearly understood, although extraction of histone proteins from the cell nucleus is thought to be one important factor. Following unmasking, postfixation, such as with paraformaldehyde, may be useful for the prevention of loss of material from the slide and for further preservation of morphology.

PROBE SELECTION

DNA or RNA molecules of specific sequence, labeled with either isotopic or nonisotopic reporter molecules, are used to detect the complementary sequence by ISH.

The choice of optimal probes for ISH must consider specificity, sensitivity, tissue penetration, stability of hybrids, and reproducibility of the technique. Probe sizes for optimal tissue penetration should be between 200 and 500 base pairs. Specific sequences of DNA or cDNA derived by reverse transcription of mRNA are cloned into vectors such as bacteriophages, plasmids, and cosmids. The amplified sequences are extracted and labeled using nick translation or random primer methods. Double-stranded DNA probes have a high level of specificity because of their length and have a sensitivity that is related to the number of incorporated reporter molecules. They require denaturation to produce single-stranded DNA before hybridization and may require cleavage into smaller sequences to allow optimal access to fixed tissues. Single-stranded DNA probes can also be generated by polymerase chain reaction (PCR) using a DNA template and an antisense primer producing single-stranded DNA, which is directly labeled during synthesis by the incorporation of nucleotide conjugated to a reporter molecule. These probes have similar advantages to the oligonucleotide probes except that they are much larger, probably in the 200- to 500-base-pair range.

Single-stranded antisense RNA probes (riboprobes) are prepared by in vitro transcription using the cDNA sequences as a template. The cDNA insert is subcloned into a transcription vector and flanked by the initiation site for two different RNA polymerases (e.g., T7, Sp6), thus enabling either the sense strand or the antisense strand to be synthesized. The sense RNA probe is usually used as a negative control. Treatment with ribonuclease A (RNase A) after hybridization with riboprobes will reduce a nonspecific background signal, because the enzyme digests single-stranded but not double-stranded RNA hybrids. Riboprobes are sensitive and useful for detection of low copy numbers of expressed genes. They may also give rise to higher background than DNA probes because of increased nonspecific binding. Oligoriboprobes may be generated in the same way as standard riboprobes by using a short DNA template or by combining single-stranded oligonucleotides with a bacteriophage promoter. Although they have the advantages of both access and stability of hybrids, they are probably more susceptible to degradation by RNases because of their short length.

With the increasing numbers of cloned and sequenced genes, oligoprobes can be generated from cDNA maps in the literature or GenBank and synthesized rapidly and inexpensively. Single-stranded DNA molecules ranging from 20 to 50 base pairs probably penetrate cells more readily and can produce excellent hybridization signals. Oligoprobes are commonly 3′ or 5′ end "tailing" labeled by using the enzyme terminal transferase with relatively few incorporated label molecules; these probes are relatively less sensitive than longer cDNA or cRNA probes. Oligoprobes are generally considered most suitable for detection of relatively abundant expressed genes, such as hormone mRNAs. The lack of sensitivity of oligoprobes can be overcome by using a cocktail of multiple oligoprobes that are complementary to different regions of the target molecules. Careful selection of oligoprobes with low homology to other nucleotide sequences is most important to ascertain the specificity of ISH. Because of their short length, they readily penetrate fixed tissues; however, if short (less than 14 base pairs), they may bind nonspecifically. The hybrids may also be more easily disrupted in posthybridization washes, leading to a false-negative result.

Peptide nucleic acids (PNAs) are synthetic analogs of DNA that hybridize with cDNAs or cRNAs with high affinity and specificity because of an uncharged and flexible polyamide backbone. Originally conceived as ligands for the recognition of double-stranded DNA, the unique physicochemical properties of PNAs have led to the development of a variety of research and diagnostic assays. Initially used as antisense and antigene reagents, the more recent applications of PNAs have involved their use as molecular hybridization probes. PNA probes are superior to traditional oligonucleotide probes. The unique physicochemical properties of PNA probes translate into unique behavior of ISH. PNAs can have the same base pairs as DNA and RNA probes; however, they are joined by a backbone of amide linkages (like proteins) instead of the sugars and phosphates of DNA and RNA. PNAs tend to hybridize more rapidly than their DNA counterparts, and they are quite effective at discriminating single-base mismatches. The primary disadvantages of PNA probes are that their properties are not yet as well understood as DNA oligonucleotides and their solubility is much lower than a corresponding DNA. They are typically quite short (usually less than 30 base pairs) and currently must be made synthetically.

REPORTER MOLECULES

Nonisotopic label methods are now commonly used for bright-field ISH. The most commonly used of these are biotin, digoxigenin, fluorescein, and dinitrophenyl. One advantage of using a fluorochrome such as hapten is that both direct fluorescent detection and indirect immunologic chromogen detection can be used with the same probe. The flexibility of these nonisotopic labels, coupled with their high morphologic resolution, has led to a dramatic increase in their use for ISH. The first nonisotopic label was biotin, because of the high sensitivity of streptavidin detection systems. However, the widespread presence of endogenous biotin and the limited success of blocking methods have stimulated the development of a range of other labels. Digoxigenin is a derivative of the cardiac glycoside digoxin and can be used for probe labeling. Because digoxigenin is not present in mammalian cells, this is a particular advantage when studying tissues such as liver or kidney, which may contain high endogenous biotin. Digoxigenin-labeled probes are widely used because there is less background and nonspecific staining than biotinylated probes. The signals can be visualized by using an antidigoxigenin antibody fragment conjugated to AP or HRP with respective substrates that yield insoluble-colored products. Nonisotopic probes are generally considered less sensitive than the corresponding isotopic probes, and the hybridization results are difficult to quantify. Other less common methods of nonisotopic probe labeling include direct conjugation to AP, labeling with bromodeoxyuridine or phenytoin, and chemical modifications including mercuration, sulphonation, and the addition of 2-acetylaminofluorene or dinitrophenol. Probes labeled with different haptens may allow the simultaneous detection of multiple nucleotide targets in a single experiment.

Isotopic labeling may be used to detect low copy sequences, to detect multiple nucleotide sequences, or further to combine with immunohistochemistry (IHC), particularly where nonisotopic alternatives are unsuccessful. Hybridization signals are detected by autoradiography, using either liquid emulsion or X-ray film, and are quantitated by using silver grain counting or semiquantitated by using densitometry. However, these applications are likely to be rare in diagnostic practice. Disadvantages of isotopic probes include biohazards and short probe half-life, and their use is time consuming. The choice of isotope usually reflects a compromise between the quality of resolution and the time of exposure. ^{32}P gives a rapid result but poor resolution; ^{3}H provides the best resolution but long exposure. ^{35}S is the most popular label because it combines reasonable specific activity with relatively high morphologic resolution. ^{33}P has recently been reported to produce superior results to ^{35}S. Other isotopes are rarely used.

DENATURATION AND HYBRIDIZATION

Once an appropriate probe has been labeled and purified, and the target nucleic acid has been exposed within the cell or tissue of interest, the probe and target must be brought together in such a way that specific hybridization can occur. For DNA detection with DNA probes, both probe and target molecules must be denatured, usually at 95° C. This can be achieved either separately or by codenaturation. The main advantage of codenaturation is that the number of practical steps is reduced. However, some argue that morphologic preservation is less optimal than with separate probe and target denaturation. Riboprobes and oligonucleotide probes are single stranded, as is cellular RNA. Therefore, denaturation is not essential for RNA detection but improves the sensitivity of riboprobe detection of RNA, possibly by removing the secondary structure of RNA probe and target.

If double-stranded DNA is heated to a temperature above its T_m (which is determined by both the length and the sequence of the DNA), the two strands separate. The temperature at which this occurs can be altered by the inclusion of organic solvents in the denaturation–hybridization solution. Formamide is commonly used, because it destabilizes the double-stranded structure of DNA at a given temperature, thus reducing the effective T_m of the hybrids. This reduces the need for high temperature incubation and consequently leads to better preservation of morphology. After the probe and target molecules have been made single stranded, all that is required for annealing to take place is either for the probe and target molecules to be brought together (for RNA detection and for separate denaturation of DNA) or for the incubation temperature to be reduced to below the T_m of the required hybrids (for DNA detection by codenaturation). At this point, the specificity (or stringency) of the hybridization reaction is determined. If hybridization is carried out at too high a temperature, no probe annealing occurs because the probe and targets remain single stranded. If hybridization is carried out at too low a temperature, probe and target molecules that are not perfectly matched will be allowed to anneal, thus reducing the specificity of the reaction. The appropriate hybridization temperature is determined by experimentation. Increasing the formamide concentration (which destabilizes mismatched hybrids) has the same effect as hybridization at a higher temperature. Other parameters that affect the specificity of the reaction are the concentration of monovalent cation (usually Na^+), the length of the probe molecules, and the probe concentration. A reduction in salt concentration increases the specificity of the reaction, as does lengthening the probe. Increasing the probe concentration drives the reaction in favor of the formation of probe–target hybrids, thus speeding up the reaction, but may also lead to nonspecific background staining. Generally, a probe concentration of 1 to 2 ng/μl is optimum for nonisotopic labeling, but this should be determined by titration experiments. However, as a rule, the time required depends on how repetitive the target sequence is; thus, highly repetitive targets, or targets present in high copy number, generally require short hybridization times (2 hours), whereas low copy number targets require overnight hybridization.

CONTROLS FOR IN SITU HYBRIDIZATION

Controls are critical for all ISH assays to assess whether the signal represents specific hybridization to the target sequence. A variety of controls can be used: (1) pretreatment of tissues with RNase or DNase, depending on the target being tested; (2) omission of the specific probes in hybridization reaction; (3) use of an unrelated or sense probe; (4) use of competition studies with unlabeled probes before adding labeled probes for hybridization; and (5) combination of ISH with immunostaining to localize the translated protein product in the same cells. Loss of target RNA or DNA may result in false-negative results, particularly for paraffin-embedded tissues. β-Actin, poly(dT), or ribosomal RNA (rRNA) and Alu DNA probe are used for the integrity of target RNA and DNA.

The probe should be characterized by Northern or Southern blot studies and by using known positive and negative tissues. Competitive hybridization with an excess of unlabeled probes or prehybridized with the complementary sequence should reduce signal intensity. Substitution of a sense probe should result in no signal. Technical problems such as nonspecific binding may arise during the assay. The application of irrelevant oligonucleotide probes may detect nonspecific binding of nucleotide sequences to specific cell types, such as neuroendocrine cells from the gastrointestinal tract.

CHROMOGENIC DETECTION OF HYBRIDS

Following hybridization, the next step is to remove the unbound hybridization probe. This is generally carried out in a saline solution in which probe–target hybrids are stable (standard saline citrate, or SSC). At this point, the specificity of the reaction can again be manipulated, although only an increase in specificity is possible at this stage. This can be done by (1) washing in solutions containing lower salt concentrations, (2) using higher formamide concentrations than those in the hybridization solution, and (3) using a higher temperature than that at which hybridization was carried out, which increases specificity by dissociating imperfectly matched hybrids. Examples of these conditions are hybridization in 60% formamide (2x SSC at 37° C) followed by washing in 60% formamide (2x SSC at 42° C) and hybridization in 50% formamide (2x SSC at 37° C) followed by washing in 50% formamide (0.1x SSC at 37° C). Formamide is added to decrease the T_m of hybrids. High temperatures, high formamide concentrations, and low ionic strength provide highly stringent conditions. In general, high degrees of specificity can be obtained by increasing the stringency.

Once the appropriate level of specificity has been achieved, the presence of probe–target hybrids can be demonstrated by detection of the probe labeling molecules. For isotopic labels, this is achieved by using dip–slide emulsion techniques. For nonisotopic labels, digoxigenin- or biotin-labeled probes can be detected by sequential incubations with mouse antidigoxigenin and goat antimouse-HRP/ diaminobenzidine (DAB) reaction or streptavidin-HRP/DAB respectively. Immunohistochemical detection may use any of the standard systems but is most often based on AP-labeled antibodies with nitroblue tetrazolium and 5-bromo-4-chloro-3-indolyl phosphate (NBT/BCIP) as chromogens, which results in a blue–black precipitate at binding sites. AP-based systems are generally more sensitive than those using peroxidase, but peroxidase substrates tend to give greater resolution. The major advantages of CISH with precipitating enzyme reactions include the stability of the resulting precipitate and thus the possibility of permanently storing cell and tissue preparations. The combination of these precipitates with routine stains, enabling the use of a standard bright-field microscope for the analysis, is an additional advantage, in particular in a setting in which histopathologic diagnostic analyses have to be performed. For optimal nucleic acid detection in situ, enzyme precipitation reactions are required that possess both a high sensitivity and the precise localization properties. Moreover, rapid staining reactions resulting in stable reaction products with contrasting colors are preferred. Despite numerous efforts, the most efficient results so far have been achieved with HRP (molecular weight 40 kDa) AP (molecular weight 100 kDa) enzymatic systems and enzyme metallography. If the biologic material examined contains endogenous enzyme activity or pseudo-peroxidase activity (such as hemoglobin in erythrocytes), this must be blocked to prevent the formation of unacceptable background. In some cases, it may be better to change the enzyme system used, rather than attempting to remove excessive endogenous enzyme activity. After performing the enzyme reactions and before embedding, the cell preparations can be lightly counterstained with, e.g., hematoxylin and/or eosin, methyl green, neutral red, or nuclear fast red for bright-field microscopic analysis. Counterstain can be omitted if reflection–contrast microscopy is used.

This approach is advantageous if surgical pathology with accurate morphologic correlation is needed, particularly in the assessment of paraffin sections. Application of CISH using a conventional ISH probe to detect gene amplification and deletion and chromosome translocation has been limited by the low ratio of signal to background staining. Interpretation of CISH is performed using a standard light microscope and permits simultaneous evaluation of gene copies and tissue morphology on the same slide. Large regions of the tissue section can be scanned rapidly in CISH using a conventional counterstain, such as hematoxylin or nuclear fast red. Amplification systems based on peroxidase-catalyzed deposition of biotinylated tyramine allow enhancement of the sensitivity of peroxidase-based systems and can be applied to AP-based detection (described later in this chapter). Routine detection of individual genes has been achieved using dinitrophenyl-labeled probes and automated SISH.

SIGNAL-ENHANCED DETECTION

Signal enhancements are approaches to improve the sensitivity of CISH. The catalyzed reporter deposition (CARD) technique is based on the deposition of activated biotinylated tyramine onto electron-rich moieties, such as tyrosine, phenylalanine, or tryptophan, at or near the sites of HRP activity. The biotin sites on the bound tyramide act as further binding sites for, e.g., streptavidin–biotin complexes or enzyme- and fluorochrome-labeled streptavidin. CARD allows between a 10- to 100-fold increase in sensitivity of ISH signals when compared to conventional avidin–biotin complex procedures without production of increased background. If biotin, digoxigenin, or dinitrophenyl or trinitrophenyl are used as haptens, which can act as further binding sites for antihapten antibodies or streptavidin conjugates, visualization of deposited tyramides can be performed directly after the CARD reaction with

bright-field microscopy. The main advantage of using CARD signal amplification for ISH is that it is performed after probe hybridization and stringent washings so that the specificity of the probe hybridization is not compromised. The practical limitations of CARD are caused by several factors. Because of its high sensitivity, CARD has the potential to amplify a nonspecific background signal, which may result in an unfavorable signal-to-noise ratio. Endogenous peroxidases in human tissue can catalyze the CARD reaction. To avoid this unwanted reaction, endogenous peroxidase must be blocked or quenched and appropriate positive and negative controls should be used. CARD has been applied successfully to detect both repetitive and single-copy DNA target sequences in cytospin and tissue specimens with high efficiency. By combining Nanogold® streptavidin and SISH with CARD, ISH sensitivity can be achieved to allow detection of single-copy sequences in formalin-fixed, paraffin-embedded section.

Branched DNA (bDNA) technology has been recently adapted to ISH for improving nucleic acid detection. To reduce potential nonspecific hybridization, non-natural nucleotides 5-methyl-2′-deoxyisocytidine and 2′-deoxyisoguanosine are included in the target, preamplifier, amplifier, and AP-conjugated label probes. AP labeled probes then catalyze the reaction of NBT/BCIP substrate. Because the original amount of the target remains unmodified, unlike the situation with target amplification methods, the main advantage is its specificity. The sensitivity of the bDNA ISH method is similar to CARD and is sufficient to detect relatively low-abundance targets, as few as one or two copies of human papillomavirus 16 (HPV-16) DNA in SiHa cells. bDNA ISH is based on the sequential hybridization of synthetic DNA probes; it does not require any DNA or RNA polymerase activity and repeated cycling through elevated temperatures. Another feature of bDNA is that bDNA ISH does not use an avidin–biotin signal amplification system and hence is not affected by binding of avidin-conjugated reporter molecules to endogenous biotin.

Rolling circle amplification (RCA) generates a localized signal using an isothermal amplification of an oligonucleotide circle, which can be performed using padlock probes as templates. The polymerase progresses continuously around the loop until the 100 base pairs have been replicated hundreds or thousands of times. Incorporating a labeled nucleotide during the RCA reaction produces a sufficient signal for easy visualization of the target. A single round of enzymatic amplification of a nucleic acid substrate leads to increased absolute amounts of measurable signal. RCA in situ used for discriminating alleles, determining gene copy number, and quantifying gene expression in single cells is an entirely new dimension to the fields of genomics, pathology, and cytogenetics. Because the procedure is technically complicated, application of RCA in situ in formalin-fixed, paraffin-embedded tissues has not been uniformly successful to date; future work is required to confirm its real potential.

DOUBLE OR TRIPLE CHROMOGENIC IN SITU HYBRIDIZATION

In performing double ISH methods for the simultaneous detection of multiple target nucleic acids, such as two mRNAs or DNA and mRNA, the two probes may be hybridized simultaneously or sequentially and the signals are detected either simultaneously or sequentially. Combinations of nonisotopic and isotopic ISH methods are mainly used for detection of two mRNAs in the same tissue sections. After histochemical detection for nonisotopic signals, the slides are subject to an autoradiographic approach for radioactive signals. A combination of two nonisotopic-labeled probes, mainly biotin and digoxigenin, conjugated to different enzymes (AP or HRP) or fluorescence is followed by respective detection systems to a simultaneous localization of multiple mRNA and genomic DNA at the same tissue sections, even in the same cells. For combined ISH–IHC, ISH is generally performed before IHC because it reduces the chances of RNase contamination.

Chromosome-specific DNA probes labeled with biotin, digoxigenin, or fluorescein can be hybridized simultaneously and then detected by enzyme cytochemistry using one AP reaction and two separate HRP reactions in sequence. For triple-color detection on single-cell preparations, the combination of the enzyme precipitates HRP–DAB (brown color), AP–fast red (red color), and HRP–tetramethylbenzidine (green color) usually results in an accurate detection of DNA targets. For ISH on tissue sections, however, this detection procedure showed some limitations with respect to both the stability of the AP–fast red and HRP–tetramethylbenzidine precipitates and the sequence of immunochemical layers in multiple-target procedures.

APPLICATIONS OF IN SITU HYBRIDIZATION

ISH methods have found many applications in basic research and in diagnostic pathology, such as identification of gene expression by the detection of mRNA, diagnosis of infectious agents, and molecular cytogenetics for detecting chromosomal abnormalities (Table 12-2).

TABLE 12-2
Details of ISH Procedure

PREPARATION OF SLIDES OR COVERSLIPS

e.g., Silane or poly-L-lysine treatment of slides

Sigma-coated coverslips

FIXATION OF MATERIAL ON SLIDE

By precipitation (e.g., ethanol)

By cross-linkage (e.g., formaldehyde)

TREATMENTS TO PREVENT BACKGROUND STAINING

Endogenous enzyme inactivation

RNase treatment

PERMEABILIZATION

Diluted acids

Detergent or alcohol

Proteases

Microwave

PREHYBRIDIZATION (OPTIONAL)

Incubation of specimen with a prehybridization solution (hybridization solution minus probe) performed at the same temperature as hybridization

Denaturation of probe and target:

- pH or heat
- Simultaneous or separate denaturation of probe and target (if double stranded)

HYBRIDIZATION

Main components of the solution:

- Denhardt's mix (ficoll, bovine serum albumin, polyvinylpyrrolidone)
- Heterologous nucleic acids (e.g., herring sperm DNA, transfer RNA, or competitor DNA)
- Sodium phosphate, ethylenediaminetetraacetic acid, sodium dodecyl sulfate, or salt

Formamide

- Dextran sulfate

POSTHYBRIDIZATION STEPS

Treatment with single-stranded specific nuclease (optional)

Stringency washes

IMMUNOLOGICAL DETECTION

Blocking step

Antibody incubation

Colorimetric substrate, fluorescence microscopy, or enzyme metallography

Counterstaining

Mounting

MICROSCOPY AND EVALUATION

Microscopic analysis of results and documentation

ISH, in situ hybridization; RNase, ribonuclease.

CHROMOGENIC AND SILVER VERSUS FLUORESCENT IN SITU HYBRIDIZATION

CISH and SISH are practical, cost-effective, and valid alternatives to fluorescent in situ hybridization (FISH) and can be easily integrated into routine testing in laboratories.

Compared to FISH, bright-field ISH offers four important advantages:
1. The histologic details of the paraffin section are generally better appreciated with a bright-field microscope.
2. The morphologic details are readily apparent using low-power objectives.
3. The probe signals are not subject to rapid fading.
4. Concomitant bright-field detection of proteins using IHC is possible.

INFECTIOUS DISEASES

ISH has been used for the identification of foreign genes or gene products, including bacteria, fungi, and viruses in tissue sections. Detection of those infectious agents with sensitive nonisotopic ISH methods provides valuable information about the etiology of the specific infectious disease, because many of the infectious agents can be readily visualized by CISH methods.

Viral infections have been widely investigated. Detection of human immunodeficiency virus (HIV), cytomegalovirus (CMV), HPV, herpes simplex virus (HSV), hepatitis C virus, Epstein-Barr virus (EBV), parvovirus B19 (PVB19), and polyomaviruses BK and JC are just some of the diagnostic applications of ISH methods (Figure 12-1). There are more than 100 types of HPV, and probes specific for the various types are available to assess infection by particular HPV types associated with neoplastic development. HPV types 16 and 18 are more likely to be associated with malignant progression. However, the role played by HPV in other lesions, including Bowen's disease, squamous cell papilloma of bronchus, and larynx, is unclear.

EBV has been implicated in the pathogenesis of various human lymphoid and epithelial tumors. It is difficult to detect viral DNA by ISH in latent infection because of the low copy number per cell. However, small nuclear RNAs encoded by the virus are highly expressed and detectable by nonisotopic ISH. EBV has been detected in some cases of Hodgkin's disease and in a variety of non-Hodgkin's lymphomas, including Burkitt lymphoma, a minority of B-cell non-Hodgkin's lymphomas, and some T-cell lymphomas, as well as in oral hairy leukoplakia. The presence of EBV in undifferentiated nasopharyngeal carcinoma can be used diagnostically to detect tumors from unknown primary sites (Figure 12-2A). ISH is useful in confirmation of infectious mononucleosis in atypical cases and of renal disease associated with EBV in patients with negative EBV serology.

Hepatitis C virus (HCV) is an attractive ISH target because IHC reagents are poor. Most studies have probed to formalin-fixed, paraffin-embedded tissues because of their availability and the excellent preservation of morphology, which allows a better localization of HCV. Few studies have applied this technique to frozen tissue. Most studies demonstrate that HCV-positive cells in liver are usually isolated with occasional clustering and less than 20% of cells are positive. HCV RNAs were shown in the cytoplasm of hepatocytes, with occasional signals detected in mononuclear cells, bile duct epithelium, and sinusoidal cells. The relationship between detection of HCV and cell damage is an important issue. The level of HCV positivity appeared to correlate with serum aminotransferase levels, suggesting that HCV might cause damage to the liver cells directly in the absence of overt morphologic changes.

ISH has been also applied to the identification of CMV in viral encephalitis and chronic encephalitis associated with acquired immunodeficiency syndrome (AIDS) and in chronic encephalitis with epilepsy. Pulmonary CMV involvement has been detected on cytologic specimens, and the extent of systemic disease has been documented where the presentation was of isolated oophoritis. CMV hepatitis has been demonstrated in liver allografts, and gastrointestinal biopsies have been used to detect infection in cardiac transplant recipients. However, for detection of CMV, there may not be a significantly greater sensitivity with ISH than with IHC. Other viruses, such as adenovirus (Figure 12-2B) and polyomavirus BK (Figure 12-2C), involved in specific human diseases can be readily detected by ISH. Other herpes viruses, including HSV, can be detected in cases of lymphadenitis and endometritis and can be demonstrated, such as human herpes virus 6 (HHV-6) in erythroderma associated with an infectious mononucleosis-like syndrome, in a variety of lymphoproliferative states and AIDS-associated retinitis. The presence of HHV-8 in Kaposi's sarcoma has been demonstrated using PCR-ISH. There is some evidence to suggest that ISH may not be as sensitive as IHC in the detection of HSV, but proper validation should be performed with the newer amplified techniques. ISH may still have an advantage over IHC in early HSV infection.

PVB19 is the etiologic agent of a range of clinical syndromes, such as postinfectious arthropathy, transient aplastic crises in patients with hemolytic disorders, chronic bone marrow failure in immunocompromised patients, and fetal hydrops. The clinical

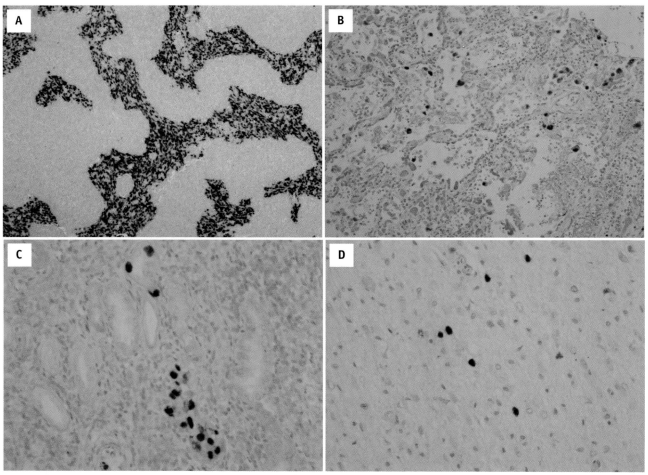

FIGURE 12-2

Detection of viruses by in situ hybridization (ISH). Examples of ISH using chromogenic methods. **A,** Detection of Epstein-Barr virus in a nasopharyngeal carcinoma metastatic to a cervical lymph node using Epstein-Barr virus-encoded small RNA oligonucleotide probes visualized by alkaline phosphatase (AP) with nitroblue tetrazolium and 5-bromo-4-chloro-3-indolyl phosphate (NBT/BCIP) as chromogen substrate. **B,** ISH for adenovirus in a lung specimen using an adenovirus complementary DNA probe with AP and NBT/BCIP. **C,** ISH positive signals for polyomavirus BK in the nuclei of tubular epithelium from a renal transplant case using a DNA probe with AP and NBT/BCIP. **D,** ISH positive cells for polyomavirus JC in a brain biopsy from a patient with progressive multifocal leukoencephalopathy.

and histopathologic patterns of PVB19-associated diseases are the result of a balance among virus, host target cells, and immune response. Identification of PVB19 by means of routine histology is seen only in lytic infections by the detection of viral inclusion bodies in cells. ISH with digoxigenin-labeled DNA probe demonstrated that lytic infections were associated with PVB19-specific target cells in formalin-fixed, paraffin-embedded tissues.

The genus *Legionella*, family Legionellaceae, causes human disease, most commonly opportunistic pneumonia in immunocompromised patients. Several methods have been used to identify these organisms in paraffin-embedded tissue sections, including various histochemical and immunohistochemical techniques. *Legionella* pneumonia is caused by the inhalation of viable organisms in fine aerosols into the lung. The organism subsequently invades the alveolar macro-

phages and other phagocytic cells. Because of slow growth and lack of suitable phenotypic tests, identification of *Legionella* spp. remains difficult. Nonradioactive ISH of whole cells with rRNA-targeted oligonucleotide probes has become a highly valuable tool for the specific detection of individual microbial cells without cultivation. *Helicobacter pylori,* the causative agent of chronic gastritis, and peptic ulcers are also associated with gastric cancer. Eradication of *H. pylori* infection may be difficult to confirm. The specificity of an ISH assay for *H. pylori* was proved by the lack of hybridization on sections with gram-negative and gram-positive bacteria other than *H. pylori,* using various controls. CISH is a highly sensitive and reliable method for detecting macrolide-resistant *H. pylori* in formalin-fixed, paraffin-embedded biopsy specimens, which represents the routine method of processing tissue obtained upon gastroscopy.

The specific identification of yeast and yeast-like organisms in tissue sections can sometimes be quite difficult because several common species have overlapping histologic features. *Blastomyces dermatitidis, Coccidioides immitis, Cryptococcus neoformans, Histoplasma capsulatum,* and *Sporothrix schenckii* can be specifically detected with ISH by using probes against specific rRNA in formalin-fixed, paraffin-embedded tissue specimens. ISH was uniformly positive with all species-specific probes yielding 100% specificity. ISH also had a higher positive predictive value (100% in all cases) compared with Grocott methenamine silver staining (83.3% to 100%). Four cases with rare organisms present (4% of cases tested) were detected by ISH but not by Grocott methenamine silver staining. These results show that ISH provides a rapid and accurate technique for the identification of fungal organisms in histologic tissue sections (Figure 12-3A,B). Aspergillosis results in significant mortality in immunosuppressed patients. Rapid diagnosis is often required to initiate appropriate therapy. The histology of the *Aspergillus* spp. may overlap with a variety of fungi, so diagnosis often relies on fungal cultures that can take weeks to complete. ISH targeting *Aspergillus* 5S rRNA identified 41 localized aspergillomas in the lung, brain, sinonasal tract, and ear, and 2 cases of invasive aspergillosis involving pleura and soft tissue of the scapular region. The diagnosis of *Pneumocystis carinii* by ISH was performed on formalin-fixed, paraffin-embedded human lung tissues and detected with the avidin–biotin peroxidase complex method. The reactions were positive in all 12 cases of *P. carinii* pneumonia but in none of the infections with other pathogenic agents, including viruses (6 cases), mycobacteria (4 cases), protozoa (4 cases), and fungi (8 cases). The reactivity and specificity of this method was comparable with that of IHC using a monoclonal antihuman *P. carinii* antibody.

GENE EXPRESSION

Gene expression is the process by which gene-coded information is converted into the structures present and operating in the cell. Expressed genes include those transcribed into mRNA and then translated into protein and those transcribed into RNA but not translated into protein (e.g., transfer RNA and rRNA).

CISH methods are powerful tools for the analysis of gene expression (Box 12-1) in normal and pathologic tissues. A major advantage of ISH is its ability to localize mRNA at the cellular level in heterogeneous tissues, thus expanding the results of other molecular techniques, such as Northern blot hybridization, for specific gene analysis. CISH methods have been of particular value for the study of mRNA-encoding oncogenes, growth factors and their receptors, hormones and their receptors, cytokines, structural proteins, and enzymes. There are many practical applications of ISH methods in tumor pathology. The correlation of oncogene expression with prognosis is being investigated in neuroblastomas and epithelial neoplasms such as colon, lung, prostate, and breast carcinomas. Detection of genes encoding cell structural proteins, including tumor-associated markers, represents potential areas of application of ISH methods in pathologic diagnosis. For example, nonisotopic ISH methods for localization of immunoglobulin light chain mRNAs in hyperplastic and neoplastic lymphoproliferative disorders, albumin mRNA for distinguishing between hepatocellular

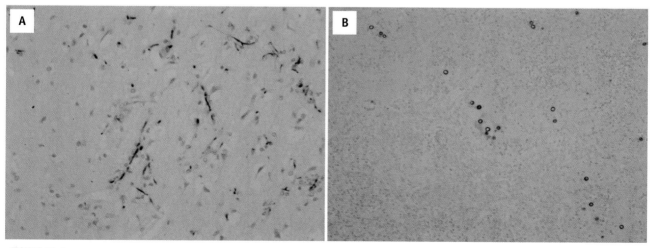

FIGURE 12-3
Detection of fungus by in situ hybridization (ISH). ISH to detect specific fungal organisms. **A,** Detection of *Aspergillus* by ISH in a brain biopsy. The organisms are detected using oligonucleotide probes targeted at the ribosomal RNA visualized by alkaline phosphatase and nitroblue tetrazolium and 5-bromo-4-chloro-3-indolyl phosphate. **B,** In situ hybridization detecting *Blastomyces* infection.

carcinomas and metastatic carcinomas to the liver (Figure 12-4A,B), and chromogranin or secretogranin mRNAs for classification of neuroendocrine tumors are used in some diagnostic pathology laboratories. ISH methods used to identify cells or tumors on the basis of their specific mRNA content are different from IHC, which depends on the protein content of cells. Thus, ISH identifies the gene products from de novo synthesis—rather than potentially nonspecific uptake of proteins by cells, which may result in false-positive immunostaining results. ISH analysis has also been used extensively in studies of endocrine tumors. For example, some small-cell lung carcinomas with few secretory granules are commonly negative for chromogranin proteins, but the mRNAs may be detected by ISH methods. Studies of gene expression in endocrine tumors, including chromogranin A, thyroglobulin, estrogen receptor proteins, parathyroid hormones, and calcitonin gene-related peptide, by ISH have contributed to our understanding of the biology and pathophysiology of various endocrine disorders.

Proliferative capacity is an important determinant of tumor biologic behavior. The expression of histone genes is a fundamental step in the process of cell proliferation. Histone H3 mRNA accumulates in the cytoplasm during S phase, then decreases as cells approach G2 phase. Histone H3 mRNA levels depend on transcriptional and post-transcriptional mechanisms, with transcription rates increasing 10-fold at the onset of S phase and being downregulated at the cessation of cell proliferation and during quiescence. The histone H3 mRNA level is a specific marker of S-phase cells. The principal advantage of histone H3 mRNA determinations by ISH is that the results are tightly coupled with de novo DNA synthesis.

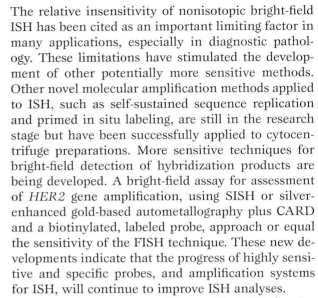

CONCLUSION

The relative insensitivity of nonisotopic bright-field ISH has been cited as an important limiting factor in many applications, especially in diagnostic pathology. These limitations have stimulated the development of other potentially more sensitive methods. Other novel molecular amplification methods applied to ISH, such as self-sustained sequence replication and primed in situ labeling, are still in the research stage but have been successfully applied to cytocentrifuge preparations. More sensitive techniques for bright-field detection of hybridization products are being developed. A bright-field assay for assessment of *HER2* gene amplification, using SISH or silver-enhanced gold-based autometallography plus CARD and a biotinylated, labeled probe, approach or equal the sensitivity of the FISH technique. These new developments indicate that the progress of highly sensitive and specific probes, and amplification systems for ISH, will continue to improve ISH analyses.

PCR with ISH can amplify specific DNA (in situ PCR) or RNA (in situ RT-PCR) sequences inside single cells or tissue sections and increases the copy numbers to levels readily detectable by conventional ISH methods. In theory, in situ PCR techniques should be reproducible like conventional PCR. In practice, however, in situ PCR can be associated with many problems, such as low amplification efficiency, poor reproducibility, and amplicon diffusion. Direct in situ PCR can be influenced by incorporation of labeled nucleotides into nonspecific PCR products resulting from mispriming. Rigorous use of controls is required to allow adequate interpretation

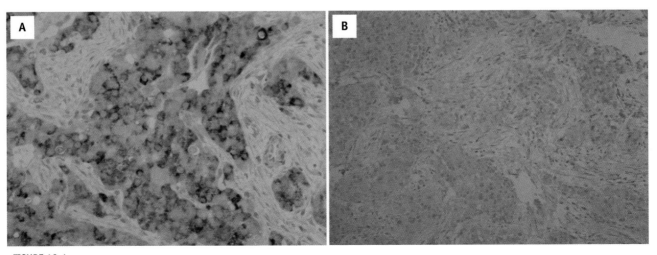

FIGURE 12-4

Detection of messenger RNAs (mRNAs) by in situ hybridization (ISH). **A,** ISH detecting albumin mRNA in a hepatocellular carcinoma metastatic to the scapula using riboprobes with alkaline phosphatase and nitroblue tetrazolium and 5-bromo-4-chloro-3-indolyl phosphate. Albumin mRNA expression is relatively specific for normal and neoplastic liver cells. **B,** The sense control probe is negative.

of in situ PCR results. The employment of in situ PCR to detect low copy number viral genes, especially HIV and HCV, has led to significant discoveries about viral infectious diseases. Although extremely versatile and sensitive, in situ PCR has limitations, with suboptimal preservation of morphology of some biologic structures and lack of reliability as a quantitative method. Clinical application of in situ PCR must await the resolution of some current limitations.

Several companies are developing automated systems for ISH. HPV, EBV, and several other ISH tests are now automated and validated on the BenchMark System of Ventana Medical Systems. Automated ISH is chosen and assigned to a specific protocol stored in the computer for each step. Reaction conditions for in situ staining are selected by varying the type, temperature, and time of all steps, including tissue pretreatment, denaturation of the probe and target sequences, hybridization, stringency, and detection. The main advantages of automated ISH are the short time of the entire procedure (on the order of a few hours), labor savings, reproducibility, and access for a broader range of laboratories. Other companies are sure to follow in the ISH automation market, a market now established in diagnostic anatomic pathology.

SUGGESTED READINGS

Basic Principles of In Situ Hybridization

Ambinder RF, Mann RB: Epstein-Barr–encoded RNA in situ hybridization: Diagnostic applications. Hum Pathol 1994;25:602–605.

Arnould L, Denoux Y, MacGrogan G, et al: Agreement between chromogenic in situ hybridization (CISH) and FISH in the determination of HER2 status in breast cancer. Br J Cancer 2003;88:1587–1591.

Baskin DG, Stahl WL: Fundamentals of quantitative autoradiography by computer densitometry for in situ hybridization, with emphasis on 33P. J Histochem Cytochem 1993;41:1767–1776.

Carr NJ, Talbot IC: In situ end labelling: Effect of proteolytic enzyme pretreatment and hydrochloric acid. Mol Pathol 1997;50:160–163.

DeLellis RA: In situ hybridization techniques for the analysis of gene expression: Applications in tumor pathology. Hum Pathol 1994;25:580–585.

Denijn M, Schuurman HJ, Jacobse KC, De Weger RA: In situ hybridization: A valuable tool in diagnostic pathology. APMIS 1992;100:669–681.

Hayden RT, Qian X, Roberts GD, Lloyd RV In situ hybridization for the identification of yeastlike organisms in tissue section. Diagn Mol Pathol 2001;10:15–23.

Hayden RT, Uhl JR, Qian X, et al: Direct detection of Legionella species from bronchoalveolar lavage and open lung biopsy specimens: Comparison of LightCycler PCR, in situ hybridization, direct fluorescence antigen detection, and culture. J Clin Microbiol 2001;39:2618–2626.

Hopman AH, Claessen S, Speel EJ: Multi-colour bright-field in situ hybridisation on tissue sections. Histochem Cell Biol 1997;108:291–298.

Jin L, Lloyd RV: In situ hybridization: Methods and applications. J Clin Lab Anal 1997;11(1):2–9.

Lisowski AR, English ML, Opsahl AC, et al: Effect of the storage period of paraffin sections on the detection of mRNAs by in situ hybridization. J Histochem Cytochem 2001;49:927–928.

Marquez A, Wu R, Zhao J, et al: Evaluation of epidermal growth factor receptor (EGFR) by chromogenic in situ hybridization (CISH) and immunohistochemistry (IHC) in archival gliomas using bright-field microscopy. Diagn Mol Pathol 2004;13:1–8.

Miller MA, Kolb PE, Raskind MA: A method for simultaneous detection of multiple mRNAs using digoxigenin and radioisotopic cRNA probes. J Histochem Cytochem 1993;41:1741–1750.

Mitsuhashi M: Technical report: Part 1. Basic requirements for designing optimal oligonucleotide probe sequences. J Clin Lab Anal 1996;10:277–284.

Nitta H, Kishimoto J, Grogan TM: Application of automated mRNA in situ hybridization for formalin-fixed, paraffin-embedded mouse skin sections: Effects of heat and enzyme pretreatment on mRNA signal detection. Appl Immunohistochem Mol Morphol 2003;11:183–187.

Oliver KR, Heavens RP, Sirinathsinghji DJ: Quantitative comparison of pretreatment regimens used to sensitize in situ hybridization using oligonucleotide probes on paraffin-embedded brain tissue. J Histochem Cytochem 1997;45:1707–1713.

Pellestor F, Paulasova P: The peptide nucleic acids, efficient tools for molecular diagnosis. 2004;13:521–525.

Pollanen R, Vuopala S, Lehto VP: Detection of human papillomavirus infection by non-isotopic in situ hybridisation in condylomatous and CIN lesions. J Clin Pathol 1993;46:936–939.

Pringle JH, Primrose L, Kind CN, et al: In situ hybridization demonstration of poly-adenylated RNA sequences in formalin-fixed paraffin sections using a biotinylated oligonucleotide poly d(T) probe. J Pathol 1989;158:279–286.

Qian X, Bauer RA, Xu HS, Lloyd RV: In situ hybridization detection of calcitonin mRNA in routinely fixed, paraffin-embedded tissue sections: A comparison of different types of probes combined with tyramide signal amplification. Appl Immunohistochem Mol Morphol 2001;9:61–69.

Qian X, Guerrero RB, Plummer TB, et al: Detection of hepatitis C virus RNA in formalin-fixed paraffin-embedded sections with digoxigenin-labeled cRNA probes. Diagn Mol Pathol 2004;13:9–14.

Qian X, Lloyd RV: Recent developments in signal amplification methods for in situ hybridization. Diagn Mol Pathol 2003;12:1–13.

Speel EJ: Robert Feulgen Prize Lecture 1999. Detection and amplification systems for sensitive, multiple-target DNA and RNA in situ hybridization: Looking inside cells with a spectrum of colors. Histochem Cell Biol 1999;112(2):89–113.

Sperry A, Jin L, Lloyd RV: Microwave treatment enhances detection of RNA and DNA by in situ hybridization. Diagn Mol Pathol 1996;5:291–296.

Steel JH, Jeffery RE, Longcroft JM, et al: Comparison of isotopic and non-isotopic labelling for in situ hybridisation of various mRNA targets with cRNA probes. Eur J Histochem 1998;42:143–150.

Temsamani J, Agrawal S: Enzymatic labeling of nucleic acids. Mol Biotechnol 1996;5:223–232.

Tubbs R, Pettay J, Skacel M, et al: Gold-facilitated in situ hybridization: A bright-field autometallographic alternative to fluorescence in situ hybridization for detection of HER-2/neu gene amplification. Am J Pathol 2002;160:1589–1595.

Weiss LM, Chen YY: Effects of different fixatives on detection of nucleic acids from paraffin-embedded tissues by in situ hybridization using oligonucleotide probes. J Histochem Cytochem 1991;39:1237– 1242.

Wilcox JN: Fundamental principles of in situ hybridization. J Histochem Cytochem 1993;41:1725–1733.

Witkiewicz H, Bolander ME, Edwards DR: Improved design of riboprobes from pBluescript® and related vectors for in situ hybridization. Biotechniques 1993;14:458–463.

Yoshii A, Koji T, Ohsawa N, Nakane PK: In situ localization of ribosomal RNAs is a reliable reference for hybridizable RNA in tissue sections. J Histochem Cytochem 1995;43:321–327.

Yulug IG, Yulug A, Fisher EM: The frequency and position of Alu repeats in cDNAs, as determined by database searching. Genomics 1995;27:544–548.

Zehbe I, Hacker GW, Su H, et al: Sensitive in situ hybridization with catalyzed reporter deposition, streptavidin-Nanogold, and silver acetate autometallography: Detection of single-copy human papillomavirus. Am J Pathol 1997;150:1553–1561.

Signal-Enhanced Detection

Christian AT, Pattee MS, Attix CM, et al: Detection of DNA point mutations and mRNA expression levels by rolling circle amplification in individual cells. Proc Natl Acad Sci USA 2001;98:14238–14243.

Hopman AH, Ramaekers FC, Speel EJ: Rapid synthesis of biotin-, digoxigenin-, trinitrophenyl-, and fluorochrome-labeled tyramides and their application for in situ hybridization using CARD amplification. J Histochem Cytochem 1998;46:771–777.

Player AN, Shen LP, Kenny D, et al: Single-copy gene detection using branched DNA (bDNA) in situ hybridization. J Histochem Cytochem 2001;49:603–612.

Speel EJ, Hopman AH, Komminoth P: Amplification methods to increase the sensitivity of in situ hybridization: Play card(s). J Histochem Cytochem 1999;47:281–288.

Trembleau A, Roche D, Calas A: Combination of non-radioactive and radioactive in situ hybridization with immunohistochemistry: A new method allowing the simultaneous detection of two mRNAs and one antigen in the same brain tissue section. J Histochem Cytochem 1993;41:489–498.

Urdea MS: Branched DNA signal amplification. Biotechnology 1994;12:926–928.

Zhou Y, Calciano M, Hamann S, et al: In situ detection of messenger RNA using digoxigenin-labeled oligonucleotides and rolling circle amplification. Exp Mol Pathol 2001;70:281–288.

Applications of In Situ Hybridization

Aksamit AJ Jr: Nonradioactive in situ hybridization in progressive multifocal leukoencephalopathy. Mayo Clin Proc 1993;68:899–910.

Bagasra O, Seshamma T, Hansen J, et al: Application of in situ PCR methods in molecular biology: I. Details of methodology for general use. Cell Vision 1994;1:324–335.

Bashir MS, Lewis FA, Quirke P, et al: In situ hybridisation for the identification of Helicobacter pylori in paraffin wax–embedded tissue. J Clin Pathol 1994;47:862–864.

Boshoff C, Schulz TF, Kennedy MM, et al: Kaposi's sarcoma–associated herpes virus infects endothelial and spindle cells. Nat Med 1995;1:1274–1278.

Chang M, Marquardt AP, Wood BL, et al: In situ distribution of hepatitis C virus replicative-intermediate RNA in hepatic tissue and its correlation with liver disease. J Virol 2000;74:944–955.

Collina G, Rossi E, Bettelli S, et al: Detection of human papillomavirus in extragenital Bowen's disease using in situ hybridization and polymerase chain reaction. Am J Dermatopathol 1995;17:236–241.

Fillet AM, Reux I, Joberty C, et al: Detection of human herpes virus 6 in AIDS-associated retinitis by means of in situ hybridization, polymerase chain reaction and immunohistochemistry. J Med Virol 1996;49:289–295.

Gaffey MJ, Ben-Ezra JM, Weiss LM: Herpes simplex lymphadenitis. Am J Clin Pathol 1991;95:709–714.

Hayashi Y, Watanabe J, Nakata K, et al: A novel diagnostic method of Pneumocystis carinii: In situ hybridization of ribosomal ribonucleic acid with biotinylated oligonucleotide probes. Lab Invest 1990;63:576–580.

Hummel M, Anagnostopoulos I, Dallenbach F, et al: EBV infection patterns in Hodgkin's disease and normal lymphoid tissue: Expression and cellular localization of EBV gene products. Br J Haematol 1992;82:689–694.

Kotelnikov V, Cass L, Coon JS, et al: Accuracy of histone H3 messenger RNA in situ hybridization for the assessment of cell proliferation in human tissues. Clin Cancer Res 1997;3:669–673.

Loriot MA, Marcellin P, Walker F, et al: Persistence of hepatitis B virus DNA in serum and liver from patients with chronic hepatitis B after loss of HBsAg. J Hepatol 1997;27:251–258.

Martinez A, Miller MJ, Quinn K, et al: Non-radioactive localization of nucleic acids by direct in situ PCR and in situ RT-PCR in paraffin-embedded sections. J Histochem Cytochem 1995;43:739–747.

Montone KT, Litzky LA: Rapid method for detection of Aspergillus 5S ribosomal RNA using a genus-specific oligonucleotide probe. Am J Clin Pathol 1995;103:48–51.

Murakami T, Hagiwara T, Yamamoto K, et al: A novel method for detecting HIV-1 by non-radioactive in situ hybridization: Application of a peptide nucleic acid probe and catalysed signal amplification. J Pathol 2001;194:130–135.

Musiani M, Zerbini M, Venturoli S, et al: Rapid diagnosis of cytomegalovirus encephalitis in patients with AIDS using in situ hybridisation. J Clin Pathol 1994;47:886–891.

Niedobitek G: Patterns of Epstein-Barr virus infection in non-Hodgkin's lymphomas. J Pathol 1995;175:259–261.

Walters C, Powe DG, Padfield CJ, Fagan DG: Detection of parvovirus B19 in macerated fetal tissue using in situ hybridisation. J Clin Pathol 1997;50:749–754.

Wu TC, Mann RB, Epstein JI, et al: Abundant expression of EBER1 small nuclear RNA in nasopharyngeal carcinoma: A morphologically distinctive target for detection of Epstein-Barr virus in formalin-fixed paraffin-embedded carcinoma specimens. Am J Pathol 1991;138:1461–1469.

13 Immunoglobulin and T-Cell Receptor Gene Rearrangement

Margaret L. Gulley

INTRODUCTION

The first molecular test of any kind to be routinely available in clinical laboratories was Southern blot analysis of the immunoglobulin *(IG)* heavy chain gene as a marker of B-cell clonality. Subsequently, T-cell receptor *(TR)* β and γ gene rearrangement testing was added to clinical test menus for ancillary diagnosis of T-cell neoplasms. In the 1990s, polymerase chain reaction (PCR) testing began to supplement Southern blot analysis for the assessment of B- and T-cell clonality. The long track record of these ancillary procedures is a testament to their utility in resolving dilemmas not otherwise decipherable by standard morphology or immunophenotyping. Despite their long history of use, B- and T-cell gene rearrangement assays remain among the most complicated assays to design, perform, and interpret.

This chapter summarizes the concepts underlying clonality assessment and reviews the technologies commonly used to distinguish monoclonal from polyclonal lymphoid processes based on *IG* and *TR* gene analysis. Automated instrumentation and commercial kits that facilitate implementation of gene rearrangement assays are discussed. Potential pitfalls and guidance for improving outcomes are discussed as they related to preanalytic, analytic, and interpretation phases of testing.

TISSUE REQUIREMENTS AND NUCLEIC ACID EXTRACTION

Nearly all gene rearrangement tests rely on extracted DNA as the substrate for analysis. Although fragments of DNA have been recovered from bodies mummified thousands of years ago and fossilized cells that lived more than a million years ago, it is important to carefully prepare and handle clinical specimens to optimize the quality of DNA used for gene rearrangement testing. This is particularly true for samples to be analyzed by the Southern blot technique, in which "degradation" (i.e., nonspecific fragmentation) of the DNA confounds interpretation of results. Southern blot analysis is thus restricted to fresh or frozen tissue from which high molecular weight DNA can be extracted. Even with DNA amplification methods such as PCR, it is often true that frozen tissue yields better outcomes than does paraffin-embedded tissue, probably because certain fixatives, such as formalin, tend to cross-link DNA, thus making it unavailable for hybridization. When preparing blood or marrow aspirates, heparin should be avoided because it interferes with certain enzymatic reactions used in molecular laboratories. Finally, it is important that the sample be representative of the lymphoid lesion; when multiple blocks or aliquots of a specimen are available, choose the one with the highest proportion of lesional cells to improve the chance of detecting a neoplastic process (Box 13-1).

PRINCIPLES OF CLONALITY

A fundamental concept unifying all cancers is clonality, whereby a malignancy arises when *one* cell among the trillions in a patient's body acquires a genetic defect or defects, triggering uncontrolled cell proliferation. In the case of lymphomas and lymphoid leukemias, chromosomal translocation is oftentimes the critical pathogenic event, although sometimes additional or alternative mechanisms appear to be required for tumorigenesis, such as deletion, mutation, or even viral infection. Regardless of which genetic defect might initiate tumor cell growth, the defect is passed to all cellular progeny within a tumor clone. Certain defects are characteristic of specific types of cancer, and these defects serve as markers of the malignancy that can be used to assist in diagnosis and in monitoring residual disease after therapy. Furthermore, knowledge of the affected biochemical pathway is used to design more effective therapies that target the underlying cause of malignant cell growth.

High-grade transformation is accompanied by the acquisition of additional genetic defects that confer a more aggressive phenotype.

Lymphomas and lymphoid leukemias commonly harbor chromosomal translocations involving the antigen receptor genes, i.e., the *IG* genes for the heavy chain, and the κ and λ light chains *(IGH, IGK, and IGL)* or the T-cell receptor genes α, β, γ, and δ *(TRA, TRB, TRG, and TRD)*. Such translocations are thought to represent errors occurring during physiologic gene rearrangement. Genes located at the reciprocal translocation breakpoint are putative oncogenes whose expression is often dysregulated by juxtaposition with the antigen receptor gene. For example, the t(8;14) translocation of Burkitt lymphoma juxtaposes the *MYC* gene on chromosome 8 with the *IGH* gene on chromosome 14, thus altering expression of the *MYC* oncogene, which, in turn, alters cell cycle regulation. Likewise, the *CCND1* gene encoding cyclin D1 is dysregulated by juxtaposition with the *IGH* gene in mantle cell lymphomas and some myelomas, and the *BCL2* gene is dysregulated by heavy or light chain gene juxtaposition in follicular lymphomas and in a subset of diffuse large-cell lymphomas.

IMMUNOGLOBULIN GENE REARRANGEMENT

In addition to any translocation that a lymphoid neoplasm may have, B-cell leukemias and lymphomas have an additional clonal marker in their rearranged *IG* genes. These genes, including *IGH, IGK,* and in some cases *IGL*, normally rearrange to encode the antigen receptor first expressed on the B-cell surface and later secreted as antibody by the terminally differentiated plasma cells.

During physiologic gene rearrangement, portions of the *IG* gene are spliced out to create a unique coding sequence made up of variable, diversity, joining, and constant regions (Figure 13-1). Because each developing B-cell splices these segments differently, polyclonal B-cell populations harbor multiple independent *IG* gene rearrangements. If a B cell acquires a genetic defect that renders it neoplastic, then that cell's particular *IG* coding sequence is inherited by all tumor cell progeny. Therefore, clonal *IG* gene rearrangement becomes a marker to distinguish monoclonal tumor cells from polyclonal reactive cells. *IG* gene rearrangement also serves as a marker, albeit imperfect, of commitment to the B-cell lineage. Information on clonality and lineage is helpful for distinguishing B-cell neoplasia from benign lymphoid hyperplasia and from a tumor of non-B-cell origin.

Southern blot analysis is considered the gold-standard assay for identifying clonal *IGH* or *IGK*

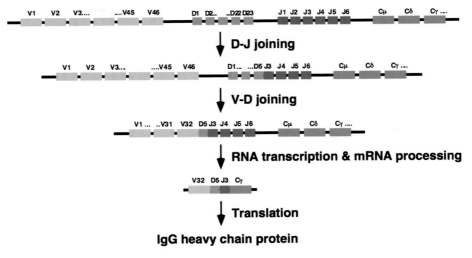

FIGURE 13-1

The immunoglobulin (Ig) heavy chain gene rearranges through a process of splicing and deletion, whereby 1 of 23 diversity (D) regions is juxtaposed with 1 of 6 joining (J) regions and then with 1 of about 46 variable (V) regions. Random nucleotides may be inserted between each splice junction to further increase diversity of the unique VDJ coding sequence. Subsequent splicing of a constant (C) segment establishes the isotype (IgM, IgD, IgG, IgA, or IgE) of the encoded heavy chain. This heavy chain complexes with κ or λ light chain protein to produce a functional antibody molecule. Note: Only the functional V, D, and J segments are displayed here; pseudogenes are not counted among the options shown here, although they may contribute to further allelic diversity among nonfunctional alleles in normal or neoplastic lymphocytes.

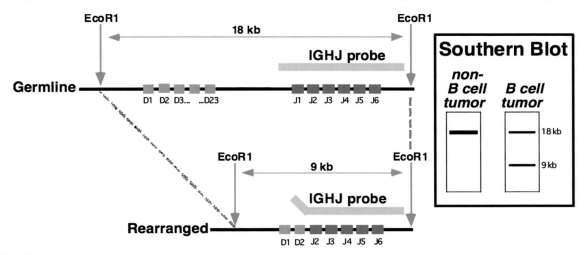

FIGURE 13-2

Southern blot analysis of an immunoglobulin heavy chain *(IGH)* gene distinguishes a monoclonal B-cell tumor from tissue lacking such a tumor. *IGH* gene arrangement involves splicing of 1 of 23 diversity (D) segments with 1 of 6 joining (J) segments, thus altering the size of the DNA fragment resulting from EcoR1 restriction enzyme digestion (green arrows). A labeled probe (pink bar) hybridizes across the J region to permit visualization of the digested fragments on Southern blots (right panel). Any B-cell tumor (leukemia, lymphoma, myeloma) harboring a monoclonal *IGH* rearrangement yields an extra band, whereas any other tissue produces only a single 18-kilobase band corresponding to the size of the germline fragment. Although normal B cells are undoubtedly present in virtually any tissue sample, their polyclonal rearrangements are invisible on Southern blots because of the diversity of their corresponding DNA fragments. On the other hand, a germline band is virtually always visible, even in lymphomas characterized by sheets of malignant B cells, because nontumor cells are present in the specimen and because the malignant cells may contain an unrearranged *IGH* allele.

gene rearrangement. (The *IGL* gene is not generally targeted because this gene is rearranged in only a third of B cells and B-cell neoplasms.) Southern analysis relies on restriction fragment size alterations in rearranged DNA compared with germline DNA, thus yielding extra bands in samples harboring clonal gene rearrangements (Figure 13-2). In theory, Southern blot analysis detects 100% of B-cell clones if the following three assumptions are met: First, high molecular weight DNA must be completely digested with restriction endonucleases. Second, the B-cell clone must exceed about 5% of cells in the tissue sample. Finally, the probe and restriction enzymes should be chosen to target portions of the gene that are consistently rearranged but are not likely to be mutated at the restriction enzyme cut sites so that extra bands are visualized only when clonal gene rearrangement is present. Probes targeting the joining region of the *IGH* or *IGK* genes work well in this regard, and it is widely accepted that extra bands must be visualized in at least two different restriction enzyme digests to interpret a case as clonal (whereas an abnormal band pattern in a single digest could be attributable to point mutation). As with all clinical laboratory tests, appropriate validation studies, quality control, and proficiency testing are essential (Box 13-2).

Because Southern blot analysis is labor intensive with a slow turnaround time, many laboratories have

---

BOX 13-2
Amplification *IGH* Relies on a Series of Assumptions

► Variable and joining regions of the gene are brought into proximity following rearrangement, allowing successful amplification of rearranged variable, diversity, and joining segments.

► Homology among the various gene segments allows consensus primers to be designed that hybridize to most of the 46 variable regions and to all 6 joining regions, thus permitting amplification of most variable, diversity, and joining combinations.

► Clonal rearrangement in tumor cells is detectable despite the polyclonal background rearrangements emanating from reactive B cells in the same tissue.

---

turned to PCR as a faster and less expensive alternative for detecting clonal *IGH* gene rearrangement. Modern PCR protocols permit detection of more than 90% of all B-cell clones by employing primers designed to maximize detection of every possible *IGH* gene rearrangement. Consensus primers can be used because of sequence homologies among subsets of segments in the *IGH* gene. The variable segments are classified into three families (frameworks 1, 2, and 3) that can be targeted by a limited number of consensus primers. Multiple primers can be combined in a multiplex PCR to distinguish monoclonal from polyclonal B-cell lesions (Figure 13-3).

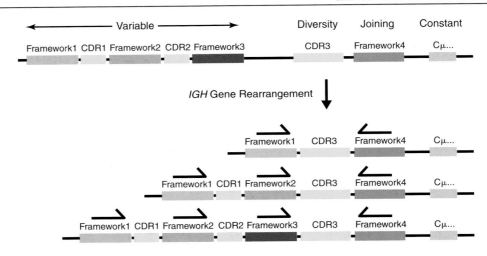

FIGURE 13-3

Polymerase chain reaction (PCR) assays can be designed to amplify across the rearranged immunoglobulin heavy chain gene. In the germline configuration depicted at the top, the variable and joining regions are too far apart (>1 kilobase) for reliable amplification. However, as depicted below, a rearranged gene juxtaposes the variable and joining segments so that PCR amplification across the spliced variable, diversity, and joining segments is feasible. To maximize detection of the many alternative variable, diversity, and joining variants while minimizing the number of primers required, a cocktail of consensus primers (shown as half arrows) targets each of four framework regions that are relatively well conserved compared to the interspersed complementary determining regions (CDR1, CDR2, and CDR3), which are quite mutation prone.

About 70% of B-cell tumors harbor clonal rearrangement detectable with framework 3 primers, and an additional 15% to 20% are detectable if framework 2 primers are added. Targeting framework 1 contributes little to the success rate, partly because product sizes are large and are not efficiently amplified, particularly in paraffin-embedded tissues. Somatic mutation also can interfere with amplification because of poor primer binding, and this is a major reason postgerminal center tumors such as follicular lymphoma and myeloma are less amenable to *IGH* amplification. To facilitate molecular diagnosis of follicular lymphoma, primers targeting *BCL2-IGH* translocation are often included. Amplification of the rearranged *IGK* gene can also be used as a supplementary test for B-cell clonality. However, lack of clonal rearrangement by all of these amplification assays does not exclude the presence of a B-cell clone. If negative by PCR, then Southern analysis can be used as a backup method (if fresh or frozen tissue is available).

Amplification tests are less labor intensive than Southern analysis. Another advantage is their suitability for use on small or fixed DNA samples, such as those derived from paraffin blocks. Amplification is not foolproof, however, and caution should be exerted when interpreting results. If no PCR product is generated, the quality of the DNA extracted from that specimen is called into question because polyclonal B cells are present in nearly all human tissues; a (larger) control sequence may be amplified to show whether amplifiable DNA is present. To reduce the possibility that DNA from a single

lymphocyte produces a seemingly clonal product, duplicate amplifications should be done to verify that the same product size is generated before concluding that a clonal population is present. Finally, use of primers targeting more than one framework often provides confirmatory data (Figure 13-4).

Although PCR is noteworthy for its ability to amplify translocation breakpoints down to a level of 1 in 1 million cells, its ability to detect clonal *IG* gene rearrangement is limited by competition from reactive lymphocytes in the sample. "Sensitivity controls" should be used to prove that the assay can detect a small clone. Typically, clones comprising 5% of cells are detectable, which is equivalent to the sensitivity achieved by Southern blot analysis. The sensitivity of the assay in a particular sample depends on myriad factors, including the relative proportion of neoplastic versus reactive lymphocytes and the sensitivity of the detection system for identifying a monoclonal population amid a polyclonal background.

Use of high-resolution capillary gel electrophoresis appears to improve visualization of very small clones above a polyclonal background. Heteroduplex analysis and melting curve analysis are alternative methods for resolving clonal populations. Results should be interpreted with caution, because a small clone does not necessarily represent a malignant clone.

Progress is being made in using *IG* or *TR* gene rearrangement as a marker of minimal residual disease. To accomplish this, the rearranged gene from a primary tumor is sequenced so that a tumor-specific junctional probe can be developed and then

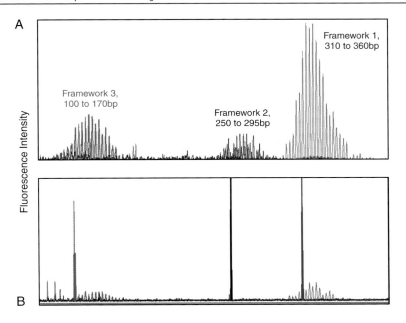

FIGURE 13-4

Immunoglobulin heavy chain *(IGH)* gene polymerase chain reaction (PCR) followed by capillary electrophoresis permits rapid evaluation of B-cell clonality. Variable region primers were labeled with a fluorochrome so that PCR products could be visualized on electropherograms. Each peak represents successful amplification of variable, diversity, and joining segments of a given length. **A,** The pattern characteristic of reactive tonsil tissue in which polyclonal B lymphocytes produce a bell-shaped spectrum of peaks. **B,** The pattern characteristic of a B-cell lymphoma in which a single peak predominates because most B lymphocytes in the tissue sample have the same clonal *IGH* gene rearrangement that characterizes the tumor clone. In cases with ambiguous peak patterns, correlation with morphology and immunophenotype to discern the proportion of atypical cells is helpful in interpreting the molecular findings.

hybridized to post-therapy DNA samples to detect rare cells with the tumor-associated gene rearrangement. This strategy is quite appealing, because it can be applied to nearly every lymphoid neoplasm, even those lacking an identifiable translocation. Furthermore, quantitative PCR technology can be used to monitor disease burden down to low levels. The drawback to this technology is that it requires labor-intensive and relatively expensive laboratory testing to identify and validate tumor-specific junctional probes for each patient.

T-CELL RECEPTOR GENE REARRANGEMENT

Just as B cells rearrange their *IG* genes, T lymphocytes rearrange their *TR* genes to encode a unique antigen receptor expressed on the cell surface. Therefore, gene rearrangement serves as a clonal marker for T-cell tumors analogous to what has been described for B-cell tumors. Again, in the case of T cells, four *TR* genes are capable of rearranging: *TRA, TRB, TRG,* and *TRD* (Figure 13-5).

During normal T-cell ontogeny, sequential gene rearrangements occur to produce a unique assemblage of coding sequences. Depending on the status of the cell from which it originated, a T-cell neoplasm may harbor clonal rearrangement of one, two, three, or all four of the *TR* genes (Figure 13-6). Molecular analysis of the *TRB* and *TRG* genes is commonly

used to distinguish monoclonal T-cell neoplasms from polyclonal reactive processes. The *TRD* gene is less than ideal because it is deleted during *TRA* gene rearrangement, and *TRA* is not ideal because it has so many possible rearrangements that current technology cannot handle the diversity (Box 13-3).

The rearranged *TRG* gene is quite amenable to PCR amplification. Nearly all T cells harbor rearrangements involving 1 of 11 variable segments. Of these segments, 8 are homologous to one another and can be targeted by a single consensus primer. In the event that one of the remaining variable segments was used, additional primers are employed in a multiplex fashion, along with several joining region primers, to detect virtually all possible *TRG* gene rearrangements. PCR products are separated by electrophoretic size, and the pattern is visualized to identify one or two major peaks indicative of a monoclonal T-cell population. A single major peak suggests monoallelic rearrangement, whereas two major peaks suggest biallelic *TRG* rearrangement in the tumor cells. In contrast, a bell-shaped distribution of peaks is indicative of polyclonal T cells. Distinguishing monoclonal from polyclonal T-cell proliferations is particularly useful in the workup of suspected cutaneous T-cell lymphoma or large granular lymphocyte leukemia.

Southern blot analysis is an alternate method for identifying clonal rearrangement of the *TR* genes. In a typical Southern blot procedure, aliquots of

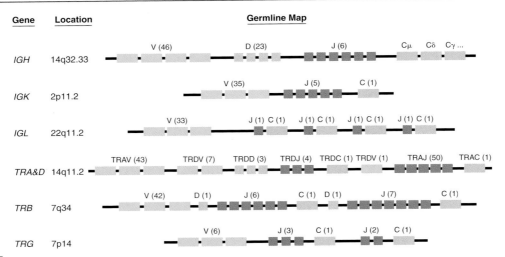

FIGURE 13-5

Structural similarities exist between the immunoglobulin *(IG)* and the T-cell receptor *(TR)* loci as shown in these maps of the germline configuration. During lymphocyte ontogeny, unique coding sequences are produced through rearrangement of the variable, diversity, joining, and constant regions of each locus. The number of functional alternatives is shown in parentheses for each cluster of elements. Note: T-cell receptor δ *(TRD)* segments are spliced out during T-cell receptor α *(TRA)* gene rearrangement. IGH, IG heavy chain gene; IGK, IG kappa light chain gene; IGL, IG lambda light chain gene; TRA, TRB, TRG and TRD, T-cell receptor alpha, beta, gamma and delta genes, respectively; V, variable; D, diversity; C, constant.

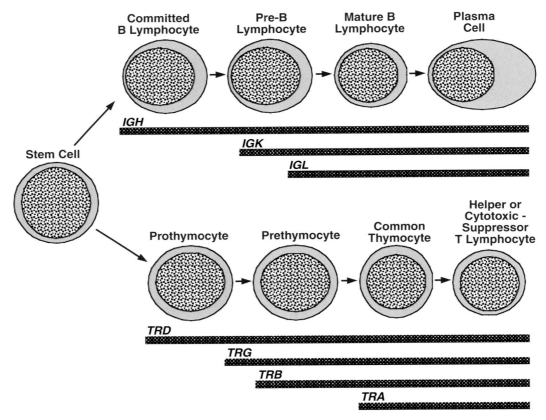

FIGURE 13-6

During lymphocyte ontogeny, a series of gene rearrangements is orchestrated to supply diverse coding sequences for antigen receptors. The immunoglobulin heavy chain *(IGH)* gene rearranges first as a hematopoietic progenitor cell commits to the B lineage. If the first *IGH* rearrangement is dysfunctional, then the other *IGH* allele rearranges. Later, one or both immunoglobulin *IGK* genes rearrange. If both *IGK* rearrangements are dysfunctional, which happens in about one third of lymphocytes, then one or both *IGL* genes rearrange to encode λ light chain protein. Even a λ-expressing cell retains its rearranged κ gene. An analogous series of gene rearrangements occurs during T-cell development, beginning with T-cell receptor δ *(TRD)* as a progenitor cell commits to the T lineage. Next, the T-cell receptor γ *(TRG)* gene rearranges. If these rearrangements are dysfunctional, then the T-cell receptor β *(TRB)* and T-cell receptor α *(TRA)* genes rearrange, in which case the cell will be an αβ T cell as opposed to a γδ T cell. About 95% of circulating T cells are αβ type, and most T-cell neoplasms are likewise αβ type. Even cells expressing αβ protein retain their *TRG* rearrangement, implying that *TRG* rearrangement characterizes virtually all T cells.

high molecular weight DNA are cut with each of several alternate restriction enzymes and the *TRB* gene is identified using a cocktail of probes spanning the two joining regions, JB1 and JB2. Germline bands are seen in all tissues, whereas extra bands are seen in tissues harboring clonal gene rearrangement.

CLINICAL UTILITY OF GENE REARRANGEMENT TESTING

Molecular testing is required in only a small fraction of all hematopathology specimens. Morphologically equivocal cases are usually examined first by immunophenotyping with or without karyotyping and then by molecular tests if the issue of clonality or lineage is still not resolved. The most helpful molecular tests include PCR and Southern blot analysis to detect antigen receptor gene rearrangement or to detect specific translocations associated with the malignancies in the differential diagnosis. Fluorescence in situ hybridization (FISH) is also quite useful to detect specific translocations or, using a break-apart probe, to show that an *IG* or *TR* locus is likely to be involved in a translocation. A list of reference laboratories offering various molecular assays for hematologic disease is found on the Association for Molecular Pathology website.

Antigen receptor gene rearrangement tests are helpful for distinguishing benign from malignant lymphoproliferations. Benign reactive lymphoid hyperplasias do not harbor monoclonal rearrangements, whereas malignant lymphoid tumors consistently harbor clonal rearrangements. Despite the incredible power of molecular analysis in identifying clonal populations, results of clonality assays should be interpreted with caution because clonality is not always synonymous with malignancy. Large granular lymphocytosis and lymphomatoid papulosis are examples of lymphoid lesions that are usually clonal even though they may regress without therapy. Because molecular studies are imperfect from both analytic and clinical perspectives, it is important that results be interpreted in correlation with morphol-

ogy, immunophenotyping, cytogenetics, and other clinicopathologic findings (Box 13-4).

A second use of gene rearrangement testing is in determining the B- versus T-cell lineage of a lymphoid proliferation. B-cell tumors virtually always harbor clonally rearranged *IG* genes, and T-cell tumors harbor clonally rearranged *TR* genes, whereas true natural killer (NK) cells have germline antigen receptor genes. A complicating factor is lineage infidelity, whereby certain tumors harbor both *IG* and *TR* gene rearrangements. Lineage infidelity is particularly common in acute lymphoblastic leukemias, although it can also be seen in more differentiated lymphoid neoplasms. Likewise, antigen receptor gene rearrangement has been reported in about 5% of acute myeloid leukemias but not in nonhematopoietic tumors. It is recommended that gene rearrangement testing be used with immunophenotyping for purposes of lineage assignment.

Another confounding variable is the presence of two separate lymphoid clones in the same biopsy sample. This can occur when two independent lymphoid malignancies coincidentally arise in the same patient or, more commonly, when a single malignancy is accompanied by a minor lymphoid clone that does not expand in a malignant fashion. Such minor lymphoid clones are poorly understood in terms of their pathobiology, and their presence can confound interpretation of gene rearrangement studies.

Distinguishing partial involvement by malignancy from a reactive cell population continues to be a problematic issue that is best dealt with by correlating the molecular findings with morphology; immunophenotyping; karyotyping, FISH, or PCR for translocation; and other clinicopathologic findings. For example, Hodgkin's lymphoma and T-cell-rich B-cell lymphomas often exhibit a minor clone consistent with the presence of a small population of malignant B cells admixed with numerous reactive inflammatory cells. In contrast, lymphoma characterized by sheets of malignant-appearing lymphocytes would be expected to yield a major clone and little, if any, evidence of polyclonal lymphocytes. If morphology suggests a major B-cell clone but no dominant peak is seen in the *IGH* assay, despite immunophenotypic evidence of lymphoid origin and control data confirming amplifiable DNA, then it is possible that the tumor is a T-cell lymphoma, an NK lymphoma, an anaplastic large-cell lymphoma, or a B-cell lymphoma for which the primer sets used were inadequate to amplify the particular rearranged *IGH* in that tumor, possibly as a consequence of somatic mutation. Molecular tests for *IGK* and *TRG* might resolve the dilemma.

A minor B-cell clone may be found in inflamed mucosa of the stomach, jejunum, salivary gland, or ocular adnexae. Although these have previously been termed *pseudolymphomas,* many are now thought to be low-grade extranodal marginal zone B-cell lymphomas of mucosa-associated lymphoid tissue (MALT lymphomas). Likewise, an ulcerative lesion of the jejunum harboring a small T-cell clone associated with morphologic evidence of celiac sprue is now thought to represent early involvement by enteropathy-type T-cell lymphoma. It appears that chronic inflammatory processes related to infection or autoimmune disease can predispose to B- or T-cell lymphoma, and gene rearrangement tests can help sort out when a neoplasm is present. The same test can be applied in follow-up biopsies in which residual disease would be expected to yield the same rearranged gene product, whereas absence of a dominant peak of that size provides some reassurance that the treatment was effective.

CONCLUSION

Molecular tests, including Southern blot analysis and PCR, are powerful tools for detecting clonal *IG* and *TR* gene rearrangements that characterize B- and T-cell neoplasms and distinguish them from reactive lymphoid lesions. Instrumentation, reagents, and strategies for designing these assays have steadily improved over the past two decades, and we expect these assays will continue to provide helpful contributions in some of the most perplexing lymphoid lesions encountered by pathologists.

SUGGESTED READINGS

Methodology, Validation, and Guidelines for Interpretation

Clinical and Laboratory Standards Institute: Immunoglobulin and T-Cell Receptor Gene Rearrangement Assays: Approved Guideline, 2nd ed, vol MM2-A2. Wayne, PA, CLSI, 2002.

Droese J, Langerak AW, Groenen PJ, et al: Validation of BIOMED-2 multiplex PCR tubes for detection of TCRB gene rearrangements in T-cell malignancies. Leukemia 2004;18(9):1531–1538.

Lassmann S, Gerlach UV, Technau-Ihling K, et al: Application of BIOMED-2 primers in fixed and decalcified bone marrow biopsies: Analysis of immunoglobulin H receptor rearrangements in B-cell non-Hodgkin's lymphomas. J Mol Diagn 2005;7(5):582–591.

McClure RF, Kaur P, Pagel E, et al: Validation of immunoglobulin gene rearrangement detection by PCR using commercially available BIOMED-2 primers. Leukemia 2006;20(1):176–179.

Sandberg Y et al: BIOMED-2 multiplex immunoglobulin/T-cell receptor polymerase chain reaction protocols can reliably replace Southern blot analysis in routine clonality diagnostics. J Mol Diagn 2005;7(4):495–503.

van Dongen JJ, Langerak AW, Brüggemann M, et al: Design and standardization of PCR primers and protocols for detection of clonal immunoglobulin and T-cell receptor gene recombinations in suspect lymphoproliferations: Report of the Biomed-2 Concerted Action BMH4-CT98-3936. Leukemia 2003;17(12):2257–2317.

van Krieken JH, Langerak AW, San Miguel JF, et al: Clonality analysis for antigen receptor genes: Preliminary results from the Biomed-2 concerted action PL 96-3936. Hum Pathol 2003;34(4):359–361.

Initial Diagnosis and Monitoring Minimal Residual Disease

Association for Molecular Pathology: Home. Available at http://www.amp.org.

Cazzaniga G, Biondi A: Molecular monitoring of childhood acute lymphoblastic leukemia using antigen receptor gene rearrangements and quantitative polymerase chain reaction technology. Haematologica 2005;90(3):382–390.

Fend F, Bock O, Kremer M, et al: Ancillary techniques in bone marrow pathology: Molecular diagnostics on bone marrow trephine biopsies. Virchows Arch 2005;447(6):909–919.

Hummel M, Oeschger S, Barth TF, et al: Wotherspoon criteria combined with B-cell clonality analysis by advanced polymerase chain reaction technology discriminates covert gastric marginal zone lymphoma from chronic gastritis. Gut 2006;55(6):782–787.

Kussick SJ, Kalnoski M, Braziel RM, Wood BL: Prominent clonal B-cell populations identified by flow cytometry in histologically reactive lymphoid proliferations. Am J Clin Pathol 2004;121(4):464–472.

van der Velden VH, Hochhaus A, Cazzaniga G, et al: Detection of minimal residual disease in hematologic malignancies by real-time quantitative PCR: Principles, approaches, and laboratory aspects. Leukemia 2003;17(6):1013–1034.

14

Monitoring of Minimal Residual Hematologic Disease

Cuihong Wei • Jeffrey H. Lipton • Suzanne Kamel-Reid

INTRODUCTION

In recent years, several advances have been made in predicting the outcome in hematologic malignancies, among them measurement of *minimal residual disease* (MRD). The term was coined to describe a scenario in which the leukemia cells are not eradicated from a patient in clinical remission but are at a level below the sensitivity of classic cytomorphologic methods. Determination of MRD is an evolving field in which the technology and result interpretation are continually being refined. Its detection relies on the presence of a leukemia-specific marker, which should be present in all leukemia cells and remain stable during disease evolution.

Historically, various techniques have been used to evaluate the malignant cell burden in leukemia, with differing levels of sensitivity (Table 14-1). Karyotyping has a sensitivity comparable to that of morphologic evaluation and can only be applied to dividing cells. Fluorescence in situ hybridization (FISH) has better sensitivity than karyotyping because it can be done on interphase nuclei and many cells can be analyzed in a short period. Flow cytometry methods, such as fluorescence-activated cell sorting (FACS) analysis, can be used to detect specific combinations of cell surface proteins that can characterize the original cell population with a sensitivity of 10^{-3}. The most sensitive method, polymerase chain reaction (PCR), appears to be the best choice to date for the detection of very low levels of MRD with a sensitivity of 10^{-5} to 10^{-6} cells.

Monitoring MRD provides independent prognostic information for treatment stratification in several types of leukemias, such as childhood acute lymphoblastic leukemia, chronic myeloid leukemia (CML), and acute promyelocytic leukemia (APL). Molecular genetic markers include fused genes associated with recurrent chromosomal translocations, such as t(9;22) *BCR/ABL* in CML, t(15;17) *PML/RARα* in APL, t(8;21) *AML1/ETO* in AML M2, and t(16;16) *CBFβ-MYH11* in AML M4Eo. Although both genomic DNA and messenger RNA (mRNA) can be used as templates for amplification, mRNA is preferable in most cases because it adds sensitivity and specificity. DNA amplification has been used to detect T-cell acute leukemia 1 deletions and immunoglobulin heavy chain–myelocytomatosis oncogene fusions, because these breakpoints cluster in a relatively small region. In most cases, however, breakpoints can occur over large intronic regions, thus necessitating the use of mRNA to enable amplification of the involved region. Specific biomarkers such as Wilms' tumor class 1 can also be used to follow MRD in hematologic malignancies such as AML. This chapter uses CML as an example to illustrate the use of real-time quantitative PCR (Q-PCR) in MRD monitoring. Because of the vast amount of information available on this disease, the correlation between molecular monitoring and clinical outcome, and the large effort in test standardization, all serve as an excellent illustrative model.

CML is associated with a reciprocal translocation t(9;22) resulting in a novel *BCR/ABL* fusion gene on chromosome 22, the Philadelphia chromosome. The *BCR/ABL* fusion protein has an elevated tyrosine kinase activity and is central to the pathogenesis of CML. This fusion protein confers a proliferative advantage and genetic instability on cells that express it. CML typically presents in chronic phase and can progress, over time, to an advanced phase. At initial diagnosis, real-time Q-PCR, karyotyping, and FISH are informative. Real-time Q-PCR will determine baseline *BCR/ABL* transcript levels, karyotyping will identify additional cytogenetic changes that may be present at diagnosis, and FISH will yield potentially prognostic information regarding the presence of a deletion on the derivative chromosome 9. Over the past 5 years, a tyrosine kinase inhibitor, imatinib mesylate, has become first-line therapy for patients with CML. The change in treatment from interferon to imatinib is based on results of the phase III International Randomized Study of Interferon versus STI571 (IRIS) trial of 1106 patients comparing imatinib (STI571) with interferon-α and low-dose cytarabine. Because of the excellent response of CML patients to imatinib, with greater than 70% of patients achieving

TABLE 14-1

Detection Limits of Techniques Used to Analyze Hematologic Malignancies

Technique	Marker	Detection Limit
Routine pathology	Cellular morphology	10^{-1} to 10^{-2}
Cytogenetics	Chromosome morphology	10^{-1} to 10^{-2}
FISH	Chromosome structure	10^{-2}
FACS analysis	Antigen profile	10^{-3}
PCR	Nucleic acid sequence or expression	10^{-5} to 10^{-6}

FACS, fluorescence-activated cell sorting; FISH, fluorescence in situ hybridization; PCR, polymerase chain reaction.

a complete cytogenetic response, molecular monitoring of MRD has become essential as a method that provides an early and sensitive indication of loss of response. Acquired resistance to imatinib can be associated with a kinase domain mutation of the *ABL* portion of the *BCR/ABL* fusion gene in about 50% of cases. The molecular mechanism for loss of response in the remainder of patients is unclear and may be associated with deregulation through the *SRC* kinase pathway. This chapter examines the methods most commonly used for monitoring MRD in the hematologic malignancies, using CML as an example.

REAL-TIME Q-PCR DETECTION METHODS

PRINCIPLES OF THE TECHNIQUE

To study fusion gene expression, mRNA must be transcribed into a single-stranded complementary DNA (cDNA) using polythymidine, random hexamers, or a fusion gene–specific reverse primer. The cDNA product is then used as a template for a PCR; this technique is usually called *reverse transcription–PCR* (RT-PCR). Real-time Q-PCR uses PCR primers and fluorescent probes to detect and quantitate fluorescent signals that increase in direct proportion to the amount of PCR product generated in a reaction. It measures not the amount of end product but its production in real time. The higher the starting copy number of the nucleic acid target, the sooner a significant increase in fluorescence is observed. The real-time PCR readout is given as the number of PCR cycles necessary to achieve a given level of fluorescence passing a threshold of the PCR (C_t). During the initial PCR cycles, the fluorescence signal emitted is usually too weak to register above the background. During

the exponential phase of the PCR, the fluorescence intensity doubles at each cycle. Following the exponential phase, a linear phase exists in which the signal still increases but is less efficient. The final plateau phase indicates that the PCR has reached saturation status. Because a C_t is proportional to the logarithm of the initial amount of the target in a sample, the quantity of one target with respect to another is reflected in the difference in cycle numbers (ΔC_t) necessary to achieve the same level of fluorescence. Therefore, real-time Q-PCR is a sensitive method for quantitation of rare transcripts and small changes in gene expression. At present, real-time Q-PCR is a preferred method of monitoring MRD in hematologic malignancies and has become standard practice.

DETECTION METHODS

There are several detection methods available on the market, so only the most widely used methods are discussed here in detail. Despite the difference in assay design among these methods, their performance is comparable except for SYBR® Green I. Although these methods have been used primarily for real-time PCR, they have been employed for other applications, such as single nucleotide polymorphism detection, loss of heterozygosity, and haplotype analysis.

DNA-Binding Dyes

The DNA-binding method involves detection of the binding of a fluorescent dye (SYBR Green I) to the minor groove of double-stranded PCR products. The unbound dye exhibits little fluorescence in solution, but during elongation increasing amounts of dye bind to the nascent double-stranded DNA, resulting in an increase in fluorescence emission upon excitation. The binding process is sequence independent. At denaturation, the SYBR Green I molecules are released and the fluorescent signal decreases in intensity to background levels. The intensity of fluorescence is monitored in real time. Figure 14-1 illustrates the SYBR Green I methodology.

The advantages of using SYBR Green I over probe-based detection include its relative simplicity and low cost. The disadvantages associated with this method include the propensity of the dye to bind to primer dimers and to nonspecific PCR products. Because such nonspecific binding could result in overestimation of the specific product, optimal design of the PCR primers is essential for accurate and specific quantification using this method. To verify the PCR specificity, a melting curve of the amplicon can be generated by plotting fluorescence as a function of temperature. A characteristic melting peak at the melting temperature of the amplicon will distinguish it from amplification artifacts.

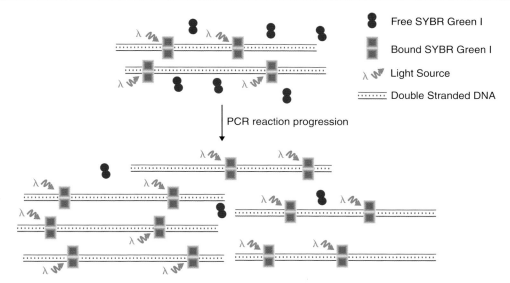

FIGURE 14-1

Fluorescent intercalating dye, SYBR Green I. Fluorescence increases with accumulation of double-stranded DNA during polymerase chain reaction (PCR).

Because of its limitations, this method is not recommended for fusion transcript quantification.

Scorpions

Scorpions are fluorogenic PCR primers with a probe element attached at the 5′ end by a PCR stopper. There are two Scorpion™ formats available: the single-oligonucleotide "stem–loop" format (or closed format; Figure 14-2A) and the two-oligonucleotide "duplex" format (or open format; Figure 14-2B). The basic elements of scorpions are the presence of a PCR primer, a PCR stopper to prevent PCR read-through of the probe element, a specific probe sequence, and a fluorescence detection system containing at least one fluorophore and one quencher. In most real-time Q-PCR assays, separate primers and probes are used to amplify and detect a target sequence. However, the Scorpion system uses a PCR primer and a probe linked to each other so that the binding of the probe to the amplicon is a unimolecular reaction (intramolecular) instead of a bimolecular one (intermolecular). In the closed format, a Scorpion primer and a normal reverse primer are required. The probe sequence is in the loop portion of a stem–loop structure that results from the annealing of complementary sequences on the 5′ and 3′ sides of the probe. In this

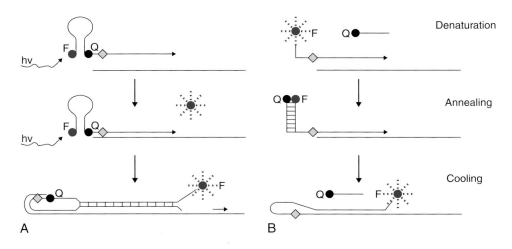

FIGURE 14-2

Schematic representation of real-time polymerase chain reaction (PCR) with Scorpion primers. **A,** In the stem–loop configuration, the quencher (black circle) forms a nonfluorescent complex with the fluorophore (blue circle). Upon extension of the amplicon, the Scorpion probe hybridizes to the newly formed complementary sequence, separating the fluorophore from the quencher restoring the fluorescence. **B,** Scorpion primers in "duplex" format. Separation of fluorophore and quencher onto different oligonucleotides improves signal intensity. The quencher oligonucleotide has the quencher at the 3′ end and is complementary to the probe sequence. Following denaturation and polymerization, intramolecular interaction of the probe and the newly generated product is more favorable than intermolecular binding between the quencher oligonucleotide and the probe. Gold diamond, PCR stopper.

configuration, the fluorophore is in close contact with the quencher, resulting in collisional quenching. In the open format, the probe element of the Scorpion primer does not have a specific secondary structure in the unhybridized form and has a fluorophore attached to its 5′ end. A separate oligonucleotide that complements the probe part of the Scorpion primer bearing a quencher at its 3′ end is required. This quencher oligonucleotide binds to the Scorpion primer to prevent fluorescence in solution or when the Scorpion primer is not bound to its intended target. After Scorpion primer extension by Taq polymerase, the amplicon containing a sequence that is complementary to the probe is denatured and renatured during each PCR cycle. Because the probe of the Scorpion primer binds to the amplified product, the quencher and the probe will be separated from each other, resulting in an increase in fluorescence. The PCR stopper prevents undesirable read-through of the probe and primer dimer formation that might lead to a displacement of the quencher and an increase in fluorescence irrelevant to the target sequence. Duplex Scorpions are considered to have significant advantage over their stem–loop counterparts, producing a more intense fluorescent signal because of the increased separation between fluorophore and quencher in the active form.

Molecular Beacons

Molecular beacons are DNA hybridization probes that have a hairpin structure: the quencher dye and the reporter dye are in close contact with each other at the end of the stem of the hairpin; the loop portion is the probe, which is complementary to the target sequence. Usually, the length of the probe portion is no more than 40 base pairs. This system comprises three components: a forward primer, a reverse primer, and a molecular beacon probe. In the free state, self-quenching occurs as the stem–loop configuration brings the dye and the quencher together. When hybridizing to the PCR product, molecular beacons open the loop of the hairpin structure and form hybrids with the complementary sequences. These hybrids have more base pairs than that of the stem in a stem–loop conformation and are thus more stable. This conformational change separates the quencher and the reporter from each other, leading to the generation of a fluorescent signal (Figure 14-3). The main drawback of molecular beacons is associated with the design of the hybridization probe, especially the stem portion.

5′-Nuclease Probes

The 5′-nuclease assay uses the 5′-nuclease activity of DNA polymerase to hydrolyze a hybridization probe bound to its target amplicon. These fluorogenic probes are typically prepared with the quencher at the 3′ terminus of single-stranded DNA and the fluorophore at the 5′ terminus. Because of the close contact of the quencher and the fluorophore, fluorescence is inhibited. The probe can be in either a sense or an antisense orientation and will be hybridized to the amplicon in a sequence-dependent manner during annealing. It remains hybridized while the Taq polymerase extends the primers and until it reaches the hybridized probe, whereupon it displaces the probe's 5′ end and holds it in a forked structure. This forked structure becomes a substrate for cleavage by Taq DNA polymerase, which has 5′-nuclease activity. Because the 5′-nuclease activity is hybridization dependent, cleavage of the probe occurs only in the presence of the target sequence. As a result of cleavage, the fluorophore and the quencher are separated and the fluorescent signal is released. This fluorescent signal is directly proportional to the amount of PCR product generated and is monitored in real time (Figure 14-4). Although extremely sensitive, the cost of this assay is relatively high because the probe is dually labeled.

Fluorescence Resonance Energy Transfer

The fluorescence resonance energy transfer (FRET) method uses two independent hybridization probes labeled with fluorescent dyes to maximize specificity. One of the probes carries a fluorophore donor at its 3′ end, and the other probe is labeled with an acceptor fluorophore at its 5′ end and is blocked at its 3′ end to prevent PCR extension. FRET occurs between a donor fluorophore and a suitable acceptor dye when the absorption spectrum of the acceptor molecule overlaps the emission spectrum of the donor fluorophore because the two molecules are in proximity. As a result of FRET, the donor fluorescence is diminished and the acceptor fluorophore is sensitized. The efficiency of the energy transfer between the donor and the acceptor molecules highly depends on the distance between the molecules. In a classic FRET-based real-time Q-PCR assay, two probes are designed to bind to a common target with a 1- to 3-base-pair gap to ensure an efficient FRET. In solution, the two dyes are far apart and FRET is weak between them, resulting in background fluorescence being emitted by the donor. During the annealing stage of PCR, a hybridization reaction allows these two probes to hybridize to a common target sequence in a head-to-tail arrangement. The proximity of the probes and their associated dyes allows a FRET reaction to occur at high efficiency. A donor fluorophore is excited by a light source and in turn excites the acceptor fluorophore. The intensity of the fluorescence from the acceptor fluorophore is increased and is proportional to the amount of amplified target DNA (Figure 14-5). Advantages of using this method include good specificity and design flexibility. Furthermore, because the probes

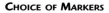

15 Molecular Detection of Circulating Tumor Cells

Karen L. Kaul

INTRODUCTION

Determination of the extent of tumor spread, or the pathologic staging of tumors, is a critical step in determining the course of therapy for patients with cancer. The presence of tumor cells from lymph node, bone marrow, and other samples indicates potential metastasis and may trigger administration of systemic treatment in place of, or in addition to, surgery. Detection of occult tumor cells is also used in monitoring response to treatment and detecting relapse of neoplasia. A variety of approaches have been used by pathologists to improve detection of circulating tumor cells, including immunohistochemical and immunofluorescent staining, flow cytometry, and more recently, molecular approaches. The goal of each of these methods is the sensitive and specific detection and differentiation of tumor cells from other cells present in the sample.

Cancer metastasis is a stepwise process, involving a series of genetic, epigenetic, and/or expression changes occurring within tumor cells. Eventually a clone of cells acquires growth advantages, survival advantages, or both, including the ability for cells to escape their local environment, enter the circulation to reach distant sites, evade immune surveillance and survive the circulatory environment, attach at the remote site, induce angiogenesis, and proliferate to form a metastatic lesion. Only a subset of the circulating cells is capable of developing into a metastatic lesion. Tumor cells enter the venous or the lymphatic circulation (or both) and thus are spread to distant tissues (such as lung, liver, or bone marrow) or local lymph nodes, respectively, before the development of clinically or radiologically detectable metastatic lesions. A significant proportion of organ-confined tumors recur following theoretically curative surgery, which argues that current approaches to cancer staging are, to some degree, inadequate. More sensitive histologic, cytologic, or molecular approaches are hoped to provide a more accurate demonstration of the presence of tumor cells in blood as a surrogate for the presence of metastases at remote sites in the body. Because the circulation is such a common conduit for metastatic spread, and blood is an easily obtainable sample, the detection of circulating tumor cells has perhaps generated the greatest amount of interest and enthusiasm. This chapter focuses on molecular and immunohistochemical approaches for the detection of circulating tumor cells. Coverage of the hundreds of articles published to date is beyond the scope of this chapter; instead, more general and technical issues are addressed. Several excellent reviews are available for more detailed reading; some of these are listed in the Suggested Readings section.

PRINCIPLES OF THE TECHNIQUE

CHOICE OF MARKERS

In general, solid tumors lack suitable common genomic alterations useful for detection of occult tumor cells, so gene expression markers are most often employed. A messenger RNA (mRNA) or protein marker, overexpressed in tumor cells relative to the background cells, can be detected using reverse transcriptase–polymerase chain reaction (RT-PCR) for mRNA targets or immunohistochemistry (IHC) or immunofluorescence for protein markers. Unfortunately, truly tumor-specific cell markers are almost nonexistent. Most studies have therefore used markers reflecting the general type of cell or organ from which the tumor originates and thus detect the presence of an expression-positive cell amid a background of theoretically nonexpressing cells, such as leukocytes. Such markers cannot distinguish a tumor from normal cells of the same cell type.

Novel molecular and protein markers are being discovered through new analytic approaches, such as expression microarray analysis. For example, differential display analysis was used to compare gene expression patterns in blood samples from normal and breast cancer patients to identify gene expression patterns correlating with the presence and absence of tumor cells. Further studies used microarray methods to define a set of 12 genes that were upregulated in breast cancer patients, although a significant degree of false-positive expression was observed. Thirteen other laboratories have used the serial analysis of gene expression method to identify genes with abundant expression in breast cancer that might serve as markers for occult tumor cells. Recently, expression analysis of circulating tumor cells has been performed, revealing cancer-specific, circulating cell expression profiles.

In addition, combinations of markers are being investigated, the goal being maximizing sensitivity and specificity for tumor cell detection and discrimination. Because tumors are heterogeneous, and no markers are universally expressed by all tumor cells, marker panels may increase the performance of molecular or histochemical studies. However, issues remain regarding definition of the ideal marker set for any tumor, and studies continue to present surprises regarding specificity of accepted tumor markers. Specificity can be particularly problematic when RT-PCR is used as a detection method because of its tremendous sensitivity. Quantitative analysis may be helpful in discriminating tumor from background positivity.

The presence of a tumor cell in the circulation does not necessarily indicate it is capable of completing the metastatic process. Further markers are needed that indicate not only the presence of tumor cells but also the biologic relevance of the detected cells. Specific details regarding expression of cell surface–binding proteins, angiogenic factors, and stromal interactions that are generated by a metastasis-competent cell are only beginning to be understood; thus, use of these types of markers remains a distant reality. Nevertheless, other indicators may be useful in assessing the ability of tumor cells to successfully complete the metastatic process. Aneusomy in circulating cells has been shown to match that of the parent tumor, and increasing genomic alterations in circulating breast cancer cells are associated with an increased risk of recurrence. The proliferative ability of these cells may be another indicator of biologic potential; expression of genes inhibiting apoptosis has also been studied.

In addition, although blood represents a convenient clinical sample, a growing number of studies suggest that assessment of bone marrow for the presence of tumor cells may yield a better predictor of disease outcome. It can be postulated that these cells have survived the circulation, have established themselves in the relatively protected environment of the marrow, and may be at an advanced step in the metastatic process relative to their precursors, who are only able to access the circulation. Nevertheless, the biology of cells in the marrow is complex, and recent studies into cancer dormancy indicate that subclinical disease in the marrow may exist for years in some patients and thus may complicate interpretation of studies of circulating tumor cells.

IMMUNOCHEMICAL DETECTION

Detection of occult tumor cells by immunodetection methods (including immunocytochemistry and immunofluorescence) has been used to study preparations of cells from bone marrow, lymph node aspirates, and peripheral blood mononuclear cells. Cells can be smeared or cytospun onto slides, and immunostaining is performed using standard approaches. Slides can be scanned visually, although thousands to millions of cells must be screened to achieve a high level of sensitivity, making this process tedious and time consuming. Image analysis facilitates these analyses, and flow cytometry has been used to achieve rapid analysis of many cells. Detection limits of about 1 tumor cell against a background of 1 million nontumor cells are typical and, to a certain degree, depend on the total number of cells examined.

Recently, two commercially available systems employing image analysis have become available for the detection of occult tumor cells, especially for breast cancer. The assay developed by ChromaVision (now owned by Clarient) as an analyte-specific reagent includes a proprietary cell stabilization buffer, immunomagnetic capture of tumor cells, and immunohistochemical staining of cells immobilized on a glass slide with a cocktail of anticytokeratin antibodies to highlight epithelial cells. The image analysis system indicates possible tumor cells on the slide, which then are reviewed cytologicially by the operator. Figure 15-1 shows the results of this approach, with cells expressing cytokeratins detectable among the background white cells cytospun onto a slide.

The immunofluorescent reagents manufactured and marketed by Veridex (a division of Johnson & Johnson) also begins with immunomagnetic selection, followed by dual-color staining for cytokeratin and Her2, 4′-6-diamidino-2-phenylindole staining of the nucleus to indicate an intact cell, and fluorescent anti-CD45 staining to highlight contaminating leukocytes that can be eliminated from the analysis. The Veridex CellSearch assay was approved by the U.S. Food and Drug Administration in 2004 for the detection of circulating breast cancer cells. Figure 15-2 shows the positive staining of tumor cells in the immunofluorescent assay. This approach has been used for detection of circulating cells from a variety of carcinomas.

REVERSE TRANSCRIPTASE–POLYMERASE CHAIN REACTION DETECTION

RT-PCR has also been widely used for detection of circulating tumor cells, as well as occult tumor cells in a variety of other sample types. Because many cells are analyzed simultaneously, this approach achieves great analytic sensitivity, with detection limits of 1 tumor cell in 10^7 background cells and beyond reported.

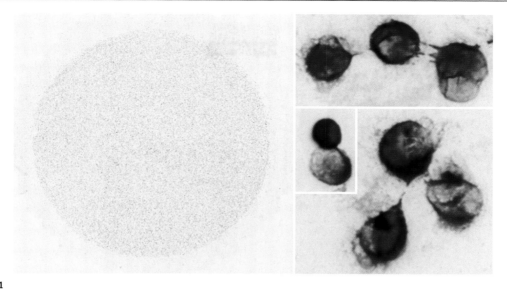

FIGURE 15-1

Immunocytochemical detection of circulating breast cancer cells in a cytospin preparation of peripheral blood from a breast cancer patient. Following immunoselection and immunostaining with a cocktail of anticytokeratin antibodies, tumor cells can be assessed by light microscopy or image analysis. (Courtesy of Clarient, Aliso Viejo, CA.)

Fundamentally, the success of this approach depends on the careful choice of an mRNA target, as described earlier, and the meticulous design of the assay. For example, pseudogenes can give rise to amplicons identical in size to those amplified from mRNA but in reality arising from contaminating DNA present in the RNA sample. Amplification reactions must be designed to detect gene transcripts rather than the gene itself by using PCR primers that span at least one intron. In addition, amplification approaches other than PCR can be used effectively.

For any of the approaches targeting RNA or protein markers of tumor cells, immunoselection can

enhance both the sensitivity and the specificity of the assay results. Positive selection offers the ability to both enrich the resultant sample for tumor cells and reduce the potential for background expression of the target to be detected in nontumor cells. However, careful consideration of the antigens used for cell capture is critical, because tumor cells will be lost if they do not express the appropriate cell surface marker for immunoselection. Conversely, negative selection can be used to remove contaminating nontumor cells, with a possible limitation being the large amount of selection reagent needed to remove the leukocytes, which

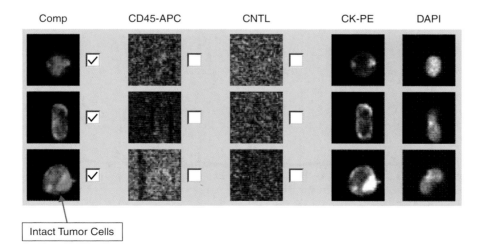

FIGURE 15-2

Immunofluorescent detection of circulating breast cancer cells. The composite image of intact circulating cells (left panel) is made up of nuclei stained with 4′-6-diamidino-2-phenylindole (DAPI) and positive cytoplasmic staining for cytokeratin, along with CD45 negativity. CK-PE, cytokeratin-phycoerythrin; Comp, composite. (Courtesy of Veridex, Warren, NJ.)

vastly outnumber the circulating cancer cells present in any sample.

Detection of positive results obtained by molecular assays has evolved dramatically over recent years, as show in Figure 15-3. Agarose or other gel electrophoresis approaches alone fail to provide adequate

sensitivity, necessitating the use of Southern blot, dot blot, or solution hybridization or autoradiographic methods. As fluorescent detection and real-time amplification methods have replaced these older methods, results are available not only more rapidly and with less work but also quantitatively. As shown in

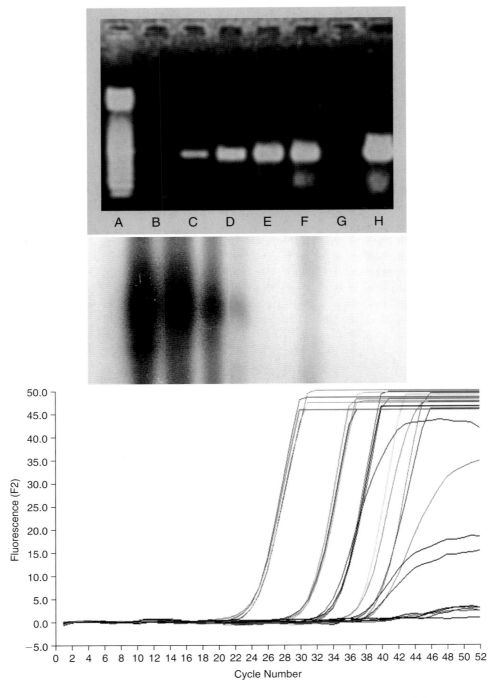

FIGURE 15-3

Evolution in signal detection of reverse transcriptase–polymerase chain reaction (RT-PCR) assays for the detection of occult tumor cells. **A,** Agarose gel showing dilutions of LNCaP cells in blood samples (lane A, molecular weight markers; lane B, 10 cells per 10 mL of blood; lane C, 100 cells; lane D, 1000 cells; lane E, 10 four cells; lane F, 10 five cells; lane G, negative control; lane H, undiluted LNCaP RNA). **B,** Autoradiographic detection of prostate-specific antigen reverse transcriptase–polymerase chain reaction (RT-PCR) amplicons using a radioactively labeled oligonucleotide probe. **C,** Real-time RT-PCR detection of LNCaP cells diluted into whole blood samples.

Figure 15-4 (using research use only reagents available from Abbott Molecular), the use of real-time PCR facilitates the quantitative analysis of RT-PCR results. This quantitative approach can be used to discriminate real positivity, caused by tumor cells from a low-level, background signal, from leukocytes, leading to increased assay specificity.

ADVANTAGES AND DISADVANTAGES

There are advantages and disadvantages to both the RT-PCR and the immunodetection approaches to identification of circulating tumor cells. RT-PCR methods probably offer the highest degree of potential sensitivity in that detection of few or even a single cell is possible, especially if the gene target is transcribed at a high level. However, the ability to visualize the cells is lost; thus, specificity may be hampered if any nontumor cell expression is present. RT-PCR approaches may be more rapid and can be performed with less expensive equipment than the image analysis systems needed by the current immunodetection methods available. Although both approaches can yield quantitative data, it is important to consider that the immunostaining methods yield results in terms of number of tumor cells and RT-PCR measures numbers of transcripts, which can vary widely between cells and from tumor to tumor. Some labs have employed quantitative assays to define a threshold value above which a positive signal indicates tumor cells and below

which nonspecific or inappropriate expression of the marker is assumed.

Many mundane issues remain to be resolved with both RT-PCR and immunodetection approaches. Sample type, volume, and collection can influence results. Rapid processing of samples to avoid target degradation is recommended, particularly for RT-PCR methods. Studies indicate that although most transcripts will decline over time, some increase and others (including glyceraldehyde 3-phosphate dehydrogenase, a housekeeping gene commonly used for assessment of sample quality) are unusually stable and therefore may not adequately reflect the quality of the RNA from the patient sample.

Lastly, assay standardization is needed so that reliable and reproducible studies can be performed in multiple laboratories. Thus, tumor cell detection approaches remain in evolution as our knowledge and technology advances. The commercial platforms are a step toward development of tools that will facilitate the large-scale clinical trials needed to better define the clinical utility of occult tumor cell detection.

APPLICATIONS

Perhaps the greatest challenge for the development and validation of molecular assays for the detection of occult tumor cells is the demonstration of clinical utility. Carefully designed assays can successfully demonstrate the presence of tumor cells in clinical samples. Determining the clinical significance of

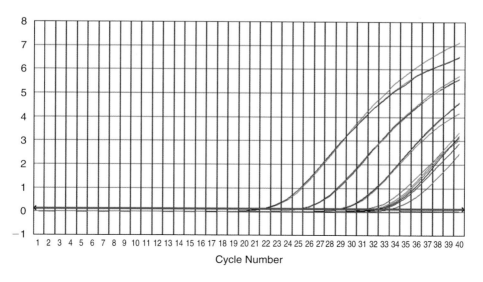

FIGURE 15-4

Real-time reverse transcriptase–polymerase chain reaction results of 10,000, 1000, 100, and 10 copies (each analyzed multiple times to demonstrate reproducibility) of cytokeratin 19 (CK19) RNA, 50 ng of Raji DNA (a cell line negative for CK19) and polyadenylated RNA (also negative for CK19). (Courtesy of Dr. Natalie Solomon, Abbott Molecular, Des Plaines, IL.)

these cells is considerably more difficult. Hundreds of studies using IHC and molecular methods to detect tumor cells have been performed. The sections that follow address some of the more common potential applications.

EARLY DETECTION

In general, detection of circulating cells can be assumed to be better suited for evaluation of a known tumor rather than for early detection of subclinical cancer primaries. Other technologies and approaches hold greater promise for early, premetastasis tumor cell detection. The study of cell-free DNA and RNA in various body fluids may prove to be an ideal method for screening and early detection of cancers. Proteomics also holds great potential.

STAGING

A general correlation between incidence of circulating cells and increased tumor stage has been demonstrated for a variety of tumor types. Unfortunately, the reverse approach does not appear to be supported by the data, such that molecular staging of cancer remains an unattained goal. This may largely be because most circulating cells are unable to complete the metastatic process and thus are biologically irrelevant, again revealing the need for markers of metastatic capability. It may also be possible that identification of circulating tumor cells provides valuable information on the systemic spread of tumor in a manner different than that used by conventional staging approaches. For example, in prostate cancer, small but aggressive tumors may shed cells into the circulation, whereas a more indolent but larger tumor may reach the surgical margin but may not shed aggressive cells into the bloodstream; in this case, circulating cells may appear to correlate poorly with traditional tumor stage but may more accurately reflect tumor aggressiveness. In addition, it is perhaps not surprising that the detection of circulating breast cancer cells has been correlated with vascular invasion in the primary tumor.

PROGNOSIS

Although a general correlation between presence of circulating tumor cells and increased tumor stage has been observed, only a few studies have demonstrated a relationship between circulating cells and cancer recurrence or progression. Correlation between circulating cells and disease-free survival following radical prostatectomy has been reported. In colorectal cancer, conflicting findings have been reported, and some reports highlight the potential correlation between cells shed at the time of surgery into blood and body fluids and risk of recurrence later. The implications of circulating tumor cells in patients with melanoma remains controversial, although a trend toward worse prognosis is evident.

Recently, a commercially available immunofluorescent detection system has been used to demonstrate that the number of circulating cells in advanced-stage breast cancer correlates with overall and disease-free survival. Prognostic information is useful, but even greater value will be realized when this approach can be used to tailor chemotherapy or if correlations to outcome and treatment response can be observed in earlier-stage patients. Clinical studies are under way.

In general, better correlation has been observed between patient outcome and molecular or IHC detection of tumor cells in the bone marrow compared to blood. It is possible that cells in the marrow are at an "advanced" stage in the metastatic continuum, having acquired the capacity to survive in the circulation, attach, and grow in the remote environment. The detection of cytokeratin-positive cells using IHC in bone marrow samples from breast cancer patients correlates with survival and outcome, as reported in a sentinel publication in this field. Similar findings have been reported for prostate cancer. In the United States, such studies can be hampered by clinical practices, which do not include bone marrow sampling as part of routine staging for many tumors.

MONITORING TREATMENT

Monitoring treatment response in patients with acute leukemia using molecular methods has become relatively routine. Few studies have examined this application for monitoring of patients with solid tumors. Decreased incidence of circulating cells has been reported in prostate cancer patients receiving androgen-deprivation treatment. A small study of breast cancer patients with clinically evident metastasis showed a significantly lower incidence of circulating cells in patients receiving chemotherapy or hormonal therapy than in patients not on treatment. Similar results were observed for lung cancer. RT-PCR has also been used to monitor interferon response in melanoma patients. Further studies are warranted.

CONCLUSION

Since the first report of RT-PCR detection of circulating cells in melanoma was published in 1991, clear establishment of the clinical relevance of occult tumor cells in blood, bone marrow, and other sites has eluded many teams of investigators. The challenges in development and validation of RT-PCR assays aimed at expression of a normal gene (rather than a mutated, translocated, or chimeric gene) are significant and have undoubtedly led to a great deal of confusion within this field. In many respects, this field parallels that of *Her2/neu* in the early days of investigation, when experimental and reagent variation complicated clear conclusions based on the various studies. Standardization of these assays is now beginning, aided by the availability of commercial platforms and kits. Carefully designed and controlled multicenter clinical studies are needed to further clarify this approach for any tumor or sample type. Recent revisions in the International Union Against Cancer staging protocol that include molecular results in some categories at this point are largely designed to facilitate data gathering.

IHC and molecular detection of tumor cells remains a promising tool for the detection of circulating tumor cells that is beginning to make the transition to clinical use. It can be anticipated that these approaches will become a standard part of patient assessment and care in the coming years. Still, significant efforts are needed before we know how to appropriately apply results to routine patient management.

SUGGESTED READINGS

Allard WJ, Matera J, Miller MC, et al: Tumor cells circulate in the peripheral blood of all major carcinomas but not in healthy subjects or patients with nonmalignant diseases. Clin Cancer Res 2004;10:6897–6904.

Bauer KD, de la Torre-Bueno J, Diel IJ, et al: Reliable and sensitive analysis of occult bone marrow metastases using automated cellular imaging. Clin Cancer Res 2000;6:3552–3559.

Benoy IH, Elst H, Philips M, et al: Real-time RT-PCR detection of disseminated tumour cells in bone marrow has superior prognostic significance in comparison with circulating tumour cells in patients with breast cancer. Br J Cancer 2006;94(5):672–680.

Benoy IH, Elst H, Van Dam P, et al: Detection of circulating tumour cells in blood by quantitative real-time RT-PCR: Effect of preanalytical time. Clin Chem Lab Med 2006;44(9):1082–1087.

Bessa X, Elizalde JI, Boix L, et al: Lack of prognostic influence of circulating tumor cells in peripheral blood of patients with colorectal cancer. Gastroenterology 2001;120(5):1084–1092.

Bessho A, Tabata M, Kiura K, et al: Detection of occult tumor cells in peripheral blood from patients with small cell lung cancer by reverse transcriptase–polymerase chain reaction. Anticancer Res 2000;20(2B):1149–1154.

Bianco FJ Jr, Powell IJ, Cher ML, Wood DP Jr: Presence of circulating prostate cancer cells in African American males adversely affects survival. Urol Oncol 2002;7:147–152.

Bianco FJ Jr, Wood DP Jr, Gomes de Oliveira J, et al: Proliferation of prostate cancer cells in the bone marrow predicts recurrence in patients with localized prostate cancer. Prostate 2001;49(4)235–242.

Bosch B, Guller U, Schnider A, et al: Perioperative detection of disseminated tumour cells is an independent prognostic factor in patients with colorectal cancer. Br J Surg 2003;90(7):882–888.

Bosma AJ, Weigelt B, Lambrechts AC, et al: Detection of circulating breast tumor cells by differential expression of marker genes. Clin Cancer Res 2002;8:1871–1877.

Braun S, Pantel K, Müller P, et al: Cytokeratin-positive cells in the bone marrow and survival of patients with stage I, II, or III breast cancer. N Engl J Med 2000;342:525–533.

Burchill SA, Perebolte L, Johnston C, et al: Comparison of the RNA-amplification based methods RT-PCR and NASBA for the detection of circulating tumour cells. Br J Cancer 2002;86(1):102–109.

Cristofanilli M, Budd GT, Ellis MJ, et al: Circulating tumor cells, disease progression, and survival in metastatic breast cancer. N Engl J Med 2004;351(8):781–791.

Cristofanilli M, Hayes DF, Budd GT, et al: Circulating tumor cells: A novel prognostic factor for newly diagnosed metastatic breast cancer. J Clin Oncol 2005;23(7):1420–1430.

Elshimani YA, Grody WW: The clinical significance of circulating tumor cells in the peripheral blood. Diagn Mol Pathol 2006;15:187–194.

Fehm T, Sagalowsky A, Clifford E, et al: Cytogenetic evidence that circulating epithelial cells in patients with carcinoma are malignant. Clin Cancer Res 2002;8:2073–2084.

Fournier MV, da Gloria Costa Carvalho M, Pardee AB: A strategy to identify genes associated with circulating solid tumor cell survival in peripheral blood. Mol Med 1999;5:313–319.

Ghossein RA, Bhattacharya S, Coit DG: Reverse transcriptase polymerase chain reaction (RT-PCR) detection of melanoma-related transcripts in the peripheral blood and bone marrow of patients with malignant melanoma: What have we learned? Cancer Res 2001;158:63–77.

Guller U, Zajac P, Schnider A, et al: Disseminated single tumor cells as detected by real-time quantitative polymerase chain reaction represent a prognostic factor in patients undergoing surgery for colorectal cancer. Ann Surg 2002;236(6):768–776.

Hermanek P, Sobin LH (eds): UICC TNM Classification of Malignant Tumors, 5th ed. New York, Springer, 1998.

Hoon DS, Wang Y, Dale PS, et al: Detection of occult melanoma cells in blood with a multiple marker polymerase chain reaction assay. J Clin Oncol 1995;13:2109–2116.

Houghton RL, Dillon DC, Molesh DA, et al: Transcriptional complementarity in breast cancer: Application to the detection of circulating tumor cells. Mol Diagn 2001;6:79–91.

Ignatoff JM, Oefelein MG, Watkin W, et al: Prostate specific antigen (PSA) reverse transcriptase polymerase chain reaction (RT-PCR) assay in preoperative staging of prostate cancer. J Urol 1997;158:1870–1875.

Kasimir-Bauer S, Oberhoff C, Schindler AE, Seeber S: A summary of two clinical studies on tumor cell dissemination and metastatic breast cancer: Methods, prognostics significance and implication for alternative treatment protocols [review]. Int J Oncol 2002;20:1027–1034.

Katz AE, de Vries GM, Begg MD, et al: Enhanced reverse transcriptase-polymerase chain reaction for prostate specific antigen as an indicator of true pathologic stage in patients with prostate cancer. Cancer 1995;75:1642–1648.

Kowalewska M, Checklinska M, Markowicz S, et al: The relevance of RT-PCR detection of disseminated tumour cells is hampered by the expression of markers regarded as tumour specific in activated lymphocytes. Eur J Cancer 2006;42(16):2671–2674.

Koyanagi K, Kuo C, Nakagawa T, et al: Multimarker quantitative real-time PCR detection of circulating melanoma cells in peripheral blood: Relation to disease stage in melanoma patients. Clin Chem 2005;51:981–988.

Lambrechts AC, Bosma AJ, Klaver SG, et al: Comparison of immunohistochemistry, reverse transcriptase polymerase chain reaction, and nucleic acid sequence-based amplification for the detection of circulating breast cancer cells. Breast Cancer Res Treat 1999;56:219–231.

Luke S, Kaul K: Detection of breast cancer cells in blood using immunomagnetic bead selection and reverse transcription–polymerase chain reaction. Mol Diagn 1998;3(3):149–155.

Marches R, Scheuermann R, Uhr J: Cancer dormancy: From mice to man. Cell Cycle 2006;5(16):1772–1778.

Martin KJ, Graner E, Li Y, et al: High-sensitivity array analysis of gene expression for the early detection of disseminated breast tumor cells in peripheral blood. Proc Natl Acad Sci USA 2001;98(5):2646–2651.

Mellado B, Del Carmen Vela M, Colomer D, et al: Tyrosinase mRNA in blood of patients with melanoma treated with adjuvant interferon. Clin Oncol 2002;20:4032–4039.

Meng S, Tripathy D, Frenkel EP, et al: Circulating tumor cells in patients with breast cancer dormancy. Clin Cancer Res 2004;10(24):8152–8162.

Mitas M, Mikhitarian K, Walters C, et al: Quantitative real-time RT-PCR detection of breast cancer micrometastasis using a multigene marker panel. Int J Cancer 2001;93:162–171.

Mocellin S, Keilholz U, Rossi CR, Nitti D: Circulating tumor cells: The "leukemic phase" of solid cancers. Trends Mol Med 2006;12:130–139.

Muller V, Hayes DF, Pantel K: Recent translational research: Circulating tumor cells in breast cancer patients. Breast Cancer Res 2006;8: 110–114.

Naume B, Borgen E, Nesland JM, et al: Increased sensitivity for detection of micrometastases in bone marrow/peripheral blood stem-cell products from breast-cancer patients by negative immunomagnetic separation. Int J Cancer 1998;78:556–560.

Olsson CA, de Vries GM, Benson MC, et al: The use of RT-PCR for prostate-specific antigen assay to predict potential surgical failures before radical prostatectomy: Molecular staging of prostate cancer. Br J Urol 1996;77:411–417.

Pantel K, Cote RJ, Fodstad O: Detection and clinical importance of micrometastatic disease. J Nat Cancer Inst 1999;91:1113–1124.

Raj GV, Moreno JG, Gomela LG: Utilization of polymerase chain reaction technology in the detection of solid tumors. Cancer 1998;82(8): 1419–1442.

Schluter K, Gassmann P, Enns A, et al: Organ-specific metastatic tumor cell adhesion and extravasation of colon carcinoma cells with different metastatic potential. Am J Pathol 2006;169(3):1064–1073.

Scoggins CR, Ross MI, Reintgen DS, et al: Prospective multi-institutional study of reverse transcriptase polymerase chain reaction for molecular staging of melanoma. J Clin Oncol 2006;24:2849–2857.

Shariat SF, Gottenger E, Nguyen C, et al: Preoperative blood reverse transcriptase–PCR assays for prostate-specific antigen and human glandular kallikrein for prediction of prostate cancer progression after radical prostatectomy. Cancer Res 2002;62(20):5974–5979.

Slade MJ, Smith BM, Sinnett HD, et al: Quantitative polymerase chain reaction for the detection of micrometastases in patients with breast cancer. J Clin Oncol 1999;17:780–789.

Smirnov DA, Zweitig DR, Foulk BW, et al: Global gene expression profiling of circulating tumor cells. Cancer Res 2005;65:4993–4997.

Smith B, Selby P, Southgate J, et al: Detection of melanoma cells in peripheral blood by means of reverse transcriptase and polymerase chain reaction. Lancet 1991;338:1227–1229.

Soeth E, Roder C, Juhl H, et al: The detection of disseminated tumor cells in bone marrow from colorectal cancer patients by a cytokeratin 20 specific nested reverse transcriptase–polymerase chain reaction is related to the stage of disease. Int J Cancer 1996;69:278–282.

Su SL, Heston WD, Perrotti M, et al: Evaluating neoadjuvant therapy effectiveness on systemic disease: Use of a prostatic-specific membrane reverse transcription–polymerase chain reaction. Urol 1997;49: 95–101.

Taback B, Chan AD, Kuo CT, et al: Detection of occult metastatic breast cancer cells in blood by a multimolecular marker assay: Correlation with clinical stage of disease. Cancer Res 2001;61:8845–8850.

Taback B, Hoon DS: Circulating nucleic acids and proteomics of plasma/ serum: Clinical utility. Ann NY Acad Sci 2004;1022:1–8.

Traweek ST, Liu J, Battifora H: Keratin gene expression in nonepithelial tissues: Detection with polymerase chain reaction. Am J Pathol 1993;142:1111–1118.

Tvasellas G, Huang A, McCullough T, et al: Flow cytometry correlates with RT-PCR for detection of spiked but not circulating colorectal cancer cells. Clin Exp Metastasis 2002;19(6):495–502.

Uciechowski P, Eder C, Böckmann B, et al: Prognostic value of genomic alterations in minimal residual cancer cells purified from the blood of breast cancer patients. Br J Cancer 2000;83(12):1664–1673.

Vogel I, Kalthoff H: Disseminated tumour cells: Their detection and significance for prognosis of gastrointestinal and pancreatic carcinomas. Virchows Arch 2001;439:109–117.

Witzig TE, Bossy B, Kiminger T, et al: Detection of circulating cytokeratin-positive cells in the blood of breast cancer patients using immunomagnetic enrichment and digital microscopy. Clin Cancer Res 2002;8:1085–1091.

Wong IHN, Yeo W, Chan A, Johnson PJ: Quantitative relationship of the circulating tumor burden assessed by reverse transcriptase–polymerase chain reaction for cytokeratin 19 mRNA in peripheral blood of colorectal cancer patients with Dukes' stage, serum carcinoembryonic antigen level and tumor progression. Cancer Lett 2001;162:65–73.

Wood DP Jr, Banerjee M: Presence of circulating prostate cells in the bone marrow of patients undergoing radical prostatectomy is predictive of disease-free survival. J Clin Oncol 1997;15:3451–3457.

Zehentner BK: Detection of disseminated tumor cells: Strategies and diagnostic implications. Expert Rev Mol Diagn 2002;2:41–48.

Zippelius A, Pantel K: RT-PCR-based detection of occult disseminated tumor cells in peripheral blood and bone marrow of patients with solid tumors: An overview. Ann NY Acad Sci 2000;906:110–123.

times, would be a major benefit in the same situation but requires each reaction site on the instrument to be independently controlled. Currently, the only such instrument appears to be the Cepheid SmartCycler. Finally, automation of as many steps as possible is preferable from both labor and reproducibility perspectives. Nucleic acid isolation, reaction setup, and even transfer to a real-time PCR instrument are all possible using a variety of robotic systems available in clinical laboratories. However, these tend to be extremely expensive, not optimized for speed, and mostly designed for batch processing rather than concurrent handling of individual samples with different processing requirements. Therefore, the available automation tools are probably not suitable for intraoperative PCR assays. One exception to this is the Cepheid GeneXpert™ which is designed specifically for rapid, point-of-care diagnostic assays. The GeneXpert automates fast nucleic acid isolation, cDNA synthesis (if necessary), and real-time PCR by combining robotics with single-use, disposable cartridges (that can be preloaded with all reagents required for a specific assay) and the real-time PCR capabilities of the SmartCycler instrument. Instruments such as the GeneXpert would therefore seem ideally suited to the requirements of an intraoperative real-time PCR assay.

POTENTIAL ADVANTAGES OF INTRAOPERATIVE POLYMERASE CHAIN REACTION ASSAYS

Intraoperative tests being performed in pathology are essentially restricted to morphologic interpretation of frozen tissue sections, tissue imprints, or needle biopsies. In most cases, this is performed using hematoxylin and eosin staining, although rapid methods for immunostaining have been reported and may be used rarely. Therefore, the biggest advantage of an alternative methodology would exist when these current methods are unable to provide an answer or when the answer is often inconclusive. PCR assays for DNA, RNA, or even microRNA targets could feasibly be developed for situations in which simple morphologic examination is inadequate. One example of this would be the identification of the tissue of origin for a tumor in the case of a patient with either a tumor of unknown origin or a history of cancer presenting with a second tumor (is it a new primary tumor or a metastasis?) These questions can typically be resolved by the pathologist using special stains, but this not feasible intraoperatively. Conversely, there is little point to developing intraoperative PCR assays for situations in which intraoperative pathology is reliably informative and accurate. However, there are many situations that fall in between the two extremes (in which intraoperative pathology is good but not perfect). In these

situations, PCR assays may be advantageous for a variety of other reasons. First, PCR assays are extremely sensitive and, in theory, can detect the desired target even if it is present in low amounts. This may be an advantage if rare cells in the specimen need to be identified in a background of other cell types but may be missed by intraoperative pathology or cytology, where sensitivity is not as good as final pathology. Second, despite considerable expertise and training, pathologic interpretation is a subjective endeavor and results can be variable and pathologist dependent. Real-time PCR assays, on the other hand, have the advantage of being completely objective, highly reproducible, and capable of standardization for use and comparison of data between different institutions. This could be a significant benefit in smaller institutions, where pathologists may not be as specialized or as experienced as those at major medical centers, as well as in multicenter clinical trials. Finally, the use of intraoperative PCR assays may reduce some of the burden for pathologists performing frozen section analysis by eliminating the need for examination of some specimens. Alternatively, a rapid PCR result may be used to assist the pathologist when the pathologic interpretation is inconclusive.

POTENTIAL DISADVANTAGES OF INTRAOPERATIVE POLYMERASE CHAIN REACTION ASSAYS

The biggest concern for many pathologists when considering molecular assays is specificity. Although the PCR reaction itself can be highly specific for amplifying the desired target and nothing else, the specificity of the assay depends more on biology and on the choice of target than the PCR reaction itself. Few things are absolute in biologic systems, and most assays have some kind of background level (either biological or technical). For example, when detecting adenocarcinoma in a lymph node, one may choose to examine expression of the carcinoembryonic antigen and design an RT-PCR assay that is highly specific for this target. However, when using this assay to analyze lymph nodes without cancer, one can find background expression in almost all lymph nodes because of the extreme sensitivity of the PCR assay. In a nonquantitative assay, this would lead to low specificity despite a highly target-specific PCR. A quantitative assay could be used to help distinguish true expression caused by cancer cells from background, but the distribution of expression values in negative and positive nodes may now overlap such that 100% accuracy cannot be achieved. Ideally, for any particular assay, one would be able to identify a PCR target in which results do not overlap between positive and negative samples. In practice, this can be extremely difficult, and few such markers have been identified to date. Thus, in many cases, one will be left with a choice of sensitivity versus specificity, positive predictive value versus negative predictive value, etc. Alternatively, a probability can be assigned to the result and used accordingly as an adjunct to pathologic evaluation. In either case, the molecular assay will only be useful when it is clinically validated so that its classification characteristics are better than or complementary to intraoperative pathology. Another disadvantage of intraoperative molecular assays, and one which may lead to reduced specificity, is their inability to distinguish a clinically relevant signal from signal caused by sample contamination. Such contamination may come from adjacent tissues, surgical instruments, or instruments used for tissue processing in the pathology suite. Because of the extreme sensitivity of PCR, even the smallest amount of contamination could potentially cause a false-positive result. Concurrent pathologic examination and implementation of process controls should reduce the incidence of false-positive tests but are unlikely to eliminate them.

Finally, the issues of speed and cost of intraoperative molecular assays need to be considered. Despite the fastest instruments available and optimized assay design, a real-time PCR assay still takes at least 30 minutes from tissue to result; this does not include freezing and sectioning of the tissue. When compared to 10 minutes or less for a hematoxylin and eosin (H&E) staining and evaluation, the molecular assay will add at least 20 minutes to the turnaround time. This may be unacceptable to the surgeon in some instances. Furthermore, these specialized and complex assays are likely to be expensive and may not be covered by insurance, particularly if they are in addition to other costs associated with intraoperative pathology rather than replacements for them. Although these costs will almost certainly drop over time, they may pose a barrier to initial acceptance of such tests.

APPLICATIONS OF INTRAOPERATIVE POLYMERASE CHAIN REACTION ASSAYS

Currently, intraoperative molecular assays are not being performed in the United States outside of small, industry-sponsored trials. Therefore, this section of the chapter discusses some of the more immediate and interesting potential applications and the pros and cons of each where appropriate.

Probably the most discussed and immediately practical application of intraoperative PCR is in the examination of lymph nodes and, in particular, sentinel lymph nodes (SLNs) for the presence of metastatic tumor cells. Regardless of the questions and controversy generated by adoption of the SLN biopsy technique, there is no doubt that one of the consequences

has been the ability of the pathologist to focus on a small number of lymph nodes and to perform a more detailed analysis of these nodes than is typically performed on nodes from extended resections. The examination of multiple sections at different levels and the use of immunohistochemical stains to enhance detection of small tumor deposits has reduced sampling error and improved sensitivity for detecting metastatic disease in SLNs. However, this process is labor intensive, is time consuming, and cannot be reliably performed in as thorough a manner intraoperatively. Instead, intraoperative pathology on SLNs is much less thorough and subject to reduced sensitivity as a result. Theoretically, a rapid molecular test using real-time RT-PCR could provide sensitivity and sampling equivalent to final pathology but do so in an intraoperative time frame. The concept underlying this approach is that tumor cells express mRNA species that the surrounding cells in the lymph node do not. Therefore, detection of these messages by RT-PCR implies the presence of tumor cells. Clearly, a tumor cell–specific mRNA would be the desired target, but in my experience few mRNAs are expressed in all tumors and not in normal tissue. Therefore, current assays rely mostly on tissue-specific markers but do not discriminate between normal and cancer cells from the tissue of tumor origin. Furthermore, because of the heterogeneity of marker gene expression in tumors, the PCR result does not correlate well with the size of the lymph node metastasis, even in a quantitative assay. Despite these limitations, an intraoperative molecular assay for SLNs remains an attractive possibility because of its potential sensitivity. Currently, SLN biopsy is routine in the United States for breast cancer and melanoma and is in the trial phases for other tumors, such as oral cancer and lung cancer. In addition, there are other tumors, such as esophageal carcinoma, for which SLN biopsy may not be applicable but for which there may still be a role for intraoperative lymph node staging. For each disease, the clinical scenario and desirable characteristics of an intraoperative assay are somewhat unique and this is discussed in more detail in the rest of this chapter.

BREAST CANCER SENTINEL LYMPH NODE ANALYSIS

CLINICAL SCENARIO

SLN biopsy is routine for early-stage breast cancer patients in the United States, and the current standard of care is to perform an axillary lymph node dissection (ALND) only if the SLN is positive. Thus, the surgeon needs to know the SLN status to determine the extent of resection. If determined intraoperatively, this decision can be made such that only one surgical procedure is required.

CURRENT ANALYSIS

Methods for intraoperative analysis of SLNs vary from institution to institution. However, the most common methods are probably to perform a touch imprint followed by a frozen section to confirm a positive result or to directly perform a frozen section examination. In either case, the examination is typically limited to one or two sections at one level with H&E staining. Methods for final pathology are again variable but involve examination of multiple sections at different levels and often include IHC for cytokeratin markers (most often AE1/AE3). Comparisons of intraoperative pathology with the final pathology report describe anywhere from 45% to 85% sensitivity of traditional intraoperative assessment; as a result, many women require a second surgery for ALND.

STATE OF THE MOLECULAR ASSAY

A rapid, real-time PCR assay for breast cancer SLN analysis was recently introduced by Veridex for use in Europe, and Food and Drug Administration clearance for the test in the United States has been achieved. The Veridex GeneSearch™ assay can be performed in 30 to 40 minutes by trained personnel and uses the Cepheid SmartCycler instrument platform, along with a kit for manual sample preparation and reaction setup. Details of the assay, including markers and assay design (quantitative versus nonquantitative or semiquantitative), were not publicly available at the time of writing, although from published work it is likely that the markers are cytokeratin 19 and mammaglobin. An alternative test is being developed in collaboration with Cepheid. This assay uses two target genes and an endogenous control gene to provide quantitative gene expression data on both markers. The assay is performed on the Cepheid GeneXpert system and is thus completely automated (RNA isolation, reverse transcription, Q-PCR, and data analysis) and can provide a negative result in 30 minutes. A positive result is typically returned in less than 25 minutes. This assay is in early trials to determine accuracy and reproducibility at multiple sites. Thus, an intraoperative molecular assay for breast cancer SLNs may be available in the United States shortly.

PROS AND CONS OF A MOLECULAR ASSAY

The biggest advantage of a molecular assay is the potential for improved sensitivity and thus the ability to complete surgical treatment in one procedure.

Clearly, specificity is also essential to avoid unnecessary ALND on some patients. Therefore, the specific characteristics of the assays available or under development will be critical to their utility and acceptance. It is unlikely that either assay will be 100% sensitive and specific in all cases, but hopefully with either the Veridex or the Cepheid assay, appropriate expression cutoffs can be set at which these criteria are met for subsets of patients. The remainder of patients would be deferred to intraoperative or final pathology. In this scenario, it should still be possible to obtain high sensitivity while maintaining specificity approaching 100% and minimizing the number of inconclusive results. This would greatly reduce the need for second procedures for ALND and could reduce the burden of intraoperative examination for pathologists (particularly in the case of negative PCR results).

LYMPH NODE SAMPLING AND COMPARISON OF HISTOLOGIC VERSUS MOLECULAR ASSAYS

The accuracy, and in particular, the sensitivity of SLN analysis by either a histologic examination or a molecular assay is determined mostly by two factors: the amount of tissue examined (sampling) and the sensitivity for identifying small tumor foci or isolated tumor cells in the tissues sampled. For histologic analysis, sensitivity could be maximized by sectioning the whole node and staining alternate sections with H&E and IHC. However, this is clearly impractical (unless the whole process can be automated) even for final pathology, let alone for intraoperative analysis. A commonly used compromise is to section the node at 1- or 2-mm intervals and then examine several sections at each level. Again, this approach is restricted to final pathology because of the time constraints associated with intraoperative analysis. For molecular assays such as RT-PCR, the sampling and sensitivity issues are more complex. Theoretically, PCR is extremely sensitive (possibly more sensitive than IHC), but as discussed earlier, the background expression levels of the mRNA markers chosen effectively limit the discriminatory capabilities of the assay. Thus, although it is possible to extract RNA from a whole lymph node and to put all of this RNA into a PCR reaction, a small metastatic focus may not be detectable (above background) in the vast excess of RNA from normal nodal tissue. One way to overcome this would be to section the node as described earlier and to analyze the RNA from each 1- to 2-mm section in individual reactions, thus reducing the background in each assay. However, as with pathology, one quickly runs into issues of practicality, cost, and timing with this approach.

When comparing histologic and molecular approaches to SLN analysis, one would like to be fair when it comes to sampling issues. For example, if you examine 20 sections from four levels by pathology, then it would seem fair to analyze the same number of adjacent sections by the molecular assay. However, for an intraoperative assay, it is not practical to examine 20 sections by histology but it is feasible to examine 20 (or 50, 100, or more) sections in a molecular assay. In fact, one of the advantages of the molecular assay for intraoperative analysis is its ability to examine more tissue without taking more time. Therefore, is it fair to restrict the molecular assay input just to produce a direct comparison? From a practical standpoint, the fairest comparison may be to use the most sensitive sampling method that is reasonably feasible for each approach. When this is done, it is likely that the molecular analysis will be more accurate than intraoperative pathology and will more closely approximate final pathology.

OTHER ISSUES

Although a rapid molecular test would appear to be beneficial to the surgeon, the patient, and the pathologist, there are some reservations on the part of all. With breast cancer often being diagnosed at an early stage when the probability of lymph node metastasis is low, some surgeons have expressed a preference to perform SLN biopsy and tumor resection followed by a separate procedure for ALND when necessary. This preference comes from a concern over efficient scheduling of operating room time and for the desire to avoid unnecessary discussions over treatment options for most patients who prove to have negative SLNs. From a patient's perspective, the choice between the ability to be done with surgery in one procedure versus the opportunity to discuss treatment and seek second opinions will be a personal one. Either way, having a definitive answer available when the patient wakes up from surgery is presumably preferable to waiting several days for final pathology for all involved. From the pathologist's perspective, there is clearly concern over the possibility of a false-positive result. Although rare, it has been suggested that benign breast cells may migrate to the lymph nodes after diagnostic procedures, such as a core biopsy, and without cancer-specific markers this could indeed be a problem for a molecular assay.

Nevertheless, for breast cancer, perhaps the biggest challenge faced by an intraoperative PCR assay is that it is being introduced when there is considerable controversy over two relevant issues. First, the need to perform ALND in the patient with a positive SLN is being questioned. If there is no proven benefit, then the need for intraoperative analysis of lymph nodes would disappear. However, the objective results, reproducibility, ability to standardize testing across institutions, and potential to reduce the workload for the pathologist may still be useful, even when speed is not essential. Second, there is much debate over the

clinical significance of micrometastatic (<0.2 mm) disease in breast cancer SLNs and the appropriate treatment for patients with such disease. This is important because it is unlikely that a molecular assay will accurately distinguish between tumor deposits less than and more than 0.2 mm. Therefore, if treatment options hinge upon this distinction, molecular assays may have limited value. On the other hand, trials are ongoing to determine the prognostic value of SLN metastasis detected by RT-PCR (most of which are presumably <0.2 mm) in SLN-negative patients. If these trials should prove positive, then a standardized and automated assay with the option for intraoperative use could be extremely valuable.

MELANOMA SENTINEL LYMPH NODE ANALYSIS

CLINICAL SCENARIO

SLN biopsy is standard practice in the treatment of melanoma, and an extended lymph node dissection is typically performed when the SLN is positive. Thus, the scenario is similar to that for breast cancer, where an accurate intraoperative analysis could limit the number of surgical procedures required to complete treatment.

CURRENT ANALYSIS

Frozen section analysis of melanoma SLNs is challenging because of the morphologic features of melanoma cells. As a result, the sensitivity compared with the final pathology is only 30% to 40%, and most institutions do not perform intraoperative analysis. Final pathology typically includes H&E analysis of sections from multiple levels, with IHC for melanocyte markers when necessary.

STATE OF THE MOLECULAR ASSAY

The literature is inundated with reports on the use of RT-PCR for staging of SLNs from melanoma patients. Most of this work, however, is aimed at improving prognostic capability in SLN-negative patients, not developing rapid assays to distinguish positive and negative nodes intraoperatively. To my knowledge, no intraoperative molecular assays for melanoma are being tested.

PROS AND CONS OF A MOLECULAR ASSAY

Because the sensitivity of frozen section is so poor for melanoma, the potential utility of a highly sensitive molecular assay is clear. Nevertheless, as with breast cancer, specificity is the main issue surrounding an intraoperative PCR test, and the preceding discussion is as relevant in melanoma as it is in breast cancer. Unlike breast cancer, however, the presence of benign melanocytic cells in lymph nodes is a relatively common finding on pathologic review and has been reported in greater than 20% of nodes in some series. This poses a major problem for a PCR-based assay because these benign nevi need to be distinguished from true metastases to avoid a significant number of false-positive results and unnecessary lymph node dissection. Unfortunately, the most common molecular markers for melanoma RT-PCR are also expressed at similar levels in normal melanocytes and therefore cannot provide this distinction. Recent papers from different groups propose that new markers (PLAB, L1CAM, GalNAc-T, and PAX3) may be able to differentiate benign from malignant melanocytes, but this remains to be verified. In the absence of melanoma-specific markers, it is unlikely that an intraoperative PCR assay will be acceptable for proceeding to a complete lymph node resection. Still, an assay with high negative predictive value possibly could be useful. Finally, if ongoing studies find that RT-PCR is prognostic even in SLN-negative patients, an argument could be made for performing the assay intraoperatively and acting on the result immediately.

ANALYSIS OF SENTINEL LYMPH NODES IN HEAD AND NECK CANCER

CLINICAL SCENARIO

Preoperative clinical staging of the neck in patients with squamous cell carcinoma of the head and neck (SCCHN) often misdiagnoses the presence or absence of lymphatic metastases. Because of the poor prognosis when these metastases are missed, the current management of the cN0 neck commonly includes routine elective neck dissection with pathologic analysis of the nodes removed. In approximately 70% of the cases, pathology is negative and the neck dissection may represent overtreatment. In an attempt to overcome this problem, SLN biopsy is being tested in a multicenter trial in the United States. If successful, SLN biopsy would potentially allow accurate staging of the neck without a complete neck dissection; in this scenario, an intraoperative analysis would be highly desirable.

CURRENT ANALYSIS

Intraoperative analysis is not typically performed on lymph nodes from SCCHN patients. However, in one small study, the sensitivity of frozen section analysis was 60% (6 of 10 patients) compared with final pathology.

STATE OF THE MOLECULAR ASSAY

As with melanoma, most research on SCCHN lymph node analysis has focused on the use of RT-PCR to predict recurrence in pN0 patients. Several potential markers have been identified and used in these studies, and these markers could form the basis of an intraoperative assay. In 2005, Ferris et al. reported a marker screen for SCCHN metastasis detection and demonstrated the feasibility of an intraoperative assay using the Cepheid GeneXpert. This work is being expanded upon, and a GeneXpert-based assay could be available for clinical testing reasonably soon.

INTRAOPERATIVE LYMPH NODE ANALYSIS IN OTHER TUMOR TYPES

In addition to the SLN applications discussed earlier, there are other possible uses of intraoperative PCR assays for lymph node staging in diseases for which SLN biopsy is not being used. For example, esophageal cancer typically spreads to lymph nodes early, and this is highly prognostic. Depending on the location of the tumor, the involvement of certain lymph nodes is considered to be almost equivalent to metastatic disease and may be the cause for a radical lymphadenectomy or the patient deemed inoperable. For example, for a distal esophageal tumor, the involvement of celiac lymph nodes is classified as M1a disease and the patient is classified as stage IVA. The same is true for a proximal tumor with cervical lymph node metastasis. Therefore, sampling of these nodes, combined with intraoperative assessment, may help determine the most appropriate surgical approach. In this regard, Japanese researchers and clinicians have published several articles describing the potential utility of intraoperative PCR assays in esophageal cancer. A similar situation exists in the staging of nonsmall cell lung cancer. Patients with suspected mediastinal (N2 and N3) lymph node metastases commonly undergo mediastinoscopy to provide definitive staging. In this case, however, the treatment decision is whether to proceed to resection of the primary tumor (if the mediastinal nodes are negative) or stop and refer the patient for neoadjuvant chemotherapy (for N2 or N3 disease). An intraoperative molecular assay for accurate assessment of mediastinal nodes could therefore be useful, and one may wish to optimize this assay for negative predictive value, because a false-negative result in this case would lead irrevocably to suboptimal treatment (assuming that neoadjuvant chemotherapy is truly more effective than postadjuvant).

ADDITIONAL APPLICATION POSSIBILITIES

Besides the possibility for intraoperative staging of lymph nodes, rapid PCR assays have potential for many other applications in cancer staging and diagnosis as long as appropriate markers can be found. Such applications could be the identification of tissue type in tumors of unknown origin or the differentiation of primary tumor from metastasis in a patient with a history of cancer. One such common scenario is a patient with history of SCCHN who presents a short time later with a squamous cell lung tumor. Treatment options for this patient could be vastly different depending on the determination of SCCHN metastasis or primary lung cancer, and this is often difficult to ascertain even with fixed tissue pathology. Although it may be possible to identify one or a few mRNA markers that could distinguish SSCHN from squamous cell lung cancer, an interesting alternative may be to use microRNA targets because these small, noncoding RNAs seem to be highly informative regarding tissue lineage and cell type. Similarly, a multiplex microRNA assay could be useful in determining the tissue of origin of a tumor metastasis when no primary tumor is evident. Although technically feasible, such an approach requires much effort to identify and validate specific microRNA targets before development of an intraoperative PCR assay can be considered. Finally, intraoperative PCR assays may find utility as diagnostic assays. For example, recent literature indicates that helical computed tomography (CT) screening for lung cancer identifies tumors at an early stage and results in much improved outcomes. However, only a small percentage of lesions identified by CT screening are malignant, and clinicians are struggling to develop the best algorithms for patient care. In high-risk cases, patients will most likely be referred to surgeons for biopsy and possible tumor resection. In this setting, an intraoperative PCR assay to help differentiate malignancy from other possible diagnoses, such as hamartoma, granuloma, or infectious disease, may be useful.

CONCLUSION

Recent advances in real-time PCR instrumentation and methods have made intraoperative PCR assays a real possibility, but this technology remains in its infancy and faces many challenges. Although PCR assays are now common in the modern molecular pathology laboratory, they are generally complex and labor-intensive assays. Performing intraoperative RT-PCR assays in 30 minutes or thereabouts poses even further problems regarding technician and instrument time, data interpretation, and quality control. In a busy molecular pathology laboratory, the logistics of running multiple intraoperative assays simultaneously or overlapping in time is difficult to imagine, particularly if the assays need to be performed manually. Therefore, I believe that the bar for introducing such assays will be set high and the first assays will have to have high clinical need and exceptional accuracy characteristics. In addition, the current health care system in the United States is only slowly adapting to the introduction of molecular pathology. The expense of these assays, lack of billing codes, and reluctance of insurance companies to cover testing when older and cheaper assays exist are challenges for molecular pathology in general and for cutting-edge assays in particular. Furthermore, although the market for molecular testing in oncology is huge, the market for intraoperative staging is relatively small and is unlikely to drive introduction of rapid assays quickly. Taking these issues into consideration, it is unlikely that intraoperative PCR assays for cancer staging will become a common occurrence in the near future.

The development and introduction of rapid molecular assays may be driven more quickly by the specialty of infectious disease. There are many scenarios in which rapid PCR assays for infectious agents could dramatically improve patient care and may result in lower care costs and reduced drug resistance. Already, assays have been introduced for methicillin-resistant *Staphylococcus aureus* and group B streptococcus, and other tests for enterovirus, avian flu, and more are in development. As the use of rapid PCR assays for the detection of infectious disease increases, instrumentation, automation, processes, and logistics will evolve to fit these specific needs. As this happens, the barriers for introduction of such tests in other specialties, including molecular pathology, should be reduced.

SUGGESTED READINGS

General

Zehentner BK: Detection of disseminated tumor cells: Strategies and diagnostic implications. Expert Rev Mol Diagn 2002;2(1):41–48.

Real-Time Polymerase Chain Reaction

Bustin SA: Absolute quantification of mRNA using real-time reverse transcription polymerase chain reaction assays. J Mol Endocrinol 2000;25(2):169–193.
Ginzinger DG: Gene quantification using real-time quantitative PCR: An emerging technology hits the mainstream. Exp Hematol 2002;30(6):503–512.

Rapid, Real-Time Polymerase Chain Reaction

Horibe D, Ochiai T, Shimada H, et al: Rapid detection of metastasis of gastric cancer using reverse transcription loop–mediated isothermal amplification. Int J Cancer 2007;120(5):1063–1069.

Raja S, El Hefnawy T, Kelly LA, et al: Temperature-controlled primer limit for multiplexing of rapid, quantitative reverse transcription–PCR assays: Application to intraoperative cancer diagnostics. Clin Chem 2002;48(8):1329–1337.

Raja S, Luketich JD, Kelly LA, et al: Rapid, quantitative reverse transcriptase–polymerase chain reaction: Application to intraoperative molecular detection of occult metastases in esophageal cancer. J Thorac Cardiovasc Surg 2002;123(3):475–483.

Breast Cancer

Backus J, Laughlin T, Wang Y, et al: Identification and characterization of optimal gene expression markers for detection of breast cancer metastasis. J Mol Diagn 2005;7(3):327–336.

Eisenberg DP, Adusumilli PS, Hendershott KJ, et al: Real-time intraoperative detection of breast cancer axillary lymph node metastases using a green fluorescent protein-expressing herpes virus. Ann Surg 2006;243(6):824–830.

Gillanders WE, Mikhitarian K, Hebert R, et al: Molecular detection of micrometastatic breast cancer in histopathology-negative axillary lymph nodes correlates with traditional predictors of prognosis: An interim analysis of a prospective multi-institutional cohort study. Ann Surg 2004;239(6):828–837.

Hughes SJ, Xi L, Raja S, et al: A rapid, fully automated, molecular-based assay accurately analyzes sentinel lymph nodes for the presence of metastatic breast cancer. Ann Surg 2006;243(3):389–398.

Zehentner BK, Dillon DC, Jiang Y, et al: Application of a multigene reverse transcription–PCR assay for detection of mammaglobin and complementary transcribed genes in breast cancer lymph nodes. Clin Chem 2002;48(8):1225–1231.

Melanoma

Kammula US, Ghossein R, Bhattacharya S, Coit DG: Serial follow-up and the prognostic significance of reverse transcriptase–polymerase chain reaction–staged sentinel lymph nodes from melanoma patients. J Clin Oncol 2004;22(19):3989–3996.

Scoggins CR, Ross MI, Reintgen DS, et al: Prospective multi-institutional study of reverse transcriptase–polymerase chain reaction for molecular staging of melanoma. J Clin Oncol 2006;24(18):2849–2857.

Takeuchi H, Morton DL, Kuo C, et al: Prognostic significance of molecular upstaging of paraffin-embedded sentinel lymph nodes in melanoma patients. J Clin Oncol 2004;22(13):2671–2680.

Talantov D, Mazumder A, Yu JX, et al: Novel genes associated with malignant melanoma but not benign melanocytic lesions. Clin Cancer Res 2005;11(20):7234–7242.

Head and Neck Cancer

Ferris RL, Xi L, Raja S, et al: Molecular staging of cervical lymph nodes in squamous cell carcinoma of the head and neck. Cancer Res 2005;65(6):2147–2156.

Garrel R, Dromard M, Costes V, et al: The diagnostic accuracy of reverse transcription–PCR quantification of cytokeratin mRNA in the detection of sentinel lymph node invasion in oral and oropharyngeal squamous cell carcinoma: A comparison with immunohistochemistry. Clin Cancer Res 2006;12(8):2498–2505.

Other Tumors

Yoshioka S, Fujiwara Y, Sugita Y, et al: Real-time rapid reverse transcriptase–polymerase chain reaction for intraoperative diagnosis of lymph node micrometastasis: Clinical application for cervical lymph node dissection in esophageal cancers. Surgery 2002;132(1):34–40.

DIAGNOSTIC MOLECULAR PATHOLOGY APPLICATIONS

17 Molecular Cytopathology
Karen S. Gustafson • Douglas P. Clark

INTRODUCTION

Clinical cytology samples offer opportunities and challenges for diagnostic molecular pathology applications. The application of molecular techniques to cytologic samples has three main goals: (1) to increase the sensitivity and specificity of screening tests for cancer; (2) to increase diagnostic accuracy; and (3) to add prognostic or predictive value. Historically, the field of cytopathology has its roots as a screening test for cervical cancer. The morphologic identification of cervical cancer precursors, in conjunction with effective therapy, remains one of the great success stories in cancer prevention. This success quickly led to a search for expanded uses of cytology for cancer screening, including sputum analysis for lung cancer, urine cytology for urothelial carcinoma, and more recently, ductal lavage for breast cancer. These morphology-based modalities have met with less success compared to cervical cytology, largely because of limits of sensitivity and specificity, particularly for early disease, and the relative inability to treat some early lesions. One major goal for molecular cytopathology remains the enhancement of these existing screening tests. In this chapter, we discuss, as two examples, the application of molecular tests such as fluorescence in situ hybridization (FISH) to urine cytology and the application of human papillomavirus (HPV) DNA testing to cervical cytology samples.

Molecular tests to enhance diagnostic accuracy in cytologic samples tend to focus on the characterization of a recognized malignancy, rather than molecular tests for malignancy. To date, the diagnosis of malignancy remains largely based on morphologic criteria, with immunocytochemistry used to further characterize the malignancy. Genetic alterations such as mutations, deletions, and translocations have been described in numerous malignancies. Molecular tests that detect these changes have the potential to significantly enhance our diagnostic accuracy in cytologic specimens; however, their application to cytologic samples has been limited. In this chapter, we

also discuss the application of molecular diagnostic tests to thyroid fine-needle aspiration (FNA) specimens for the detection of genetic alterations that may potentially improve diagnostic accuracy.

Perhaps the most important development in medicine that will profoundly affect molecular cytopathology is the advent of targeted therapeutics for cancer. *Targeted therapeutics* typically refers to the development of a drug, often a small molecule or an antibody-based therapy, that blocks a specific molecule that is abnormally activated in the cancer cell. Because human tumors are heterogeneous, particularly in their response to these novel targeted therapeutics, careful patient selection will be crucial. Molecular characterization of the initial tumor sample, such as that obtained through an FNA biopsy, will provide information that is essential for the oncologist to choose the appropriate therapy. Pathologists are well aware of the increasing need for the analysis of Her2 overexpression in breast carcinomas as a means to predict responsiveness to Herceptin® (Genetech) therapy. This example is likely to be just the first of many in which detection of a particular biomarker in the tumor is predictive of its response to a targeted therapy. In addition to these predictive markers, oncologists are increasingly eager to monitor their patients for an early response to therapy. Such monitoring will ideally be performed using minimally invasive sampling techniques, such as FNA. Molecular cytopathology will likely play an important role in the clinical development and practical applications of targeted therapeutics. However, findings to date are limited to investigational studies and early clinical trials; therefore, specific examples are not discussed in this chapter.

GYNECOLOGIC CYTOPATHOLOGY

Cervical carcinoma is the second most common cancer among women worldwide, with estimates of 470,000 new cases and 233,000 deaths annually.

However, in the United States, cervical carcinoma incidence and mortality rates have decreased by about 70% over the past five decades, with approximately 9,700 new cases and 3,700 deaths estimated for 2006. This marked reduction primarily results from cytology-based cervical cancer screening programs using the Papanicolaou (Pap) test. The Pap test has been a successful and effective screening test for cervical cancer because (1) established morphologic criteria exist for the precursor intraepithelial lesions; (2) the progression from intraepithelial lesions to invasive cervical cancer usually occurs over a prolonged period of 10 to 20 years; and (3) women undergo repeat testing as part of routine health care maintenance. In recent years, advances in our understanding of the pathogenesis of cervical carcinoma and the development of new technologies have led to improvements in the diagnosis and management of cervical neoplasia.

Most invasive cervical cancers are squamous cell carcinomas (~80%); the remainder are endocervical adenocarcinomas and, much less commonly, small cell carcinomas. The Pap test is primarily a screening test to detect invasive squamous cell carcinoma and its precursor squamous intraepithelial lesions (SILs). With adequate sampling of the squamocolumnar junction and transformation zone of the cervix, atypical endocervical cells, adenocarcinoma in situ, and endocervical adenocarcinoma may also be detected. The Pap test is not considered a screening test for endometrial carcinoma; however, when atypical endometrial cells or endometrial adenocarcinoma is encountered, reporting is warranted. Interpretation of atypical glandular cells or more significant glandular lesions of endocervical and/or endometrial origin that are directly sampled or spontaneously exfoliated continue to be challenging and evolving areas in Pap test interpretations. Thus, given the primary role of cytologic screening in the detection of precursor SILs and cervical squamous cell carcinoma, the discussion that follows focuses on the molecular pathogenesis and testing related to cervical squamous neoplasia.

PATHOGENESIS OF CERVICAL SQUAMOUS CELL CARCINOMA

Role of the Human Papillomavirus in Cervical Carcinogenesis

HPVs are nonenveloped viruses with a double-stranded circular DNA genome consisting of approximately 8000 base pairs (Figure 17-1). The HPV genome contains a noncoding upstream regulatory region (URR) that regulates viral DNA replication and transcription of the early open reading frames (ORFs; E1 to E7) that encode proteins involved in viral replication and cellular transformation and two late ORFs (L1 and L2) that encode

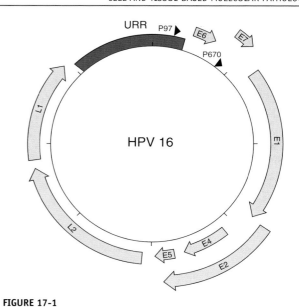

FIGURE 17-1

Organization of the HPV 16 genome. The noncoding upstream regulatory region (URR) is involved in regulation of viral replication and transcription. The six early open reading frames (E1 to E7) and two late open reading frames (L1 and L2), indicated by shaded arrows, are expressed from either the early (p97) or the late (p670) promoter.

proteins that form the viral capsid. Polymerase chain reaction (PCR)–based assays with DNA sequencing have been used to identify more than 100 HPV genotypes that, by definition, have less than 90% DNA sequence homology. Approximately 40 of the genotypes infect the anogenital mucosa. These anogenital types are classified as low-risk and high-risk HPV types based on the potential for inducing malignant transformation. The low-risk types, such as HPV 6 and 11, are mainly found in benign genital warts and low-grade squamous intraepithelial lesions (LSILs). The high-risk HPV types while also producing low-grade lesions are, by definition, associated with the development of precancerous high-grade squamous intraepithelial lesions (HSILs) and invasive squamous cell carcinoma. Studies have shown that most women with LSILs are also infected with high-risk HPV types. Approximately 15 high-risk HPV types have been identified. The two most common are HPV 16 and 18, which cause more than 50% and 10% to 20% of squamous cell carcinomas, respectively. DNA-based assays that use type-specific PCR primers and probes have detected high-risk HPV DNA in more than 99% of invasive squamous cell carcinomas worldwide. These findings provide convincing molecular evidence that high-risk HPV is the main etiologic factor and a necessary cause for the development of cervical squamous cell carcinoma and its precursor SILs. In the subsequent discussion, HPV refers to high-risk types unless otherwise specified.

HPV-induced cervical carcinogenesis is characterized by a multistep process from the time of HPV infection to the development of invasive squamous cell carcinoma, with a latency period of up to 15 years (Figure 17-2). HPV is sexually transmitted, and it infects the basal cells through microlesions in the mucosal surface or at the cervical transformation zone. Most HPV infections are subclinical and are cleared by the host immune system within 12 months. The morphologic changes recognized as SILs on cytology and cervical intraepithelial neoplasias (CINs) on histology develop in a subset of cases and occur as a result of interactions between viral and host proteins. LSIL (CIN 1) occurs in the setting of transient HPV infections where the viral oncoproteins E6 and E7 reprogram the cell cycle machinery within the suprabasal cells to result in productive viral infections. In these cases, the HPV genome is maintained in an episomal form and viral gene expression is tightly regulated in a differentiation-dependent manner to result in the release of virions from terminally differentiated squamous cells. With clearance of HPV by the immune system, most of these lesions will spontaneously regress. However, with persistent HPV infections at the transformation zone, increased expression of the HPV E6 and E7 oncoproteins results in the proliferation of basal and parabasal epithelial cells and the development of HSILs (some

CIN 2 and CIN 3). The mechanisms that lead to altered viral gene expression are not completely understood but may include viral integration into host genomic DNA. Integration of the HPV genome often results in disruption of the viral E2 ORF and, therefore, loss of E2-mediated repression, with consequent overexpression of HPV E6 and E7. The uncontrolled cellular proliferation induced by HPV E6 and E7 overexpression, together with other non-HPV risk factors such as external mutagens or genetic predisposition, promotes the accumulation of additional genetic and epigenetic alterations, with eventual progression to invasive squamous cell carcinoma.

Human Papillomavirus and the Cell Cycle

Progression through the cell cycle is tightly regulated through interactions between cellular proteins, including the cyclins, cyclin-dependent kinases (CDKs), CDK inhibitors, and the tumor suppressor protein p53, to ensure DNA integrity before replication, chromosome segregation, and cell division. The HPV E6 and E7 oncoproteins interact with a number of cellular proteins that function to regulate cell cycle progression and apoptosis, thereby inducing cell cycle alterations and uncontrolled proliferation (Figure 17-3). A major function of the HPV E7 oncoprotein is to activate the cell cycle at the G1- to S-phase transition through its ability to bind and

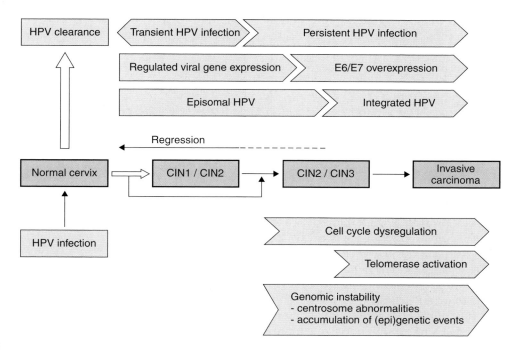

FIGURE 17-2

Human papillomavirus (HPV)–induced cervical carcinogenesis. With persistent HPV infection, there is an increased risk for the development of cervical intraepithelial neoplasia (CIN 2 or CIN 3) as a result of molecular events, such as integration of the HPV genome into the host genomic DNA, that leads to the overexpression of HPV E6 and E7 oncoproteins. The cell cycle dysregulation that occurs with HPV E6 and E7 overexpression leads to uncontrolled proliferation and genomically unstable cells. In addition, the activation of telomerase contributes to the immortalized phenotype that allows accumulation of additional genetic and epigenetic alterations, which promote the progression to invasive cervical carcinoma.

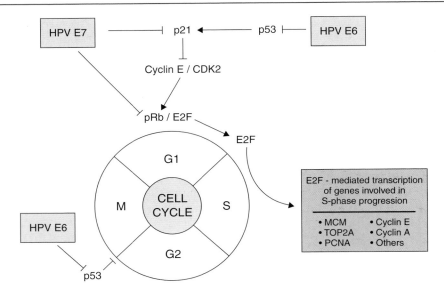

FIGURE 17-3

Effects of human papillomavirus (HPV) on the cell cycle. In normal cells in the G1-phase of the cell cycle, the hypophosphorylated form of retinoblastoma (pRb) interacts with E2F to prevent entry into S-phase. The interaction of HPV E6 with p53 leads to abrogation of the G1/S and G2/M cell cycle checkpoints. CDK, cyclin-dependent kinase; MCM, minichromosome maintenance; PCNA, proliferating cell nuclear antigen; TOP2A, topoisomerase IIα.

degrade the retinoblastoma (pRb) tumor suppressor family of proteins through a proteasome-dependent pathway. The E7–pRb interaction leads to the release of the E2F cellular transcription factors and increased expression of several proteins involved in DNA synthesis and cell cycle progression, including the minichromosome maintenance (MCM) proteins, topoisomerase IIα (TOP2A), proliferating cell nuclear antigen, and cyclins A and E. Constitutive activation of E2F-mediated genes leads to entry and transit through S phase. In addition, the inactivation of the CDK inhibitors p21 and p27 by HPV E7 promotes cell cycle progression.

Dysregulation of the cell cycle triggers an antiproliferative response within the host cell, which involves the activation of the tumor suppressor protein p53. In normal cells, p53 functions to regulate the G1/S and G2/M cell cycle checkpoints. Consequently, in response to inappropriate activation of the cell cycle and DNA damage, p53 induces the expression of cellular factors that mediate cell cycle arrest and apoptosis. One of the main functions of the HPV E6 oncoprotein is to bind p53 through the cellular ubiquitin ligase, E6-associated protein, and target it for degradation through the ubiquitin–proteasome pathway. Thus, abrogation of cellular defense mechanisms caused by functional loss of p53 contributes to uncontrolled cell cycle progression and genomic instability. Another important function of the HPV E6 oncoprotein is to induce expression of the catalytic subunit of telomerase, human telomerase reverse transcriptase. Telomerase functions to maintain telomeric DNA sequences at the ends of chromosomes

to allow continued DNA replication and cellular proliferation. Thus, transcriptional activation of telomerase by HPV E6 plays an important role in extending cellular life span and immortalization.

Together, the complex interactions of HPV E6 and E7 with host cellular proteins involved in cell cycle regulation lead to uncontrolled cellular proliferation. Studies using HPV E6- and E7-transformed keratinocytes and cervical cancer cell lines have demonstrated that expression of HPV E6 and E7 oncoproteins is required for cellular transformation and maintenance of the malignant phenotype.

Genomic Instability Induced by Human Papillomavirus

The uncontrolled cellular proliferation induced by HPV E6 and E7 overexpression that is characteristic of CIN 2 and CIN 3 (primarily CIN 3) can result in genomically unstable cells that are at increased risk for the accumulation of additional genetic and epigenetic alterations, which further promote the development of invasive cervical carcinoma. Both numeric and structural chromosomal abnormalities are often associated with HPV-induced cervical carcinogenesis. Numeric chromosomal abnormalities, or aneuploidy, as demonstrated by both gains and losses of chromosomes, may occur as the result of mitotic defects associated with abnormal centrosome numbers. The HPV E6 and E7 oncoproteins induce abnormal centrosome numbers that can cause the formation of multipolar mitoses and asymmetric cell divisions to result in chromosomal gains or losses. Chromosomal alterations that may contribute to the development of a malignant phenotype have been identified in HPV-transformed keratinocytes and invasive cervical cancer tissues. For example, gains in the long arm of chromosome 3 (3q) have often been detected in invasive carcinomas. This region is of interest because it harbors sequences for the structural RNA component of the telomerase complex. Allelic losses at chromosome 11q22-q24, as demonstrated by loss of heterozygosity, have been detected in invasive carcinomas, which suggests the presence of one or more tumor suppressor genes in this area. The tumor suppressor gene *IGSF4/TSLC1*, which is localized to 11q23.2, has recently been shown to be often silenced in both HSILs (CIN 2 and CIN 3) and invasive carcinomas as a result of promoter hypermethylation. This example highlights that loss of tumor suppressor gene function can occur not only through genetic mutation or deletion but also through aberrant DNA methylation, as discussed later.

Epigenetic alterations, including DNA methylation and post-translational modifications of histones, lead to changes in chromatin structure and gene expression. Interactions between the HPV E6 and E7 oncoproteins and the cellular proteins that mediate these epigenetic modifications, including DNA methyltransferases, histone deacetylases, and histone acetyltransferases, have been identified. Aberrant DNA methylation of tumor suppressor genes is a common epigenetic change in many types of cancer, including cervical squamous cell carcinoma, which can contribute to tumorigenesis by inactivating genes that function in important cellular pathways, including cell cycle, apoptosis, DNA repair, and cell–cell adhesion. The methylation profiles of several candidate tumor suppressor genes, as well as genes discovered through global demethylation and expression microarray analysis, demonstrate that selective genes (e.g., *IGSF4*, *DAPK1*, *RARB*, *SPARC*, and *TFPI2*) are often methylated in invasive cervical carcinoma. Furthermore, studies using both cytologic specimens and cervical tissues have shown that several of these genes are methylated in precursor SILs (CINs), with methylation detected more often in HSILs (CIN 2 and CIN 3) than in LSIL (CIN 1). Identification of additional genes that are aberrantly methylated in cervical carcinogenesis and elucidation of the mechanisms involved in these epigenetic changes are active areas of research aimed at better understanding the pathogenesis of cervical carcinoma.

DIAGNOSTIC AND PREDICTIVE MARKERS FOR HIGH-GRADE SQUAMOUS INTRAEPITHELIAL LESIONS

Based on our current understanding of the pathogenesis of cervical carcinoma, the goal of cervical cancer screening is to detect and treat HSILs (CIN 2 and, in particular, CIN 3). The Bethesda System 2001

(TBS 2001) represents a standardized system for reporting cytologic abnormalities in Pap tests in which the two-tiered classification of SILs into LSILs and HSILs reflects the finding that these lesions represent biologically distinct HPV-induced changes, as discussed earlier. In addition, TBS 2001 includes the equivocal categories of atypical squamous cells of undetermined significance (ASC-US) and atypical squamous cells, cannot exclude HSIL (ASC-H), which represent abnormal findings that are quantitatively or qualitatively insufficient for a diagnosis of LSIL and HSIL, respectively. Several studies that have used TBS 2001 for Pap test interpretations and correlation with histologic outcomes have demonstrated that each of these cytologic categories is associated with a defined risk of underlying CIN 2 and CIN 3.

Of the 50 million to 60 million Pap tests performed each year in the United States, nearly 4 million tests will show abnormal cytologic findings, with approximately 300,000 cases of HSILs and more than 3 million cases with mildly abnormal cytologic findings of LSIL. The current management guidelines for women with an HSIL on a Pap test include referral to colposcopy with biopsy and a definitive excisional procedure. However, initial management strategies for women with Pap tests with results of atypical squamous cells and LSIL have been more problematic, largely because of the tendency for these lesions to spontaneously regress together with the moderate sensitivity and limited reproducibility of Pap tests. Importantly, approximately 10% to 20% of women with mildly abnormal findings on a Pap test will have underlying CIN 2, CIN 3, or invasive cancer (CIN 2/3+) on cervical biopsy follow-up. Determining which women with mildly abnormal Pap tests have underlying CIN 2/3+ and require further evaluation and treatment constitutes a major challenge to avoid overtreatment of patients and unnecessary costs to the health care system.

Despite its success as a screening test for cervical cancer, a single conventional Pap test has only a moderate sensitivity (60% to 70%) for the detection of HSILs. The use of liquid-based Pap test preparations (ThinPrep®, Cytyc; SurePath®, TriPath Imaging) has led to an improved sensitivity (70% to 80%) for the detection of HSILs and allows the performance of ancillary molecular testing on a residual specimen. As discussed later, the use of HPV DNA testing as an adjunct to the Pap test has greatly improved the sensitivity for CIN 2/3+ detection to greater than 96% and has become an integral part of cervical cancer screening. Although HPV DNA testing is useful in assessing the risk of underlying CIN 2/3+ in selected populations, its utility is limited in women with mild cytologic abnormalities, such as LSILs, where the prevalence of HPV is high. As such, the identification of additional molecular tests with increased specificity for the detection of underlying CIN 2/3+ would be of value. Several candidate biomarkers under investigation are discussed here.

Human Papillomavirus DNA Testing

Given the etiologic role of HPV in cervical carcinoma and precursor CINs, HPV DNA testing has emerged as a useful adjunct to Pap tests for determining the risk of associated CIN 2/3+ in selective populations. Data from the National Cancer Institute (NCI)–sponsored ASC-US/LSIL Triage Study (ALTS), a large multicenter, randomized clinical trial with 2-year follow-up, and from several other large clinical screening studies have led to the development of evidence-based recommendations for the management of women undergoing cytology screening for cervical cancer. Examples of recommended uses for HPV DNA testing as an adjunct to the Pap test and the rationale for testing are discussed. The discussion is limited primarily to examples in which HPV DNA testing is useful as an adjunct to cervical cytology for the initial management of women with abnormal cytologic findings and for those women undergoing cervical cytology for screening, because a detailed discussion of uses in subsequent management algorithms and in special circumstances is beyond the scope of this chapter.

USE IN PRIMARY SCREENING FOR WOMEN 30 YEARS AND OLDER In 2003, a consensus workshop sponsored by the NCI, the American Society for Colposcopy and Cervical Pathology (ASCCP), and the American Cancer Society was convened to develop guidance for the use of HPV DNA testing as an adjunct to cytology for primary cervical cancer screening. The interim guidance that was established states that HPV DNA testing may be added to the Pap test for screening in women 30 years and older. Consistent with the fact that HPV is sexually transmitted, the prevalence of HPV infections is highest (25% to 30%) among sexually active women in their early 20s and drops to approximately 5% to 15% after age 30 as the number of new sexual partners is diminished. Accordingly, detection of HPV in women 30 years old more often represents persistent HPV infections and, consequently, is associated with an increased risk of CIN 2/3+. Given the decreased prevalence of HPV infection in women 30 years old and the high sensitivity (>95%) of HPV DNA testing for CIN 2/3+ when used with a Pap test, several large clinical screening studies have reported a negative predictive value of 99% to 100% for CIN 2/3+ in women with concurrent negative Pap tests and negative HPV DNA tests. Therefore, when such results are obtained in primary screening tests in women over 30 years of age, the risk of CIN 2/3+ is extremely low (approximately 1 in 1000) and repeat screening with a Pap test and an HPV DNA test can safely be extended to 3 years. In women who have a negative Pap test but a positive HPV DNA test, a repeat Pap test and repeat HPV DNA testing in 6 to 12 months is recommended. Since most HPV infections will be cleared by the immune system within this time period and increased risk for CIN 2/3+ occurs with persistent HPV infection, referral to colposcopy is not initially recommended.

USE FOR WOMEN WITH ASC-US ON A PAP TEST In 2001, a consensus conference was sponsored by ASCCP to develop guidelines for the management of women with cervical cytologic abnormalities. The management guidelines that were developed recommend the use of reflex HPV DNA testing as the preferred approach for the initial management of women with ASC-US on a Pap test. Women with ASC-US on a Pap test and a positive HPV DNA test should be referred for colposcopic evaluation. Women with ASC-US on a Pap test and a negative HPV DNA test should be followed with a repeat Pap test in 12 months.

ASC-US is the most common abnormal cytologic interpretation on a Pap test with approximately 2 million to 3 million cases annually. In these equivocal cases, the atypical cells may represent either reactive changes or an HPV-induced lesion. Importantly, a small but significant percentage of women with ASC-US will have underlying CIN 2/3+, and identifying those women who require further evaluation constitutes a major challenge. Given the etiologic role of HPV in cervical carcinogenesis, HPV DNA testing can be used to identify women with ASC-US who have an increased risk of CIN 2/3+. The ALTS and other large studies provide strong evidence for use of reflex HPV DNA testing to triage women with ASC-US to colposcopy. Using this management strategy, the sensitivity of HPV DNA testing for underlying CIN 2/3+ was 96% and the percentage of women with ASC-US that were referred to colposcopy was 56%. Thus, the use of HPV DNA testing to triage women with ASC-US reduces the number of unnecessary colposcopic examinations and the risk of overtreatment of these women.

USE FOR WOMEN WITH ASC-H, LSIL, OR HSIL ON A PAP TEST According to the ASCCP 2001 consensus guidelines, women with ASC-H, LSIL, or HSIL on a Pap test should be referred for colposcopic examination. The ALTS demonstrated that 86% of women with ASC-H cytology tested positive for HPV DNA. Moreover, during the 2-year follow-up period, underlying CIN 2/3+ was detected in 50% of women. Given the high prevalence of HPV and the significant risk of underlying CIN 2/3+, immediate colposcopy is recommended for the initial management of women with ASC-H on a Pap test. Similarly, the high HPV prevalence and increased risk of CIN 2/3+ associated with LSIL or more severe lesion on a Pap test warrants immediate referral to colposcopy regardless of HPV DNA test results.

Molecular Methods for Detection of Human Papillomavirus DNA

The three basic molecular testing methods available for the detection of HPV DNA are (1) signal amplification (e.g., Hybrid Capture® 2, or HC2; Digene); (2) direct probe methods (e.g., in situ hybridization); and (3) target amplification (e.g., PCR-based techniques). The methods, together with the advantages and disadvantages of each, are discussed in the sections that follow.

SIGNAL AMPLIFICATION The HC2 test is approved by the U.S. Food and Drug Administration (FDA) for the detection of HPV DNA. It has been clinically validated in several studies, including the ALTS. The method is based on nucleic acid hybridization and signal amplification using chemiluminescent detection and a microtiter plate platform (Figure 17-4). To detect high-risk HPV DNA, DNA isolated from the residual liquid-based Pap test is mixed with a cocktail of RNA probes specific for 13 high-risk HPV genotypes (16, 18, 31, 33, 35, 39, 45, 51, 52, 56, 58, 59, and 68) and RNA:DNA hybrids form in solution. The solution is then added to the well of a microtiter plate, and the RNA:DNA hybrids are "captured" onto the surface by immobilized antibodies that specifically recognize RNA:DNA hybrids. Alkaline phosphatase–conjugated antibodies that specifically recognize RNA:DNA hybrids are added to the well. Each antibody molecule is linked to several alkaline phosphatase molecules and several antibody molecules bind to each target RNA:DNA hybrid, which

results in substantial signal amplification. Excess unbound DNA, nonhybridized probes, and antibodies are removed, and the chemiluminescent substrate is added. A luminometer is used to detect the emitted light as relative light units, and a semiquantitative measure of viral load is determined.

The major strengths of the HC2 test are that it provides standardized, objective results and that it is the method approved by the FDA. Importantly, the high sensitivity of the HC2 test for the detection of HPV in clinically relevant disease (i.e., CIN 2/3+) has been clearly demonstrated in the ALTS, as well as other studies. The established test performance and clinical validation make the HC2 test the preferred assay for HPV detection. A drawback of the current HC2 test is that the system uses a pool of RNA probes for several HPV genotypes and does not detect the presence of a specific genotype. Next-generation tests that can identify specific genotypes (e.g., HPV 16 and 18) may become commercially available in the future; however, the utility of HPV type–specific assays will require further investigation.

DIRECT PROBE METHODS The Inform® HPV System (Ventana Medical Systems) is a commercially available system that uses in situ hybridization (ISH) with a cocktail of DNA probes designed to detect 12 high-risk HPV genotypes (16, 18, 31, 33, 35, 39, 45, 51, 52, 56, 58, and 66). The DNA probes, which are labeled with a dye, are applied directly to target tissue and bind to specific HPV sequences. A dye-specific primary antibody detects the probes bound to the

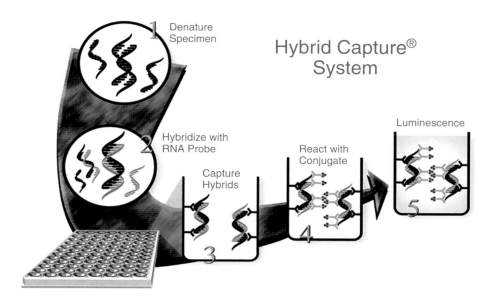

FIGURE 17-4

Basic steps of the Hybrid Capture 2 test. DNA in the specimen is denatured and then hybridized in solution with a cocktail of RNA probes that recognize specific HPV types. The RNA:DNA hybrids are captured onto the surface of a microtiter plate well by immobilized antibodies that specifically recognize RNA:DNA hybrids. Alkaline phosphatase–conjugated antibodies specific for RNA:DNA hybrids react with captured RNA:DNA hybrids. A chemiluminescent substrate is added, and the emitted light is detected using a luminometer. (Courtesy of Dr. Attila Lorincz, Digene, Gaithersburg, MD.)

target sequences. This is followed by application of a biotinylated secondary antibody against the primary antibody. Streptavidin-conjugated alkaline phosphatase is then used as the chromogenic enzyme, which, when substrate is added, produces a colorimetric readout that can be visualized. One advantage of a direct probe method, such as ISH, is that it allows one to correlate HPV detection with the morphology of the positive stained cells. However, this test requires interpretation by a pathologist; thus, the analysis may be more subjective and time consuming. Moreover, the utility of ISH as an adjunct to the Pap test requires that the atypical cells of interest be present on the slide; thus, sampling issues may be more significant than they are in other detection methods. The analytic sensitivity for the detection of HPV is generally lower than that of other methods and, although in-house clinical validation studies have been performed at individual institutions, ISH has not been used in large multicenter studies. Therefore, we do not know how this test performs compared to the HC2 test.

TARGET AMPLIFICATION Detection of HPV DNA by PCR methods has been widely used to define genotypes and study the natural history of HPV infection and the relationship to cervical carcinoma. Many home-brew assays have been used in these studies. The Roche Linear Array HPV genotyping test (Roche Molecular Systems) is a commercially available PCR-based HPV detection and genotyping kit; however, it is not yet readily available in the United States. Many assays used in previous studies use a two-step process that includes PCR amplification with biotin-labeled consensus primers that bind to highly conserved regions within the HPV L1 ORF and subsequent hybridization of the PCR product to a line blot with type-specific oligoprobes. Streptavidin-linked alkaline phosphatase can then be used as the chromogenic detection system. Advantages of PCR-based assays include a flexible technology that permits detection of specific HPV types, viral load quantitation, and mutation analysis. PCR-based assays have a high analytic sensitivity, which may be important for some applications. As with other PCR-based assays, drawbacks include the lack of interlaboratory standardization and an increased risk of contamination that can lead to false-positive results. In addition, although most home-brew PCR-based detection systems have been validated within individual laboratories, their performance has not been clinically validated in large clinical trials. Of particular concern is the finding that PCR-based methods have an increased analytic sensitivity for HPV detection compared to other methods, such as the HC2 test. This increase in sensitivity could, therefore, lead to the detection of clinically irrelevant HPV infections and result in overtreatment and unnecessary costs.

Surrogate Biomarkers of HPV–induced Cervical Disease: Detection by Immunocytochemical Methods

HPV DNA testing will continue to play an increasingly important role as a diagnostic and prognostic molecular test to aid in the management of women with cervical disease; however, its lack of specificity for CIN 2/3+ limits its utility in populations for which the prevalence of HPV is high, such as in women with mildly abnormal Pap tests (LSIL). Therefore, ongoing efforts have been aimed at identifying additional biomarkers that can better predict the risk of underlying CIN 2/3+. The dysregulated cell cycle progression induced by HPV E6 and E7 overexpression leads to the altered expression of several downstream molecules involved in cellular proliferation. Molecular techniques, such as complementary DNA (cDNA) expression microarrays, have been used to identify genes differentially expressed in normal squamous epithelium or CIN 1 compared to CIN 2/3+. Using this approach, several genes upregulated in CIN 2/3+ have been identified as potential candidate biomarkers. Antibodies directed against these candidate proteins have been developed to investigate protein expression in both cervical tissue and cytologic specimens using immunoperoxidase staining techniques. Although in general studies have shown similar results using both tissue and cytologic samples, the interpretation of immunocytochemical stains in cytologic specimens can present unique challenges and limitations that should be acknowledged. Specifically, the optimization and validation of immunocytochemical stains should be performed using cytologic material; the methodology developed for tissue sections may not necessarily be directly applicable to cytologic specimens because the differences in fixation and preparation are variables that can affect epitope recognition and antibody binding. Even with ideal immunocytochemical optimization, the interpretation of staining in cytologic specimens poses several additional challenges compared to those with tissue sections. Because a positive result requires the staining to be present in cytologically abnormal cells, one must be able to simultaneously visualize and interpret both cytologic and staining features on the same slide. Factors such as positive staining in both the nuclear and the cytoplasmic compartments and staining in metaplastic cells and benign endocervical cells in cytologic specimens may preclude an accurate interpretation. Furthermore, cytologic preparations often lack the architectural context that histologic tissue sections provide and do not permit evaluation of serial sections, which can make interpretations more challenging. Despite these limitations, significant progress has been made toward the development of useful immunocytochemical-based biomarkers.

The use of p16^{INK4a} (p16) overexpression as a marker of HPV-induced cervical disease has been examined in both cervical tissues and cytologic specimens. In the cell cycle, p16 normally functions to inhibit cell cycle progression from G1- to S-phase by regulating levels of active cyclin D and CDK. In the absence of CDK activity, unphosphorylated pRb remains bound to E2F, thus preventing transcriptional activation of E2F-mediated genes. Because the expression of p16 is regulated by a pRb-dependent negative feedback loop, the continuous degradation of pRb mediated by HPV E7 leads to increased levels of p16 protein that can be detected in CINs and invasive carcinoma. Studies using tissue sections and immunohistochemical staining for p16 expression have demonstrated a good correlation between the severity of the cervical lesion associated with high-risk HPV and the staining for p16, with little to no staining in normal epithelium. Diffuse, strong nuclear and/or cytoplasmic staining for p16 was detected in 38% to 88% of CIN 1, 56% to 100% of CIN 2, and 100% of CIN 3 and invasive carcinomas. The findings suggest that immunostaining for p16 may serve as a potential biomarker of cervical neoplasia associated with persistent HPV infection and may be applicable to cytologic specimens for screening or triage of patients. Studies performed using liquid-based cytologic specimens have generally demonstrated a similar correlation between the detection of p16 overexpression and the severity of cervical lesions, although direct comparisons of results are difficult, partly because of the lack of standardization in how p16 overexpression is defined (i.e., the required number of positive cells and staining intensity). Furthermore, although some studies use a commercially available kit optimized to detect p16 in cytologic specimens (CINtec™ p16^{INK4a} Cytology Kit; Dako), the use of other antibody clones or immunocytochemical protocols can hinder direct comparisons. Despite these limitations, the findings overall are encouraging and the potential utility of p16 immunostaining in cervical cytology continues to be an active area of investigation.

Gene expression profiling studies have also identified *MCM2* and *TOP2A* as genes that are overexpressed in CINs and invasive carcinoma. These genes are induced by E2F transcription factors during the G1- to S-phase transition of the cell cycle and function during S-phase progression. The MCM2 protein functions as part of the prereplicative complex that is essential for DNA replication. The TOP2A protein is an enzyme that functions to introduce temporary double-stranded breaks into the DNA that are also necessary for DNA replication. Thus, overexpression of these proteins can serve as a potential molecular biomarker of the cell cycle dysregulation that is induced by HPV E6 and E7 overexpression in CIN

2/3+. ProEx™ C (TriPath Imaging) is a commercially available reagent optimized for use with cytologic specimens that contains a mixture of monoclonal antibodies directed against the MCM2 and TOP2A proteins. ProEx C can be used with standard immunocytochemical techniques and applied to liquid-based cytologic preparations to detect expression of these proteins within the nucleus of cytologically abnormal cells. Validation studies have defined positive ProEx C staining as moderate to intense nuclear staining in at least one cytologically abnormal cell. Initial validation studies have demonstrated that the ProEx C immunocytochemical assay can be integrated into a clinical cytology laboratory and that it demonstrates excellent staining and scoring reproducibility. Retrospective studies have suggested that ProEx C may aid in the interpretation of challenging cytologic cases and may increase the positive predictive value of liquid-based cytology for biopsy-proven CIN 2/3+ in cervical cancer screening programs. Although ProEx C and p16 both show promise as surrogate biomarkers of CIN 2/3+, one advantage to ProEx C is that staining is confined to the nucleus, whereas staining of the nucleus, cytoplasm, or both occurs with p16 overexpression. Similar to immunocytochemical staining for p16, positive staining with ProEx C may occasionally be detected in metaplastic cells and benign endocervical cells, and careful correlation with morphology is necessary for accurate interpretation. The utility of ProEx C or similar products as a diagnostic or prognostic biomarker awaits further evaluation in large clinical trials with histologic follow-up.

Aberrant DNA Methylation of Tumor Suppressor Genes as a Molecular Biomarker of HPV-induced Cervical Disease: Detection by Methylation-specific PCR

Epigenetic silencing of tumor suppressor genes by promoter methylation occurs often in virtually all human tumors, including cervical squamous cell carcinoma. Aberrant DNA methylation promotes tumor progression by inactivating genes that function in key cellular pathways, including cell cycle, apoptosis, DNA repair, and cell–cell adhesion. Determination of the methylation status of several tumor suppressor genes in a broad range of primary tumors has demonstrated that tumor-type and gene-specific methylation profiles can be identified for most malignancies. The methylation status of several candidate tumor suppressor genes has been examined in cervical cancer and precursor CINs using both cervical tissues and cytologic specimens. In addition, treatment of cervical carcinoma cell lines with epigenetic modifying drugs to induce global demethylation followed by cDNA microarray analysis has led to the identification of novel genes that are methylated in cervical carcinoma. Using these approaches, several genes, including *IGSF4, DAPK1, RARB, TWIST, SPARC,* and *TFPI2,* appear to be methylated often in invasive cervical carcinoma. Furthermore, the findings that many of these genes are methylated more often in CIN 2 and CIN 3 than in CIN 1 suggests that detection of aberrant DNA methylation may serve as a potential diagnostic or prognostic biomarker of cervical neoplasia. In a large study that examined 20 candidate tumor suppressor genes in histologic and cytologic specimens, *DAPK1, TWIST,* and *RARB* were determined to be an optimal panel of hypermethylated genes, where at least one of three genes was methylated in 57% of CIN 3 and 74% of invasive carcinomas but only 5% of CIN 1. Although findings to date show promising results, additional studies that identify an optimal panel of tumor suppressor genes with increased sensitivity and specificity and subsequent testing in large clinical trials with histologic follow-up are needed to determine the utility of aberrant DNA methylation as a biomarker.

Most methods developed to detect DNA methylation of the promoter sequences of tumor suppressor genes use methylation-sensitive endonuclease digestion or sodium bisulfite treatment of DNA followed by subsequent PCR amplification. Most studies that have examined the methylation profiles in cervical carcinogenesis have used methylation-specific PCR (MSP). MSP is a sensitive and specific detection method whereby primer design exploits sequence differences between methylated and unmethylated DNA following bisulfite treatment. In standard MSP, the presence or absence of methylated alleles is determined by evaluating PCR products by gel electrophoresis. More recently studies have used quantitative MSP (e.g., MethylLight), a procedure in which standard MSP is combined with real-time quantitative PCR techniques that use fluorogenic TaqMan probes. Advantages of quantitative MSP over standard MSP include increased sensitivity and specificity, high throughput, and the ability to quantitate methylated DNA in the sample.

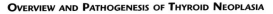

THYROID CYTOPATHOLOGY

OVERVIEW AND PATHOGENESIS OF THYROID NEOPLASIA

It has been estimated that 4% to 7% of the adult population has a palpable thyroid nodule and up to 70% may develop nonpalpable nodules. Thyroid FNA has emerged as the most useful test for the management of patients with a clinically significant thyroid nodule. Diagnostic accuracy of FNA, based on morphologic analysis alone, is high for lesions that are either definitively benign or definitively malignant. However, a significant percentage of thyroid FNAs (approximately 15%) fall into an indeterminate or "suspicious" category that has a risk of malignancy ranging from 15% to 60%. Clearly, the identification of molecular diagnostic tests that could be used as an adjunct to thyroid FNA to improve the diagnostic accuracy for thyroid carcinomas would be extremely useful in the management of these patients to avoid repeat FNAs, delays in diagnosis, and unnecessary surgical procedures.

Studies of the pathogenesis of thyroid cancer have revealed several potential molecular markers. The most common type of thyroid cancer, papillary thyroid carcinoma (PTC), often contains one of three major categories of genetic alterations: *BRAF* mutations, *RET/PTC* translocations, or *RAS* mutations. Although these genetic abnormalities may seem disparate, they all converge on a single signal transduction pathway within the cell, the mitogen-activated protein kinase (MAPK) pathway. This pathway normally transduces signals from growth factors, cytokines, and hormones from outside the cell to the nucleus using cell membrane receptor tyrosine kinases. Downstream cytoplasmic effectors in this pathway, including RAS, RAF, MEK and ERK proteins, ultimately regulate cell differentiation, survival, and proliferation. Constitutive activation of this pathway may be induced by point mutations in *RAS* or *BRAF* or as a result of translocations involving the *RET* gene.

MOLECULAR MARKERS OF PAPILLARY THYROID CARCINOMA

B-type Raf Mutations

Mutation of the gene for B-type raf (BRAF) kinase is the most common known mutation in thyroid cancer. This gene encodes a serine–threonine kinase involved in the MAPK signal transduction pathway. Most *BRAF* mutations in PTC occur at a single nucleotide (T1799A), which results in the replacement of the amino acid valine with glutamate (V600E). This point mutation results in the constitutive activation of BRAF kinase and leads to the oncogenic activation of the MAPK pathway. A meta-analysis of the prevalence of *BRAF* mutations in thyroid lesions demonstrates that it is present in 44% of PTC and some anaplastic thyroid carcinomas but not in medullary thyroid carcinoma, follicular thyroid carcinoma, adenomas, or adenomatous hyperplasia. In addition, among histologic variants of PTC, the prevalence of *BRAF* mutations is unevenly distributed, with mutations detected in 77% of the tall cell variant of PTC, 60% of conventional PTC, and only 12% of the follicular variant of PTC (FVPTC). The relatively low prevalence of *BRAF* mutations observed in FVPTC may reflect biologic differences related to this histologic variant. However, given the high interobserver variability in the diagnosis of FVPTC, this diagnostic category may also include some nonmalignant follicular lesions that could partly account for the lower prevalence.

Although *BRAF* mutational analysis has a modest sensitivity (56% of PTCs are negative), the specificity for PTC is extremely high; therefore, it may be useful as an adjunct to thyroid FNAs for the evaluation of suspicious thyroid nodules. Results from retrospective or small prospective studies have demonstrated that use of *BRAF* mutational analysis with FNA cytology correctly identifies PTC in approximately 8% of all suspicious thyroid FNAs. Widespread application of *BRAF* mutational analysis to thyroid FNAs is technically feasible but may require further refinement to enable the detection of rare mutant alleles in a background of abundant wild-type alleles. Other intriguing applications of *BRAF* mutation assays relate to the prognostic or therapeutic relevance of *BRAF* mutations. There is some evidence to show that the presence of the V600E amino acid substitution correlates with increased risk of recurrence and lack of radioactive iodine avidity in recurrent tumors. Interestingly, several small molecule inhibitors of BRAF kinase activity or other MAPK pathway targets may ultimately prove useful in patients whose tumors harbor *BRAF* mutations and are unresponsive to traditional therapy.

Molecular Methods for Detection of B-type Raf Mutations

The finding that most *BRAF* mutations occur at a single base within the gene allows for the development of clinically useful molecular diagnostic tests. Potential molecular techniques that can be used to detect *BRAF* mutations include all technologies that detect point mutations in DNA. *BRAF* mutations have been detected in thyroid FNA samples using the Mutector™ kit (TrimGen), which is commercially available and uses a proprietary primer extension-based technology and a colorimetric detection system. Other technologies applied to thyroid FNAs for the detection of *BRAF* mutations include real-time LightCycler™ PCR (Roche) with fluorescence resonance energy transfer probes, and allele-specific LightCycler PCR with melting curve analysis. Detection of *BRAF* mutations by these methods requires that the mutant DNA represent at least 5% of the total DNA, which may be a limiting factor if the FNA specimens are from predominantly cystic thyroid nodules or if there are few lesional cells.

Receptor Tyrosine Translocations

Another genetic alteration found in up to 40% of PTCs involves the activation of the receptor tyrosine (RET) kinase as a result of chromosomal translocation. Specifically, the kinase domain of *RET* is fused to the 5′ region of one of a heterogeneous set of genes, which are collectively referred to as *RET/PTC translocations*. The mechanism for cellular transformation most likely involves the activation of the *RET* gene in cells where it is normally not expressed, along with the fact that the RET kinase is constitutively active in these cells. To date, more than 10 fusion partners have been identified in PTC, which creates challenges for a comprehensive diagnostic test. Fortunately, just two translocations, *RET/PTC1* and *RET/PTC3,* are the most common in sporadic PTC. The two *RET* fusion partner genes are both located on the long arm of chromosome 10, along with *RET.* Most *RET/PTC1* and *RET/PTC3* fusions are generated by chromosomal inversions. The breakpoints for these two translocations are quite variable and are scattered over a relatively large genomic intronic region, which presents challenges for the development of molecular diagnostic tests. Consequently, most PCR-based methods for detecting *RET/PTC* translocations have relied on RT-PCR using messenger RNA for the fusion proteins rather than genomic DNA as a template. Applications of this assay to suspicious thyroid FNAs have been relatively few; however, one study found that the detection of *RET/PTC* rearrangements refined the diagnosis of PTC in 60% of FNA samples with indeterminate results. Another study found that the combination of testing for *BRAF* mutations and *RET/PTC* translocations refined the diagnosis of PTC in 33% of the indeterminate thyroid FNAs. Widespread application of these tests to FNA samples will require both analytic validation of the *RET/PTC* assay, perhaps in combination with a test for *BRAF* mutations, and clinical validation in large, prospective clinical trials.

RAS Mutations

Mutations in the *RAS* oncogenes occur in a small subset of thyroid cancers. Specifically, mutations in codon 61 of *NRAS* are most common, but mutations in *KRAS* and *HRAS* have also been identified. *NRAS* mutations have been identified in approximately 5% of PTC and in about 43% of FVPTC. In addition, *RAS* mutations may be mutually exclusive with other genetic alterations found in *BRAF* and *RET* genes. Unfortunately, detection of *RAS* mutations as a biomarker will likely have a lower specificity for malignancy than *BRAF* mutations or *RET/PTC* rearrangements because *RAS* mutations are also found in adenomas and some adenomatoid nodules.

MOLECULAR MARKERS OF FOLLICULAR AND MEDULLARY THYROID CARCINOMAS

Other less common thyroid cancers contain specific genetic alterations. A chromosomal translocation that creates a fusion protein between the thyroid transcription factor (PAX8) and the nuclear receptor peroxisome proliferator-activated receptor-γ was initially detected in approximately 50% of follicular thyroid carcinomas. Recently, it has also been found in a subset of follicular adenomas, raising the possibility that it is a transforming event in the pathway of follicular carcinogenesis. Although this translocation can be detected by FISH or RT-PCR, follicular carcinomas are uncommon, which has hindered the introduction of such molecular diagnostic tests into routine clinical practice. Another uncommon thyroid cancer, medullary thyroid carcinoma, often contains germline mutations in the *RET* gene, particularly in patients with multiple endocrine neoplasia type 2 syndromes; however, somatic detection of these mutations does not currently have a diagnostic role in patients with clinical nodules.

URINARY CYTOPATHOLOGY

OVERVIEW AND PATHOGENESIS OF UROTHELIAL NEOPLASIA

The American Cancer Society estimated that there would be more than 60,000 new cases of bladder cancer in the United States in the 2006. Most of these patients were expected to present with superficial urothelial carcinomas (UCs) that are treated by transurethral resection of the tumor. Recurrence of UCs in such patients is common (50% to 80%), and some low-grade tumors will recur as high-grade UCs. Postoperative cytologic screening of voided urine and bladder washings, combined with cystoscopy, represents the cornerstone of surveillance programs for recurrent bladder cancer. The reported sensitivity of urine cytology for UCs varies tremendously in the literature. A recent meta-analysis suggests an overall sensitivity of 48%. This number is significantly less for low-grade UCs, but clinical detection of these indolent lesions is less imperative, because these low-grade neoplasms are often exophytic lesions that are readily identified by cystoscopy. The addition of molecular tests for genetic abnormalities associated with urothelial carcinoma may significantly increase the sensitivity of urine cytology.

Although multiple genetic alterations are associated with urothelial carcinogenesis, there is increasing evidence to suggest that low-grade and high-grade UCs are distinct lesions that emerge from two different molecular pathways. Most UCs are low-grade papillary UCs (70% to 80%) that tend to recur but rarely progress to muscle-invasive UCs. Low-grade lesions often display loss of all or part of chromosome 9 and often contain activating

mutations in the *HRAS* gene (30% to 40%) and *FGFR3* gene (about 70%). In contrast, high-grade UCs, which represent approximately 20% to 30% of UCs, progress from dysplasia and flat carcinoma in situ to invasive tumors that are clinically more aggressive. High-grade UCs typically contain mutations of *TP53* and loss of heterozygosity of chromosome 9, often at the 9p21 locus that contains the tumor suppressor gene *CDKN2A* (p16). In addition, UCs often contain numeric chromosomal alterations (aneuploidy), as well as amplification and overexpression of specific oncogenes, which correlate with increased risk of progression and aggressive behavior. It is also possible that the specific patterns of aneuploidy or deletion may correlate with recurrence or progression.

MOLECULAR MARKERS OF UROTHELIAL CARCINOMAS

The knowledge of chromosomal alterations associated with UCs has fueled the development of molecular diagnostic assays for use with urine samples. In fact, one of the few molecular cytology tests with FDA approval is the UroVysion™ (Abbott Molecular) FISH test for bladder cancer. This FISH assay employs a probe set that includes centromeric probes for chromosomes 3, 7, and 17 to detect aneuploidy of these chromosomes, along with a locus-specific probe (LSI 9p21) to detect loss of the tumor suppressor gene *CDKN2A* (p16) (Figure 17-5). The UroVysion protocol defines a positive test result as the detection of at least 4 of 25 morphologically abnormal cells with gains of at least 2 chromosomes, loss of 9p21 signals in at least 12 of 25 abnormal cells, or both. In reports comparing the accuracy of FISH and routine cytology for the detection of recurrent UCs, FISH consistently outperforms routine cytology. In one meta-analysis, the sensitivity of UroVysion for high-grade UCs was 96% compared with 71% for routine cytology. The sensitivity of both FISH and routine cytology is reduced for low-grade UCs, but this may not be clinically important given the indolent nature of these lesions. Recent studies have also suggested that UroVysion may provide predictive information, in addition to contributing to the detection of existing disease. Results from one study suggested that FISH results may stratify patients into low- and high-risk groups for recurrence within 29 months. In addition, another study suggested that a positive UroVysion test may predict response to bacillus Calmette-Guérin treatment. Interestingly, aneuploidy of specific chromosomes within the set tested by the UroVysion assay may provide additional prognostic information;, however, more studies are necessary to establish their value.

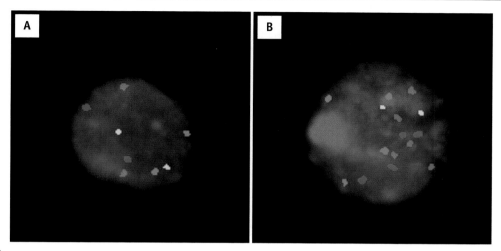

FIGURE 17-5

Application of FISH to urinary cytology. FISH images using the UroVysion probe set from a normal urothelial cell **(A)** and an aneuploid, high-grade urothelial carcinoma cell **(B)** containing multiple copies of chromosomes 3, 7, and 17. Probe color description: CEP 3, red; CEP 7, green; CEP 17, aqua; LSI 9p21, yellow. (Courtesy of Dr. Kevin C. Halling, The Mayo Clinic and Foundation, Rochester, MN.)

CONCLUSION

The application of molecular tests to cytologic samples will continue to play an important role in cytopathology as the demand for additional clinically useful diagnostic and predictive molecular markers increases. Identification and implementation of clinically useful molecular tests can have a significant impact on patient management, as demonstrated by the use of HPV DNA testing in cervical cytology. HPV DNA testing has become integrated into most clinical laboratories and is now a part of routine clinical practice. Similarly, FISH is increasingly used to enhance the sensitivity of cytology-based bladder cancer surveillance programs.

Given the tremendous potential for molecular diagnostics to enhance cytologic analysis, what challenges have prevented its widespread application? Several factors have contributed to its limited use thus far, including small sample size, sample heterogeneity, preanalytic processing variability, lack of validated assays, and lack of integration with clinical management schemes. The small number of cells in a cytologic sample, relative to an entire tumor resection specimen, does create challenges, but sensitive molecular techniques such as PCR or whole genome amplification techniques should make this surmountable. Tumors are never homogeneous collections of cells and usually contain inflammatory cells, blood vessels, and normal cells from the surrounding tissues. This heterogeneity is most extreme in screening samples, such as cervical samples or sputum, in which the neoplastic cells may represent only 0.1%, or less,

of the entire sample. The FNA technique itself may enrich for neoplastic cells, but even these samples often contain contaminating blood and other cellular elements. Careful preanalytic analysis should take place to ensure that the sample type is perfectly matched to the sensitivity and specificity of the diagnostic test to avoid the "garbage in–garbage out" phenomenon. In addition, preanalytic processing must be carefully coordinated with the molecular test. Fixation methods and timing may profoundly affect the outcome of a molecular test and should be carefully standardized. The assay itself should also be analytically validated to ensure reproducibility. Commercially produced diagnostic kits or analyte-specific reagents typically meet these standards, but research protocols or home-brewed protocols may be deficient. Development of such validated clinical assays from preliminary research discoveries remains a major bottleneck in the application of molecular diagnostic tests. Finally, a molecular test should not simply provide additional descriptive data of questionable utility. Instead, it should clearly add value to the cytologic sample that addresses a specific clinical need and, ideally, clearly fit into a clinical management scheme.

As our understanding of the molecular pathogenesis of disease processes increases and more molecular tests become integrated into the clinical cytopathology laboratory, cytologic specimens may prove to be the ideal vehicle for translating scientific discoveries into clinically useful molecular diagnostics. FNA may be recognized as the preferred method to sample tumors in a minimally invasive, cost-effective manner for molecular testing. In addition, exfoliated cellular samples may become the foundation for molecular biomarker–based early cancer detection strategies.

SUGGESTED READINGS

Bossuyt PM, Reitsma JB, Bruns DE, et al: Standards for reporting of diagnostic accuracy. Toward complete and accurate reporting of studies of diagnostic accuracy: The STARD initiative. Am J Clin Pathol 2003;119(1):18–22.

Pepe MS, Etzioni R, Feng Z, et al: Phases of biomarker development for early detection of cancer. J Natl Cancer Inst 2001;93(14):1054–1061.

Gynecologic Cytopathology

Duenas-Gonzalez A, Lizano M, Candelaria M, et al: Epigenetics of cervical cancer: An overview and therapeutic perspectives. Mol Cancer 2005;4:38.

Solomon D, Schiffman M, Tarrone R: Comparison of three management strategies for patients with atypical squamous cells of undetermined significance. J Natl Cancer Inst 2001;93:293–299.

Wright TC Jr, Cox JT, Massad LS, et al: 2001 consensus guidelines for the management of women with cervical cytological abnormalities. JAMA 2002;287:2120–2129.

Wright TC Jr, Schiffman M, Solomon D, et al: Interim guidance for the use of human papillomavirus DNA testing as an adjunct to cervical cytology for screening. Obstet Gynecol 2004;103:304–309.

Thyroid Cytopathology

Santoro M, Melillo RM, Carlomagno F, et al: Minireview: RET: Normal and abnormal functions. Endocrinology 2004;145(12):5448–5451.

Xing M: BRAF mutation in thyroid cancer. Endocr Relat Cancer 2005;12(2):245–262.

Urinary Cytopathology

Jones JS: DNA-based molecular cytology for bladder cancer surveillance. Urology 2006;67(3 Suppl 1):35–45.

18 Molecular Diagnosis of Infectious Agents in Tissue

Randall T. Hayden • Gary W. Procop

INTRODUCTION

The ability to detect and characterize infectious pathogens in anatomic pathology specimens can be of critical importance because of both primary diagnostic purposes and implications for treatment and prognosis. Infection can present as a primary pathogenic process, with injury caused by either the organism itself or the host immune response. In other cases, particular infections are associated with the presence or genesis of neoplasia. In such cases, the presence of organism can be an indicator of the need for preemptive therapy to prevent malignant transformation (e.g., human papillomavirus and cervical carcinoma). In other circumstances, identification of a particular agent may represent a key diagnostic feature (human herpes virus 8 in Kaposi's sarcoma). In some instances, direct treatment of an infectious process may prevent the onset of malignancy (*Helicobacter pylori* and gastric lymphoma).

The detection and characterization of such pathogens has long relied upon morphologic examination, together with the use of cytochemical stains, such as Grocott-Gomori's methenamine silver (GMS), tissue Gram, and periodic acid Schiff (PAS). The diagnosis of infection by histopathology alone, however, can be challenging, with limitations in sensitivity and in the ability to identify organisms with a high degree of taxonomic precision. Diagnosis may be hampered by low numbers of organisms, by artifactual distortion, by the presence of necrosis or other degenerative processes, or by other ongoing processes, such as dense cellular inflammatory infiltrates, which may mask the typical morphologic appearance of some agents. Many diagnoses of viral infections rely on the identification of characteristic intracellular inclusions. These may be absent, atypical in appearance, or otherwise lacking in specificity. Some organisms may lack typical staining characteristics or structural features because of factors such as intercurrent drug therapy, subspecies level variations in genomic makeup or phenotypic expression, or variations in staining reagents, tissue processing, or laboratory techniques used. Organisms may be detected, but classification to the genus or species level may be impossible when based solely on morphology. Finally, some agents are invisible when routine cytochemical stains are used. Although adjunctive culture may be of use, these techniques often require prolonged processing and incubation times and rely on cumbersome and time-consuming methods for identification. In many cases, infection may be unsuspected before specimen submission, obviating the use of culture. Identification of organisms in situ, while retaining surrounding histopathology, can also help differentiate pathogens from nonpathogenic colonizing organisms or contaminants. Such differentiation is often not possible when relying solely on culture as a diagnostic modality.

Increasingly, molecular diagnostics has been seen as a way to increase our ability to rapidly and accurately detect infections in fixed tissues and cellular material. Such techniques include probe-based, signal amplification methods, and tools such as polymerase chain reaction (PCR), that are based on direct target amplification. These methods, as described in earlier chapters, can be highly sensitive and specific. Since their advent, they have increasingly made their way from the research laboratory into mainstream clinical diagnostics. As more assays have been developed and published, and more commercial reagents, tests, and platforms have become available, greater ease of use, reduced processing time, and improved standardization have all contributed to improve the utility of such methods for routine clinical diagnostic use. Although caveats remain in the interpretation of results generated by such tests, their impact has been seen across a range of taxonomically diverse organisms, with implications for diagnosis and treatment of patients. Although a detailed exploration of all such applications is beyond the scope of this chapter, the following sections outline some examples of the more common or clinically significant uses of these powerful techniques.

HUMAN PAPILLOMAVIRUS

BACKGROUND

Human papillomavirus (HPV) is a member of the family *Papovaviridae*. It is a nonenveloped double-stranded DNA virus with a closed circular genome and icosahedral capsid symmetry. The virus has a worldwide geographic distribution and is endemic throughout the human population, with other species affecting various animals in a species-specific manner. The virus exhibits various periods of incubation, latency, and spontaneous resolution, as well as symptomatic infection. Population prevalence varies depending on geography, age, socioeconomic group, and anatomic site. The virus infects squamous epithelial cells throughout the body with a range of neoplastic and non-neoplastic sequelae.

HPV is typed based on the sequence of the L1 capsid protein open reading frame. Individual types are distinguished by having less than 90% homology within this sequence, subtypes having 90% to 95% homology. Viral types have been closely associated with various anatomic sites of involvement and disease states, as well with the risk for malignant transformation. Thus, plantar warts are associated with types 1 and 2; flat warts are linked with types 3 and 10; recurrent respiratory papillomatosis is tied to types 6 and 11; and focal epithelial hyperplasia is associated with types 13 and 32.

The genital tract provides the most widely recognized association between HPV and neoplasia. HPV has been associated with genital warts and penile carcinoma, as well as with epithelial dysplasia and malignancy of the vulva and uterine cervix. Screening for evidence of HPV infection and dysplasia through the use of the Pap smear has resulted in a marked decline in the frequency of cervical carcinoma in regions where these measures have been implemented. It is clear that HPV types can be risk stratified with respect to the frequency of progression to malignancy when detected in cervical epithelial cells (Table 18-1). Thus, HPV types 16, 18, 31, and 45 have the highest association with cervical carcinoma, whereas types 6, 11, and 42 to 44 have a low degree of association with malignancy. The ability to detect and type viruses in cervical scrapings has long been promoted as a potential adjunct or even a replacement for the conventional Pap smear. The latter, although proved highly effective, may result in many unnecessary procedures, because patients with low-risk viruses and atypical findings on morphologic examination are followed with colposcopy and biopsy.

TABLE 18-1

HPV and Cervical Carcinoma: Risk Associations with Viral Types

Association with Malignancy	HPV Types
High risk	16, 18, 31, 45
Medium risk	33, 35, 39, 51, 52, 56–59, 68
Low risk	6, 11, 26, 42–44, 53–55, 62, 66

HPV, human papillomavirus.

DIAGNOSTIC APPLICATIONS

Because of the difficulty of recovering HPV in culture, together with the need for viral typing, molecular diagnostic methods have become the primary means for obtaining this information. Although HPV has been associated with numerous neoplastic and non-neoplastic conditions at various anatomic sites, the predominant clinical application of such testing is in the screening and diagnostic evaluation of cytology and biopsy samples of the cervical squamous epithelium. Based on the nearly 100% association of HPV with cervical squamous dysplasia and malignancy, and on the high predictive value of individual HPV types, the routine laboratory detection of HPV in clinical specimens has become an integral part of national guidelines for cervical cancer screening programs. Several methods have been used for this purpose, including both signal and target amplification methods (Table 18-2).

Signal amplifications are perhaps most widely used. They include two commercialized methods: Hybrid Capture® 2 (HC2, Digene) and in situ hybridization (ISH) using the Inform® system (Ventana Medical Systems). HC2 is the only test currently cleared by the U.S. Food and Drug Administration (FDA) for screening of clinical samples for HPV. This test can be performed only on liquid-based cytology specimens and relies on the detection of RNA probes binding to HPV-specific DNA targets. The probe cocktails can identify most common high- and low-risk viral types, although it is unable to differentiate individual viral types. The Inform system is a chromogenic, ISH test, classified as an analyte-specific reagent. This test also relies on probe cocktails specific to the most common high- and low-risk HPV types. The reagents can be used manually or can be adapted to the Bench-Mark® Automated Slide Staining System (Ventana Medical Systems). Table 18-2 compares the various

TABLE 18-2

Detection and Typing of HPV in Cervical Specimens: Comparison of Methods

Method	Advantages	Disadvantages
SIGNAL AMPLIFICATION		
Southern blot	High specificity.	Not commonly used for this application. Requires technical expertise and has a prolonged turnaround time and lower sensitivity.
ISH	Works on cytologic preparations or on paraffin-embedded tissue, thus allowing morphologic localization. Commercial reagents available (Inform® method); processing can be automated.	Has lower sensitivity compared to Hybrid Capture® 2 in some studies but can be improved with secondary amplification methods (tyramide amplification).
Hybrid capture	Commercialized, U.S. FDA-cleared method (Hybrid Capture 2). Widely used; can be run directly from liquid Pap samples. Can provide quantitative data.	Instrumentation requirements. No ability to perform on tissue sections. No morphologic link with positive results.
TARGET AMPLIFICATION		
PCR	Highly sensitive. Flexible technology. Easily available reagents.	Can be used on disrupted tissue but has no ability to maintain morphologic relationships. Potential for contamination, false-positive results. Some commercial reagents available as research use only devices. Not yet in wide use.

FDA, Food and Drug Administration; HPV, human papillomavirus; ISH, in situ hybridization; PCR, polymerase chain reaction.

performance characteristics of these methods. ISH has the capability to detect HPV from biopsy specimens, as well from liquid-based cytologic specimens. HC2 offers the potential for quantitative results, which may have prognostic implications. Studies available for comparing relative sensitivity, specificity, and predictive value of results achieved by these two methods are limited.

Numerous other methods have been described in the literature, consisting of user-defined methods, both for ISH (Figure 18-1) and PCR-based tests, some using commercially available reagents (probes or primers) and some describing those developed by individual investigators. PCR or other target amplification methods may offer a higher degree of sensitivity than some signal amplification methods; however, the relative advantage or disadvantage in terms of clinical predictive value is uncertain. Furthermore, these methods, as well as other user-defined methodologies, require a higher degree of expertise to develop, validate, and perform on an ongoing basis. They are less amenable to automation than the commercialized methods and suffer from lower numbers of users; this makes it harder to assess their relative performance and their optimal role in diagnostic algorithms.

HERPES VIRUSES

BACKGROUND

Members of the family *Herpesviridae* consist of enveloped, double-stranded DNA viruses with icosahedral capsid symmetry. There are nine member of this family that have been shown to infect humans, including herpes simplex 1 and 2 (HSV-1 and HSV-2), cytomegalovirus (CMV), varicella-zoster virus (VZV), Epstein-Barr virus (EBV), and human herpes viruses 6A, 6B, 7, and 8 (HHV-6 to HHV-8). These viruses all have high seroprevalence among adult populations worldwide. They are characterized by lifelong latency, which can result in re-emergence of symptomatic disease when patients are immunocompromised or otherwise undergo significant stress. Initial infection with these viruses typically occurs in childhood. When primary infection occurs later in life, it may present with more severe clinical findings. Findings in immunocompromised patients with reactivated or primary infection are of most concern and may manifest in individual end-organ infections throughout the body, as well as with multiorgan system or disseminated disease, sometimes life threatening. Primary

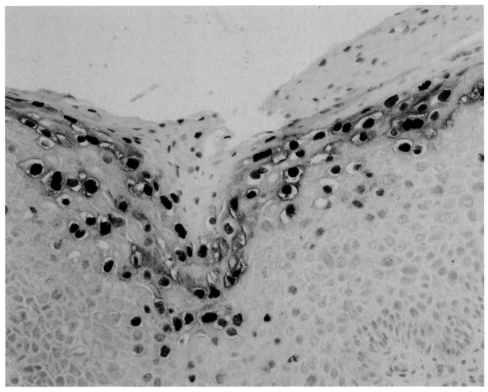

FIGURE 18-1

In situ hybridization for the detection of human papillomavirus in a case of low-grade cervical dysplasia. (Courtesy of Dr. Ann Marie Nelson, Armed Forces Institute of Pathology, Washington, DC.)

sites of infection vary depending on the host factors and the viral species. Manifestations include severe infections of the central nervous system, gastrointestinal tract, respiratory tract, liver, blood and bone marrow, genitourinary tract, skin, and mucous membranes (Table 18-3). Infections (particularly with EBV and HHV-8) have been linked to conditions of hyperplasia, neoplasia, and frank malignancy. The detection and characterization of these viruses can have critical importance for diagnosis, prognosis, and treatment of critically ill patients.

PROGNOSTIC FACTORS

Although the simple detection and identification of causative herpes viruses is of primary importance and can be of high clinical impact, there are other issues to be considered in correlating such findings to a patient's condition and in using such findings to direct clinical care. Because these viruses are commonly found in the general population as latent infections, their detection does not always correspond to clinical disease; thus, end-organ localization in tissue, as well as specific localization within hyperplasic or neoplastic cells, can help support disease causality. In addition, viral load or percentage of cells infected may have clinical importance. The examination of

tissue specimens can therefore provide significant useful information beyond that achieved with assessment of blood and other body fluids.

The identification and characterization of herpes viruses, as with other viruses, has gained additional importance as our understanding of the pathophysiology of such infections has improved and as therapeutic agents have been developed to help ameliorate both viral infections and neoplastic conditions that they may trigger. For example, the identification of a viral species causing pneumonitis or hepatitis has become increasingly critical in directing the appropriate antiviral regimen and in some cases in deciding upon appropriate modulation of a patient's immunosuppressive therapy when such findings are in the context of transplant or treatment with cytotoxic agents. In addition, the genotypic analysis of herpes viruses can demonstrate polymorphisms, which are linked with resistance to commonly used antiviral agents.

DIAGNOSTIC APPLICATIONS

Detection, identification, and further characterization of herpes viruses, as for other viruses, have traditionally been the realm of culture-based methodologies. Such techniques can be extremely useful. When

TABLE 18-3

Herpes Viruses: Clinical Features

Virus	Site of Latency	Disease Manifestations
Herpes simplex 1, 2	Trigeminal ganglion	Oropharyngeal herpes, herpes labialis, disseminated mucocutaneous disease, keratitis, genital herpes, systemic disease (immunocompromised)
Varicella-zoster virus	Dorsal root ganglia	Varicella, herpes zoster, pneumonia, hepatitis, encephalitis
Epstein-Barr virus (EBV)	Lymphocytes	Infectious mononucleosis, X-linked lymphoproliferative syndrome, chronic active EBV, post-transplant lymphoproliferative disease, lymphoma (Hodgkin's, non-Hodgkin's, Burkett's), leiomyosarcoma, nasopharyngeal carcinoma
Cytomegalovirus (CMV)	Myeloid cells	CMV mononucleosis, congenital CMV infection, pneumonitis, gastroenteritis, hepatitis, encephalitis, retinitis
Human herpes virus 6A, 6B, 7	Monocyte macrophages, T lymphocytes	Fever, rash, bone marrow suppression, meningitis, encephalitis, pneumonitis
Human herpes virus 8	Lymphocytes	Fever, rash, Kaposi's sarcoma, primary effusion lymphoma, plasma cell form of multicentric Castleman's disease

grown in culture, viruses can be identified with a high degree of confidence through the use of cytopathic effect and immunofluorescent methods (high analytic specificity). However, these methods often have limitations in terms of sensitivity, particularly with low viral loads or with viruses that are more difficult to propagate in vitro. In particular, culture of EBV and HHV-6, HHV-7, and HHV-8 may be difficult to achieve and may require cocultivation with umbilical cord lymphocytes. VZV and CMV are characterized by slow growth in vitro, requiring several days to weeks (in the case of CMV) to propagate using conventional cell culture–based assays. Moreover, detection of these viruses in culture does not maintain morphologic relationships, nor does it provide good information on viral load in a given tissue or anatomic site. Routine histopathology can also be highly useful. Many of these viruses demonstrate intranuclear or intracytoplasmic inclusions that can be detected on hematoxylin and eosin–stained slides. These inclusions are useful guideposts but may lack both sensitivity and specificity and, again, may not accurately reflect viral load in a given site of infection.

The use of molecular diagnostic techniques has vastly improved our ability to detect, identify, and quantify herpes viruses in tissue. Whereas target amplification methods, such as PCR, can have an extremely high degree of sensitivity and specificity, methods that maintain morphology, notably ISH, have been the most widely used among anatomic pathologists (Figure 18-2). ISH techniques offer added advantages over PCR in terms of ease of use, availability of fully automated platforms, and availability of commercially prepared reagents. As of this writing, commercially prepared probes were available for all herpes viruses except HHV-6 and HHV-7 (Table 18-4). This wide availability and amenability to the use of automated techniques allows such assays to be run in a variety of clinical laboratory settings and permits the application of a common technology to all similar agents. When paired with secondary signal amplification techniques, in situ methods can have a high degree of sensitivity approaching that of target amplification methods—again while maintaining morphologic relationships, both within individual cells and in the context of surrounding anatomy.

Molecular diagnostic techniques can also be used to help predict susceptibility to commonly used antiviral therapeutics. Such methods have most commonly been applied to CMV, although they may be used for other herpes viruses. Phenotypic methods for characterizing antiviral susceptibility depend on culture-based plaque reduction assays. Genotypic methods are aimed at detecting polymorphisms in the viral genome that correspond to pharmacologic targets for antiviral agents. Resistance to drugs including acyclovir, gancyclovir, foscarnate, and cidofovir can be monitored by looking for genetic polymorphisms in the phosphotransferase and DNA polymerase genes (UL97 and UL54 in the CMV genome). Currently, these methods require a large quantity of input viral genome and are most successfully applied to viral culture isolates; however, direct application to tissue samples may be feasible.

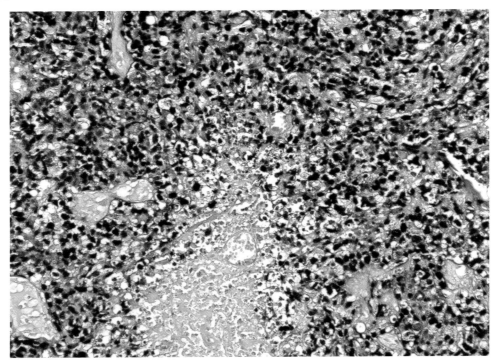

FIGURE 18-2

In situ hybridization for the detection of Epstein-Barr virus, probe cocktail directed against EBER1 to 3. High-power view showing strong nuclear staining in neoplastic cells of extranodal T- and natural killer lymphoma, nasal type.

TABLE 18-4

Molecular Targets for Detection of Herpes Viruses in Tissue

Virus	Commercial ISH Probes Available	Common Genetic Targets (ISH and PCR)
Herpes simplex 1, 2	X	Thymidine kinase, DNA polymerase, DNase
Varicella-Zoster virus	X	DNA polymerase, single-stranded DNA-binding protein, glycoprotein E, glycoprotein B
Epstein-Barr virus	X	EBER, EBNA, BamH1 W
Cytomegalovirus	X	Glycoprotein B, DNA polymerase, immediate early
Human herpes virus 6A, 6B		U67, glycoprotein 105, DNA polymerase, large tegument protein
Human herpes virus 7		Transactivator protein, large tegument protein
Human herpes virus 8	X	T0.8, T1.1, ORF 65, ORF 73, cyclin D

DNase, deoxyribonuclease; EBER, Epstein-Barr virus-encoded small RNAs; EBNA, Epstein-Barr virus nuclear antigen; ISH, in situ hybridization; ORF, open reading frame; PCR, polymerase chain reaction.

BACTERIAL AND MYCOBACTERIAL INFECTIONS

BACKGROUND

The kingdom Bacteria is vast, consisting of microorganisms that vary in their ability to grow on commonly used media. The bacteria that fail to grow on artificial media (e.g., *Tropheryma whipplei*), require cell culture for growth (e.g., *Chlamydia trachomatis*), are extremely fastidious in nature (e.g., *Bartonella* spp.), or grow slowly (e.g., *Mycobacterium tuberculosis*) are all candidates for detection by molecular methods. The number of bacteria in these categories is too great to comprehensively delineate in this section, so clinically important examples are given in Table 18-5. These examples focus on use of molecular

---

TABLE 18-5

Examples of Molecular Detection of Bacteria and Mycobacteria in Tissue

Disease State	Bacteria	Techniques and Targets
Endocarditis	Any, ranging from typical (*Staphylococcus aureus*) to fastidious and less common (*Tropheryma whipplei*)	Species-specific PCR (e.g., *sa442* gene PCR for *S. aureus*) vs. broad-range PCR (e.g., 16S rRNA gene). DNA sequencing following broad-range PCR for species identification.
Sexually transmitted diseases	*Neisseria gonorrhoeae, Chlamydia trachomatis*	Species-specific targets or unique 16S rRNA gene sequences. In situ hybridization in histologic sections for *Chlamydia*.
Community-acquired pneumonia	*Legionella* spp., *Chlamydophila pneumoniae, Mycoplasma pneumoniae*	Species-specific targets (e.g., *mip* gene sequences for *Legionella pneumophila*–specific PCR) or unique 16S rRNA gene sequences.
Tuberculosis	*Mycobacterium tuberculosis*	Species-specific targets (e.g., *IS6110* insertion sequences for *M. tuberculosis*–specific PCR) or unique *rpoB* gene or 16S rRNA gene sequences.
Diseases caused by nontuberculous mycobacteria	*M. kansasii, M. avium, M. intracellulare, M. marinum, M. gordonae, M. leprae, M. ulcerans,* and others	Species-specific PCR (e.g., *IS2404* insertion sequences for *M. ulcerans*–specific PCR), multiplex PCR, or broad-range PCR (e.g., *rpoB* or 16S rRNA gene). Postamplification analysis for differentiation following broad-range PCR.

PCR, polymerase chain reaction; rRNA, ribosomal RNA.

---

methods to identify the causative bacterial agents of endocarditis and many of the most clinically significant mycobacteria, including *M. tuberculosis*, as well as some nontuberculous mycobacteria, in both tissue and cytologic preparations.

PROGNOSTIC FACTORS

The first step in the successful targeted therapy of any infection is the detection and identification of the etiologic agent or agents of disease. Detection allows initiation of empirical therapy directed against the most likely causes of disease, whereas identification of the pathogen affords more specific, directed therapy. In both examples given here, specific identification of the causative agent is particularly important in guiding therapy. Such information often cannot be gained based solely on morphologic examination or on the results of microbiologic culture.

In cases of endocarditis, only limited information about the bacterial cause of the infection may be derived based on morphologic examination. Gram-positive cocci in a heart valve in histologic section could represent acute endocarditis (e.g., *Staphylococcus aureus*) or subacute endocarditis caused by coagulase-negative *Staphylococcus* spp., *Enterococcus* spp., or *Streptococcus* spp. The characteristic chaining of the streptococci and enterococci is not usually evident in histologic section, and all that may be seen are aggregates of gram-positive cocci. There are numerous antimicrobial therapeutic considerations given such a

broad differential, such as oxacillin resistance in the *Staphylococcus* spp., vancomycin resistance in the *Enterococcus* spp., and penicillin resistance in the *Streptococcus* spp. This clearly demonstrates the potential value of accurate and specific identification in allowing clinicians to rapidly optimize therapy.

The presence of acid-fast bacilli, whether in tissue or cytologic specimens, raises the concern of tuberculosis, a serious communicable disease. Although tuberculosis may be of foremost concern, nontuberculous mycobacteria are also important human pathogens, which in many cases are most effectively treated with different antimicrobial agents compared with those used against *M. tuberculosis*. It is important that infections caused by *M. tuberculosis* be confirmed or excluded first so that patients with potentially life-threatening and highly communicable disease may be immediately isolated and started on a multidrug antituberculous regimen. In addition, public health specialists must track and test contacts of infected individuals to help control the spread of the microorganism. If *M. tuberculosis* is initially excluded, positive identification of acid-fast bacilli must still be completed, both to assure the clinician (i.e., as a quality assurance check to confirm that a false negative did not occur) and to aid in the selection of appropriate antimycobacterial therapy. For example, acid-fast bacilli in lung tissue in association with a necrotizing granuloma may represent *M. tuberculosis, M. kansasii,* or *M. avium* or *M. intracellulare,* each of which has a different clinical implication and treatment profile.

DIAGNOSTIC APPLICATIONS

As is the case with other microorganisms described in this chapter, diagnostic tools that have been used to identify bacteria in tissue include ISH, species-specific and broad-range PCR, and DNA sequencing (Table 18-6).

ISH for bacteria uses labeled probes to detect specific nucleic acid sequences, confirming the identity of the microorganism in question. These may be either DNA oligonucleotide probes or peptide nucleic acid probes. The feasibility of ISH for the detection and identification of bacteria in tissue has been well demonstrated. Examples of bacteria that have been detected with such methods include *H. pylori*, *C. trachomatis*, and *Legionella pneumophila*. Another application has been the use of this technology to differentiate filamentous bacteria (i.e., *Actinomyces*

from *Nocardia*). The latter has proved an important application, often definitively demonstrating the presence of suspected microorganisms in areas of pathologic change. A variety of species-specific oligonucleotide and peptide nucleic acid hybridization probes have been described for the rapid identification of bacteria and yeast in blood culture bottles that signal positive. Any of these bacteria may be associated with endocarditis, so with these same well-defined probes it may be possible to definitively identify the causes of endocarditis using ISH. The application of such techniques to the diagnosis of infections in fixed tissue sections offers promise but has not yet been widely adopted. For example, ISH techniques have been developed for the identification of mycobacteria in tissue or in cytologic specimens that contain acid-fast bacilli and in cultures that grow acid-fast bacilli, but these applications

TABLE 18-6
Detection of Bacteria and Mycobacteria: A Comparison of Methods

Method	Advantages	Disadvantages
SIGNAL AMPLIFICATION		
Southern blot	High specificity.	Not commonly used for this application. Requires technical expertise and has a prolonged turn-around time and a lower sensitivity.
ISH	Works on cytologic preparations or on paraffin-embedded tissue, thus allowing morphologic localization. Commercial reagents are not available for histologic applications, but reagents are available for microbiologic applications (i.e., *S. aureus* and *Candida albicans* FISH); processing can be automated.	Has a lower sensitivity compared to nucleic acid amplification methods but can be improved with secondary amplification methods (tyramide amplification).
TARGET AMPLIFICATION		
PCR	Highly sensitive, flexible technology, easily available reagents. May be organism specific or broad range, and can be used with postamplification analysis (e.g., DNA sequencing).	Can be used on disrupted tissue but has no ability to view bacteria in the context of histopathology. Potential for contamination, false-positive results. Some commercial reagents available as ASRs. Not yet in wide use.
POSTAMPLIFICATION ANALYSIS		
Melting curve analysis	Limited differentiation of related bacteria and mycobacteria.	Differentiation capability is limited; decreased assay sensitivity for the target with lower melting temperatures (i.e., those with less than 100% complementarity between the target and the hybridization probe).
DNA sequencing	Ability to differentiate a variety of bacteria or mycobacteria following a broad-range PCR.	Cost requirement for expensive equipment and DNA sequencing expertise. Mixed sequences and clinically useless results are expected from polymicrobial infections.
Microarrays	Ability to differentiate a variety of bacteria or mycobacteria following a broad-range PCR. Can differentiate bacteria in polymicrobial infections.	Cost requirement for expensive equipment and DNA microarray expertise.

ASR, analyte-specific reagent; FISH, fluorescence in situ hybridization; ISH, in situ hybridization; PCR, polymerase chain reaction.

protein gene sequencing can also be performed; this allows identification of specific mutations that have been tied to various subtypes of human spongiform encephalopathy, including rare inherited forms of these diseases. Western blot can be performed on fresh or frozen tissue, so triaging tissue appropriately at the time of biopsy or autopsy to accommodate this is required.

PHAKOMATOSES

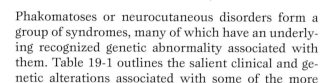

Phakomatoses or neurocutaneous disorders form a group of syndromes, many of which have an underlying recognized genetic abnormality associated with them. Table 19-1 outlines the salient clinical and genetic alterations associated with some of the more common syndromes in this group. In many of these cases, the diagnosis is based on the presence of a constellation of clinical findings. In cases in which the phenotype is ambiguous, genetic testing (usually DNA based) can be done. This is generally not part of routine laboratory testing and is relegated to a few large centers across the country.

NEURODEGENERATIVE DISEASE

The diagnosis of most neurodegenerative diseases is based on a combination of clinical presentation and morphologic findings. Most morphologic findings are nonspecific and need to be interpreted in the context of the disease process. An example of this is neurofibrillary tangles. Neurofibrillary tangles are classically

---

TABLE 19-1

Phakomatoses with Genetic Basis

Neurofibromatosis Type 1

Incidence: 1:3000–5000

Clinical criteria:

- At least six café-au-lait spots > 5 mm in diameter in prepubertal individuals or > 15 mm in postpubertal individuals
- At least two neurofibromas of any type or one plexiform neurofibroma
- Axillary and/or inguinal freckling
- Optic nerve glioma
- Dysplasia of the sphenoid wing or thinning of the cortex of a long bone
- First-degree relative with NF1 by these criteria

Pattern of inheritance: Autosomal dominant

Chromosome: 17q12

Gene/protein: Neurofibromin

Neurofibromatosis Type 2

Incidence: 1:50,000

Clinical criteria (at least one listed feature):

- Bilateral vestibular schwannoma
- A first-degree relative with NF2 and one vestibular schwannoma
- Two of the following: meningioma, schwannoma of another nerve, glioma of any type, posterior subcapsular lens opacity, cerebral calcification
- Two of the following: one vestibular schwannoma, multiple meningiomas, schwannoma of another nerve, glioma of any type, subcapsular lens opacity, cerebral calcification

Pattern of inheritance: Autosomal dominant

Chromosome: 22q12

Gene/protein: Merlin (schwannomin)

Tuberous Sclerosis

Incidence: 1:6000

Clinical criteria:

- Definitive: One primary feature, two secondary features, or one secondary plus two tertiary features
- Provisional: One secondary and one tertiary feature or three tertiary features
- Suspect: One secondary feature or two tertiary features
- Primary features: Facial angiofibroma, multiple subungual fibromas, cortical tuber,* subependymal nodule or giant cell tumor,* multiple retinal nodules, multiple calcified exophytic subependymal nodules by neuroimaging
- Secondary features: Affected first-degree relative, cardiac rhabdomyoma(s), retinal achromia, cortical tuber(s) by neuroimaging, noncalcified subependymal nodules by neuroimaging, shagreen patch, forehead plaque, pulmonary lymphangioleiomyomatosis,* renal angiomyolipoma, renal cysts*
- Tertiary features: Hypomelanotic macules, "confetti" skin lesions, renal cysts by imaging, dental enamel pits, hamartomatous rectal polyps,* bone cysts by imaging, pulmonary lymphangioleiomyomatosis by imaging, cerebral white matter heterotopia by neuroimaging, gingival fibromas, hamartomas of other organs,* infantile spasms

Pattern of inheritance: Autosomal dominant

Chromosomes: 9q34 or 16p13.3

Gene/protein: TSC1 gene, hamartin (9q), and TSC2 gene, tuberin (16p)

(Continued)

TABLE 19-1

Phakomatoses with Genetic Basis—cont'd

Von Hippel-Lindau

Incidence: 1:36,000

Clinical criteria (all listed features):

- Capillary hemangioblastoma of the cerebellum or retina
- Renal cell carcinoma, pancreatic islet cell tumor, endolymphatic sac tumor, pheochromocytoma, or family member with VHL disease

Pattern of inheritance: Autosomal dominant

Chromosome: 3p25-26

Gene/protein: VHL gene, pVHL

Ataxia Telangiectasia

Incidence: 1:40,000

Clinical criteria:

- Cerebellar degeneration
- Immunodeficiency (sinonasal and pulmonary infections)
- Sensitivity to radiation
- Mucocutaneous and conjunctival telangiectasias
- Myoclonus, choreoathetosis, loss of speech

Pattern of inheritance: Autosomal recessive

Chromosome: 11q22-23

Gene/protein: ATM gene

Cowden's Disease

Incidence: Rare

Clinical criteria:

- Tricholemmomas
- Thyroid nodules
- Breast cancer
- Lhermitte-Duclos disease (dysplastic gangliocytoma of the cerebellum)
- Mental retardation, epilepsy

Pattern of inheritance: Autosomal dominant

Chromosome: 10q23

Gene/protein: PTEN/MMAC1, protein that regulates phosphatidylinositol 3'-kinase

Gorlin Syndrome

Incidence: 1:50,000–1:150,000

Clinical criteria:

- Basal cell carcinomas
- Odontogenic keratocysts of jaw

- Medulloblastomas, meningiomas
- Intracranial calcification, macrocephaly, agenesis of the corpus callosum, and hydrocephalus
- Ovarian fibromas
- Skeletal malformations

Pattern of inheritance: Autosomal dominant

Chromosome: 9q22.3

Gene/protein: PTCH gene, PTCH protein

Li-Fraumeni Syndrome

Incidence: Rare

Clinical criteria:

- For the full syndrome (all listed features):
- Sarcoma before age 45
- First-degree relative with any tumor before age 45
- Another first- or second-degree relative with cancer before age 45 or sarcoma at any age
- For the variant (at least one listed feature):
- Three separate primary cancers, one arising before age 45
- Childhood cancer or Li-Fraumeni-related tumors before age 45 and first- or second-degree relative with any cancer arising before age 60
- CNS tumors, including astrocytoma, medulloblastoma, embryonal tumor, meningioma, schwannoma, ependymoma, and choroid plexus papilloma

Pattern of Inheritance: Autosomal dominant

Chromosome: 17p13

Gene/protein: TP53 gene

Turcot's Syndrome

Incidence: Rare

Clinical criteria:

- High-grade glioma (type 1) and medulloblastoma (type 2)
- Adenomatous polyps and colon carcinomas

Pattern of inheritance: Most autosomal dominant

Chromosomes: 5q21 (APC gene), 3p21 (hMLH1), 2p21 (hMSH2), 7p22

Gene/protein: Type 1 with germline mutations of DNA mismatch repair genes hMLH1, hMSH2, or hPMS2; type 2 germline mutations of the APC gene

* Histologically confirmed.

associated with Alzheimer's disease. In reality, neurofibrillary tangles can be seen in small numbers in elderly individuals who have no history of dementia. Neurofibrillary tangles can also be encountered in a host of other central nervous system pathologies, both neoplastic and non-neoplastic. Even within

the setting of neurodegenerative disease, the distribution of tangles is important. Progressive supranuclear palsy is another neurodegenerative disorder marked by the formation of neurofibrillary tangles. The tangles in progressive supranuclear palsy are typically located in subcortical gray matter locations, including globus pallidus, subthalamus, substantia nigra, midbrain reticular formation, and pons. This is in contrast to the cortical-based tangles that mark Alzheimer's disease.

The underlying etiology of many common neurodegenerative disorders is not well understood. Genetic alterations have been described in several of these diseases (Table 19-2). For example, presenilin gene abnormalities are associated with familial cases of Alzheimer's disease. Genetic testing is offered by some laboratories specifically looking at mutations in some of these genes. Most of this testing at this point should not be used as the sole diagnostic test in the evaluation of patients. Patients with early-onset Alzheimer's disease (less than 65 years of age) comprise less than 10% of all patients with Alzheimer's disease. Three genes have been identified by linkage analysis of affected families that are associated with familial cases: the presenilin 1 gene, the presenilin 2 gene, and the amyloid-β precursor protein gene. A variety of mutations within these genes have been associated with Alzheimer's disease, with mutations in the presenilin 1 gene being the most common. Testing for the diagnosis or risk assessment of Alzheimer's disease continues to be somewhat investigational and needs to be done in association with appropriate genetic counseling.

An additional group of neurodegenerative disorders, which represent so-called trinucleotide repeat disorders, are worth mentioning. Testing is done by a simple PCR-based assay. These disorders fall into two distinct classes: those that are polyglutamine repeat disorders in which the expanded repeat is translated into an expanded polyglutamine tract, which results in the formation of protein aggregations within the cell, and those in which the trinucleotide repeat is present in an untranslated region of a gene. Table 19-3 summarizes some of the more common trinucleotide repeat disorders to affect the nervous system. All disorders associated with trinucleotide repeats generally have unusual inheritance features, including anticipation. Anticipation is defined by increasing severity or early onset of disease in successive generations of an affected family, often accompanied by a rise in the number of repeat units. These disorders are also marked by incomplete penetrance in that individuals known to carry mutation may show no symptoms. For most disorders, two major mechanisms of trinucleotide mutations have emerged: a loss of normal function, possibly related to an alteration in DNA sequence or methylation of the gene, and a gain of function because of abnormal regulation of gene expression or changes in protein structure.

Huntington's disease is a prototypical example of a trinucleotide repeat neurodegenerative disorder. The disease has an autosomal dominant pattern of inheritance and is associated with mutations on the short arm of chromosome 4. Clinically, the patients present in adulthood with a movement disorder, usually characterized by chorea, akinesia and rigidity,

---

TABLE 19-2

Neurodegenerative Disorders

Disease	Chromosome	Genetic Abnormality
Alzheimer's disease	14q24.3	Presenilin 1
	1q31-q41	Presenilin 2
	21q21.3	Amyloid precursor protein
	19q13.2	Apolipoprotein E4
Parkinson's disease	4q21.3-q22	Park 1 (autosomal dominant) α-synuclein gene (Greek and Italian families)
	6q25-q27	Park 2 (autosomal recessive) parkin gene, associated with juvenile onset
	4p14	Park 5 mismutation, UCHL1 gene
Frontotemporal lobar degeneration	17q21-22	*Tau* gene mutations (p301L) in frontotemporal dementia and parkinsonism linked to chromosome 17
Amyotrophic lateral sclerosis	21q22.1	Cu/Zn superoxide dismutase 1 gene (autosomal dominant)
Spinal muscular atrophy type 1 (Werdnig-Hoffmann disease)	5q13	SMN1 gene (autosomal recessive)
Neurodegeneration with brain iron accumulation type 1 (Hallervorden-Spatz disease)	20p13	PANK2 gene (autosomal recessive)

TABLE 19-3
Trinucleotide Repeat Disorders

Disorder	Chromosome	Gene and Product	Repeat	Number of Repeat Units
Fragile X syndrome	Xq27.3	FMR1/FMR1 protein	CGG	~44 ≥200
FRAXE mental retardation	Xq27	FRAXE	GCC	130 ≥700
Myotonic muscular dystrophy	19q13.3	DM/myotonin protein kinase	CTG	50 ≥200 (congenital > 700)
Kennedy's disease (spinal bulbar muscular atrophy	Xq11.2-q12	AR/androgen receptor	CAG	40–62
Huntington's disease	4p16.3	HO/huntington	CAG	37–121
Dentatorubropallidoluysian atrophy	12p13.31	DRPLA/atrophin 1	CAG	49–88
Spinocerebellar ataxia 1	6p23	SCA1/ataxin 1	CAG	40–81
Spinocerebellar ataxia 2	12q24.1	SCA2/ataxin 2	CAG	33–64
Spinocerebellar ataxia 3 (Machado-Joseph disease)	14q32.1	SCA3/ataxin 3	CAG	54–86
Spinocerebellar ataxia 6	19q13	SCA6/α1A-voltage-dependent calcium channel subunit	CAG	20–31
Spinocerebellar ataxia 7	3p14-21.4	SCA7/ataxin 7	CAG	37 ≥200

emotional disturbances, changes in personality, and dementia. The repeat involves a CAG triplet, which codes for the amino acid glutamine, that normally varies between 5 and 34 triplet repeats. Expansion of the repeat in excess of 37 triplets is associated with Huntington's disease. The number of triplet repeats is inversely correlated with the age of onset of the disease. Patients with juvenile onset of the disease have inherited the disease gene predominantly from the father; this may be because the expansion of the repeat appears likely during spermatogenesis. Detection by use of a simple PCR reaction can be performed and may be useful for genetic counseling. Presymptomatic testing should include extensive counseling before and after the test, informed consent of the proband, maintenance of the confidentiality of the test results, and exclusion of testing for those below 18 years.

METABOLIC DISEASE

A large group of metabolic disorders is defined by specific enzyme deficiencies or abnormalities that have been tied to specific genes in chromosome sites. As a group, these are relatively rare diseases and generally are not encountered in routine surgical

neuropathology practice in most hospitals. The diagnosis of these disorders can be made in one of several ways. The most definitive diagnosis rests on demonstrating evidence of an enzyme deficiency or the genetic defect underlying the disorder. It is beyond the scope of this chapter to discuss in detail each of these disorders. Some of the more common entities are summarized in Table 19-4.

NEUROMUSCULAR DISORDERS

Although the diagnosis of many of the more common neuromuscular disorders, including inflammatory myopathies and denervation atrophy, are primarily morphologic based, a growing number of less common disorders appear to have a genetic underpinning. Testing for these genetic abnormalities is becoming available in large centers and reference laboratories. Table 19-5 summarizes the genes and chromosomal locations of some of the more common neuromuscular disorders known to have a genetic basis. The discussion in this section focuses on Duchenne and Becker muscular dystrophies as prototypical types of dystrophic processes marked by known gene abnormalities and use of molecular testing in confirmation of their diagnoses.

TABLE 19-4
Metabolic Disorders

Disease	Enzyme or Protein	Locus
Sphingolipidoses		
GM1 gangliosidosis, Morquio type C	β-Galactosidase	3p21.33
GM2 Gangliosidoses		
Tay-Sachs disease	Hexosaminidase A	15q23-24
Sandhoff's disease	Hexosaminidase A and B	5q13 (Hex B)
GM2 activator deficiency	Hexosaminidase A and B	5q31.3-32.1
Niemann-Pick A and B	Sphingomyelinase	11p15.1-p15.4
Gaucher's disease	Glucocerebrosidase	1q21
	Glucosylsphingosine	
Krabbe's disease	Galatocerebrosidase	14q24.3-32.1
	Psychosine	
Metachromatic leukodystrophy	Arylsulfatase A	22q3.31-tes
	Galactosylsphingosine	
Fabry's disease	α-Galactosidase	Xq22.1
Farber's granulomatosis	Ceramidase	8p22-p21.3
Mucopolysaccharidoses		
Hurler Scheie (MPS I)	α-L-iduronidase	4p16.3
Hurler-Scheie		
Hunter (MPS II)	Iduronate sulfatase	Xq28
Sanfilippo A (MPS III-A)	Heparan N-sulfatase	17q25.3
Sanfilippo B (MPS III-B)	α-N-acetyl gluosaminidase	17q21
Sanfilippo C (MPS III-C)	Acetyl-CoA: α-glucosaminide acetyl-transferase	14
Sanfilippo D (MPS III-D)	N-acetylglucosamine-6-sulfatase	12q14
Morquio A (MPS IV-A)	Galactose-6-sulfatase	16q24.3
Morquio B (MPS IV-B)	β-Galactosidase	3p21.33
Maroteaux-Lamy (MPS VI)	Arylsulfatase B	5q13-q14
Sly (MPS VII)	β-Glucuronidase	7q21.11
MPS IX	Hyaluronidase	3p21.2-p21.3
Glycoproteinoses		
Sialidosis	Acid sialidase	6p21.3
α-Mannosidosis	α-Mannosidase	19p13.2q12
β-Mannosidosis	β-Mannosidase	4q22-q25
Fucosidosis	α-Fucosidase	1p34
Aspartylglucosaminuria	Aspartylglucosaminidase	4q32-q33
Schindler's disease	α-N-acetylgalactosaminidase	22q13
Peroxisomal Disorders		
Zellweger spectrum (ZS; NALD, IRD)	Pex1	7q21-22
	Matrix protein import	
Rhizomelic chondrodysplasia punctata	Pex7	6q22-q24
	PTS2 receptor	
D-bifunctional protein deficiency	17 β-Hydroxysteroid dehydrogenase	5q2
Adult Refsum's disease	Phytanoyl-CoA hydroxylase	10pter-p11.2

(Continued)

TABLE 19-4

Metabolic Disorders—cont'd

Disease	Enzyme or Protein	Locus
X-linked adrenoleukodystrophy	VLCFA transport (ALDP) ATP-binding cassette, subfamily D	Xq28
Amino Acid Disorders		
Phenylketonuria	Phenylalanine hydroxylase	12q24.1
Nonketotic hyperglycinemia	Glycine cleavage system	9p22
Homocystinuria	CBS	21q22.3
Urea cycle disorders	Five enzymes of the urea cycle	Multiple
Maple syrup urine disease	Branched-chain ketoacid dehydrogenase (four proteins)	19q13.1-q13.2, 6p22-p21
Propionic and methylmalonic acidemia	Propionyl-CoA carboxylase methylmalonyl-CoA mutase	13q, 3q21-q22, 6p21
Urea Cycle Disorders		
Carbamoyl phosphate deficiency	Carbamoyl phosphate synthetase	2q35
Ornithine transcarbamylase deficiency	Ornithine transcarbamylase	Xp21.1
Argininosuccinate synthetase deficiency	Argininosuccinate synthetase (citrullinemia)	9q34
Argininosuccinic aciduria	Arginosuccinate lyase (AL-argininosuccinase)	7cen-q11.2
Argininemia	Arginase deficiency	6q23
Miscellaneous		
Ceroid lipofuscinosis	CLN1 (infantile)	1p32
	CLN2 (late infantile)	11p15
	CLN3 (juvenile)	16p12
	CLN4 (adult)	Unknown
Leigh's syndrome		Many electron transport chain genes (most nuclear DNA), pyruvate carboxylase
Myoclonic epilepsy with ragged-red fibers		Mutations 8344, 8356 tRNA lysine
Mitochondrial encephalopathy with lactic acidosis and stroke-like episodes		Mutations 3243, 3271 tRNA leucine
Kearns-Sayre syndrome: progressive external ophthalmoplegia		Multiple mtDNA deletions and duplications
Leber's hereditary optic neuropathy		G11778A, 63460A, T14494C mutations
Leukodystrophies		
Adrenoleukodystrophy	Adrenoleukodystrophy protein	Xq28 (>400 mutations identified)
Alexander's disease	GFAP gene protein	17q21
Canavan's disease	Aspartoacylase	17p13-ter
Pelizaeus-Merzbacher	Proteolipid protein	Xq22 (approximately 40 mutations identified)

ALDP, adrenoleukodystrophy protein; ATP, adenosine triphosphate; CBS, cystathionine beta-synthase; CLN, neuronal ceroid lipofuscinosis; CoA, coenzyme A; GFAP, glial fibrillary acidic protein; IRD, infantile Refsum disease; mtDNA, mitochondrial DNA; NALD, neonatal adrenoleukodystrophy; tRNA, transfer RNA; VLCFA, very long-chain fatty acid.

TABLE 19-5

Neuromuscular Disorders

Disease	Gene	Locus
Duchenne muscular dystrophy	Dystrophin	Xp21
Becker muscular dystrophy	Dystrophin	Xp21
Emery-Dreifuss muscular dystrophy	Emerin	Xq28
Facioscapulohumeral	?	4q35-qter
Oculopharyngeal	?	14q11-q13
Myotonic	Myotonic protein kinase	19q13.2-13.3
Limb-Girdle		
Type 1A	?	5q22.3-q31.3
Type 1B	?	1q11-q21
Type 1C	Caveolin-3	3p25
Distal (Miyoshi)	Dysferlin	2p13
Congenital		
Merosin-negative	Erosin, α-2-laminin	6q2
Merosin-positive	?	?
Limb-Girdle		
Type 2A	Calpain 3	15q15.1-21.1
Type 2B	?	2p13
Type 2C	γ-Sarcoglycan	13q12
Type 2D	α-Sarcoglycan	17q21
Type 2E	β-Sarcoglycan	4q12
Type 2F	δ-Sarcoglycan	5q33-34
Type 2G	?	17q11-q12
Central core myopathy	Ryanodine receptor	19q13.1
Pompe's (type 1 glycogenoses)	Acid maltase	17q21-23
McArdle's (type 5 glycogenoses)	Myophosphorylase	11q13
Charcot-Marie-Tooth	PMP22 gene (duplication)	CMT1: 17p11.2
	Myclin protein 0 gene (point mutation)	1q22-33
	LITAF gene (point mutation)	16p12-13
	EGR2 gene (point mutation)	10q21-22
	Connexin 32 gene (>200 mutations)	CMTX: Xq13
	Five subtypes corresponding to five genes designated A, B, C, D, E	CMT2: 1p36, 3q13, 7p14

The muscular dystrophies used to be classified based on clinical phenotype through the pattern of inheritance. Duchenne muscular dystrophy and its counterpart Becker muscular dystrophy are X-linked recessive disorders associated with an abnormality in the dystrophin gene and protein. The incidence of Duchenne dystrophy is approximately 1:33,000 to 35,000 male births, and approximately one third of these cases arise as the result of a new mutation. An affected individual typically presents at birth and becomes symptomatic early in life with proximal muscle weakness, development of an inability to ambulate by the end of the first decade, and death usually by the end of the second or early third decades. Affected individuals often experience impaired motor development, abnormal gait, difficulty climbing stairs, and a classic Gower sign. On examination, these individuals often have enlarged calf, gluteal, vastus lateralis, deltoid, and infraspinatus muscles because of fibrofatty infiltration of the tissue. Myocardial involvement is relatively common, and patients may develop a dilated cardiomyopathy. Becker

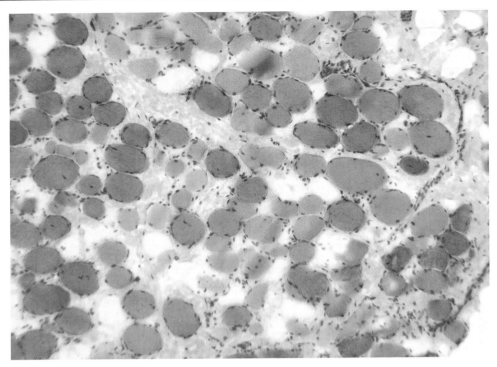

FIGURE 19-12
Hematoxylin and eosin–stained section of skeletal muscle in a 4-year-old boy with Duchenne muscular dystrophy. The biopsy is marked by some variation in muscle fiber size and increased fibrosis. (Original magnification, 100x.)

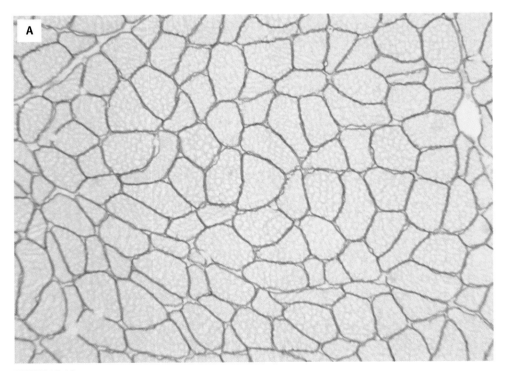

FIGURE 19-13
Immunohistochemical staining of a normal muscle **(A)** and muscle of Duchenne muscular dystrophy.

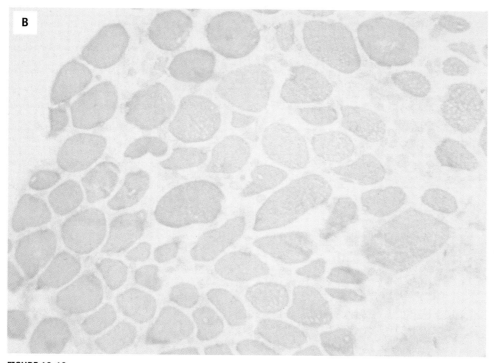

FIGURE 19-13
Cont'd, **(B)** with dystrophin (amino-terminus) antibody. (Original magnification, 200x.)

muscular dystrophy has an incidence of approximately 1:30,000 male births and typically presents later in life with proximal muscle weakness.

Morphologically, both processes are marked by a prominent variation in muscle fiber size, fibrofatty replacement of muscle tissue, muscle fiber splitting, and increased numbers of muscle fibers that contain centralized nuclei (Figure 19-12). Scattered degenerating and regenerating muscle fibers are often observed. Occasional foci of chronic inflammation are also noted.

Confirmation of the diagnosis rests in demonstrating abnormalities associated with the dystrophin protein gene. This can be done by a variety of methodologies. Most simply, antibodies are available that allow immunohistochemical or immunofluorescence evaluation for the dystrophin protein (Figure 19-13). Classically, in Duchenne dystrophy, there is an absence of dystrophin protein. Less commonly, dystrophin protein may be present but is nonfunctional. In contrast, Becker muscular dystrophy is characterized by a decreased amount of dystrophin or a partially inactive dystrophin protein. In addition, more definitive testing would involve western blot analysis or DNA deletion testing using multiplex PCR technology. In approximately 65% of patients with Duchenne or Becker muscular dystrophy, the underlying genetic defect results from deletion mutations clustered in two regions of the dystrophin gene. Testing

directed at these two regions yields the best results. Testing can also be used to help identify the carrier of the disease. Prenatal and carrier testing can also be performed using DNA analysis. The general approach to evaluating a suspected case is to begin with immunohistochemical or immunofluorescence evaluation for screening. This allows for a fairly quick answer if straightforward. In questionable cases, additional molecular-based testing can be done.

SUGGESTED READINGS

Vascular Disease

Joutel A, Vahedi K, Corpechot C, et al: Strong clustering and stereotyped nature of *NOTCH3* mutations in CADASIL patients. Lancet 1997;350:1511–1515.
Kalimo H, Rochoux MM, Viitanen M, et al: CADASIL: A common form of hereditary arteriopathy causing brain infarcts and dementia. Brain Pathol 2002;12:371–384.
Markus HS, Martin RJ, Simpson MA, et al: Diagnostic strategies in CADASIL. Neurology 2002;59:1134–1138.
Ruchoux MM, Maurage CL: CADASIL: Cerebral autosomal dominant arteriopathy with subcortical infarcts and leukoencephalopathy. J Neuropath Exp Neurol 1997;56:947–964.

Brain Tumors

Bello MJ, Leone PE, Vaquero J, et al: Allelic loss at 1p and 19q frequently occurs in association and may represent early oncogenic events in oligodendroglial tumors. Int J Cancer 1995;64:207–210.
Burger PC, Minn AY, Smith JS, et al: Losses of chromosomal arms 1p and 19q in the diagnosis of oligodendroglioma: A study of paraffin-embedded sections. Mod Pathol 2001;14:842–853.

Cai DX, Banerjee R, Scheithauer BW, et al: Chromosome 1p and 14q FISH analysis in clinicopathologic subsets of meningioma: Diagnostic and prognostic implications. J Neuropathol Exp Neurol 2001;60:628–636.

Cairncross JG, Ueki K, Zlatescu MC, et al: Specific genetic predictors of chemotherapeutic response and survival in patients with anaplastic oligodendrogliomas. J Natl Cancer Inst 1998;90:1473–1479.

Daston MM, Scrable H, Nordlund M, et al: The protein product of the neurofibromatosis type 1 gene is expressed at highest abundance in neurons, Schwann cells, and oligodendrocytes. Neuron 1992;8:415–428.

Eberhart CG, Kratz J, Wung Y, et al: Histopathological and molecular prognostic markers in medulloblastoma: C-myc, N-myc, TrkC, and anaplasia. J Neuropathol Exp Neurol 2004;63:441–449.

Grotzer MA, Janss AJ, Fung K, et al: TrkC expression predicts good clinical outcome in primitive neuroectodermal tumors. J Clin Oncol 2000;18:1027–1035.

Ino Y, Betensky RA, Zlatescu MC, et al: Molecular subtypes of anaplastic oligodendroglioma: Implications for patient management at diagnosis. Clin Cancer Res 2001;7:839–845.

Jaeckle KA, Ballman KV, Rao RD, et al: Current strategies in treatment of oligodendroglioma: Evaluation of molecular signatures of response. J Clin Oncol 2006;24:1246–1252.

Kelley TW, Tubbs, RR, Prayson RA: Molecular diagnostic techniques for the clinical evaluation of gliomas. Diagn Mol Pathol 2005;14:1–8.

Kleihues P, Cavenee WK: Tumours of the Nervous System. Lyon, France, IARC Press, 2000.

Kraus JA, Koopmann J, Kaskel P, et al: Shared allelic losses on chromosomes 1p and 9q suggest a common origin of oligodendroglioma and oligoastrocytoma. J Neuropathol Exp Neurol 1997;56:1098–1104.

Libermann TA, Nusbaum HR, Razon N, et al: Amplification, enhanced expression and possible rearrangement of EGF receptor gene in primary human brain tumours of glial origin. Nature 1985;313:144–147.

Libermann TA, Razon N, Baral AD, et al: Expression of epidermal growth factor receptors in human brain tumors. Cancer Res 1984;44:753–760.

Perry A, Fuller CE, Judkins AR, et al: INI1 expression is retained in composite rhabdoid tumors, including rhabdoid meningiomas. Mod Pathol 2005;18:951–958.

Prayson A, Castilla EA, Hartke M, et al: Chromosome 1p allelic loss by fluorescence in situ hybridization is not observed in dysembryoplastic neuroepithelial tumors. Am J Clin Pathol 2002;118:512–517.

Reardon DA, Rich JN, Friedman HS, et al: Recent advances in the treatment of malignant astrocytoma. J Clin Oncol 2006;24:1253–1265.

Reifenberger J, Reifenberger G, Liu L, et al: Molecular genetic analysis of oligodendroglial tumors shows preferential allelic deletions on 19q and 1p. Am J Pathol 1994;145:1175–1190.

Rorke LB, Packer RJ, Biegel JA: Central nervous system atypical teratoid (rhabdoid tumors of infancy and childhood): Definition of an entity. J Neurosurg 1996;85:56–65.

Shinojima N, Tada K, Shiraishi S, et al: Prognostic value of epidermal growth factor receptor in patients with glioblastoma multiforme. Cancer Res 2003;63:6962–6970.

Smith JS, Perry A, Borell TJ, et al: Molecular subtypes of anaplastic oligodendroglioma: Implications for patient management at diagnosis. Clin Cancer Res 2001;7:839–845.

Viskochil D, Buchberg AM, Xu G, et al: Deletions and a translocation interrupt a cloned gene at the neurofibromatosis type 1 locus. Cell 1990;62:187–192.

Infections

Budka H, Aguzzi A, Brown P, et al: Neuropathological diagnostic criteria for Creutzfeldt-Jakob disease (CJD) and other human spongiform encephalopathies (prion diseases). Brain Pathol 1995;5:459–466.

DeBiasi RL, Tyler KL: Polymerase chain reaction in the diagnosis and management of central nervous system infections. Arch Neurol 1999;56:1215–1219.

Figueroa ME, Rasheed S: Molecular pathology and diagnosis of infectious diseases. Am J Clin Pathol 1991;95:S8–S21.

Green AJE, Thompson EJ, Stewart GE: Use of 14-3-13 and other brain-specific proteins in CSF in the diagnosis of variant Creutzfeldt-Jakob disease. J Neurol Neurosurg Psych 2001;70:744–748.

Hsich G, Kenney K, Gibbs CJ, et al: The 14-3-3 brain protein in cerebrospinal fluid as a marker for transmissible spongiform encephalopathies. New Engl J Med 1996;335:924–930.

Jackson GS, Collinge J: The molecular pathology of CJD: Old and new variants. J Clin Pathol: Mol Pathol 2001;54:393–399.

Lemstra AW, van Meegan MT, Vreyling JP, et al: 14-3-3 testing in diagnosing Creutzfeldt-Jakob disease: A prospective study of 112 patients. Neurology 2000;55:514–416.

Naber SP: Molecular pathology: Diagnosis of infectious disease. New Engl J Med 1994;331:1212–1215.

Parchi P, Castellani R, Capellari S, et al: Molecular basis of phenotypic variability in sporadic Creutzfeldt-Jakob disease. Ann Neurol 1996;39:767–778.

Piccardo P, Dloughy SR, Lievens PMJ, et al: Phenotypic variability of Gerstmann-Straussler-Scheinker disease is associated with prion protein heterogeneity. J Neuropathol Exp Neurol 1998;57:979–988.

Prusiner SB: Shattuck Lecture: Neurodegenerative diseases and prions. New Engl J Med 2001;344:1516–1526.

Tompkins LS: The use of molecular methods in infectious diseases [review]. New Engl J Med 1992;327:1290–1297.

Versalovic J, Woods CR, Georghiou PR, et al: DNA-based identification and epidemiologic typing of bacterial pathogens. Arch Pathol Lab Med 1993;117:1088–1098.

Phakomatoses

Ball S, Arolker M, Purushotham AD: Breast cancer, Cowden disease and PTEN-MATCHS syndrome. Eur J Surg Oncol 2001;27:604–606.

Clifford SC, Maher ER: Von Hippel-Lindau disease: Clinical and molecular perspectives. Adv Cancer Res 2001;82:85–105.

Gareth D, Evans R, Sainio M, et al: Neurofibromatosis type 2. J Med Genet 2000;37:897–904.

Gutmann DH, Aylsworth A, Carey JC, et al: The diagnostic evaluation and multidisciplinary management of neurofibromatosis 1 and neurofibromatosis 2. JAMA 1997;278:51–57.

Hamilton SR, Liu B, Parsons RE, et al: The molecular basis of Turcot's syndrome. N Engl J Med 1995;332:839–847.

Kleihues P, Cavenee WK: Pathology and Genetics of Tumours of the Nervous System. Lyon, France. IARC Press, 2000, pp 216–241.

Louis DN, von Demling A: Hereditary tumor syndromes of the nervous system: Overview and rare syndromes. Brain Pathol 1995;5:145–151.

Narayanan V: Tuberous sclerosis complex: Genetics of pathogenesis. Pediatr Neurol 2003;29:404–409.

Varyley JM: Germline TP53 mutations and Li-Fraumeni syndrome. Hum Mutat 2003;21:313–320.

von Deimling A, Krone W, Menon AG: Neurofibromatosis type 1: Pathology, clinical features and molecular genetics. Brain Pathol 1995;5:153–162.

Neurodegenerative Disease

Blacker D, Tanzi RE: The genetics of Alzheimer disease: Current status and future prospects. Arch Neurol 1998;55:294–296.

Everett CM, Wood NW: Trinucleotide repeats and neurodegenerative disease. Brain 2004;127:2385–2405.

Gasser T: Advances in the genetics of movement disorders: Implications for molecular diagnosis. J Neurol 1997;244:341–348.

Ghetti B, Hutton ML, Wszolek ZK: Frontotemporal dementia and parkinsonism linked to chromosome 17 associated with Tau gene mutations (FTDP-17T). In Dickson DW (ed): Neurodegeneration: The Molecular Pathology of Dementia and Movement Disorders. Basel, ISN Neuropath Press, 2003, pp 86–102.

Hedreen JC, Roos RAC: Huntington's disease. In Dickson DW (ed): Neurodegeneration: The Molecular Pathology of Dementia and Movement Disorders. Basel, ISN Neuropath Press, 2003, pp 229–241.

Houlden H, Baker M, Adamson J, et al: Frequency of tau mutations in 3 series of non-AD degenerative dementias. Ann Neurol 1999;46:243–248.

Ince PG, Tomkins J, Slade JY, et al: Amyotrophic lateral sclerosis associated with genetic abnormalities in the gene encoding Cu/Zn superoxide dismutase: Molecular pathology of five new cases, and comparison with previous reports and 73 sporadic cases of ALS. J Neuropathol Exp Neurol 1998;57:895–904.

Kim TW, Tanzi RE: Presenilins and Alzheimer's disease. Current Opinion Neurobiol 1997;7:683–688.

Majoor-Krakauer D, Willems PJ, Hofman A: Genetic epidemiology of amyotrophic lateral sclerosis. Clin Genet 2003;63:83–101.

Mann DMA, McDonagh AN, Snowden J, et al: Molecular classification of the dementias. Lancet 2000;355:626.

Ogino S, Wilson RB: Genetic testing and risk assessment for spinal muscular atrophy (SMA). Hum Genet 2002;111:477–500.

Orrell RW, Figlewicz DA: Clinical implications of the genetics of ALS and other motor neuron diseases. Neurology 2001;57:9–17.

Polymeropoulos MH, Lavedan C, Leroy E, et al: Mutation in the α synuclein gene identified in families with Parkinson's disease. Science 1997;276:2045–2047.

Robitaille Y, Lopes-Cendes I, Becher M, et al: The neuropathology of CAG repeat diseases: Review and update of genetic and molecular features. Brain Pathol 1997;7:901–926.

Wilson RB: Frataxin and frataxin deficiency in Friedreich's ataxia. J Neurol Sci 2003;207:103–105.

Zabar Y, Kawas CH: Epidemiology and clinical genetics of Alzheimer's disease. In Clark CM, Trojanowski JQ (eds): Neurodegenerative Dementias: Clinical Features and Pathological Mechanisms. New York, McGraw-Hill, 2000, pp 79–94.

Metabolic Disease

Agamanolis DP: Disorders of amino acid metabolism. In Golden JA, Harding B (eds): Pathology and Genetics: Developmental Neuropathology. Basel, ISN Neuropath Press, 2004, pp 303–310.

Agamanolis DP: Metabolic and toxic disorders. In Prayson RA (ed): Neuropathology. Philadelphia, PA, Elsevier, 2005, pp 339–420.

Baumgartner MR, Saudubray JM: Peroxisomal disorders. Semin Neonat 2002;7:85–94.

Bernier FP, Boneh A, Dennett X, et al: Diagnostic criteria for respiratory chain disorders in adults and children. Neurology 2002;59:1406–1411.

DiMauro S: Lessons from mitochondrial DNA mutations. Semin Cell Dev Biol 2001;12:397–405.

Goebel HH, Sharp JD: The neuronal ceroid-lipofuscinoses: Recent advances. Brain Pathol 1998;8:151–162.

Goebel HH: The neuronal ceroid-lipofuscinoses. J Child Neurol 1995;10:424–437.

Gould SJ, Valle D: Peroxisome biogenesis disorders: Genetics and cell biology. Trends Genet 2000;16:340–345.

Gray RGF, Preece MA, Green SH, et al: Inborn errors of metabolism as a cause of neurological disease in adults: An approach to investigation. J Neurol Neurosurg Psych 2000;69:5–12.

Matalon R, Michals K, Kaul R: Canavan disease: From spongy degeneration to molecular analysis. J Ped 1995;127:511–517.

Messing A, Goldman JE, Johnson AB: Alexander disease: New insights from genetics. J Neuropathol Exp Neurol 2001;60:563–573.

Moser HW, Powers JM, Smith KD: Adrenoleukodystrophy: Molecular genetics, pathology and Lorenzo's oil. Brain Pathol 1995;5:259–266.

Seitelberger F: Neuropathology and genetics of Pelizaeus-Merzbacher disease. Brain Pathol 1995;5:267–273.

Smeitink J, van der Heuvel L, DiMauro S: The genetics and pathology of oxidative phosphorylation. Nat Rev 2001;2:342–352.

Neuromuscular Disorders

Bodensteiner JB: Congenital myopathies. Muscle Nerve 1994;17: 131–144.

Bornemann A, Goebel HH: Congenital myopathies. Brain Pathol 2001;11:206–217.

DiMauro S, Tsujino S, Shanske S, et al: Biochemistry and molecular genetics of human glycogenoses: An overview. Muscle Nerve 1995;18(Suppl 3): S10–S17.

Hoshino S, Ohkoshi N, Watanabe M, et al: Immunohistochemical staining of dystrophin-fixed paraffin-fixed embedded sections of Duchenne/Becker muscular dystrophy and manifesting carriers of Duchenne muscular dystrophy. Neuromusc Dis 2000;10:425–429.

Ionasescu VV: Charcot-Marie-Tooth neuropathies: From clinical description to molecular genetics. Muscle Nerve 1995;18:267–275.

Kubisch C, Wicklein EV, Jentsch TJ: Molecular diagnosis of McArdle's disease: Revised genomic structure of the myophosphorylase gene and identification of novel mutation. Hum Mutation 1998;12:27–32.

Mansfield ES, Robertson JM, Lebo RV, et al: Duchenne/Becker muscular dystrophy carrier detection using quantitative PCR and fluorescence-based strategies. Am J Med Genet (Neuropsych Genetics) 1993;48:200–208.

Matsuo M: Duchenne/Becker muscular dystrophy: From molecular diagnosis to gene therapy. Brain Dev 1996;18:167–172.

Multicenter Study Group: Diagnosis of Duchenne and Becker muscular dystrophies by polymerase chain reaction: A multicenter study. JAMA 1992;267:2609–2615.

Prayson RA: Muscle and peripheral nerve pathology. In Silverberg SG, DeLellis RA, Frable WJ, et al (eds): Principles and Practice of Surgical Pathology and Cytopathology, 4th ed. Philadelphia, PA, Churchill Livingstone, 2006, pp 2213–2265.

Raben N, Nichols RC, Boerkoel C, et al: Genetic defects in patients with glycogenosis type II (acid maltase deficiency). Muscle Nerve 1995;18(Suppl 3):S70–S74.

Tsujino S, Shanske S, DiMauro S: Molecular genetic heterogeneity of myophosphorylase deficiency (McArdle's disease). N Engl J Med 1993;329:241–245.

Vallat JM, Tazir M, Magdelaine C, et al: Autosomal-recessive Charcot-Marie-Tooth diseases. J Neuropathol Exp Neurol 2005;64:363–370.

20 Molecular Pathology of the Cardiovascular System

Carmela D. Tan • E. Rene Rodriguez

INTRODUCTION

In this chapter, we present a summary of the diseases of the cardiovascular system for which molecular genetic defects have been documented in humans. It is clear at this time that genetic defects have been found in genes that encode or regulate proteins present practically in all cellular compartments of the cardiac myocyte. These compartments include sarcolemmal (membrane) proteins, cytoskeletal proteins, contractile myofilaments, proteins that regulate contraction, proteins involved in mechanical transduction, ion channels, nuclear membrane proteins, energy metabolism, and mitochondrial proteins. Defects in extracellular matrix proteins are also devastating to the cardiovascular system.

The impact of these defects is noticeable from development through adulthood and senility. In some cases, genetic defects affect cardiac development of the very young. But in other instances, the effects of a single mutation may become manifest early in life or adolescence in one member of the family but in another member of the same family it will not produce disease until adulthood. This clearly indicates that there potentially are modifying genes that influence the expression of a given phenotype.

In an ideal environment, a patient with cardiovascular disease could be assessed comprehensively based on clinical and genetic evaluation. In this situation, one could address the phenotype of the individual and correlate this with clinical course and outcome. This information could also provide an assessment of the patient's relative risk of serious cardiovascular events. In this manner, the appropriate lifestyle changes, along with pharmacologic or surgical interventions, could be instituted at a stage at which the worse pathology is avoided and when it prevents devastating and more costly consequences.

In the following sections, we present current knowledge of molecular genetic defects found in diseases that affect the cardiac muscle and the vascular tree, as well as some defects known to occur during development that produce congenital heart malformations. Little was known at the time of this writing about single nucleotide polymorphisms (SNPs) affecting cardiovascular development and disease states; therefore, SNPs are not discussed in the chapter. Lastly, we address some of the most common viral agents that produce heart disease, because these are also targets for molecular diagnostics.

CARDIOMYOPATHIES

The traditional descriptive and functional classification of cardiomyopathies has been challenged in recent years as the genetic basis of several "idiopathic" cardiomyopathies has been discovered. An updated classification emphasizing etiopathogenesis was proposed recently in a scientific statement issued by the American Heart Association. This classification introduces the ion channelopathies (see the next section) as a primary cardiomyopathy and takes into consideration the novel achievements in molecular cardiology. The genetic causes of cardiomyopathy can be divided into mutations of genes encoding sarcomeric proteins, structural–cytoskeletal proteins, cell junction proteins, and energy-producing proteins.

HYPERTROPHIC CARDIOMYOPATHY

Hypertrophic cardiomyopathy (HCM) is characterized by impaired left ventricular filling and reduced ventricular compliance with or without left ventricular outflow tract obstruction. This is because of a marked increase in left ventricular mass with often asymmetric thickening of the interventricular septum. The histologic hallmark of this disorder is myocyte and myofibrillar disarray, often accompanied by interstitial fibrosis and, well known but often forgotten, small intramural coronary artery dysplasia. The prevalence of HCM is about 1:500. It is the most common cause of sudden death in young individuals and athletes in the United States. Clinical presentation is variable, with complaints of exertional dyspnea, chest pain, and heart failure symptoms. Other patients are relatively asymptomatic with normal life expectancy. The disease is inherited as an autosomal dominant trait with age-dependent penetrance.

HCM is genetically heterogeneous with most mutations found in genes that encode sarcomeric proteins (Table 20-1). As the basic contractile unit of striated muscles, the sarcomere is organized into distinct domains where thick and thin filaments interact (Figure 20-1). The thick filament is predominantly made of myosin heavy chain, myosin binding protein C, and myosin essential and regulatory light chains. The thin filament is composed of actin, the heterotrimer troponin, and tropomyosin (Figure 20-2). The sarcomeres are delineated by the Z-discs, which anchor the thin filaments and cytoskeletal proteins. The major component of the Z-disc is α-actinin-2, which is arranged in homodimers that provide organizational structure for the insertion of actin, titin,

TABLE 20-1
Molecular Genetics of the Hypertrophic Cardiomyopathy Phenotype

Gene	Description	Chromosome Locus	Exons	Amino Acids
Myofilaments				
MYH7	β-Myosin heavy chain	14q11.2	40	1935
MYBPC3	Cardiac myosin-binding protein C	11p11.2	35	1274
MYL2	Ventricular regulatory myosin light chain	12q23-q24.3	7	166
MYL3	Ventricular essential myosin light chain	3p21.3-p21.2	7	195
TNNT2	Cardiac troponin T	1q32	16	295
TNNI3	Cardiac troponin I	19p13.4	8	210
TNNC1	Cardiac troponin C	3p	6	161
TPM1	α-Tropomyosin	15q22.1	10	284
ACTC	α-Cardiac actin	15q14	6	377
MYH6	α-Myosin heavy chain	14q11.2-q12	39	1939
Z-Disc				
TTN	Titin	2q24.3	363	26,926
ACTN2	α-Actinin 2	1q42-q43	21	894
CSRP3	Muscle LIM protein	11p15.1	6	194
TCAP	Telethonin	17q12-q21.1	2	167
LDB3	LIM domain-binding 3 (also known as ZASP, or Z-band alternatively spliced protein)	10q22.2-q23.3	16	727
Costamere				
VCL	Vinculin	10q22.1-q23	22	1066*
Calcium Homeostasis				
PLN	Phospholamban	6q22.1	2	52
Glycogen Storage Diseases				
PRKAG2	γ2 Regulatory subunit of adenosine monophosphate–activated protein kinase	7q36.1	16	569
LAMP2	Lysosome-associated membrane protein 2	Xq24	9	410
Lysosomal Storage Disorder				
GLA	α-Galactosidase A	Xq22.1	7	429

* A variant called metavinculin has an additional exon in the 3′ coding region and is a longer isoform of vinculin expressed in cardiac muscle.

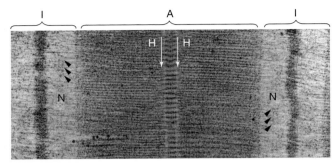

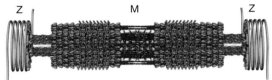

FIGURE 20-1

The sarcomere. The upper panel shows a transmission electron micrograph of a human cardiac sarcomere. The boundaries of the sarcomere are the two Z-discs, which are dark and electron dense. On each side of the Z-discs, an area of electron-lucent material with fine filaments runs perpendicular to the Z-disc. These represent actin filaments, which insert into the Z-disc. The area that encompasses a Z-disc and the adjacent electron-lucent area of actin filaments from two sarcomeres is designated the I band. In the middle of this electron-lucent actin-rich area, some subtle electron-dense streaks run parallel to the Z-disc and are named the N-disc. In this area, some proteins interact with titin, actin, and α-actinin. The midportion of the sarcomere comprises the A band. Within the A band, several areas have specific patterns of electron density. A middle line, or M band, bisects the A band. Adjacent to the M band, two lighter electron-lucent areas are designated the H band. The M band corresponds to the insertion site of the tails of the thick filaments into a matrix of proteins that keeps them organized and in register. Within the M band, a subtle electron-dense core of proteins corresponds to myomesin and other proteins that anchor the thick filaments. The larger dark areas that flank the M and H bands are the actual rows of thick filaments. In the middle third of these areas, some vertical striations correspond to electron-dense myosin binding protein C.

The lower portion of the figure shows a simplified illustration of the sarcomere. The M band shows the tails of the thick filaments interacting with a light brown lattice of myomesin molecules. The thick filaments extend from the M band, with the heads (green) protruding away from the axis of the filament. Myosin binding protein C is visible as small blue subunits that cover about one third of the length of the thick filament. The thin filaments (red) are made of several proteins (Figure 20-2).

The yellow coils shown at the level of the Z-disc represent intermediate filaments of desmin, which connect adjacent myofibrils to each other and to the sarcolemma.

nebulette, and other proteins (Figure 20-3). α-Actinin-2 cross-links actin and titin from adjacent sarcomeres. Titin is a giant protein that spans half a sarcomere (approximately 1 μm) from the Z-disc to the M band. Sometimes referred to as the third myofilament, titin has elastic properties responsible for generating passive tension and maintaining the central position of the thick filament in the sarcomere. It also acts as a binding site for several other sarcomeric proteins. The Z-disc is also believed to function in signal transduction and has been proposed as the site of the cardiac stretch receptor. Some Z-disc-associated

proteins involved in sensing mechanical stretch include muscle LIM protein (MLP) and T-cap or telethonin (Figure 20-3). Telethonin also binds the potassium channel subunit minK, suggesting a role in the regulation of ion channels through a mechanoelectric feedback loop.

Z-discs of neighboring sarcomeres are connected and held in parallel alignment by the intermediate filament desmin. Desmin also links Z-discs to the sarcolemma through the costamere and to the nuclear envelope. Costameres are circumferential, vinculin-rich, rib-like bands representing sites of myofibril–sarcolemma association. Costameres are multiprotein complexes that serve as transmitters of contractile force to the sarcolemma and extracellular matrix. Metavinculin, an isoform of vinculin, is a membrane-associated protein localized to the costameres, intercalated discs, and T tubules. It anchors actin filaments and has a role in the maintenance of the myocyte architecture.

The molecular pathogenesis of sarcomeric gene mutations is incompletely understood. Studies of animal models indicate that cardiac hypertrophy probably occurs from dominant-negative effects of mutant myofilament proteins. However, functional studies of mutant proteins have shown both increased and decreased protein activity. Hearts of mice deficient in MLP develop severe cardiomyopathy. Ultrastructural examination demonstrated more dispersed and misaligned Z-discs, and T-cap dislocation was evident on immunohistochemical staining. In addition to providing structural and mechanical stability of the sarcomere, Z-discs are important binding sites for transcription factors, calcium signaling proteins, kinases, and phosphatases. This indicates a broader role for Z-disc proteins in intracellular signaling cascades that lead to myocardial hypertrophy and heart failure. Although mutations in different sarcomeric genes with different in vitro functional effects can result in a clinical hypertrophic phenotype, it is even more perplexing that mutations in the same sarcomeric gene can produce different phenotypes, e.g., mutations in actin have been detected in both cardiomyopathy (hypertrophic and dilated phenotypes) and skeletal myopathy (nemaline and actin myopathies).

The diagnosis of HCM is usually made on echocardiography in a patient with unexplained cardiac hypertrophy. Rarely, the diagnosis is based on confirmation of an HCM-associated gene in patients who do not fulfill the clinical diagnostic criteria. About 50% to 70% of index cases will have a detectable mutation in one of the sarcomeric genes. Mutations are more often present in younger patients than in the elderly group. The most commonly involved genes are β-myosin heavy chain (MHY7) and myosin binding protein C (MYBPC3), which account for 30% to 50%

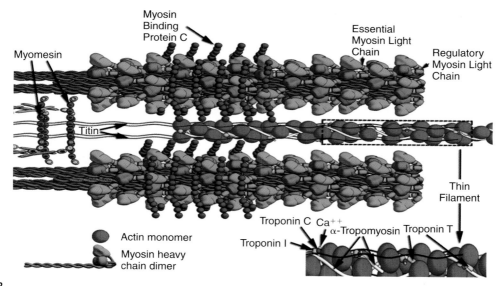

FIGURE 20-2

The thick and thin filaments. Myosin (lower left corner) is the monomer that forms the thick filament. Myosin heavy chains form a duplex through their rod domains. They have a "hinge" region, which bends, and at the end of this hinge region is the myosin head, which interacts with actin. The light chains of myosin (regulatory [pink] and essential [orange] chains) are located near the hinge region. The thick filament is made of multiple dimers of myosin (lower left corner), which are organized by overlapping helically around the long axis of the filament. The most medial portion of the thick filament consists mainly of the rod portion of multiple dimers, which "insert" in the lattice formed by myomesin and other molecules in the M band (dark orange). Myosin binding protein C is represented by the blue spherical monomers. Between the thick filaments, one thin filament (red) is illustrated. This is composed of monomers of actin (red spheres) and a helical coil of α-tropomyosin. The troponins (I, C, and T) form clusters spaced along the course of the α-tropomyosin. Running parallel to the thick and thin filaments is a giant protein appropriately named titin, which spans half a sarcomere (about 1 μm). This protein is believed to play a role in sensing stretch.

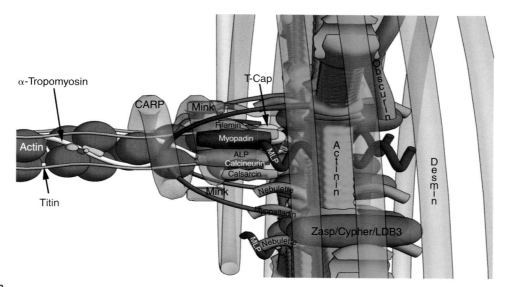

FIGURE 20-3

Thin filament at the Z-disc. This region of the sarcomere is a rather sophisticated structure that serves mechanical and regulatory functions. It also allows the organization of six thin filaments around one thick filament. Multiple proteins are present at the Z-disc. T-cap is a capping protein present at the end of the titin molecules. Filamin is the capping protein at the end of the thin filament. CARP extends away from the Z-disc and, along with nebulette and filamin, may form the visible N-disc seen on electron microscopy. Other proteins present here include α-actinin-associated LIM protein, calcineurin, calsarcin, minK, myopadin, myopalladin, muscle LIM protein, and ZASP/Cypher/LDB3. Some of these proteins are thought to form part of the cardiac stretch-sensing mechanism, which may, in turn, mediate signal transduction to adapt to hypertrophic stimuli. The core of the organization of the Z-disc is α-actinin. Many proteins identified in the Z-disc are thought to interact with α-actinin. Mutations in several of these proteins have been described in patients with dilated and hypertrophic cardiomyopathies.

of genotyped patients; thin filament and Z-disc protein mutations are much less common, comprising approximately 5% and 4%, respectively. Mutations in MHY7 are almost always a missense mutation, with 70% located in the globular head and neck region of the protein. On the other hand, mutations in MYBPC3 are predominantly nonsense mutations distributed along the entire gene. Patients with myofilament gene mutations present at a younger age with greater extent of hypertrophy than those who are genotype negative. Mutations have also been associated with distinct septal morphology based on contour and location and extent of hypertrophy. Reverse septal curvature is associated with mutations in myofilament proteins, sigmoidal septal curvature with Z-disc proteins, and apical septal hypertrophy with cardiac actin. Recently, a mutation in the promoter region of phospholamban (PLN) gene, has been reported in a family with a benign form of apical HCM. Phospholamban is a key regulator of sarcoplasmic reticulum calcium cycling. Muscle relaxation is initiated by sequestration of calcium from the cytosol into the sarcoplasmic reticulum, mediated by the sarcoplasmic reticulum Ca^{2+}-ATPase (SERCA2a) pump. Phospholamban reversibly inhibits SERCA2a. An increase in activity of phospholamban is associated with HCM and a decrease in activity with dilated cardiomyopathy (DCM).

The concept of malignant versus benign HCM mutations is controversial. In a cohort of 389 patients with HCM, sequencing results revealed no significant differences in age at diagnosis, degree of hypertrophy, or family history of sudden death between cases with or without mutations in myofilament genes. Moreover, most mutations were private, and previously implicated malignant and benign mutations were found to be rare (2.8%) in this cohort of unrelated individuals. In addition, 3% of patients were found to carry two different mutations, either in two different genes or in the same gene, and were associated with a more severe form of disease. The conclusions that can be drawn from several studies support the necessity of performing entire gene sequencing of at least the eight most commonly involved genes (MYH7, MYBPC3, TNNT2, TNNI3, TPM1, MYL2, MYL3, and ACTC) in the diagnosis of HCM. Sequence analysis of these genes is commercially available as clinical tests. Genetic testing is also suggested for screening family members who may carry an identified mutation in the index case for the purpose of appropriate clinical follow-up and recommendations for participation in recreational physical activities and sports. At present, prognostication and risk stratification based on identified disease-causing mutation must be practiced with caution.

In patients with HCM who do not show mutations in myofilament and Z-disc genes, other differential diagnoses can be considered, such as adult-onset glycogen storage diseases and a cardiac variant of Fabry's disease. A subset of familial HCM patients have conduction abnormalities, particularly progressive atrioventricular block, Wolff-Parkinson-White (WPW) syndrome, and atrial fibrillation, which have been attributed to mutations in the genes encoding the γ2 regulatory subunit of adenosine monophosphate–activated protein kinase (PRKAG2) and lysosome-associated membrane protein 2 (LAMP2). Adenosine monophosphate–activated protein kinase (AMPK) functions in the regulation of gene expression, ion channel gating kinetics, and key metabolic pathways, including glucose metabolism. Mutations in PRKAG2 cause constitutive activation of AMPK associated with increased glycogen content of skeletal muscle cells in animal models. Affected patients develop severe cardiac hypertrophy with supraventricular tachyarrhythmias and progressive atrioventricular block that necessitate aggressive control of arrhythmias and pacemaker insertion. The histopathology of PRKAG2 mutations shows glycogen accumulation in myocytes without myocyte disarray. Mutations in LAMP2 are responsible for Danon disease, an X-linked dominant lysosomal glycogen storage disease characterized by a triad of HCM, skeletal myopathy, and mental retardation. Skeletal myopathy is mild in most cases and can easily be overlooked. WPW syndrome is present in 35% of cases, and mental retardation is seen in 70%. A DCM phenotype is sometimes observed. Affected males are usually symptomatic before the age of 20, with generally poor prognosis; female carriers develop cardiomyopathy later in adulthood. Pathologic analysis of muscle tissue shows autophagic vacuoles containing glycogen. Skeletal muscle testing, including measurement of serum creatine kinase levels and evaluation for WPW syndrome, can aid in the identification of these patients. Clinical testing is available for direct gene sequencing of PRKAG2 and LAMP2. A cardiac variant of Fabry's disease has recently been recognized to present as late-onset, unexplained left ventricular hypertrophy in adult males and female carriers of this X-linked lysosomal storage disorder. A decreased α-galactosidase A enzyme activity in blood or cultured cells in males is diagnostic, but this assay is unreliable for testing female carriers. Genetic analysis of the α-galactosidase A gene serves as a confirmatory test for males and a better screening test for suspected female carriers.

DILATED CARDIOMYOPATHY

DCM is the most common clinical phenotype of heart muscle disease, characterized by systolic dysfunction and dilated ventricles. DCM affects 36.5 per 100,000 individuals in the United States. The histologic features of DCM are nonspecific and consist of myocardial hypertrophy and degeneration with variable amounts of interstitial fibrosis. Heart failure as a sequelae of myocarditis (viral, giant cell myocarditis, sarcoidosis), toxin-induced injury (alcohol, drugs), infiltrative diseases (hemochromatosis, glycogen storage disease), and autoimmune processes often acquires a dilated phenotype. Most DCM patients, however, do not have a readily identifiable cause of cardiac dysfunction and fall into the idiopathic category. About a third of the idiopathic group are considered familial, with autosomal dominant mode of inheritance being the most common. Autosomal recessive, X-linked, and mitochondrial transmission are also seen in a few pedigrees.

The genes involved in DCM include not only the sarcomeric proteins but also intermediate filaments, nuclear membrane and cytoskeletal proteins, phospholamban, and ion channel proteins (Table 20-2). Most of these susceptibility genes were originally implicated in HCM. Variation in phenotypic expression and penetrance of these single gene defects underscores the complex pathogenesis of cardiomyopathy. For instance, mutations in troponin I have been discovered in patients with HCM, restrictive cardiomyopathy, and autosomal recessive DCM. Even if the protein structure is known, it is difficult to predict the functional consequence and phenotype from the position and type of mutation. Correlation between genotype and phenotype is further complicated by the effects of other modifier genes and environmental influences on the phenotypic expression of disease among carriers of the same gene mutation.

Numerous pathogenetic mechanisms have been proposed to explain the functional deficits in DCM in relation to the mutant proteins. Mutations in the myofilament proteins are believed to result in impaired force generation by the sarcomere through disruption of actin–myosin interaction or change in myofilament calcium-binding affinity. Alteration in intracellular calcium homeostasis mediated by mutations that lead to increased activity or expression of phospholamban is associated with depressed cardiac contractility. Mechanical stress induced by volume or pressure overload is known to activate several signal transduction pathways that direct myocyte hypertrophy and survival. Mutations in titin and other Z-disc proteins (believed to be responsible for mechanical stretch sensing) often lead to impaired interaction between the protein components of this complex; this, in turn, can affect Z-disc formation, decrease stretch-regulated response and muscle cell signaling, and activate cell death pathways, leading to progressive heart failure.

Force generated by the sarcomere must be effectively transmitted within and between myocytes and to the extracellular matrix. This is accomplished through the complex network of cytoskeletal proteins, membrane-associated proteins, and intercalated disc proteins. Desmin, the predominant intermediate filament in cardiac muscle, forms an elaborate cytoskeleton by surrounding the Z-discs and interconnecting them to one another and to the cytoplasmic organelles, sarcolemma, and nuclear envelope. Desmin is also increased in the intercalated disc, particularly in the desmosomes. Desmin-related myopathy in humans presents a wide phenotypic spectrum of neuromuscular derangement with or without cardiac involvement. A subgroup of pure cardiac phenotype in the absence of myopathy has been described that includes DCM and restrictive cardiomyopathy with atrioventricular block. Structural studies show accumulation of electron-dense granulofilamentous aggregates in the cytoplasm, which is detected best by transmission electron microscopy and immunoelectron microscopy. These electron-dense bodies contain desmin, αB-crystallin, and other proteins. Most of these disorders are caused by mutations in desmin, but some are associated with mutations in αB-crystallin. αB-crystallin is a molecular chaperone and a member of the small heat-shock protein family. It is colocalized with desmin and associates with titin at the I-band region. It stabilizes desmin by preventing aggregation and protects the cell in general by assisting in normal protein folding and restoring proteins to their native conformation after exposure to heat, ischemia reperfusion, or other conditions of cellular stress. Mutations in the desmin gene are proposed to result in loss of desmin function, accumulation of insoluble toxic aggregates, and Z-disc disorganization that lead to myocyte degeneration. Transgenic mice expressing mutant αB-crystallin also show accumulation of misfolded proteins and αB-crystallin in cardiomyocytes.

A second type of intermediate filaments is involved in familial DCM. The lamin proteins (A, B, C) are intermediate filaments located in the nuclear lamina, a filamentous structure associated with the inner nuclear membrane. The nuclear lamina maintains the nuclear shape and structure and plays a role in transcriptional regulation, nuclear pore positioning and function, and heterochromatin organization. It binds to the chromatin, several nuclear envelope proteins, and transcription factors. The lamin A/C gene, LMNA, encodes two isoforms, lamin A and C, produced by alternative splicing. Lamin A and C are expressed exclusively in differentiated cells. Mutations in LMNA are associated with a range of clinical phenotypes, mostly affecting skeletal and cardiac muscle, peripheral nervous tissue, adipose tissue, and bone. Cardiac involvement is manifested as DCM often complicated by conduction system disease and variable skeletal myopathy. Mutations in lamin A and C are thought to result in increased

TABLE 20-2

Molecular Genetics of the Dilated Cardiomyopathy Phenotype

Gene	Description	Chromosome Locus	Exons	Amino Acids
AUTOSOMAL DOMINANT				
Myofilament Proteins				
MYH7	β-Myosin heavy chain	14q11.2	40	1935
MYH6	α-Myosin heavy chain	14q11.2-q12	39	1939
MYBPC3	Cardiac myosin-binding protein C	11p11.2	35	1274
ACTC	α-Cardiac actin	15q14	6	377
TNNT2	Cardiac troponin T	1q32	16	295
TNNI3	Cardiac troponin I	19p13.4	8	210
TNNC1	Cardiac troponin C	3p	6	161
TPM1	α-Tropomyosin	15q22.1	10	284
Z-Disc-Associated Proteins				
TTN	Titin	2q24.3	363	26,926
ACTN2	α-Actinin 2	1q42-q43	21	894
CSRP3	Muscle LIM protein	11p15.1	6	194
TCAP	Telethonin	17q12-q21.1	2	167
LDB3	LIM domain-binding 3 (also known as ZASP, or Z-band alternatively spliced protein)	10q22.2-q23.3	16	727
Membrane-Associated Protein				
VCL	vinculin	10q22.1-q23	22	1066*
Intermediate Filaments				
DES	Desmin	2q35	9	470
LMNA	Lamin A/C	1q21	12	664/572**
Chaperone Protein				
CRYAB	αB-Crystallin	11q22.3-q23.1	3	175
Dystrophin-Associated Protein Complex Components				
SGCB	β-Sarcoglycan	4q12	6	318
SGCD	δ-Sarcoglycan	5q33	9	290
DTNA	α-Dystrobrevin	18q12.1-q12.2	21	743
Calcium Regulatory Protein				
PLN	Phospholamban	6q22.1	2	52
Nuclear Protein				
TPMO	Thymopoietin/lamina-associated polypeptide 2	12q22	8	694
Ion Channel Proteins				
SCN5A	Voltage-gated sodium channel	3p21-24	28	2015
ABCC9	SUR2A regulatory subunit of Kir6.2, an inwardly rectifying cardiac K_{ATP} channel	12p12.1	38	1549
AUTOSOMAL RECESSIVE				
TNNI3	Cardiac troponin I	19p13.4	8	210
X-LINKED DOMINANT				
LAMP2	Lysosome-associated membrane protein 2	Xq24	9	410

TABLE 20-2

Molecular Genetics of the Dilated Cardiomyopathy Phenotype—cont'd

Gene	Description	Chromosome Locus	Exons	Amino Acids
X-LINKED RECESSIVE				
DMD	Dystrophin	Xp21	79	3685
TAZ/G4.5	Taffazin	Xq28	11	292
EMD/STA	Emerin	Xq28	6	254
XK	Putative membrane transport protein XK	Xp21.2-p21.1	3	444

* A variant called metavinculin has an additional exon in the 3′ coding region and is a longer isoform.
** Lamin A (664 amino acids) and C (572 amino acids) are produced by alternative splicing in exon 10.

fragility and decreased mechanical stiffness of the nuclear envelope. Structural changes observed are fractures with leakage of lamins and chromatin into the cytoplasm, nuclear membrane blebs, and nuclear pore clustering. Interestingly, disruption of desmin attachment at the nuclear–cytoskeletal interface and disorganization of the desmin filament network was evident in LMNA knockout mice. A novel mechanism of defective force transmission in DCM is put forth because of the loss of nuclear anchoring with altered cytoskeletal tension. In addition to its mechanical function, effects on chromosomal organization, gene regulation, and transcription may be expected. Recently, a mutation in another inner nuclear membrane protein called lamina-associated polypeptide 2 has been reported in a family with DCM and shown to exhibit decreased binding to lamin in vitro. Mutations in lamin-binding proteins may cause functional defects similar to those caused by lamin mutation by altering lamin's interaction with other proteins. LMNA mutation appears to be one of the more common causes of familial DCM, the other being the β-MHC gene, with an estimated prevalence of 0.5% to 5% of all DCM patients. More importantly, carriers had a reported worse prognosis and higher risk of sudden death, probably related to tachyarrhythmias. Supraventricular arrhythmia, conduction disease, and skeletal muscle involvement are clinical predictors of mutations in LMNA. Conduction system defects are progressive, with half of the patients dying suddenly before heart failure becomes overt. Sequence analysis of the entire coding region is available as a clinical test in some centers.

The dystrophin-associated protein complex (DAPC) (Figure 20-4) is located in the sarcoplasmic membrane, where it links the cytoskeleton to the extracellular matrix, maintains structural and functional integrity of the sarcolemma during contraction and relaxation,

and transmits force generated in the sarcomeres to the extracellular matrix. This multifunctional complex is also involved in cell survival signaling cascades through its interactions with calmodulin, Grb2, and neuronal nitric oxide synthase. In skeletal and cardiac muscle cells, the DAPC is concentrated over costameres. DAPC consists of three multiprotein components—dystroglycan, sarcoglycan, and cytoplasmic complexes. The dystroglycans (α and β) are transmembrane proteins that interact with laminin-2 in the extracellular matrix and bind to dystrophin on the cytoplasmic side of the sarcolemma. The sarcoglycan complex is composed of transmembrane proteins α-, β-, γ-, and δ-sarcoglycan and sarcospan. The cytoplasmic components consist of syntrophins, α-dystrobrevin, and dystrophin. Dystrobrevin binds to dystrophin and intermediate filament proteins syncoilin and desmuslin or synemin, which in turn bind to desmin. Dystrobrevin and dystrophin together anchor four syntrophin molecules, which bind to several other proteins, including neuronal nitric oxide synthase. Dystrophin also binds directly to actin, and through its association with dystroglycan, a link between the cytoskeleton and the extracellular matrix is formed. Mutations in the various proteins of the DAPC are known to cause several types of muscular dystrophy and account for a small number of familial DCMs. Mutation in one of the DAPC components often results in less stable protein complexes, which are reduced in number within the sarcolemma. The plasma membrane becomes fragile and leaky with increased susceptibility to contraction-induced damage.

The dystrophinopathies are caused by mutations in the Duchenne muscular dystrophy (DMD) gene, which encodes dystrophin. A spectrum of clinically manifested diseases includes asymptomatic patients with increased serum creatine phosphokinase and myoglobulinuria, isolated myopathy, DMD, Becker

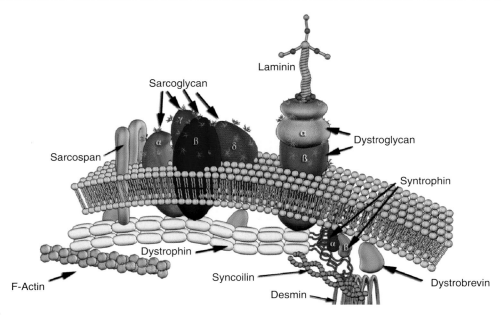

FIGURE 20-4

Dystrophin-associated protein complex (DAPC). Multiple proteins form a scaffold that links the cellular cytoskeleton to the extracellular matrix. This large multimeric complex is composed of transmembrane proteins (dystroglycans, sarcoglycans, and sarcospan) and the intracellular component of dystrobrevin and syntrophin, which interacts with the carboxyl-terminal domain of dystrophin. In the sarcoplasmic domain, the amino-terminus of dystrophin binds to F-actin. The intermediate filaments of the sarcoplasm (desmin) also interact with DAPC. Dystroglycan has two subunits. One traverses the sarcolemma (β-subunit), and the other subunit (α) works as a receptor for laminin-2 in the extracellular space. The sarcoglycans are glycosylated transmembrane proteins, which may play a role in stabilizing the DAPC.

muscular dystrophy (BMD), and X-linked DCM without significant skeletal muscle symptoms. In DMD, subclinical and clinical cardiac involvement affects 90% of patients detected through electrocardiography and echocardiography, but overt heart failure occurs in only 10% to 20% of cases. Fibrofatty replacement of the myocardium with initial selective posterobasal scarring progressively involves the lateral free wall of the left ventricle. Respiratory complications are the most common cause of death in DMD patients. On the other hand, BMD has a later-onset muscular weakness and an estimated 50% incidence of cardiac involvement that progresses to DCM. The right ventricle is also noted to be more often involved. Cardiomyopathy and arrhythmias are the most common causes of death in BMD. X-linked DCM is a rapidly progressive cardiomyopathy that affects adolescent or young male patients. Most patients die within 2 years after presentation. Female carriers of mutations in DMD gene are also at risk of developing DCM, although DCM manifests much later and sometimes with milder symptoms and slower progression. Poor genotype–phenotype correlation of cardiac involvement in the dystrophinopathies reflects the complexity of the dystrophin gene in its organization and regulation of expression in cardiac and skeletal muscles. The dystrophin gene is the largest gene found in humans, spanning about 1.5% of the X chromosome. It has 79 exons and eight promoters. Multiple isoforms are generated through alternative splicing and combination with specific tissue promoters. Molecular genetic testing of the DMD gene is performed for establishing diagnosis of probands, carrier testing in females, and prenatal diagnosis. About 60% of mutations in the DMD gene are deletions of one exon or more; in another 5% to 10%, gross duplications are responsible for the disease. These mutations can be detected by multiplex polymerase chain reaction (PCR), Southern blot analysis, or fluorescence in situ hybridization (FISH). The remaining one third of cases have small deletions, insertions, or point mutations that require mutation scanning through denaturing gradient gel electrophoresis or rapid and thorough sequence analysis by single condition amplification or the internal primer method.

Dystrophin is one of at least five genes encoding proteins of diverse functions that have been identified in familial DCM with X-linked inheritance pattern (Table 20-2). X-linked DCM is often associated with skeletal muscle involvement and accounts for approximately 5% to 10% of familial DCM. Sequence analysis of these genes, except XK, is clinically available.

Emery-Dreifuss muscular dystrophy (EDMD) is characterized by slowly progressive weakness and

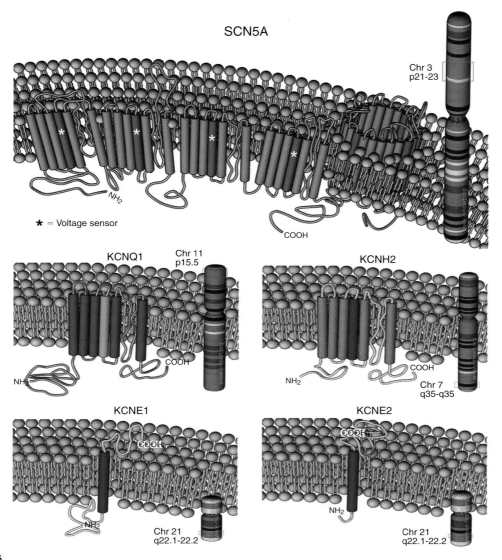

FIGURE 20-6

The cardiac ion channels. The three-dimensional structure of the ion channels and the chromosomal location of the gene encoding them are shown. The sodium channel encoded by the SCN5A gene is a large protein with four sets of six transmembrane domains. Each of the sets has a specific domain that acts as a voltage sensor (*). The sarcoplasmic loops act as gates to the movement of ions. The potassium channels are encoded as smaller α-subunits of six transmembrane domains (KCNQ1 and KCNH2) and accessory β-subunits (KCNE1 and KCNE2). These subunits form multimers, which in turn become organized as cylindric channels through the sarcolemma, with a central opening for ions to pass through.

potassium channel pore-forming α-subunit protein with six transmembrane segments. The β-subunit protein called minK-related peptide 1 encoded by KCNE2 coassembles with KCNH2. MinK-related peptide 1 mutations have been implicated in drug-associated LQTS. Mutations in yet another potassium channel gene, KCNJ2, which encodes the Kir2.1 protein, are correlated with Andersen-Tawil syndrome (ATS) or LQT7. ATS is a rare autosomal dominant disorder characterized by periodic paralysis, cardiac arrhythmias, and dysmorphic features affecting craniofacial and limb development. Confirmation of clinical diagnosis of ATS requires analysis of the entire coding sequence.

Approximately 60% of ATS individuals have a pathogenic KCNJ2 mutation.

Mutations in the sodium and calcium channels result in a gain-of-function abnormality because of impaired channel inactivation leading to persistent inward current. The cardiac sodium channel gene, SCN5A, encodes for the pore-forming protein subunit with four homologous domains, each of which has six transmembrane segments. Unlike potassium channels which have accessory β-subunits, a single α-subunit serves as the functioning unit of sodium channels. A defective cardiac calcium channel encoded by CACNA1 is linked with LQT8 or

TABLE 20-4
Molecular Genetics of Inherited Arrhythmogenic Syndromes

Gene	Description*	Chromosome Locus	Clinical Syndrome	Exons	Amino Acids
Long QT Syndrome, Autosomal Dominant (Romano-Ward Syndrome)					
KCNQ1 (KVLQT1)	I_{ks} potassium channel α-subunit	11p15.5	LQT1	19	676
KCNH2 (HERG)	I_{kr} potassium channel α-subunit	7q35-36	LQT2	16	1159
SCN5A	Voltage-gated sodium channel	3p21	LQT3	28	2015
ANK2	Ankyrin B	4q25-27	LQT4	46	3957
KCNE1 (MinK)	I_{ks} potassium channel β-subunit	21q22.1-22.2	LQT5	3	129
KCNE2 (MiRP1)	I_{kr} potassium channel β-subunit	21q22.1-q22.2	LQT6	3	123
KCNJ2 (Kir2.1)	I_{k1} potassium channel α-subunit	17q23.1-q24.2	LQT7 (Andersen-Tawil syndrome)	2	427
CACNA1	Calcium channel α-subunit	12p13.3	LQT8 (Timothy syndrome)	50	2138
Long QT Syndrome, Autosomal Recessive (Jervell-Lange-Nielsen Syndrome)					
KCNQ1 (KVLQT1)	I_{ks} potassium channel α-subunit	11p15.5	JLN1	19	676
KCNE1 (MinK)	I_{ks} potassium channel β-subunit	21q22.1-q22.2	JLN2	3	129
Catecholaminergic Polymorphic Ventricular Tachycardia					
RyR2	Ryanodine receptor	1q42-q43	CPVT1, autosomal dominant	105	4967
CASQ2	Calsequestrin	1p13.3-p11	CPVT2, autosomal recessive	11	399
SCN5A	Voltage-gated sodium channel	3p21	Brugada syndrome	28	2015
Short QT Syndrome					
KCNH2 (HERG)	I_{kr} potassium channel α-subunit	7q35-q36	SQT1	16	1159
KCNQ1 (KVLQT1)	I_{ks} potassium channel α-subunit	11p15.5	SQT2	19	676
KCNJ2 (Kir2.1)	I_{k1} potassium channel α-subunit	17q23.1-q24.2	SQT3	2	427
Progressive Cardiac Conduction Disease					
SCN5A	Voltage-gated sodium channel	3p21	PCCD	28	2015
Idiopathic Ventricular Fibrillation					
SCN5A	Voltage-gated sodium channel	3p21	VF	28	2015
Familial Atrial Fibrillation					
KCNQ1 (KVLQT1)	I_{ks} potassium channel α-subunit	11p15.5	ATFB1	19	676
KCNE2 (MiRP1)	I_{kr} potassium channel β-subunit	21q22.1-q22.2	ATFB1	3	123
Sick Sinus Syndrome					
SCN5A	Voltage-gated sodium channel	3p21	SSS1, autosomal recessive	28	2015
HCN4	I_f hyperpolarization-activated cation channel	15q24-q25	SSS2, autosomal dominant	8	1203

*I_{kr}, rapidly activating delayed rectifier outward potassium current; I_{ks}, slowly activating delayed rectifier outward potassium current; I_{k1}, rectifier inward potassium current; I_f, pacemaker current.

Timothy syndrome. This syndrome is characterized by multiorgan dysfunction including lethal arrhythmias, congenital heart disease (CHD), syndactyly, immune deficiency, intermittent hypoglycemia, cognitive abnormalities, and autism. Mutations in CACNA1 appear to arise de novo; thus, the inheritance pattern is usually sporadic. Genetic testing for Timothy syndrome is by targeted mutation analysis for known exon 8 mutations of CACNA1.

Loss-of-function mutation in ANK2 was described in a large family with type 4 LQTS for which the prolonged QT interval is associated with sinus bradycardia and atrial fibrillation. ANK2 encodes for ankyrin-B, a structural protein responsible for the proper expression and membrane localization of ion channels and transporters. It interacts with membrane-associated transporters and ion channels, including sodium–potassium adenosine triphosphatase, sodium/calcium exchanger, anion exchanger, and voltage-gated sodium channels. It also interacts with calcium-release channels of the T-tubule–sarcoplasmic reticulum membrane in the cardiac myocytes, including inositol 1,4,5-triphosphate receptor and RyR. The phenotype of patients harboring mutations in the ANK2 gene has been expanded to include sick sinus syndrome, idiopathic ventricular fibrillation, catecholaminergic polymorphic ventricular tachycardia (CPVT), and sudden death.

Mutations in the ion channel proteins account for 50% to 75% of patients with inherited LQTS. Clinical correlation and molecular analysis of LQTS gene mutations imply that the electrocardiographic repolarization pattern, time to first cardiac event, triggers for arrhythmic events, and frequency of lethal events might be genotype specific. Arrhythmic events in LQT1 are usually related to exercise. Auditory stimuli may also elicit syncopal episodes in patients with LQT2, and cardiac events during sleep most commonly occur in LQT3. Most LQT1 patients become symptomatic before the age of 10, but LQT2 and LQT3 patients remain at risk of experiencing onset of cardiac events later in life. The rate of lethal events is highest in LQT3 patients. Genotype–phenotype correlation studies can provide guidance to a gene-specific approach to therapy by identifying the triggers associated with high risk for cardiac arrhythmic events and optimal response to medical therapy with beta-blockers.

The diagnosis of LQTS is usually made using clinical history, family history, and electrocardiogram (ECG) findings based on established criteria that generate a clinical score of low, intermediate, or high probability of having LQTS. However, clinical diagnostic criteria have only 38% sensitivity in identifying carriers of mutated gene. In addition, borderline cases with inconclusive clinical scores may need genetic testing to establish the diagnosis, stratify risks, and make therapeutic decisions. Because of the variable expression and reduced penetrance of LQTS, genetic testing of family members of a proband may be warranted. Up to half of gene carriers are asymptomatic, and 4% to 5% of gene carriers experience sudden death as the sentinel episode. Genetic testing for LQTS requires analysis of the entire coding regions and intronic splice junction sites for the five most commonly involved channel-encoding genes. A negative genetic test in a patient with phenotypically definite LQTS should not rule out the diagnosis because the mutation is unknown in approximately 25% of patients. In patients with atypical presentation and negative genetic testing for classic LQTS, other differential diagnosis should be considered, e.g., catecholaminergic polymorphic tachycardia, ATS, and ARVD.

CATECHOLAMINERGIC POLYMORPHIC VENTRICULAR TACHYCARDIA

CPVT is a malignant syndrome that manifests at an early age with poor clinical outcome. More than half of patients experience their first episode of syncope or cardiac arrest by age 20. When left untreated, the cumulative mortality rate reaches 30% to 50% by age 35. Similar to LQT1 and ARVD, CPVT can be precipitated by exercise, stress, or emotions.

Autosomal dominant mutations in the cardiac RyR2 gene have been identified in patients with CPVT. RyR2 is a tetrameric channel that regulates the release of stored calcium ions from the sarcoplasmic reticulum. It is a large protein that interacts with other proteins, including junctin, triadin, calmodulin, FK-506-binding proteins, protein kinases, phosphatases, and calsequestrin, to form a macromolecular complex. A second gene involved in the recessive form of the syndrome is the CASQ-encoded calsequestrin 2, which is a calcium-binding protein that serves as the major calcium reservoir within the sarcoplasmic reticulum of cardiac myocytes. Calsequestrin is anchored to the RyR2 complex by triadin and junctin, where it is speculated to participate in RyR2 gating. Abnormal calcium ion leak into the cytosol through defective RyR2 receptors, decreased calcium binding by CASQ2, or disrupted interactions of CASQ2 with RyR2 complex lead to increased intracellular calcium and delayed afterdepolarizations that trigger CPVT.

Heterozygous RyR2 mutation is identified in approximately 50% and homozygous CASQ2 mutation in 1% to 2% of probands by genetic screening. The risk of cardiac event at a young age has been shown to be higher in males with RyR2 mutations. Clinical testing is available in a few research-oriented laboratories by mutation scanning followed by sequence analysis of abnormal fragments. This method, however, will not be able to detect large intragenic deletions and exon skipping.

BRUGADA SYNDROME

Brugada syndrome is characterized by right bundle branch block, ST elevation in the right precordial leads (V1 to 3), ventricular arrhythmia, and increased risk of sudden death. The syndrome is transmitted with an autosomal dominant pattern with marked male predominance. Usually, it presents in the fourth decade of life with sudden cardiac death caused by ventricular fibrillation or with syncope caused by polymorphic ventricular tachycardia.

Genetic heterogeneity is suggested in this disorder because only 20% of patients with Brugada syndrome have been shown to harbor loss-of-function mutations in the sodium channel gene SCN5A (Figure 20-6). The missense mutations in Brugada syndrome tend to cluster around the linker between the third and the fourth domains and the carboxyl-terminus, which are important regions critical to inactivation of the channel. Premature termination of the mutant protein, altered processing with retention in the endoplasmic reticulum, and altered gating kinetics explain the phenotypic expression of this syndrome. Interestingly, fever is a known precipitant of ventricular arrhythmic episodes with certain Brugada syndrome–associated sodium channel mutations. Silent gene carriers are identified by using class I sodium channel blockers to unmask characteristic ECG changes; however, it is unknown if a positive test is associated with increased risk of sudden death. Multivariate analysis had identified a history of syncope and the inducibility of a sustained ventricular arrhythmia during electrophysiologic study as predictors of future sudden death or ventricular fibrillation.

Sudden unexpected death during sleep in previously healthy young Asian men, also known as sudden unexpected nocturnal death syndrome (SUNDS), appears to exhibit a characteristic Brugada ECG pattern. In Southeast Asia, this is known by several names, including *bangungut* in the Philippines, *non-laitai* in Laos, *lai-tai* in Thailand, and *pokkuri* in Japan. Mutations in SCN5A have been found in a proportion of probands, suggesting that SUNDS may be a similar phenotype to Brugada syndrome usually diagnosed in individuals of European descent.

SHORT QT SYNDROME

Short QT syndrome is a familial electric disease characterized by short QT interval, episodes of syncope, paroxysmal atrial fibrillation, and risk of lethal arrhythmia. Severity of disease is variable and can range from being asymptomatic to experiencing palpitations, dizziness, recurrent syncope, and sudden death in infancy. Autosomal dominant inheritance was suggested. Gain-of-function mutations in the three potassium ion channels involved in repolarization have been identified—KCNH2 (HERG), KCNQ1 (KVLQT1), and KCNJ2 (Kir2.1). Extensive genotype–phenotype correlation data are not available. However, genetic screening may hold promise of risk stratification and appropriate pharmacologic approach with antiarrhythmics that block the HERG channel, causing QT prolongation in this clinically and genotypically heterogeneous disease.

HERITABLE DISORDERS OF THE BLOOD VESSELS

Heritable disorders that affect major arteries present as life-threatening conditions with aortic dissection, arterial aneurysm, and rupture. Identification of individuals predisposed to these catastrophic events is important for prophylactic intervention. Ascending aortic aneurysms are clinically distinct from descending thoracic and abdominal aortic aneurysms. Cystic medial degeneration is often found in ascending aortic aneurysms of several heritable disorders. These disorders include Marfan syndrome (MFS), vascular Ehlers-Danlos syndrome (EDS), nonsyndromic familial aortic dissection and aneurysm, and bicuspid aortic valve (BAV).

Mutant connective tissue matrix proteins are thought to alter the structure and integrity of the extracellular matrix by exerting a dominant-negative effect that structurally weakens the vascular wall. In addition to providing structural support to cells and tissues, matrix macromolecules are also now known to act as repository for storage and release of growth factors such as TGF-β, bone morphogenetic proteins, fibroblast growth factors, and insulin-like growth factors. By regulating growth factor bioavailability, the extracellular matrices act as temporal and spatial modulators of signaling events involved in morphogenesis and tissue homeostasis and repair.

MARFAN SYNDROME

The prototype of the heritable connective tissue disorder is MFS. It presents as an autosomal dominant trait with variable manifestations in the ocular, skeletal, and cardiovascular systems. It affects 1 in every 5000 live births with variable penetrance. Clinical diagnosis is based on a set of criteria known as the *Ghent nosology*. Affected individuals have bilateral ectopia lentis, tall stature, long slender limbs,

In summary, although many molecular defects have been found to produce pathology in the cardiovascular system, this is, for pathologists, a new and exciting field virtually unexplored. The value of the traditional observation of the pathology in medical biopsies and surgical specimens synergizes with the molecular diagnostics to provide better service to our patients, better understanding of the pathophysiology of cardiovascular diseases, and continued advancement of science.

SUGGESTED READINGS

Cardiomyopathies

Arbustini E, Diegoli M, Fasani R, et al: Mitochondrial DNA mutations and mitochondrial abnormalities in dilated cardiomyopathy. Am J Pathol 1998;153:1501–1510.

Gerull B, Heuser A, Wichter T, et al: Mutations in the desmosomal protein plakophilin-2 are common in arrhythmogenic right ventricular cardiomyopathy. Nat Genet 2004;36:1162–1164.

Knoll R, Hoshijima M, Hoffman HM, et al: The cardiac mechanical stretch sensor machinery involves a Z disc complex that is defective in a subset of human dilated cardiomyopathy. Cell 2005;111:943–955.

Maron BJ, Towbin JA, Thiene G, et al: Contemporary definitions and classification of the cardiomyopathies: An American Heart Association Scientific Statement from the Council on Clinical Cardiology, Heart Failure and Transplantation Committee; Quality of Care and Outcomes Research and Functional Genomics and Translational Biology Interdisciplinary Working Groups; and Council on Epidemiology and Prevention. Circulation 2006;113:1807–1816.

Richard P, Charron P, Carrier L, et al: Hypertrophic cardiomyopathy: Distribution of disease genes, spectrum of mutations, and implications for a molecular diagnosis strategy. Circulation 2003;107:2227–2232.

Richard P, Villard E, Charron P, et al: The genetic bases of cardiomyopathies. J Am Coll Cardiol 2006;48:A79–A89.

Sim KG, Hammond J, Wilcken B: Strategies for the diagnosis of mitochondrial fatty acid β-oxidation disorders. Clin Chim Acta 2002;323:37–58.

Tan CD, Ratliff NB, Young JB, et al: Nonischemic Cardiomyopathies. In Topol EJ (ed): Textbook of Cardiovascular Medicine. Philadelphia, PA, Lippincott Williams & Wilkins, 2007, pp 1406–1427.

Taylor MR, Fain PR, Sinagra G, et al: Natural history of dilated cardiomyopathy due to lamin A/C gene mutations. J Am Coll Cardiol 2003;41:771–780.

Van Driest SL, Vasile VC, Ommen SR, et al: Myosin binding protein C mutations and compound heterozygosity in hypertrophic cardiomyopathy. J Am Coll Cardiol 2004;44:1903–1910.

Villard E, Duboscq-Bidot L, Charron P, et al: Mutation screening in dilated cardiomyopathy: Prominent role of the β-myosin heavy chain gene. Eur Heart J 2005;26:794–803.

Inherited Arrhythmogenic Syndromes

Bellocq C, van Ginneken AC, Bezzina CR, et al: Mutation in the KCNQ1 gene leading to the short QT-interval syndrome. Circulation 2004;109:2394–2397.

Grant AO: Electrophysiological basis and genetics of Brugada syndrome. J Cardiovasc Electrophysiol 2005;16(Suppl 1):S3–S7.

Mohler PJ, Splawski I, Napolitano C, et al: A cardiac arrhythmia syndrome caused by loss of ankyrin-B function. Proc Natl Acad Sci USA 2004;101:9137–9142.

Plaster NM, Tawil R, Tristani-Firouzi M, et al: Mutations in Kir2.1 cause the developmental and episodic electrical phenotypes of Andersen's syndrome. Cell 2001;105:511–519.

Sarkozy A, Brugada P: Sudden cardiac death and inherited arrhythmia syndromes. J Cardiovasc Electrophysiol 2005;16(Suppl 1):S8–20.

Schwartz PJ, Priori SG, Spazzolini C, et al: Genotype–phenotype correlation in the long-QT syndrome: Gene-specific triggers for life-threatening arrhythmias. Circulation 2001;103:89–95.

Splawski I, Timothy KW, Sharpe LM, et al: Ca(V)1.2 calcium channel dysfunction causes a multisystem disorder including arrhythmia and autism. Cell 2004;119:19–31.

Tester DJ, Arya P, Will M, et al: Genotypic heterogeneity and phenotypic mimicry among unrelated patients referred for catecholaminergic polymorphic ventricular tachycardia genetic testing. Heart Rhythm 2006;3:800–805.

Tester DJ, Will ML, Haglund CM, et al: Compendium of cardiac channel mutations in 541 consecutive unrelated patients referred for long QT syndrome genetic testing. Heart Rhythm 2005;2:507–517.

Vatta M, Dumaine R, Varghese G, et al: Genetic and biophysical basis of sudden unexplained nocturnal death syndrome (SUNDS), a disease allelic to Brugada syndrome. Hum Mol Genet 2002;11:337–345.

Zareba W, Moss AJ, Schwartz PJ, et al: Influence of genotype on the clinical course of the long-QT syndrome: International Long-QT Syndrome Registry Research Group. N Engl J Med 1998;339:960–965.

Heritable Disorders of Blood Vessels

Garg V, Muth AN, Ransom JF, et al: Mutations in NOTCH1 cause aortic valve disease. Nature 2005;437:270–274.

Guo DC, Hasham S, Kuang SQ, et al: Familial thoracic aortic aneurysms and dissections: Genetic heterogeneity with a major locus mapping to 5q13-14. Circulation 2001;103:2461–2468.

Guo DC, Pannu H, Tran-Fudulo V, et al: Mutations in smooth muscle alpha-actin (ACTA2) lead to thoracic aortic aneurysms and dissections. Nat Genet 2007;39:1488–1493.

Hahn RT, Roman MJ, Mogtader AH, et al: Association of aortic dilation with regurgitant, stenotic and functionally normal bicuspid aortic valves. J Am Coll Cardiol 1992;19:283–288.

Loeys BL, Schwarze U, Holm T, et al: Aneurysm syndromes caused by mutations in the TGF-βreceptor. N Engl J Med 2006;355:788–798.

Pannu H, Fadulu VT, Chang J, et al: Mutations in transforming growth factor-βreceptor type II cause familial thoracic aortic aneurysms and dissections. Circulation 2005;112:513–520.

Pepin M, Schwarze U, Superti-Furga A, et al: Clinical and genetic features of Ehlers-Danlos syndrome type IV, the vascular type. N Engl J Med 2000;342:673–680.

Robinson PN, Arteaga-Solis E, Baldock C, et al: The molecular genetics of Marfan syndrome and related disorders. J Med Genet 2006;43:769–787.

Vaughan CJ, Casey M, He J, et al: Identification of a chromosome 11q23.2-q24 locus for familial aortic aneurysm disease, a genetically heterogeneous disorder. Circulation 2001;103:2469–2475.

Zhu L, Vranckx R, Khau Van KP, et al: Mutations in myosin heavy chain 11 cause a syndrome associating thoracic aortic aneurysm/aortic dissection and patent ductus arteriosus. Nat Genet 2006;38:343–349.

Congenital Heart Diseases

Baldini A: Dissecting contiguous gene defects: Tbx1. Curr Opin Genet Dev 2005;15:279–284.

Basson CT, Bachinsky DR, Lin RC, et al: Mutations in human TBX5 [corrected] cause limb and cardiac malformation in Holt-Oram syndrome. Nat Genet 1997;15:30–35.

Clark KL, Yutzey KE, Benson DW: Transcription factors and congenital heart defects. Annu Rev Physiol 2006;68:97–121.

Garg V, Kathiriya IS, Barnes R, et al: GATA4 mutations cause human congenital heart defects and reveal an interaction with TBX5. Nature 2003;424:443–447.

Gelb BD, Tartaglia M: Noonan syndrome and related disorders: Dysregulated Ras-mitogen activated protein kinase signal transduction. Hum Mol Genet 2006;15(Spec 2):R220–R226.

Metcalfe K, Rucka AK, Smoot L, et al: Elastin: Mutational spectrum in supravalvular aortic stenosis. Eur J Hum Genet 2000;8:955–963.

Sarkozy A, Conti E, Seripa D, et al: Correlation between PTPN11 gene mutations and congenital heart defects in Noonan and LEOPARD syndromes. J Med Genet 2003;40:704–708.

Satoda M, Zhao F, Diaz GA, et al: Mutations in TFAP2B cause Char syndrome, a familial form of patent ductus arteriosus. Nat Genet 2000;25:42–46.

Schott JJ, Benson DW, Basson CT, et al: Congenital heart disease caused by mutations in the transcription factor NKX2-5. Science 1998;281:108–111.

Ware SM, Peng J, Zhu L, et al: Identification and functional analysis of ZIC3 mutations in heterotaxy and related congenital heart defects. Am J Hum Genet 2004;74:93–105.

Warthen DM, Moore EC, Kamath BM, et al: Jagged 1 (JAG1) mutations in Alagille syndrome: Increasing the mutation detection rate. Hum Mutat 2006;27:436–443.

Yagi H, Furutani Y, Hamada H, et al: Role of Tbx1 in human del22q11.2 syndrome. Lancet 2003;362:1366–1373.

Viral Myocarditis

Baboonian C, Treasure T: Meta-analysis of the association of enteroviruses with human heart disease. Heart 1997;78:539–543.

Calabrese F, Rigo E, Milanesi O, et al: Molecular diagnosis of myocarditis and dilated cardiomyopathy in children: Clinicopathologic features and prognostic implications. Diagn Mol Pathol 2002;11:212–221.

Calabrese F, Thiene G: Myocarditis and inflammatory cardiomyopathy: Microbiological and molecular biological aspects. Cardiovasc Res 2003;60:11–25.

Feldman AM, McNamara D: Myocarditis. N Engl J Med 2003;343:1388–1398.

Fujioka S, Kitaura Y, Ukimura A, et al: Evaluation of viral infection in the myocardium of patients with idiopathic dilated cardiomyopathy. J Am Coll Cardiol 2000;36:1920–1926.

Kuhl U, Pauschinger M, Noutsias M, et al: High prevalence of viral genomes and multiple viral infections in the myocardium of adults with "idiopathic" left ventricular dysfunction. Circulation 2005;111:887–893.

Pauschinger M, Kallwellis-Opara A: Frontiers in viral diagnostics. Ernst Schering Res Found Workshop 2006;55:39–54.

21 Molecular Pulmonary Pathology

Samuel Yousem · Sanja Dacic

INTRODUCTION

Recent advances in molecular biology have improved our understanding of the biology and etiology of neoplastic and non-neoplastic lung diseases, resulting in the development of novel molecular approaches for detection, diagnosis, and prognosis. Two major areas of molecular testing in pulmonary pathology include lung neoplasia and infectious diseases. Although our understanding of the pathogenesis of interstitial lung diseases has improved in recent years, no diagnostic or prognostic clinical molecular testing is available at this time. Some brief examples of current clinical applicators are given later, followed by more detailed discussion of selected topics outlined in Table 21-1.

In the current era of promising adjuvant and targeted therapies, an early diagnosis of lung cancer and prediction of a prognosis could be improved by information on genetic characteristics of the tumors. The backbone of clinical molecular testing is polymerase chain reaction (PCR) manipulation of nucleic acids. PCR provides rapid and reliable identification of various nucleic acid sequences, including mutations and polymorphisms. Mutations often occur in cancer, causing the molecular alterations that are reflected in chromosomal or nucleotide sequence abnormalities. For example, the discovery of mutations of the tyrosine kinase (TK) domain of the epidermal growth factor receptor (EGFR) in lung adenocarcinomas and their prediction of patients' sensitivity to tyrosine kinase inhibitors (TKIs) has resulted in an enormous amount of clinical interest. In addition, it seems that amplification of the EGFR gene may influence sensitivity to TKI therapy. Therefore, many laboratories are testing EGFR gene status in lung adenocarcinomas by fluorescence in situ hybridization (FISH) for amplification and by PCR direct sequencing for mutations. The main advantage of these techniques is that they can be performed on formalin-fixed, paraffin-embedded tissue at relatively low cost.

Necrotizing and non-necrotizing granulomas are common in lung specimens, but the etiology cannot always be determined with certainty based on morphology alone. Until recently, the diagnosis of mycobacterial infections depended on insensitive Ziehl-Neelsen stains and slow, labor-intensive microbiologic cultures. Several sensitive and specific PCR-based techniques have definitely improved and accelerated the diagnosis and treatment of mycobacterial infections, especially using formalin-fixed, paraffin-embedded material when fresh tissue has not been sent for cultures and in cases with atypical histology. Several simple and standardized commercial kits are used in the routine microbiology laboratory, but in molecular anatomic pathology "home-brew" PCR tests on paraffin-embedded tissue are available and may offer a less costly alternative.

In immunocompromised individuals, including transplant recipients and AIDS patients, cytomegalovirus (CMV) is an important pathogen. The most important diagnostic challenge with CMV infection is to distinguish latent or low-level persistent infection from clinically significant reactivation. Several types of amplification assays are available for CMV detection and quantitation, including reverse transcriptase–PCR (RT-PCR), branched-chain amplification, and nucleic acid sequence–based amplification (NASBA). The application of molecular testing to determine viral load, which is usually done on peripheral blood but can be done on tissue or cytology, is important because viral load can be correlated with disease versus latency. In contrast to CMV, Epstein-Barr virus (EBV) infection is most often diagnosed on a tissue sample. Chromogenic in situ hybridization (CISH) and FISH have been used for localization of EBV DNA sequences. The FISH technique has also been applied to visualization of specific viral RNAs within the nuclei of cells latently infected with EBV. Each of these applications in infectious diseases and molecular assays is discussed in more detail in other chapters of this book.

The distinction between benign reactive mesothelial cells and malignant mesothelial cells is a common and difficult diagnostic problem in pulmonary pathology and cytology (Table 21-1). Unfortunately, no generally accepted immunohistochemical or molecular

TABLE 21-1
Pulmonary Molecular Diagnostics Examples

Lung Cancer

EGFR status in adenocarcinoma
- EGFR gene amplification → FISH
- EGFR gene mutations → DNA sequencing

Infections

Mycobacterium tuberculosis and other mycobacteria
- PCR-based commercial and "home-brew" assays

CMV
- RT-PCR
- NASBA and branched-chain amplification

EBV
- FISH
- CISH or silver in situ hybridization

Lymphangioleiomyomatosis

TSC1 and TSC2 gene mutations

Mesothelioma

FISH for p16/CDKN2A gene deletions

LUNG CANCER

PATHOBIOLOGY AND PATHOGENESIS

Based on current knowledge, lung cancers carry multiple genetic and epigenetic alterations, indicating inactivation of tumor suppressor genes and activation of oncogenes that can be correlated with the sequential morphologic changes during the multistep carcinogenesis. The carcinogenesis sequence for non-small-cell lung carcinoma, particularly squamous cell carcinoma, has been relatively well defined (Figure 21-1). Sequential molecular changes have been defined on microdissected target tissues using methods such as loss of heterozygosity (LOH), comparative genomic hybridization (CGH), and FISH. It has been shown that squamous metaplasia may progress to dysplasia and subsequently to carcinoma in situ and invasive carcinoma. Early events include LOH at 3p and 9p in squamous metaplasia and dysplasia, followed by p53 and mutations in carcinoma in situ. It has been demonstrated that the frequency of 3p allelic losses increases progressively along the preinvasive–invasive progression model of lung carcinogenesis, suggesting that multiple tumor suppressor genes may be located on 3p. In contrast to squamous cell carcinoma, relatively little is known about the development of other histologic types of lung carcinoma. Atypical adenomatous hyperplasia, which is detectable on high-resolution computed tomography (CT) scan, is considered the preinvasive lesion of the nonmucinous type of bronchioloalveolar carcinoma and invasive adenocarcinoma. It is believed that K-ras mutations and LOH at chromosomes 3p and 9p represent early events in lung adenocarcinoma carcinogenesis, followed by LOH at 17p, mutations of p53, and telomerase activation in invasive adenocarcinoma (Figure 21-2). No characteristic morphologic precursor lesion has been

markers distinguish between these two diagnostic possibilities. Homozygous deletions of p16/CDKN2A have often been reported in mesothelioma. Recent studies have shown that dual-color FISH for p16/CDKN2A and chromosome 9 centromere has the potential to become an ancillary diagnostic test in the cytologic diagnosis of malignant mesothelioma. A commercial kit for p16/CDKN2A FISH analysis (LSI p16/CEP9 Dual Color Probe, Abbott Molecular) is available, and the efficacy and accuracy of this approach can be further validated on larger series of patients with suspicious cytology.

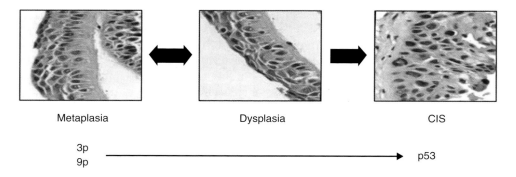

Metaplasia   Dysplasia   CIS

3p
9p ────────────────────────────────────→ p53

FIGURE 21-1

Sequential morphologic and molecular abnormalities in the multistep development of squamous cell carcinoma of the lung. Squamous metaplasia may progress to dysplasia and subsequently to carcinoma in situ (CIS) and invasive squamous cell carcinoma. Loss of heterozygosity at 3p and 9p in squamous metaplasia and dysplasia is followed by p53 and mutations in CIS.

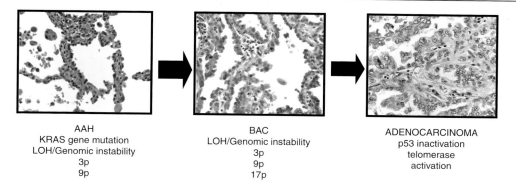

AAH
KRAS gene mutation
LOH/Genomic instability
3p
9p

BAC
LOH/Genomic instability
3p
9p
17p

ADENOCARCINOMA
p53 inactivation
telomerase
activation

FIGURE 21-2

Sequential morphologic and molecular abnormalities in the multistep development of adenocarcinoma of the lung. Atypical adenomatous hyperplasia (AAH) is considered the precursor lesion of the nonmucinous type of bronchioloalveolar carcinoma (BAC), which may progress into invasive adenocarcinoma. K-ras mutations and loss of heterozygosity (LOH) at 3p and 9p are early events detectable in AAH, and LOH at 17p, p53 mutations, and telomerase activations are seen in invasive adenocarcinoma.

defined for small-cell lung carcinoma. Recent studies suggest that these tumors may arise directly from molecularly abnormal, but morphologically normal, hyperplastic or dysplastic respiratory epithelium or reserve cells with neuroendocrine differentiation embedded in such epithelia.

PROGNOSTIC AND PREDICTIVE MARKERS

As briefly introduced earlier, the development of small-molecule inhibitors of EGFR has resulted in many studies trying to define characteristics and mechanistic principles of EGFR action in lung carcinoma that would predict an individual patient's clinical response to treatment. It is clear from the experience with targeted therapy for breast cancer that new, standardized assay procedures for assessing and predicting the effects of therapeutic agents must be developed. Following the breast cancer model with the Her2/neu oncogene, the status of the EGFR has been explored by immunohistochemistry and FISH. Although in general a good correlation exists between EGFR protein expression as determined by immunohistochemistry and gene amplification as determined by FISH, these methods have not been completely able to predict patient responses to EGFR inhibitors. In addition, the impact of EGFR status on patient survival as assessed by these two methods is controversial. Recently, Lynch et al. identified specific mutations in the EGFR gene, which better correlated with clinical responsiveness to the TKI gefitinib. These deletions, insertions, and missense point mutations are mostly limited to exons 18 to 21 of the TK domain of EGFR (Figure 21-3). The most common are in-frame deletions in exon 19 (44%), followed by missense point mutations at L858R in exon 21 (41%). The mutations cause conformational changes of the receptor, which result in

increased gene activation and TKI sensitivity. Because of this discovery, some academic and commercial molecular pathology laboratories have introduced PCR-based DNA mutational analysis of exons 18 to 21 of the TK domain of the EGFR gene in their clinical practice, using fresh, frozen, or formalin-fixed, paraffin-embedded tissue. In studies, it has been suggested that EGFR mutations were somewhat limited to lung cancer, and initially no mutations were identified in other types of cancer. However, rare missense mutations in exons 19 and 21 were recently detected in colorectal carcinoma. The deletions in exon 19 seen in lung cancer have also been detected in squamous cell carcinoma of the head and neck.

EGFR mutations are strikingly prevalent in adenocarcinomas arising in individuals who have never smoked and in women. Studies repeatedly have shown that tobacco's mode of action on DNA is unlikely to produce EGFR mutations. This supports the concept that the pathogenesis of lung cancers arising in smokers and nonsmokers is different. This is further confirmed by the observation that K-ras mutations, which are clearly associated with smoking tobacco, tend to occur in adenocarcinomas without EGFR mutations. Ethnic variation in K-ras mutations has also been observed in East Asian patients whose adenocarcinomas have a 48% mutation rate; other ethnicities, including Caucasians in the United States, have only a 12% rate. Polymorphic variations in the EGFR gene, including a CA repeat in intron 1 or single nucleotide polymorphisms in the promoter region, have been identified in several ethnic groups. It remains to be determined whether these polymorphisms contribute to the higher mutational rate in these ethnic groups. The role of gender in the frequency of EGFR abnormalities is not well understood, although it is postulated that

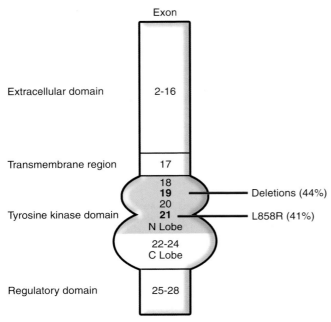

FIGURE 21-3

Frequencies of epidermal growth factor receptor (EGFR) gene mutations in lung adenocarcinomas. EGFR is a member of tyrosine kinase (TK) receptors that are composed of an extracellular domain, a transmembrane region, a TK domain, and a regulatory domain. Deletions, insertions, and missense point mutations detected in lung adenocarcinomas and responsible for patient responsiveness to TK inhibitors are limited to exons 18 to 21 of the TK domain of EGFR. The most common are deletions of exon 19 (44%) and point mutation L858R of exon 21 (41%). Other mutational types include rare missense mutations of exons 18 to 21 (6%), mutation G719X in exon 18 (4%), and exon 20 insertions (5%).

sex hormones or environmental factors may play a role.

EGFR mutations strongly correlate with the clinical response to TKIs, but the correlation is not absolute and recent clinical trials have demonstrated that the survival benefit cannot be explained solely by the observed mutations. The issue is even more complicated because patients who initially responded to TKIs may develop recurrent disease resistant to further TKI therapy. Molecular analysis of biopsies from relapsed tumors in patients initially treated with TKIs may provide the answer to questions about the significance of second mutations and may lead to the discovery of other possible mutations or other genetic alterations responsible for patients' relapse or drug resistance.

So should both amplification and mutation for EGFR be analyzed? A recent study looked at EGFR gene amplification and protein expression and its relationship to the EGFR gene mutations and survival in patients treated with TKIs. In addition, the genetic status of EGFR-related genes was explored. Cappuzzo et al. evaluated EGFR status in tumor samples from 102 patients with non-small-cell lung carcinoma treated with gefitinib using FISH, DNA

sequencing, and immunohistochemistry. The study showed that gefitinib was most effective in non-small-cell lung carcinoma patients with a high EGFR gene copy number, high protein expression, or EGFR mutations. Because only high EGFR gene copy number determined by FISH correlated with prolonged survival, the authors recommended EGFR FISH analysis as a clinical test for selecting patients for TKI therapy.

EGFR is a member of a family of TKs that includes Her2. Somatic mutations targeting the same region in exon 20 of the Her2 TK domain have been reported in lung adenocarcinomas, with a predilection for Asian women and nonsmokers. These findings indicate that our understanding of EGFR-related signaling pathways should be expanded to improve the selection of patients most likely to benefit from targeted therapies. It seems that a combination of clinical tests will be used to assess the status of a panel of markers in selection of patients for TKI therapies.

SINGLE TUMOR WITH INTRAPULMONIC SPREAD VERSUS INDEPENDENT PRIMARY

The TNM classification of patients with synchronous carcinomas of the lung has always been difficult and somewhat suboptimal. The reported incidence of synchronous tumors of the lung ranges from 0.5% to 2%, which is probably a result of different interpretations of the accepted definitions and criteria. The American Joint Committee on Cancer staging system classifies a second focus of cancer within the same lobe as T4, whereas a second focus in another lobe is classified as M1. This classification is based on criteria proposed more than 30 years ago. Essentially, a diagnosis of multiple primary lung carcinomas is made chiefly when the morphology is different. If the morphology is the same, the tumor can be diagnosed as either a metastasis or a separate primary carcinoma, with distinctly different prognostic implications. A clinicopathologic distinction between the two groups is not always possible, and it may not be genetically or prognostically valid. LOH analysis with multiple microsatellite markers has been used to study clonality in multiple lung cancers. This approach is directed to stochastic tumor-associated genetic alterations during carcinogenesis and enables calculation of the statistical likelihood of dependent versus independent origin. Clonal tumor cells often show similar patterns of LOH when multiple genes and chromosomal loci are analyzed. However, the interpretation of results can be complicated by genetic intratumoral heterogeneity. Some studies using an LOH approach suggest that the results of molecular analysis can have an impact on staging and subsequently on treatment and prognosis. At the University of Pittsburgh, an LOH study of synchronous adenocarcinomas of the lung was performed to define two molecular groups: molecularly homogenous (presumably intrapulmonary metastases) and molecularly heterogenous (presumably independent primary tumors). Because this distinction could be prognostically important, we looked at the survival of both molecular groups, but surprisingly there was no statistically significant difference in survival; perhaps the overall prognosis for either group is poor. Hence, implementation of molecular information into the staging and treatment decisions of this subset of lung cancer patients may be confounded by the lack of correlation between a tumor's genetic profile and established prognostic factors. However, this same approach has been successfully used to distinguish primary lung carcinoma and metastatic disease, particularly in patients with a history of squamous cell carcinoma of the head and neck presenting with solitary or multiple lung nodules, a distinction that clearly has prognostic impact.

DIAGNOSTIC MARKERS AND APPLICATIONS

Advances in molecular technologies and expanding knowledge about lung carcinogenesis have resulted in numerous studies searching for diagnostic markers of early lung carcinoma. The status of tumor suppressor genes and oncogenes involved in lung carcinogenesis has been explored using various molecular techniques, mostly PCR-based assays. Although the impact of translating results from new technologies to early diagnosis and survival has not been completely determined, these technologies offer novel approaches to early diagnosis of this deadly disease. As noted throughout this text, molecular changes of tumor suppressor genes can be identified by a variety of methods, including LOH analysis, CGH, array CGH, and FISH. LOH studies have provided clues to the localization of tumor suppressor genes involved in lung carcinogenesis, but they have generally failed to define a specific diagnostic or prognostic gene for lung cancer. Alterations of chromosomes 3p, 9p21, 13q14, and 17p13 are often observed, even in the early precursor dysplastic lesions. These changes are progressive; advanced tumors often show complete or partial loss of chromosomal arms, and precursor lesions tend to show more focal losses. Most of these molecular alterations indicate smoking-related damage and may not necessarily indicate an increased risk for development of invasive carcinoma. At present, it is unlikely that any of these markers will be incorporated into daily clinical practice as specific diagnostics. Array CGH is a promising tool that is helping define quantitative genomic events, but the technology is associated

with significant cost and is not yet available as a routine cancer diagnostic tool. Gene expression profiling is identifying predictive and discriminating genes that have to be further validated in larger groups of patients and is identifying biologically distinct subtypes of lung carcinomas that are not recognized by traditional diagnostic methods and classification criteria. Proteomic analysis and testing of epigenetic changes are further contributing to our understanding of the biology of lung cancer, but clear diagnostic applications are lacking.

One good example of an oncogene important in lung carcinogenesis that could potentially be used for early detection and prevention of non-small-cell carcinoma is K-ras. K-ras mutations are predominantly G to T transversions typical of tobacco smoking in their occurrence. K-ras mutations occur almost exclusively in adenocarcinoma; about 30% of these tumors harbor K-ras mutations. K-ras mutations have been reported in atypical adenomatous hyperplasia, indicating its role in early lung adenocarcinoma carcinogenesis. Because K-ras mutations in lung adenocarcinoma are identified at codons 12 and 13, it is possible to develop a simple and rapid PCR-based assay for detection of these mutations in sputum or bronchoalveolar lavage (BAL) fluid samples. It has been shown that mutations at K-ras codon 12 can be detected up to 4 years before the clinical diagnosis of cancer in about 50% of the patients whose tumors harbor these mutations. Unfortunately, K-ras mutations were also detected in sputum of the patients whose tumors were negative for such mutations or in individuals who have no clinically detectable disease. These results are not surprising, because K-ras mutations are associated with smoking tobacco and occur in individuals with high risk for lung cancer who usually have widespread precancerous lesions harboring these mutations. Clearly, this test would not solve the problem of early detection of adenocarcinoma of the lung in nonsmokers, who represent a significant proportion of lung cancer patients in recent years.

Allelic losses on 3p and 9p are also common in early lung cancer but do not offer discrimination between histologic subtypes of lung carcinoma and have been described in histologically normal or metaplastic bronchial mucosa in healthy current or former smokers. Mutations of p53 are common in lung cancer, and frequency of mutations is similar for the different histologic subtypes. The large spectrum of p53 "hot spots" makes mutational analysis of the p53 gene less suitable for clinical testing. These mutations most likely represent direct DNA damage from carcinogens found in cigarette smoke. Based on these observations, it is unlikely that either p53 protein expression or mutational analysis will be incorporated into daily clinical practice.

Recent evidence suggests that aberrant gene methylation can be an early event in lung carcinogenesis and may represent a potential marker for early detection and monitoring or chemoprevention. PCR-based methylation assays are technically improving, resulting in a long list of methylated genes in lung cancer that could potentially be used as a screening markers in clinical specimens such as sputum, BAL, or blood. In lung cancer, DNA methylation most often plays a role in inactivation of the FHIT gene at 3p14.2, the RASSF1 gene at 3p21.3, and the CDKN2A (p16^{INK4A})/ARF locus at 9p21. RASSF1A hypermethylation is significantly associated with onset of smoking at an earlier age, adenocarcinoma histology, and adverse survival in patients with stage 1 or 2 disease. The cyclin-dependent kinase inhibitor p16 regulates the phosphorylation status of the Rb protein, which is altered in almost all small-cell carcinomas yet only 15% to 30% of non-small-cell lung carcinomas. Methylation of p16^{INK4A} has been demonstrated in 75% of cases of carcinoma in situ that are adjacent to invasive squamous cell carcinoma of the lung. There is an increasing frequency of this event during disease progression from basal cell hyperplasia (17%), to squamous metaplasia (24%), to carcinoma in situ and invasive carcinoma (50% to 75%). The significance of aberrant methylation detected in clinical specimens should be interpreted with caution and with other clinical and radiographic findings, because aberrant methylation can be also detected in cancer-free long-term tobacco smokers.

CONCLUSION

At present, molecular testing of lung carcinoma is best established as a predictive tool for patient response to targeted therapies (Table 21-2). Molecular techniques associated with this application, FISH and DNA mutational analysis, are relatively inexpensive and readily available in many molecular laboratories. An expanding knowledge of lung carcinogenesis has resulted in a search for diagnostic and prognostic biomarkers of lung carcinoma. At present, it seems that no single biomarker is sensitive and specific enough to be used in clinical practice for diagnostic or prognostic purposes. Gene expression profiling or other methods of multiple marker analysis may define a "panel" of genes rather than a single gene that will allow innovative approaches to screening, prevention, diagnosis, therapy, and clinical follow-up. Although K-ras seems to be a good marker for early diagnosis of lung adenocarcinoma, the major limitation is the low frequency of K-ras mutations in primary lung cancers. It is uncertain what will be the best method for screening analysis, but certainly the current complementary DNA array chips are too expensive for routine clinical use. Microarray technologies need to be

---

TABLE 21-2

Lung Carcinoma Molecular Features

Pathobiology and Pathogenesis

Morphologic and molecular carcinogenesis sequence
- Squamous cell carcinoma (metaplasia → dysplasia → carcinoma)
- Adenocarcinoma (atypical adenomatous hyperplasia → bronchioloalveolar carcinoma → invasive adenocarcinoma)

Early events in squamous carcinogenesis
- LOH at 3p and 9p

Early events in adenocarcinoma carcinogenesis
- K-ras mutations
- LOH at 3p and 9p

Prognosis and Predictive Markers

EGFR gene mutations (exons 18–21)

EGFR amplification

Diagnostic Markers and Applications

PCR-based lung cancer screening assays in sputum and BAL
- 3p, 9p21, 13q14, and 17p13 microsatellite alterations
- K-ras and p53 DNA mutations
- FHIT, RASSF1, CDKN2A (p16^{INK4A})/ARF methylation

---

more fully developed, and current variances in tissue collection, sample preparation, probes, and chip processing should be standardized and reproducible before clinical utility can be assessed. An alternative would be to test the significance of potential biomarkers proposed by large-scale analyses using available, cheaper, and automated methods such as immunohistochemistry, FISH, and RT-PCR.

DIFFUSE PARENCHYMAL DISEASES OF THE LUNG: LYMPHANGIOLEIOMYOMATOSIS

PATHOBIOLOGY AND PATHOGENESIS

Lymphangioleiomyomatosis (LAM) is a rare disease of young women that is characterized by a proliferation of abnormal smooth muscle-like cells (LAM cells), which leads to cystic lung lesions, lymphatic abnormalities, and abdominal tumors (angiomyolipomas). LAM occurs sporadically or with the tuberous sclerosis complex (TSC), an autosomal dominant syndrome characterized by hamartoma-like tumor growths. The TSC1 and TSC2 genes have been implicated in etiology of LAM. TSC1 mutations can be identified in 27% of patients with TSC, and 73% have mutations in TSC2. Mutations and LOH across TSC1 and TSC2 loci in TSC-associated lesions indicate that TSC1 and TSC2 are tumor suppressor genes. The TSC1 gene is located on chromosome 9q34 and contains 23 exons. It encodes the 130-kDa, ubiquitously expressed protein hamartin, which is a highly evolutionary conserved protein with a low similarity with other known proteins (Figure 21-4). Hamartin is postulated to play a role in the reorganization of the actin cytoskeleton by interacting with the ezrin–radxin–moesin family of actin-binding proteins, the small G-protein Rho, and cell division protein kinases. The TSC2 gene is located on chromosome 16p13.3. It encodes the 198-kDa, ubiquitously expressed protein tuberin that plays a role in cell growth and proliferation, transcriptional activation, and endocytosis (Figure 21-4).

Hamartin and tuberin form heterodimers that regulate cell proliferation. The complex is a key regulator of the AKT pathway and participates in several other signaling pathways, including the mitogen-activated protein kinase, adenosine monophosphate–activated protein kinase, b-catenin, calmodulin, mammalian target of rapamycin (mTOR)/S6 kinase, cyclin-dependent kinase, and cell cycle pathways.

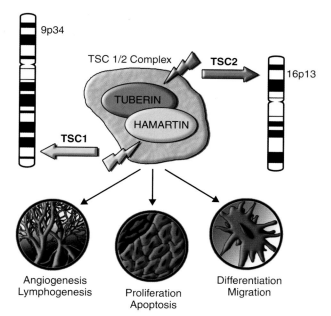

FIGURE 21-4

Biologic effects of the tuberous sclerosis complex (TSC). The TSC1 gene is located on chromosome 9q34 and contains 23 exons. It encodes the 130-kDa, ubiquitously expressed protein hamartin, with a postulated role in actin cytoskeleton reorganization. The TSC2 gene is located on chromosome 16p13.3. It encodes the 198-kDa, ubiquitously expressed protein tuberin that plays a role in cell growth and proliferation, transcriptional activation, and endocytosis. Based on the clinical overlap between TSC1- and TSC2-affected patients, it was postulated that the two genes participate in the same biochemical pathways that regulate cell growth, proliferation, survival, migration, differentiation, and angiogenesis.

PROGNOSTIC AND PREDICTIVE MARKERS

The phenotypes caused by mutations in TSC1 and TSC2 genes were initially considered identical; however, as more genotypic–phenotypic data has become available, it appears that TSC1 mutations produce a less severe phenotype than TSC2 mutations. There are some exceptions, because some missense TSC2 mutations are associated with milder disease phenotypes. The penetrance of TSC1 and TSC2 mutations is believed to be 100%. However, TSC is characterized by extreme variability in clinical findings; therefore, results from molecular genetic testing cannot be used to predict phenotype. Although only 2.3% of individuals with TSC will develop pulmonary LAM, TSC1 and TSC2 somatic mutations have been detected in individuals with sporadic pulmonary LAM. This is probably related to the complex role of TSC1 and TSC2 in LAM development.

DIAGNOSTIC MARKERS AND APPLICATIONS

Although clinical molecular testing is available to exclude or confirm a clinically suspected association of LAM with TSC, molecular genetic testing of TSC1 and TSC2 genes is difficult because of the numerous disease-causing mutations (more than 300 TSC1 and 800 TSC2 mutations to date) and the large size of each gene. The presence of somatic mosaicism in 10% to 25% of cases further complicates the interpretation of the possible results. TSC1 mutations are primarily small deletions, insertions, and nonsense mutations that could be detected by sequence analysis of the entire coding region, selected exons, or targeted mutational analysis. In contrast, TSC2 mutations include large deletions and rearrangements that cannot be detected by sequence analysis. These abnormalities could be identified by genomic microarray analysis (SignatureChip®, Signature Genomic Laboratories) using FISH-validated bronchioloalveolar carcinomas or by targeted single FISH probes. One tested region on the SignatureChip covers approximately 200 kilobases of the genomic DNA. Because of the size of the tested area, these two methods cannot detect most TSC2 gene deletions or duplications.

CONCLUSION

Because sporadic and TSC-associated LAM are rare diseases, it is difficult to predict much of a future for molecular testing in patients with LAM. Screening for LAM in patients with TSC remains controversial. High-resolution CT is likely to be the most sensitive tool for recognizing LAM, but it could be costly and unwise to screen all women with TSC for evidence of LAM until early successful therapies are available. At present, no prognostic molecular factors

TABLE 21-3

Lymphangioleiomyomatosis Molecular Features

Pathobiology and Pathogenesis

Tumor suppressor genes

- TSC1 (9q34) encodes hamartin
- TSC2 (16p13.3) encodes tuberin

Hamartin–tuberin complex regulates cell proliferation and several signaling pathways, including AKT and mTOR/S6 kinase

Prognosis and Predictive Markers

TSC1 mutations are associated with less severe phenotype

Mutations cannot predict phenotype

Diagnostic Markers and Applications

The numerous TSC1 and TSC2 mutations make molecular genetic testing difficult

TSC1 mutations detectable by sequence analysis

- Small deletions
- Insertions
- Nonsense mutations

TSC2 mutations detectable by genomic microarray analysis

- Large deletions
- Rearrangements

in patients with TSC would predict which individuals with TSC are at the greatest risk of developing lung disease. The evidence that the hamartin–tuberin complex inhibits the mTOR protein suggested that rapamycin and similar drugs may be potential therapies for LAM and tuberous sclerosis. Clinical trials of rapamycin in LAM are under way. The prognosis and outcome of patients with LAM are variable and unpredictable, and it is uncertain why some patients decline rapidly and others remain stable for years. It is likely that genetic variation in modifier genes in related pathways is responsible for this clinical variation. Hence, identification of gene polymorphisms may allow prediction of patients' clinical outcome. Molecular studies with detailed clinical correlations are still needed to improve treatment and outcome of patients with LAM (Table 21-3).

SUGGESTED READINGS

Lung Carcinoma

Beer DG, Kardia SL, Huang CC, et al: Gene-expression profiles predict survival of patients with lung adenocarcinoma. Nat Med 2002;8(8):816–824.

Belinsky SA, Palmisano WA, Gilliland FD, et al: Aberrant promoter methylation in bronchial epithelium and sputum from current and former smokers. Cancer Res 2002;62(8):2370–2377.

Cappuzzo F, Hirsch FR, Rossi E, et al: Epidermal growth factor receptor gene and protein and gefitinib sensitivity in non-small-cell lung cancer. J Natl Cancer Inst 2005;97(9):643–655.

Lynch TJ, Bell DW, Sordella R, et al: Activating mutations in the epidermal growth factor receptor underlying responsiveness of non-small-cell lung cancer to gefitinib. N Engl J Med 2004;350(21): 2129–2139.

Mao L, Hruban RH, Boyle JO, Tockman M, Sidransky D: Detection of oncogene mutations in sputum precedes diagnosis of lung cancer. Cancer Res 1994;54(7):1634–1637.

Paez JG, Janne PA, Lee JC, et al: EGFR mutations in lung cancer: Correlation with clinical response to gefitinib therapy. Science 2004;304(5676):1497–1500.

Palmisano WA, Divine KK, Saccomanno G, et al: Predicting lung cancer by detecting aberrant promoter methylation in sputum. Cancer Res 2000;60(21):5954–5958.

Tomida S, Koshikawa K, Yatabe Y, et al: Gene expression–based, individualized outcome prediction for surgically treated lung cancer patients. Oncogene 2004;23(31):5360–5370.

Wistuba, II, Lam S, Behrens C, et al: Molecular damage in the bronchial epithelium of current and former smokers. J Natl Cancer Inst 1997;89(18):1366–1373.

Lymphangioleiomyomatosis

Carsillo T, Astrinidis A, Henske EP: Mutations in the tuberous sclerosis complex gene TSC2 are a cause of sporadic pulmonary lymphangioleiomyomatosis. Proc Natl Acad Sci USA 2000;97:6085–6090.

Henske EP: Metastasis of benign tumor cells in tuberous sclerosis complex. Genes Chromosome Cancer 2003;38:376–381.

Johnson SR: Lymphangioleiomyomatosis. Eur Respir J 2006;27: 1056–1065.

Sancak O, Nellist M, Goedbloed M, et al: Mutational analysis of TSC1 and TSC2 genes in a diagnostic setting: Genotype–phenotype correlations and comparison of diagnostic DNA techniques in tuberous sclerosis complex. Eur J Human Genet 2005;13:731–741.

Strizheva GD, Carsillo T, Kruger WD, et al: The spectrum of mutations in TSC1 and TSC2 in women with tuberous sclerosis and lymphangiomyomatosis. Am J Respir Crit Care Med 2001;163:253–258.

von Slegtenhorst M, de Hoogt R, Hermans C, et al: Identification of the tuberous sclerosis gene TSC1 on chromosome 9q34. Science 1997;277:805–808.

Molecular Dermatopathology

Alexander J.F. Lazar • Jason W. Nash • Hafeez Diwan

INTRODUCTION

The field of dermatopathology spans an astonishingly diverse array of inflammatory, infectious, and neoplastic conditions. Hundreds of specific diagnoses can be made, but the sheer volume of diagnostic considerations can complicate definitive assessment. Rigorous clinicopathologic correlation will always be invaluable; nevertheless, adjunct molecular methods are making early and important contributions to the analysis of biopsy material. Although numerous genetic syndromes have prominent cutaneous findings, these are not discussed here because skin biopsies are generally not necessary for diagnosis of these germline or hereditary conditions. We focus in this chapter on the application of molecular techniques to skin biopsies involving primarily neoplastic and infectious conditions. Because many diseases described in other chapters involve the skin secondarily, we limit our discussion to diseases occurring primarily in the skin, with additional, brief consideration of diseases that secondarily involve the skin but for which interpretation is strongly influenced by the cutaneous context.

Cutaneous ailments are relatively common, the skin is uniquely accessible to clinical examination, and biopsy is readily accomplished. Thus, skin biopsies are among the most common encountered in most pathology practices. Although the armamentarium of useful molecular testing in the skin is limited, these approaches are being increasingly applied to skin pathology, often adapted from findings in analogous noncutaneous tumors. This chapter discusses some assays in use and indicates those likely to gain more widespread use.

MELANOCYTIC NEOPLASIA

MELANOMA

Melanoma has long been subclassified into multiple clinicopathologic subtypes, including superficial spreading, nodular, acral lentiginous, lentigo maligna,

mucosal, and ocular or uveal types. This classification scheme, although somewhat arbitrary and at times difficult to precisely apply, has clinical utility because there are differences in behavior, incidence, and presentation among the groups. More recently, molecular epidemiology has reinforced the biologic underpinnings of some of these diseases. In particular, mucosal, acral, ocular, chronic sun-exposure, and intermittent sun-exposure melanomas seem to have varying and rather distinct genetic profiles. An in-depth discussion of the molecular pathogenesis of melanoma is beyond the scope of this chapter; instead, we focus on receptor tyrosine kinases and the downstream *NRAS/BRAF/ERK* and phosphatidylinositol 3′-kinase (PI3K)/*PTEN* pathways depicted in Figure 22-1. The tyrosinase kinase *KIT* (CD117) is depicted in the figure because it has been recently reported to have activating mutations in a subset of melanoma cases, although other members of this receptor family are also involved in activating downstream effectors. In general, intermittent sun-exposure melanomas (probably the most common subset in Caucasians) are associated with *BRAF*-activating (70%) or *NRAS*-activating (20%) mutations. These mutations are essentially mutually exclusive in individual cases given that *BRAF* functions downstream of *NRAS*. Mucosal, acral, and chronic sun-exposure melanomas tend to lack mutations in both *NRAS* and *BRAF* and are associated with mutations or genetic amplification of *KIT* in up to 40% of cases. Loss of *PTEN* (usually by methylation suppression) results in increased phosphatidylinositol 3′-kinase signaling and is often seen with *BRAF* mutations, probably because *NRAS* activates phosphatidylinositol 3′-kinase but *BRAF* does not. We focus on these particular signaling pathways and proteins because therapeutic agents that inhibit these pathways are in clinical trials in multiple institutions.

Mutations in *BRAF* result predominantly in V600E amino acid substitution in exon 15, but other exons are encountered less often (Figure 22-2). *NRAS* mutations are present virtually exclusively in exon 2 and inhibit the deactivating guanine triphosphatase function of this protein, resulting in downstream *ERK* activation (Figure 22-3). Mutations in *KIT* are seen predominantly in exons 11, 13, and 17 but tend to be point mutations leading to in-frame amino acid

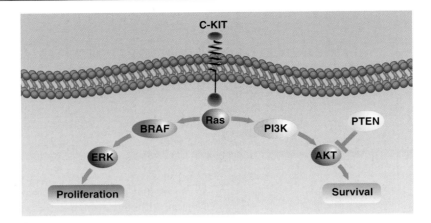

FIGURE 22-1

A simplified schematic diagram of the relationships of key cell cycle regulatory proteins implicated in melanoma pathogenesis. Although other tyrosinase kinase receptors are involved, *c-Kit* is depicted here. (Adapted from Curtin JA, Fridlyand J, Kageshita T, et al: Distinct sets of genetic alterations in melanoma. N Engl J Med 2005;353(20):2135–2147.)

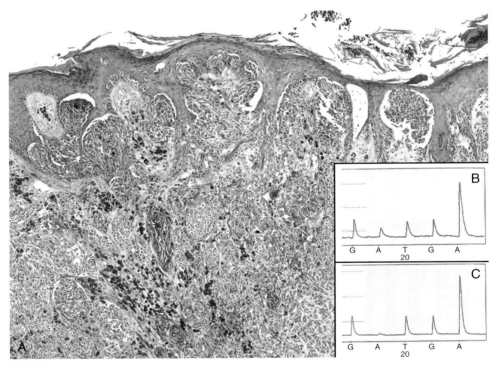

FIGURE 22-2

Superficial spreading melanoma **(A)**, with insets showing *BRAF* V600E–activating mutation in exon 15 **(B)**, compared with control wild-type sequence **(C)** demonstrated using DNA pyrosequencing. (Courtesy of Dr. Dan Jones, University of Texas M.D. Anderson Cancer Center, Houston, TX.)

substitutions, rather than the deletions and insertions commonly encountered in gastrointestinal stromal tumors (Figure 22-4).

Genetic amplification of the *KIT* locus at 4q12 is also encountered with or without an associated activating mutation. Of the *KIT* aberrations described in melanoma, about half are amplification or increased copy number and half are point mutations. *PTEN* loss is usually not by mutation but rather by

methylation suppression of the promoter. *NRAS*, *BRAF*, and *KIT* are assayed by polymerase chain reaction (PCR) amplification of the relevant exons and can be screened by single-strand conformation polymorphisms analysis, but they are confirmed by either traditional Sanger sequencing or pyrosequencing of the DNA amplicons.

Manual microdissection to enrich for tumor cells can be helpful. Pyrosequencing is sensitive but

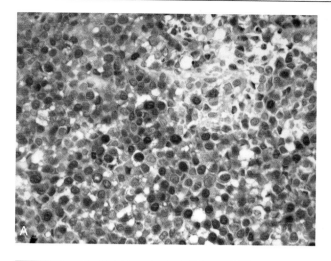

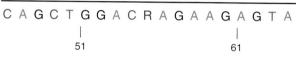

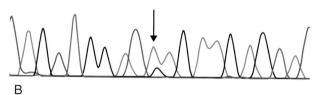

B

FIGURE 22-3

Increased activated phosphorylated ERK (mitogen-activated protein kinase) nuclear accumulation on immunohistochemistry **(A)** associated with an upstream activating Q61R mutation in exon 2 of *NRAS* **(B).** (Courtesy of Dr. Dan Jones, University of Texas M.D. Anderson Cancer Center, Houston, TX.)

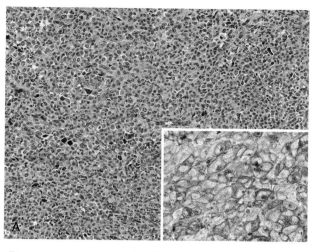

Reverse   L576P

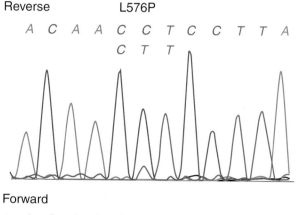

Forward

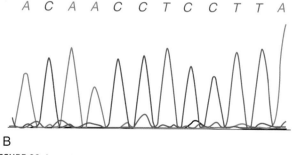

B

FIGURE 22-4

Metastatic acral-lentiginous melanoma **(A),** with inset showing strong immunoreactivity with *c-Kit* (CD117). Forward and reverse sequencing of exon 11 revealed an L576P-activating mutation in *KIT* **(B),** also encountered in gastrointestinal stromal tumors. (Courtesy of Dr. Dan Jones, University of Texas M.D. Anderson Cancer Center, Houston, TX.)

functions most efficiently when looking for point mutations involving a known and limited set of codons, as depicted for *BRAF* mutation in Figure 22-2. *KIT* is often examined in a staged assay in gastrointestinal stromal tumors, where exon 11 is examined first, followed by exon 9 and then the remaining relevant exons; this may need to be modified for detection of the point mutations apparently common in melanoma (exons 11, 13, and 17), but additional series are needed to determine the frequency and distribution of the mutations.

It is not known whether mutations in any of these genes lead to increased sensitivity to the pathway-specific agents being tested in clinical trials. Gastrointestinal stromal tumors have some mutations demonstrated in melanoma, and some of these respond to imatinib mesylate. However, results can be complicated, as demonstrated by patients who responded to one *BRAF* inhibitor but did not correlate with the mutational status of this gene, perhaps because the agent (sorafenib) had an inhibitory profile beyond *BRAF.* This molecular

characterization and application of targeted therapeutic agents marks the beginning of rational therapy in melanoma, where effective treatments for metastatic disease are generally lacking, and perhaps represents the initial steps in pathway-specific, individualized therapy. Application of these molecular assays to prospective clinical trials will be critical to establish efficacy and to define the populations that will benefit from any particular treatment. It is likely that combinations of therapeutic agents will be used to achieve the greatest efficacy possible.

SENTINEL LYMPH NODES FOR MELANOMA

Although there is still debate as to whether sentinel lymph node biopsy in melanoma should be a universal standard of care, it is widely employed by surgeons, given its proven utility for accurate disease staging and prognosis. Thus, these samples are commonly encountered by pathologists.

Many regimens have been employed for the analysis of sentinel lymph nodes, and most use multiple tissue levels stained by hematoxylin and eosin and supplemented with immunohistochemistry for standard melanocytic markers. PCR-based methods have been attempted for melanocytic markers and greatly increase the detection of "positive" lymph nodes, primarily in the setting of clinical trials. However, the methodology appears to be overly sensitive, because specificity of predicting a more adverse clinical outcome is reduced when positive lymph nodes are defined in this manner. This could be because RT-PCR in this context detects events that are not clinically relevant. In addition, benign intracapsular nevi are noted in 2% to 5% of sentinel lymph nodes (Figure 22-5) and represent a potential source of false positivity because the RT-PCR-based assays currently do not discriminate between benign and malignant melanocytes. The prevalence of intracapsular nevi is particularly disquieting because the metastatic rate in sentinel lymph nodes is usually less than 20%, given the expanded criteria often employed for selecting patients to whom this procedure is offered. Thus, the standard of care for sentinel lymph node evaluation is likely to remain examination of multiple levels and immunohistochemistry, and RT-PCR-based testing will need to await further validation (perhaps after robust markers for differentiation of intracapsular nevi and melanoma are discovered).

SPITZ NEVUS AND MELANOMA

Distinguishing between Spitz nevus or Spitz nevus with atypical features and melanoma is a process often wrought with anguish in dermatopathology. There are overlapping features, both histologic and immunophenotypic, and even respected experts have only partial agreement when considering actual individual cases with known outcome data. This rightfully creates concern for the clinicians managing these cases. Because many cases occur in children, even mitotic figures, while helpful, cannot always clearly differentiate melanoma and Spitz nevi in equivocal cases, although mitoses deep in a lesion or at the edges are always a concerning feature. In general, the older a

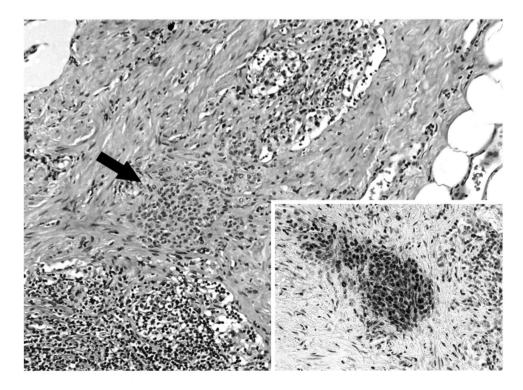

FIGURE 22-5

Lymph node with intracapsular collection of benign melanocytes. Inset shows immunoreactivity of the melanocytes with anti-*MART1* antibody on immunohistochemistry. Intracapsular nevi complicate polymerase chain reaction–based assessment of sentinel lymph nodes for metastatic melanoma.

patient is, the more likely a lesion is to be a melanoma mimicking Spitz nevus; nevertheless, Spitz nevi definitely occur in older adults. A final complication is the observation that in the rarely encountered examples of "spiztoid" melanoma in children the disease may not always behave in such a uniformly aggressive manner as in adults.

In this complex milieu, comparative genomic hybridization studies have indicated that melanomas are often associated with aberrations involving chromosomes 6, 7, 9, and 10, and a subset of Spitz nevi shows gains or amplification at the short arm of chromosome 11 containing the *HRAS* locus. Some Spitz nevi also contain activating mutations in *HRAS*. Gains in 11p have not been noted in melanoma, and melanomas show mutations in *NRAS* rather than in *HRAS*, as noted earlier. Unfortunately, these distinguishing features are encountered in only a subset of Spitz nevi, and this testing has not been validated prospectively in larger series with appropriate follow-up. Given that misdiagnosis of a melanoma can have devastating consequences, many dermatopathologists and clinicians recommend complete excision of all Spitz nevi. Molecular testing, such as comparative genomic hybridization, to resolve this important and often vexing differential diagnosis requires further investigation before it can be applied routinely in clinical practice.

MELANOMA—FACT SHEET

Definition

▶ A highly malignant tumor of melanocytic differentiation primarily involving skin and sometimes mucosal sites, characterized by a tendency to metastasis even with small primary tumors.

Incidence and Location

▶ Incidence has rapidly risen over the last several decades, and lifetime risk is now at least 1 in 60 people in the United States.

▶ Fifth most common cancer in men and sixth in women, with 58,000 new cases in total annually.

▶ Incidence appears to be doubling every few decades across the world in Caucasian populations, but the rate may be slowing with application of preventive screening and behavior.

Morbidity and Mortality

▶ Approximately 7700 deaths occur from melanoma per year in the United States.

▶ Mortality may be decreasing because of screening and early intervention.

Gender, Race, and Age Distribution

▶ Slight male predominance.

▶ Incidence of sun-exposure-related melanoma is much higher in Caucasians.

▶ Age of onset ranges from children to elderly, but onset is primarily in midadult life.

Clinical Features

▶ Early signs of cutaneous melanoma are melanocytic lesions showing asymmetry, irregular borders, variation in color, increasing diameter, and rapid evolution over time.

▶ Regional lymph nodes are the most common initial site of metastasis.

Prognosis and Treatment

▶ Risk of death correlates strongly with the thickness of the lesion (Breslow measurement).

▶ Metastasis portends a poor prognosis.

▶ Surgical intervention is the best hope for cure, because chemotherapy and radiation are generally ineffective in modifying overall mortality in metastatic disease.

▶ Sentinel lymph node biopsy provides important staging information.

SEBACEOUS NEOPLASIA AND THE MUIR-TORRE SYNDROME

Most genetic syndromes that involve the skin are assayed from peripheral blood lymphocytes or perhaps buccal swabs and are not discussed in this chapter. An exception to this general rule is the Muir-Torre syndrome. Described simultaneously by two observers in 1967–1968, this syndrome is the association of sebaceous neoplasia with internal malignancy, often in a hereditary setting. Sebaceous neoplasia can sometimes be the initial presenting feature; thus, careful surveillance can be employed to great benefit if the syndrome is detected in this fashion. Sebaceous lesions associated with this syndrome include sebaceous adenoma, sebaceoma, and sebaceous carcinoma. The sebaceous lesions can be multiple and sometimes exhibit keratoacanthoma-like or cystic architecture. Benign sebaceous lesions are more often associated with this syndrome than are frank sebaceous carcinomas. Keratoacanthomas can sometimes be associated with the syndrome, but these often show at least focal sebaceous differentiation. The internal malignancies most commonly documented as occurring with this syndrome are colon (>70% lifetime risk), bladder and renal pelvis, endometrium, ovarian, and breast. Hematolymphoid and mesenchymal malignancies are rarely reported.

The Muir-Torre syndrome is known to be a subset of the hereditary nonpolyposis colon cancer (HNPCC) syndrome and to be caused by germline-inactivating mutation of DNA mismatch repair genes *MLH1* and *MSH2* and less commonly *MSH3, MSH6, PMS1,* and *PMS2.* HNPCC is estimated to account for approximately 1% to 3% of colonic carcinoma, and the Muir-Torre syndrome is a small subset of all HNPCC. Somatic loss of the remaining mismatch repair allele leads to microsatellite instability (MSI). In MSI, areas of mononucleotide and binucleotide repeats experience primarily deletions and sometimes insertions, leading to variability in the length of microsatellites. MSI is seen in the tumors associated with this syndrome and can be demonstrated by a PCR-based assay using 10 (or most often a subset of 5 or 6) microsatellites established by an expert National Cancer Institute panel (Figure 22-6). Although these microsatellites have only been well validated in colonic carcinoma, they appear to be sensitive and specific for tumors in other tissues as well, such as endometrial or sebaceous tumors. Instability detected in at least 30% of markers (compared to non-neoplastic tissue) defines MSI in the tumor. If no markers show variability, then the tumor is designated as microsatellite stable. Having at least one marker, but less than 30% designates instability in low MSI. This does not seem to correlate with loss of mismatch repair proteins and is of unclear significance.

Recent reports indicate that using immunohistochemistry to examine for loss of mismatch repair proteins (primarily hMLH1, hMSH2, and hMSH6) is highly specific but only perhaps 85% to 90% sensitive for MSI, as designated by the PCR-based gold standard test. Interestingly, although HNPCC as a whole shows equivalent rates of *MLH1* and *MSH2* involvement, the Muir-Torre syndrome shows a 9 or 10:1 predominance of *MSH2* involvement over *MLH1*. This may indicate that hMSH2 loss more readily gives rise to cutaneous sebaceous neoplasia. Colonic and endometrial carcinomas show somatic loss of *MLH1* transcription by methylation suppression of the promoter at both alleles in 10% to 15% of *sporadic* cases. This does not appear to be the case in sebaceous tumors, where loss of a mismatch repair proteins demonstrated by immunohistochemistry implies a germline deficit and personal and potentially heritable increased cancer risk. These results can guide germline testing, because loss of either hMLH1 or hMSH2 by immunohistochemistry can screen for a variety of inactivating mutations distributed throughout virtually all exons. The PCR-based MSI testing is often used both for confirmation of immunohistochemical results and for further

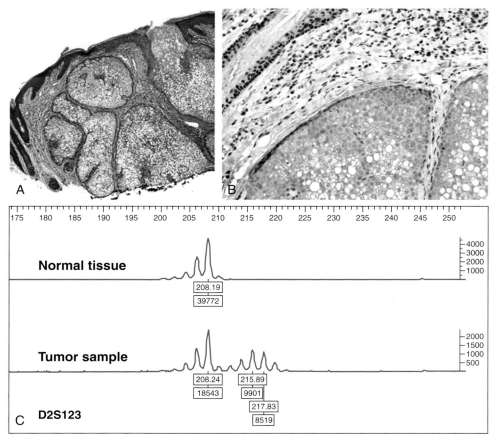

FIGURE 22-6

Sebaceous adenoma (**A**) associated with the Muir-Torre syndrome. Immunohistochemistry showed loss of *MSH2* within tumor nuclei in contrast to retained nuclear reactivity in surrounding non-neoplastic cells (**B**). Microsatellite instability is confirmed at one microsatellite locus by sizing chromatography of the D2S123 locus amplicons that reveal increased variability in the tumor tissue. (Courtesy of Dr. Raja Luthra, University of Texas M.D. Anderson Cancer Center, Houston, TX.)

examination of suspicious cases, because the sensitivity of immunohistochemical testing is not perfect. Recent data indicates that sebaceous neoplasia may be associated with inactivating mutations in the *WNT* signaling pathway and in particular the *LEF1/TCF3* transcription factor in a significant proportion of lesions, but this does not correlate with the mismatch repair status of the tumor.

OTHER SKIN ADNEXAL TUMORS

Cutaneous adnexal neoplasms (those showing follicular, sebaceous, apocrine, or eccrine differentiation) are relatively uncommon, with their malignant counterparts being even more so. Treatment options are limited, consisting primarily of surgical approaches with or without radiotherapy and, more recently, sentinel lymph node biopsy. Chemotherapeutic regimens are not well established for such neoplasms, given their rarity, and demonstrate only variable success rates. Effective therapeutic options are limited in the fortunately rare setting of metastatic disease.

Some adnexal neoplasms show histologic overlap with neoplasms arising in other organ systems, in particular breast, bowel, and salivary gland. Tumors of sweat (or apocrine) gland origin specifically share many features with breast ductal adenocarcinomas. Demonstration of immunohistochemical reactivity has been reported in some sweat gland tumors for estrogen receptor, progesterone receptor, and gross cystic disease fluid protein-15, further demonstrating the degree of overlap or homology of these tumors with those of breast origin. In many instances, the degree of morphologic overlap makes clinical correlation necessary to exclude the possibility of an origin from any extracutaneous site and to ensure adequate treatment and staging. The extensive similarity among these tumors suggests that diagnostic and treatment strategies applicable to breast carcinomas may have relevant application. As an example of this, hidradenocarcinomas have been reported to overexpress the HER2 protein, as demonstrated by immunohistochemistry, in a fashion analogous to breast carcinoma, and amplification of the *HER2* locus demonstrated by fluorescence in situ hybridization (FISH) has been reported in a metastatic hidradenocarcinoma (Figure 22-7).

Based on these findings, alternative therapeutic options, including antiestrogen treatment with tamoxifen, have been employed in some cases, demonstrating estrogen receptor immunoreactivity with some anecdotal success. In the setting of amplification of the *HER2* locus, trastuzumab has been employed, in addition to an existing adjuvant

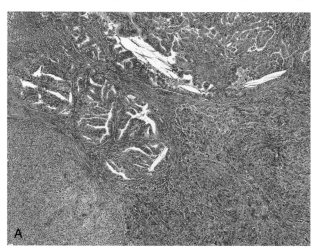

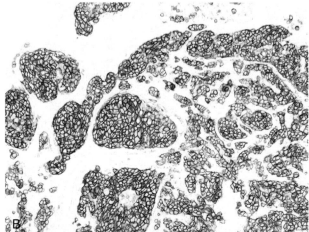

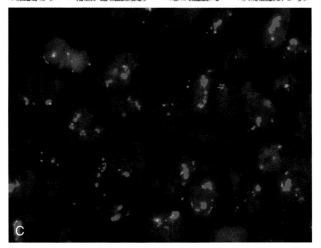

FIGURE 22-7

A hidradenocarcinoma can be seen arising in the context of a benign hidradenoma (**A,** lower left corner). This lesion metastasized to lymph nodes and the malignant cells showed intense membranous staining with *HER2* on immunohistochemistry **(B).** The *HER2* locus at chromosome 17q (red probe) showed approximately 2.5-fold amplification on fluorescence in situ hybridization analysis **(C).** The green signal is the chromosome 17 centromeric probe. (Courtesy of Dr. Nour Sneige, University of Texas M.D. Anderson Cancer Center, Houston, TX.)

regimen of chemotherapy and radiotherapy. Although these findings appear to be rare in most adnexal neoplasms, screening by immunohistochemistry followed by techniques such as FISH to detect gene amplifications of the *HER2* locus can be employed. There appears to be a rational basis for screening certain malignant eccrine and apocrine skin tumors using molecular techniques commonly employed for breast carcinoma.

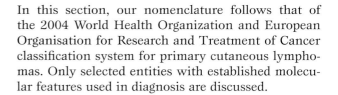

MESENCHYMAL TUMORS: DERMATOFIBROSARCOMA PROTUBERANS

Although most soft tissue sarcomas that sometimes involve the skin are discussed in another chapter, dermatofibrosarcoma protuberans (DFSP) is briefly discussed here because it characteristically involves the dermis. This tumor is composed of fibrous spindle cells that adopt a storiform architecture and are diffusely reactive for CD34 by immunohistochemistry (Figure 22-8B,C). This lesion is based in the dermis but often shows subcuticular involvement infiltrating and surrounding single adipocytes, producing a characteristic "Swiss cheese" pattern. The tumor usually arises on the trunk and can be seen in a wide age range. These tumors show a strong tendency for local recurrence, and complete excision is necessary to reduce this complication. With time, fibrosarcomatous differentiation composed of fascicles of spindle cells with prominent mitoses can sometimes be seen, representing a higher-grade transformation associated with some increased risk of local recurrence and the possibility of metastasis. Given the characteristic histologic features and diffuse, strong immunoreactivity for CD34 in DFSP, this diagnosis is usually readily made, but considerable confusion results with more cellular dermatofibromas or benign fibrous histiocytomas that are centered in the dermis but can sometimes involve the subcutis. In addition, the pediatric variant of DFSP, giant cell fibroblastoma, is periodically encountered and can be a diagnostic challenge (Figure 22-8A).

DFSP is associated with a translocation involving chromosomes 17 and 22 that results in a fusion gene with the strong *COL1A1* promoter, driving overexpression of platelet-derived growth factor (*PDGF*β). Demonstration of the fusion transcript by PCR is complicated because *COL1A1* has 52 exons and virtually any intron can be involved as the breakpoint, requiring many PCR reactions to cover all possible chimeric gene structures (Figure 22-8E,F). Fortunately exon 2 of *PDGF*β is employed in virtually all

fusion events. FISH using dual-color break-apart probes for the *PDGF*-β locus has also been employed (Figure 22-8D). The pediatric variant of DFSP, giant cell fibroblastoma, tends to show rearrangement of the *PDGF*β locus, but a fusion transcript with *COL1A1* is sometimes not identified, perhaps implying that alternative fusion partners can drive the expression of *PDGF*β. This test is unlikely to be routinely employed for cases with characteristic features because the histology and diffuse, strong expression of CD34 on immunohistochemistry are characteristic, but it is helpful in instances that are unusual clinically or histologically. These techniques will also find application in cases in which the initial presentation or recurrence shows extensive fibrosarcomatous transformation and histologic and immunohistochemical features are less characteristic, because CD34 expression is often absent in fibrosarcomatous areas. In addition, because imatinib mesylate may be employed to treat surgically intractable or metastatic cases caused by inhibition of the PDGFβ receptor, molecular testing could be used to support the therapeutic efficacy of this agent.

HEMATOPOIETIC MALIGNANCIES

In this section, our nomenclature follows that of the 2004 World Health Organization and European Organisation for Research and Treatment of Cancer classification system for primary cutaneous lymphomas. Only selected entities with established molecular features used in diagnosis are discussed.

CUTANEOUS T-CELL LYMPHOMAS

Mycosis Fungoides

The diagnosis of early mycosis fungoides remains one of the most difficult and controversial areas of dermatopathology. Although more advanced cases tend to show the characteristic features of epidermotropism, Pautrier-type microabscesses, and lymphocytic nuclear atypia, early patch-stage cases often show infiltrates with only minimal lymphocytic atypia or epidermal involvement (Figure 22-9). In addition, numerous, overlapping inflammatory conditions mimic mycoses fungoides. Correlation with the clinical features such as the presentation in older adults, characteristic truncal involvement, recalcitrance to topical treatments, and persistence for many months or years is helpful. Studies indicate that mycoses fungoides is often biopsied multiple times over several years before this disease is definitively established or often even raised as a diagnostic consideration.

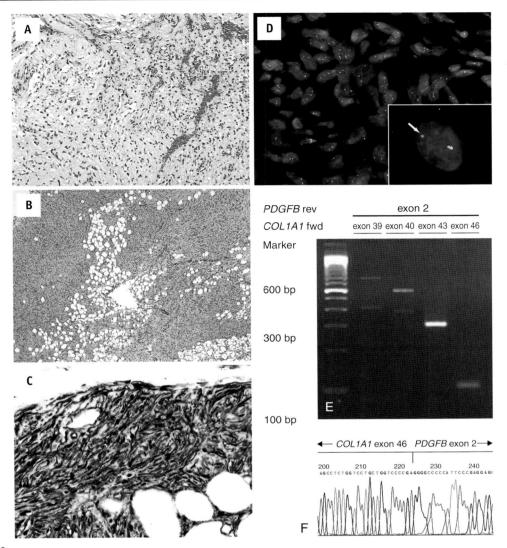

FIGURE 22-8

Giant cell fibroblastoma **(A)** and dermatofibrosarcoma protuberans **(B)** with characteristic diffuse and strong immunoreactivity for CD34 within dermatofibrosarcoma protuberans **(C)**. **(D)** A fluorescence in situ hybridization image depicting rearrangement at the *PDGF-β* locus. where the telomeric probe (red/orange) is often lost and sometimes the centromeric probe reveals multiple copy numbers or amplification. Multiplex polymerase chain reactions yielded products with multiple primer sets that can amplify across the fusion transcript **(E)**, but DNA sequencing confirmed direct junction of exon 46 of *COL1A1* and exon 2 of *PDGF-β* **(F)**. (Courtesy of Dr. Delores Lopez-Terrada, Texas Children Hospital, Houston, TX.)

Immunohistochemical analysis can be helpful because the infiltrates usually consist primarily of CD4-positive T cells, with a few CD8-positive forms admixed, and the epidermotropic forms are usually predominantly CD4 positive. Some authors find utility in loss of CD7 or other T-cell markers as a surrogate indicator of clonality in the infiltrate, although this is often difficult to demonstrate. Direct T-cell receptor clonality studies can be extremely helpful in the assessment of mycosis fungoides. Demonstration of clonality in the appropriate clinical setting can strongly support this diagnosis in any otherwise histologically equivocal biopsy. Unfortunately, some mimics of mycosis fungoides can sometimes also show clonality, and the growing list of inflammatory conditions often associated with clonal T-cell infiltrates includes lichen planus, pityriasis lichenoides et varioliformis acuta (PLEVA or Mucha Habermann disease), pityriasis lichenoides chronica, and lichen sclerosus. Although clonality studies can be performed by Southern blot, this requires more DNA than usually present in these samples; thus, the biopsies today use amplification by PCR. The detection methods include polyacrylamide gel electrophoresis, single-strand conformation polymorphism analysis, gradient gel electrophoresis using either temperature or denaturing, or heteroduplex analysis. Currently, the state of the art has been reached by automatic capillary electrophoresis with fluorescent DNA probes (GeneScan™), because this method is highly

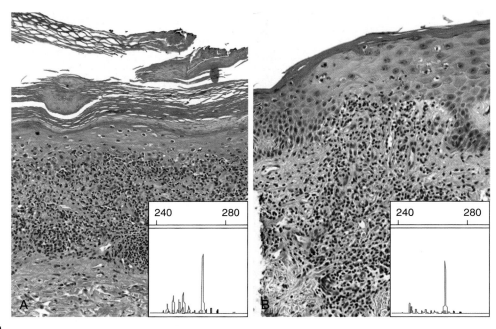

FIGURE 22-9

Two skin biopsies taken from different sites at different times with a lichenoid infiltrate and minimal epidermotropism **(A** and **B).** Although the histologic features are not diagnostic on their own, a diagnosis of mycoses fungoides was established, given the more characteristic clinical features and presence of a persisting identical T-cell receptor gene rearrangement depicted in the insets. (Courtesy of Dr. Dan Jones, University of Texas M. D. Anderson Cancer Center, Houston, TX.)

sensitive and offers facile direct comparison of samples from a patient taken from different locations or at different times. Maintenance of a single clone over time and space is quite characteristic of mycosis fungoides and not generally seen in inflammatory disorders, including those showing clonality in a single lesion, although more study is needed. These remarks generally hold true for all described variants of mycoses fungoides.

In the end, the diagnosis of mycoses fungoides is based on clinical, histologic, immunophenotypic, and molecular findings. In general, if three of these four features are highly supportive and the third is not inconsistent, one is on firm ground for suggesting the diagnosis. What is important to note is that there is no need to be aggressive about early diagnosis in unclear situations, because the early clinical course is most often indolent and usually declares itself over many years (and most cases remain indolent). Even in the cases that eventually progress, there is no current evidence that early aggressive intervention fundamentally alters the natural history of the disease, perhaps because none of the early treatments are curative.

Other T–Cell Lymphomas

T-cell clonality studies can be useful for establishing the diagnosis of other cutaneous T-cell lymphomas, such as Sézary syndrome, subcutaneous panniculitis-like T-cell lymphoma, angioimmunoblastic T-cell lymphoma, and other nodal T-cell lymphomas that can involve the skin secondarily. In the case of subcutaneous panniculitis-like T-cell lymphoma, molecular studies may aid in the differential diagnosis of lupus panniculitis and other reactive panniculitides. Interestingly, when this disease is derived from γ/δ T cells, it appears to have a much worse prognosis than seen when it expresses α/β T-cell receptors.

Anaplastic large-cell lymphoma is associated with multiple rearrangements of the *ALK* locus at 2p23. Primary cutaneous anaplastic large-cell lymphoma usually lacks both this rearrangement and any nuclear (or cytoplasmic) expression of the ALK protein by immunohistochemistry. This latter assay can be a less expensive screen to determine whether additional molecular analysis will be helpful, because expression of ALK protein implies the presence of a translocation and can be further investigated by either FISH- or PCR-based methods. In general, the finding of an *ALK* rearrangement in anaplastic large-cell lymphoma involving the skin implies systemic disease that secondarily involves the skin—a condition associated with a more guarded clinical outcome. Anaplastic large-cell lymphoma generally has a clonal T-cell receptor gene rearrangement, and this can be helpful in differentiating this disease from exuberant reactive lymphoid infiltrates, such as an insect bite reaction that can show prominent admixed CD30-positive-activated cells. Clusters of CD30-positive

Definition

▶ A cutaneous T-cell lymphoma, usually of helper (CD4) T cells, characterized by a long clinical course, with some cases progressing to extensive tumor burden and profound immunodeficiency.

Incidence and Location

▶ This is a rare disease, with annual incidence in the United States of less than 0.5 per 100,000 people. Nonetheless, it is the most common primarily cutaneous T-cell lymphoma.
▶ Early involvement is usually in truncal areas.

Morbidity and Mortality

▶ Death from this disease is rare and usually results from opportunistic infection in the setting of immunosuppression late in the disease course.
▶ Involvement of the skin early in the disease course is both an irritating (can be profoundly pruritic) and a cosmetic issue.

Gender, Race, and Age Distribution

▶ There is a male predominance of approximately 2:1.
▶ The disease is more common in blacks and less commonly affects Asians and Hispanics.
▶ It most commonly arises in the fourth to sixth decades but can be seen rarely in children.

Clinical Features

▶ The disease usually begins as nonspecific erythematous patches involving the trunk. With time, these can evolve to plaques and even tumors. Bone marrow or lymph node involvement is a late and ominous complication.
▶ Patients usually succumb to infection, often with unusual organisms, because of profound immunosuppression rather than tumor-related organ failure.

Prognosis and Treatment

▶ Severity of disease, likelihood of progression, and outcome correlate with percentage of body surface involvement and progression from patch, to plaque, to tumor involvement. Less than 10% involvement is associated with approximately normal life expectancy.
▶ Treatment varies given the range of disease severity, from topical steroids and ultraviolet light therapy to topical and systemic chemotherapy, radiation, photophoresis, and bone marrow transplantation in severe cases.

cells tend to favor a CD30-positive lymphoproliferative disorder. Anaplastic large-cell lymphoma can usually be readily distinguished from lymphomatoid papulosis with the clinical history of crops of lesions that resolve spontaneously in the latter, although the morphologic features do overlap. Lymphomatoid papulosis can also be seen with mycoses fungoides, creating a complex clinical picture. Lymphomatoid papulosis and mycosis fungoides can show identical T-cell clones in a patient, perhaps indicating that they are related disorders.

CUTANEOUS B-CELL LYMPHOMAS

Primary Cutaneous Follicular Center Lymphoma

Although follicular lymphoma is covered in other chapters, a few remarks are warranted here regarding this disease in the skin. Primary cutaneous follicular lymphoma is most common in the head and neck region. It consists of a dermal and sometimes subcuticular nodular infiltrate of lymphocytes with expanded follicles, particularly the germinal centers. It is usually an indolent disease that will respond well to injected steroids or local excision, but it can recur. Local irradiation is sometimes employed therapeutically. The analysis of this disease in the skin is complicated because not all cases are associated with the characteristic translocation between chromosomes 14 and 18 involving the *IGH* and *BCL2* loci. There is disagreement in the literature concerning the prevalence of both this translocation and the aberrant nuclear overexpression of BCL2 in follicular center cells that retain their characteristic BCL6 and CD10 reactivity on immunohistochemistry in cutaneous primary tumors. Most authorities do agree that demonstration of the translocation should prompt clinical staging to exclude systemic disease. The translocation can be demonstrated by either FISH- or RT-PCR-based amplification of the fusion transcript. One can also use studies to demonstrate clonal immunoglobulin heavy chain rearrangements by PCR. Neither κ- nor λ-light chains are usually expressed highly enough to be of value in evaluating clonality by immunohistochemistry. Immunohistochemistry can be of use in this diagnosis, particularly coexpression of cytoplasmic BCL2 and CD10 or nuclear BCL6, defining an aberrant follicular center cell population. Some authorities maintain that cutaneous disease without the characteristic translocation should not be considered a true lymphoma, but others vehemently disagree. Yet others view the cutaneous lesions lacking the translocation as possible precursor lesions where the translocation may eventually arise; thus, early eradication may be efficacious as a preventive procedure.

Cutaneous Marginal Zone B-Cell Lymphoma (MALT-Like)

Cutaneous marginal zone B-cell lymphoma is a low-grade cutaneous lymphoma that commonly involves the head and neck. Systemic disease can be associated with a translocation involving chromosomes 11 and 18. Interestingly, this disease in Europe is sometimes associated with *Borrelia burgdorferi* exposure or infection, but this association is rarely noted in the North American literature. The disease tends to show lymphoplasmacytic differentiation. Therefore, immunohistochemistry to demonstrate κ- or λ-light chain restriction can often be used as a surrogate for clonality studies—something that is usually more difficult to demonstrate in follicular lymphoma. Light chain restriction can also be demonstrated by in situ hybridization (ISH) studies, but this offers few advantages (some authorities suggest increased sensitivity) over immunohistochemistry in this context. Other techniques include FISH or RT-PCR for detection of the fusion transcript. Dual-color fusion FISH probes are often employed. A small subset of marginal zone lymphomas can be demonstrated to have one of several chromosomal translocations, including t(14;18)(q32;q21) *IGH/MALT1,* t(11;18)(q21;q21) *API2/MALT1,* and t(3;14)(p14;q32) *FOXP1/IGH.* Demonstration of immunoglobulin heavy chain clonality may be more sensitive for making this diagnosis when the characteristic histologic features are present.

Mantle Zone Lymphoma

Primary cutaneous mantle zone lymphoma is exquisitely rare, and demonstration of the characteristic translocation between chromosomes 11 and 14 is needed to establish the diagnosis. Immunohistochemistry for cyclin D1 can also be helpful, but molecular confirmation is probably needed given the rarity of this condition in the skin. Clearly, this diagnosis should prompt staging to exclude systemic disease with secondary cutaneous involvement.

Other B-Cell Lymphomas

Cutaneous diffuse large B-cell lymphoma is encountered in the skin, and there is a "leg type" that occurs on the lower extremities and appears to have a worse prognosis. By gene expression analysis, primary cutaneous disease appears distinct from systemic diffuse large B-cell lymphoma; thus, demonstration of a translocation characteristic of systemic disease should prompt careful staging. Immunoglobulin cells are clonally rearranged in cutaneous diffuse large B-cell lymphomas, but further specific molecular features remain to be discovered. Burkitt lymphoma can be encountered in the skin and, again, because of the rarity of the diagnosis, should be confirmed by molecular methods that detect the 8;14 *IGH/MYC* translocation, as detailed in Chapter 25. Chronic lymphocytic leukemia or small cell lymphoma can also involve the skin, but this is virtually always secondary to a known diagnosis or can be readily diagnosed with additional systemic evaluation.

CUTANEOUS INFECTIONS

INTRODUCTION

The diagnosis of cutaneous infections is a multistep process. The options available to clinicians are microbiologic assessment (e.g., tissue culture),

histopathologic diagnosis, or both. Sometimes immediate evaluation using frozen section is used to examine for infectious organisms in the setting of an immunocompromised patient. Use of this technique may allow prompt empirical antimicrobial treatment without the need to wait for definitive culture results, which may take weeks in the case of fungal culture.

Skin biopsy can provide valuable information regarding infections and is a common procedure. Light microscopy can detect fungi, bacteria, and viral changes—e.g., caused by human papillomavirus (HPV) or herpes viruses—by a simple and thorough evaluation of formalin-fixed, paraffin-embedded tissue on hematoxylin and eosin stain. If deemed necessary, one can resort to special studies—e.g., Gram stains, Grocott methenamine silver for fungi, a Fite study for mycobacteria, and immunohistochemistry for herpes simplex virus (HSV) or varicella-zoster virus (VZV). Despite these efforts, an infectious etiology may remain elusive, with potentially harmful ramifications to the patient.

Therefore, in the interstices of current clinical practice, there is much room for diagnostic strategies that are both fast and accurate and that require minimal tissue. This is a strong attraction of molecular diagnostic techniques in the evaluation of cutaneous infections.

In general, these techniques provide better, often greatly improved, sensitivity and specificity over traditional stains and microbiologic culture. This is not always true, however, and sometimes (as in Kaposi's sarcoma) it is simply not necessary to resort to molecular techniques. The greater cost of these techniques can be offset by the increased accuracy, speed, and ability to use small amounts of tissue. Indeed, it is anticipated that costs will further decrease over time, perhaps markedly. Here we discuss some molecular methods that can be brought to bear specifically in the context of skin biopsies. A more general discussion of methods applicable to infectious diseases can be found in Chapter 18.

MYCOBACTERIAL INFECTIONS

Rapid diagnosis of mycobacterial infections poses a significant challenge. Light microscopy can provide valuable clues, such as granulomatous inflammation in most mycobacterial infections or a perineural location and foamy histiocytes in the case of leprosy. But to visualize the organisms, a Ziehl-Nelson or Fite study is usually performed. Often there are few mycobacteria and one has to painstakingly evaluate the stained tissue sections at high magnification (at least 400×, if not at 1000× under oil immersion). In the end, inability to identify the organisms does not effectively exclude infection. In many cases, there is no choice but to wait for microbiologic cultures results, which can involve extended waits (with the exception of certain faster-growing atypical mycobacteria). In contrast, detection of specific mycobacterial genes by PCR-based methods is quick, sensitive, and specific and can be performed on skin biopsies, including formalin-fixed, paraffin-embedded tissue. For *Mycobacterium tuberculosis,* this procedure may be more sensitive than culture. Another advantage is that *M. tuberculosis* can be readily differentiated from atypical mycobacteria such as *Mycobacterium ulcerans.* One method used is amplification and sequencing of hypervariable regions of the 16S ribosomal RNA gene (Figure 22-10). This technique allows ready differentiation of various species of mycobacteria (including *M. tuberculosis, Mycobacterium fortuitum,* and *Mycobacterium kansasii*). Other methods can be applied to fresh or formalin-fixed biopsies as well.

The use of PCR-based methods extends to *Mycobacterium leprae,* even after initiation of therapy. A caveat is that detection of *M. leprae* DNA does not always correlate with active disease. But the ability to use PCR-based methods when other methodologies fail and the ability to detect the organism in the early phases, even when characteristic histologic features are not well developed, allow specific diagnosis and timely treatment to be initiated.

A possible complication of the use of PCR is that formalin-fixed, paraffin-embedded tissue may not be an optimal source for several reasons, including DNA degradation in archival tissue. Some authors recommend not using tissue blocks that have been archived for more than 5 years. But this problem is rarely encountered, because this diagnostic consideration is usually raised in a timely fashion and rebiopsy is usually an option if required.

Another molecular diagnostic technique that can be used for detection of *M. leprae* and *M. tuberculosis* is ISH. This technique differs from PCR in that it can be used to demonstrate the presence of the organisms *directly* in sections of tissue without the need for tissue digestion or DNA extraction steps. This technique is probably more specific for active disease than is PCR amplification, but it is also less sensitive. Because these techniques have been elaborately described in earlier chapters of this book, at this juncture we only note that unlike PCR, which amplifies the *genetic* material of the microorganism being probed, ISH is an example of *signal* amplification, in which the genetic material is probed, and the signal detected is amplified by chemical or immunologic means and detected either by light (CISH™ or SISH™) or fluorescence microscopy (FISH). However, only a few species can be probed by hybridization; so, in our opinion, PCR amplification and sequencing of the 16S ribosomal RNA is currently a more robust methodology.

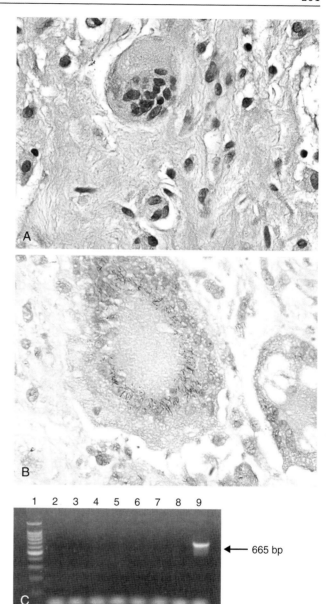

FIGURE 22-10

(A) Dermal granulomatous inflammation highlighting giant cells—microorganisms cannot be appreciated. **(B)** A Fite stain highlights the bacillary forms within the giant cell in the center. **(C)** Polymerase chain reaction amplification of *Mycobacterium tuberculosis* by acid-fast bacilli by primers (designed based on alignment of numerous 16S ribosomal DNA sequences). Lane 1 shows the standard migration ladder, and lane 9 shows *M. tuberculosis*. Findings were confirmed by DNA sequencing. (Reproduced with permission from Han XY, Pham AS, Tarrand J, et al: Rapid and accurate identification of mycobacteria by sequencing hypervariable regions of the 16S ribosomal RNA gene. Am J Clin Pathol 2002;118:796–801 © American Society for Clinical Pathology.)

Another application of PCR is in the detection of genetic microbial resistance to antimycobacterial therapy. Real-time or traditional PCR can be employed to determine the presence of point mutations that confer resistance in *M. tuberculosis* to rifampin, isoniazid, ethambutol, and streptomycin. Rifampin resistance in *M. leprae* can also be evaluated using PCR-based methods.

OTHER BACTERIAL INFECTIONS

Treponema Pallidum

A spectrum of lesions spans the primary, secondary, and tertiary stages of syphilis, and an astute diagnostician can often arrive at a reasonably accurate working diagnosis of syphilis pending confirmatory studies. The studies include dark-field examination of scrapings from genital lesions (which are more useful early in disease than the serology described later). On skin biopsy, the presence of plasma cells or lichenoid dermal infiltrates with plasma cells and neutrophils or granulomatous inflammation in various combinations can indicate the possibility of syphilis in the appropriate clinical setting (Figure 22-11). But to make the diagnosis with confidence, special studies are required because the inflammatory findings are not specific. A Warthin-Starry stain using silver impregnation of organisms is traditionally used to detect the spirochetes, but it is notoriously difficult to interpret and is technically demanding to perform. As a result, some laboratories employ immunohistochemistry using an antitreponemal antibody; this has proved to be of considerable benefit, but a negative result does not necessarily prove the absence of the microorganism and one is usually obligated to caution the clinician that "correlation with serologic studies is recommended."

Serologic studies are extremely useful, but there can be false-positive results (the rapid plasma reagin test can be positive in collagen vascular diseases, infectious mononucleosis, pregnancy, etc., and the fluorescent treponemal–antibody absorption test can also be falsely positive in collagen vascular diseases). Additional problems with the serologic testing of *active*

syphilis include the inability to detect early infection, reinfections (serology will not indicate if there is reinfection or "hangover" of antibodies from the original infection), or late stages of the disease (the sensitivities of serology for primary, secondary, and tertiary syphilis are 84%, 100%, and 96%, respectively). The use of PCR circumvents this, because it can be used directly on cutaneous lesions of primary, secondary, and tertiary syphilis. Primers directed to the DNA polymerase I antigen *(polA)* are probably more specific than targets such as *tpf1, tmpA, tmpB,* and the 47-kDa gene; in contrast to *polA,* these latter genes definitely require confirmation by DNA sequencing. All of this is not to imply that traditional serologic methods should not be employed; rather, one should be cognizant of the inherent limitations and thus the role for PCR-based methodologies.

Lyme Disease

The diagnosis of *Borrelia burgdorferi* rests upon the clinical picture, serology, and culture (taken from the border of the expansile erythema chronicum migrans lesion). A chronic form of this skin lesion, acrodermatitis chronica atrophicans, is described in Europe but rarely encountered in North America. The clinical presentation of the skin lesions are classic, but the biopsy findings are nonspecific and diagnosis requires additional confirmation. Microbial culture can take several weeks and requires 6 weeks of incubation and monitoring before it can be deemed definitely negative. Serology, detecting immunoglobulin M and G to *Borrelia,* is useful, but there are false-negative tests earlier in the disease process, and there can be false-positive tests (e.g., in infectious mononucleosis). Furthermore, these tests only indicate exposure to *Borrelia* and thus are of limited use in endemic areas. In principle, *B. burgdorferi* is an attractive target for amplification by PCR in either traditional or

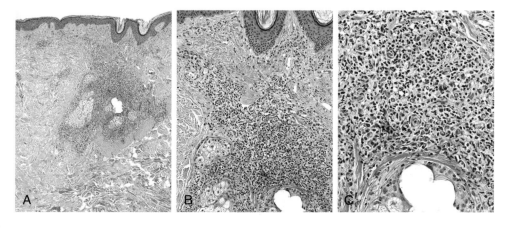

FIGURE 22-11

Secondary syphilis at progressively higher magnifications **(A–C)** shows a perivascular and periadnexal mixed lymphocytic infiltrate with prominent plasma cells. The histologic findings are somewhat suggestive but entirely nonspecific and require confirmatory studies.

TABLE 23-3

Genes Commonly Affected by CpG-Island Methylation

Gene	Sensitivity	Specificity	Function
MLH1	72%	98%	DNA mismatch repair protein
CDKN2A	90%	81%	Cell cycle inhibitor
CRABP1	99%	80%	Cellular retinoic acid–binding protein
IGF-2	97%	89%	Insulin-like growth factor 2
CACNA1G	98%	92%	Voltage-dependent calcium channel
NEUROG1	98%	82%	Transcription factor
RUNX3	97%	93%	Transcription factor
SOCS1	72%	93%	Negative regulation of cell signaling

Some pathologists, clinicians, and basic scientists have suggested that CRCs be classified according to the presence or absence of MSI and CIMP for prognostic, as well as therapeutic, purposes (Table 23-4).

Using these molecular alterations, many groups have attempted to develop screening methods to detect premalignant lesions (e.g., *APC* or *KRAS* mutations). The goal would be to develop a highly sensitive, specific, and inexpensive stool or blood screening test. Although much progress has been made, these screening tests are years from clinical use because of their high costs and low sensitivity. In addition, attempts have been made to develop a molecular-based prognostic test. Certain microarray gene signatures are associated with poor prognosis or resistant to certain chemotherapeutic agents; however, currently it is not practical to perform these tests on all CRCs. Research is under way to develop inexpensive microarray chips that would make this possible.

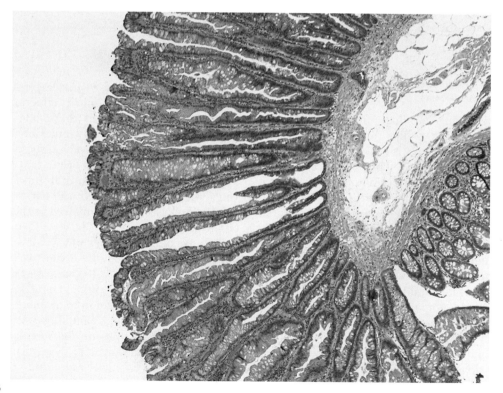

FIGURE 23-6

Sessile serrated polyp or adenoma. These serrated lesions are distinguished from hyperplastic polyps by their large size, predominantly right-sided location, prominent dilatation at the base, growth along the muscularis mucosae, and mild epithelial atypia.

TABLE 23-4

Colon Cancer Stratified by CIMP and MSI Status[a]

Feature	Group 1	Group 2	Group 3	Group 4
CIMP	+/−	+/−	+++	+++
MSI	+/−	1++	+/−	+++
Associated genetic syndrome	FAP	HNPCC[b]	?	?
Precursor lesion	TA	TA	SSP > TA	SSP >> TA
Ploidy	An >> Dip	Dip >> An	Dip > An	Dip >> An
Location	Left >> Right	Right >> Left	Right > Left	Right >> Left
Histology	Dirty necrosis, tumor budding	Poor differentiation, tumor-infiltrating lymphocytes, Crohn's-like reaction	Poor differentiation, mucinous, serration	Poor differentiation, mucinous, serration, circumscribed, tumor-infiltrating lymphocytes
Gender	M > F	M > F	F > M	F > M
Incidence	75–80%	~2%	~5%	10–15%
Clinical outcome	Variable	Possibly improved	Poor (limited data)	Possibly improved
Mutated genes	*APC, KRAS, TP53*	*MLH1, MSH2, MSH6, or PMS2*	*BRAF (V600E)*	*BRAF (V600E)*
5-FU treatment	Responsive	Resistant	Partially responsive (limited data)	Resistant (limited data)

[a] CIMP, CpG-island methylator phenotype; FAP, familial adenomatous polyposis; FU, fluorouracil; HNPCC, hereditary nonpolyposis colon cancer; MSI, microsatellite instability; SSP, sessile serrated polyp; TA, tubular adenoma.
[b] Group 2 consists of exclusively HNPCC/Lynch syndrome patients.

INFLAMMATORY BOWEL DISEASE–ASSOCIATED DYSPLASIA OR CARCINOMA

Patients with long-standing idiopathic IBD are among the highest risk groups for developing CRC. Patients with ulcerative colitis (UC) have a 0.3% annual risk of developing CRC. The incidence of CRC in patients with Crohn's disease is more difficult to assess; however, those with extensive colonic involvement seem to have a similar risk as UC patients. Besides the presence of chronic inflammation, many factors influence the development of CRC in IBD patients, including age at onset, extent of disease, duration of disease, and family history of CRC. Whereas both sporadic and IBD-associated CRCs can develop through adenomatous polyps, patients with IBD also develop flat dysplastic lesions. Sporadic and IBD-associated CRCs develop through mutations or silencing of similar genes; however, some significant differences in the sequence of genetic alterations are perhaps related to the presence of the chronic inflammatory background in IBD patients. Mutations in *TP53* are a relatively early finding in IBD patients

and can even be found in histologically normal colonic mucosa. The chronic production of reactive oxygen species is thought to be one the principle mechanisms leading to early mutations in *TP53*. Aneuploidy also occurs relatively early, whereas mutations in *APC* and *KRAS* occur late in neoplastic progression. In addition, chronic inflammation activates the antiapoptotic NF-κB pathway, which in animal models of IBD is involved in the development of CRC.

Because of the high risk of CRC development, IBD patients are enrolled in extensive colonoscopic screening programs 8 to 10 years after diagnosis. It is recommended that 40 random mucosal biopsies be taken throughout the colon to evaluate for dysplasia. Even with this thorough sampling protocol, flat areas of dysplasia can be missed. The Vienna classification recognizes five categories of dysplasia: negative, indefinite, low-grade, high-grade, and invasive carcinoma. Similar to the diagnosis of dysplasia in Barrett's esophagus, there is significant interobserver variation in the diagnosis of dysplasia, particularly at the lower end of the spectrum. Endoscopic detection of dysplastic foci is also more difficult in IBD patients than in patients with Barrett's esophagus. Therefore, a search is needed for molecular markers to predict patients who harbor dysplastic lesions and those who will progress to invasive carcinoma.

Immunohistochemical analysis of mucosal biopsies for p53 has been investigated as a tool to identify high-risk patients. Mutations in *TP53* commonly lead to mutant protein that is resistant to degradation and thus accumulates in the cell. Therefore, increased p53 expression by immunohistochemistry can be a surrogate for identifying *TP53* mutations. Some studies have shown a correlation between immunohistologic detection of p53 expression and progression to dysplasia; however, these studies are retrospective, limited, and do not provide a high degree of specificity. Studies measuring DNA content by flow cytometry found a high rate of aneuploidy in random biopsies obtained from patients with long-standing, extensive UC. Aneuploidy correlated directly with dysplasia and was thought to indicate a high-risk colon. More recently, analysis of DNA fingerprints using inter-simple sequence repeat PCR and arbitrarily primed PCR has been used to identify UC patients who have a high likelihood of developing dysplasia or carcinoma. These PCR reactions are used to determine the presence of genomic instability. Using this technique, patients who progressed to dysplasia had evidence of genomic instability even in nondysplastic mucosa, whereas normal controls and UC patients without dysplasia did not. These findings suggest that analysis of a few biopsies by this method may help identify patients who will progress to dysplasia or carcinoma. Analysis of telomere length by in situ confocal microscopy performed on random biopsies was also able to separate UC progressors from nonprogressors. Telomere length is significantly shorter in biopsies of nondysplastic mucosa from patients with dysplasia than from UC patients without dysplasia and from normal controls. Short telomeres can contribute to genomic instability because of their tendency to fuse, resulting in cycles of chromatin bridge breakage and fusion. Despite these advances, no current molecular test can provide a simple and cost-effective way of identifying at-risk patients.

STOMACH

Gastrointestinal Stromal Tumors

The discovery of the pathogenesis and activating mutations of GI stromal tumors (GISTs) is one of pathology's greatest success stories, because GISTs are the paradigm for molecular-based diagnosis and treat-ment of solid tumors. Although 50% to 70% of GISTs arise in the stomach, it is important to note that GISTs may occur anywhere in the GI tract, as well as other intra-abdominal locations such as the mesentery and omentum. Also, variations among GISTs of different anatomic locations exist. Histologically, epithelioid variants of GISTs are more common in the stomach, whereas collagen condensation (so-called skenoid fibers) is more typical of GISTs originating in the small bowel. More importantly, their behavior is different: multivariate analysis of more than 1000 stromal tumors at the Armed Forces Institute of Pathology showed that tumor location was an independent predictor of outcome. Most GISTs arising in the stomach are benign, but half of small bowel GISTs are best categorized as malignant or aggressive. As data continues to be collected on these relatively rare tumors, GISTs may eventually be categorized independently based on their location of origin.

In 1983, Mazur and Clark proposed the ambiguous term *stromal tumor* to describe these lesions. By the late 1990s, the mystery of the GIST began to unfold when they were shown to share both immunophenotypic and genetic characteristics with the interstitial cells of Cajal, also known as the pacemaker cells of the gut. Strong *KIT* expression was shown to be present in interstitial cells of Cajal, as well as hematopoietic stem cells, mast cells, and melanocytes. Hirota et al. were the first to report the expression of c-Kit protein (CD117 antigen) as a result of activating mutations in the *KIT* proto-oncogene within GISTs, thus providing a powerful diagnostic tool by which GISTs could be differentiated from smooth muscle tumors and other spindle cell neoplasms of the GI tract by their immunoreactivity.

c-Kit is a transmembrane tyrosine kinase receptor normally regulated by binding of the c-Kit ligand (also known as the stem cell factor or kit ligand) to the extracellular portion of the receptor. Ligand binding results in homodimerization of two c-Kit molecules. This structural change results in activation and stimulation of multiple intracellular signaling pathways, including those that upregulate cell proliferation and downregulate apoptosis. Mutations of *KIT* result in ligand-independent (spontaneous) receptor activation. Around the same time that these activating *KIT* mutations were first being described as the driving force behind the neoplastic growth of GISTs, a new drug, STI571, was emerging. Now known by its trade name, Gleevec™ (Novartis), or imatinib, STI571 was originally designed to specifically target and inhibit the Abl tyrosine kinase present in most chronic myelogenous leukemia patients. Eventually, it was realized that imatinib was able to inhibit the activity of several tyrosine kinase families, including c-Kit, thus providing a treatment option for GISTs.

In 2002, the U.S. Food and Drug Administration approved the use of imatinib for patients with metastatic GISTs. The natural history of GISTs is characteristic, with recurrence at the resection site, intra-abdominal spread, and ultimately liver metastasis, whereas lymph node metastasis is rare. Predicting which GISTs will metastasize is not always straightforward, because even morphologically low-grade GISTs have been shown to reoccur many years after resection. Therefore, consensus guidelines for GIST prognosis established during a National Institutes of Health– and National Cancer Institute–sponsored workshop (2002) categorized these lesions by "risk of progression" rather than as simply benign or malignant. Tumor size and mitotic rate were the two dominant factors used for risk stratification. Early studies had shown that the type of *KIT* mutation might have some effect on prognosis; however, results are conflicting and may not have accounted for progression because of secondary mutations in Kit. This is not to say that screening for kinase mutations in suspected GISTs is not important. The presence of a mutation provides confirmation of the diagnosis at the molecular level. Furthermore, the type of kinase mutation predicts the clinical response to treatment with imatinib.

Mutations in *KIT* are found in approximately 80% of GISTs. The most common mutation in all anatomic locations occurs in exon 11, but mutations are also well documented in exons 9, 13, and 17. Although point mutations, deletions, and insertions have all been described, observed *KIT* mutations are invariably inframe. Although the result is only a slightly altered protein structure, the mutant kinase isoform results in the constitutive tyrosine activity seen in these tumors. A subset of GISTs (7% to 8%) have a normal *KIT* gene but have activating mutations in the gene for the related tyrosine kinase receptor, platelet-derived growth factor-α (*PDGFR*-α). *PDGFR*-α mutations have been found in exons 12, 14, and 18. The remaining GISTs have no detectable mutations in either *KIT* or *PDGFR*-α. Although only accounting for approximately 10% of cases, GISTs with wild-type *KIT* or *PDGFR*-α are common in the pediatric population and in type I neurofibromatosis (NF1) patients. Corless et al. have proposed that GISTs be classified molecularly, especially because the mutation status predicts clinical response to imatinib (Table 23-5).

Although *KIT* and *PDGFR*-α are highly homologous, histologic and clinical differences between GISTs are driven by mutations in these two kinases. Unlike *KIT*-mutated GISTs, *PDGFR*-α-mutated GISTs often have low expression levels of c-Kit and therefore can be weak or negative by immunohistochemical staining with anti-CD117. Distinct histologic features of *PDGFR*-α-mutated GISTs include an epithelioid phenotype, myxoid stroma, multinucleated giant cells, and rhabdoid cells. Finally, these tumors almost exclusively

TABLE 23-5
Molecular Classification of GISTs

Sporadic GISTs *KIT* Mutation	Response to Imatinib
Exon 11	Best response to imatinib
Exon 9	Intermediate response to imatinib
Exon 13	Sensitive to imatinib in vitro, clinical responses observed
Exon 17	Sensitive to imatinib in vitro, clinical responses observed
PDGFR-α Mutation	
Exon 12	Sensitive to imatinib in vitro, clinical responses observed
Exon 14	Sensitive to imatinib in vitro, no documented clinical response (too rare)
Exon 18	D842V has poor response to imatinib; other mutations are sensitive
Wild Type	
	Poor response to imatinib

GIST, gastrointestinal stromal tumor; *PDGFR*-α; platelet-derived growth factor-α.

occur in the stomach. Denaturing high-performance liquid chromatography, a highly sensitive method for detection of both deletions and point mutation, followed by sequencing may be warranted in CD117-negative gastric tumors highly suspicious by histologic examination for GIST, because imatinib remains a treatment option for some *PDGFR*-α-mutated GISTs (Table 23-5 and Figure 23-7).

Although mutations of *KIT* and *PDGFR*-α are mutually exclusive in primary, untreated GISTs, treated GISTs can acquire additional mutations and can lose their c-Kit positivity by immunohistochemistry. These additional mutations may play a role in drug resistance to imatinib. As additional tyrosine kinase inhibitors become available, the need for mutation testing will increase, because drug options may be tailored to both primary and treated GISTs for optimal therapeutic effect.

HEREDITARY DIFFUSE GASTRIC CANCER

Although even rarer than GISTs, hereditary diffuse gastric cancer (HDGC) is an equally interesting story in the field of molecular diagnostics. Germline mutations of the E-cadherin gene, *CDH1,* are highly penetrant,

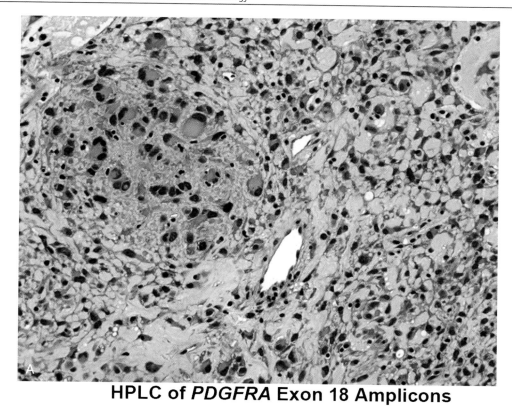

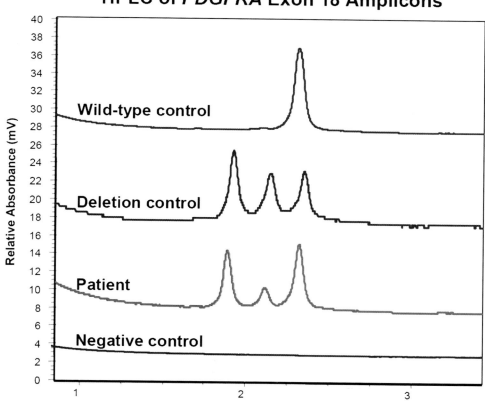

FIGURE 23-7

Platelet-derived growth factor-α (*PDGFR*-α)–mutated gastrointestinal stromal tumor. **(A)** Hematoxylin and eosin section of a gastric mass showing a predominantly epithelioid neoplasm in a myxoid stromal background. Numerous multinucleated giant cells with focal rhabdoid features are also present. Immunostaining with CD117 was negative. **(B)** High-performance liquid chromatography showing evidence of *PDGFR*-α exon 18 deletion (courtesy of Heinrich-Corless Laboratories, Oregon Health & Sciences University); confirmed by sequencing (*PDGFR*-α exon 18; deletion DIMII 842–845).

with a specific phenotype of diffuse, signet-ring cell morphology. Molecular diagnostics is warranted for early detection in carriers and provides the potential for genetic counseling in other family members.

About 2% to 8% of all gastric cancers arise from inherited gastric cancer syndromes. Although both intestinal and diffuse types of hereditary gastric cancer exist, most families with autosomal dominant familial gastric cancer develop diffuse, poorly differentiated (linitis plastica) tumors. *Hereditary diffuse gastric cancer* is the term given to families predisposed to this morphologically distinct form of gastric cancer.

In 1999, the International Gastric Cancer Linkage Consortium (IGCLC) met to define the criteria for a diagnosis of HDGC (Table 23-6). Using these strict criteria, approximately one third of HDGC families have been found to carry a germline mutation in the tumor suppressor gene *CDH1* on chromosome 16q22.1 that encodes the E-cadherin protein. To date, more than 50 *CDH1* mutations have been described in diverse ethnic populations. These mutations span the entire coding region of the E-cadherin gene, with few repeat sites in different families. This differs from the reported range of somatic mutations in sporadic diffuse gastric cancer, which tend to cluster at the exon 7 to 9 region. Furthermore, there is a heterogeneous nature to the documented mutations in hereditary gastric cancer, including point mutations, deletions, and insertions.

The *CDH1* mutation is highly specific for families who meet the IGCLC criteria for HDGC and has not been described in families with inherited intestinal-type gastric cancer. This is not a surprising finding, considering E-cadherin's role as a cell adhesion and signaling molecule essential to cell differentiation and normal epithelial cell architecture.

Gastric cancers that occur in *CDH1* mutation carriers have abnormal or absent E-cadherin expression. However, decreased expression of E-cadherin is not specific to HDGC. Loss of E-cadherin has been well documented in sporadic diffuse gastric cancer and lobular breast cancer. In HDGC families, the most common malignancy other than diffuse gastric cancer is lobular breast cancer. Therefore, Brooks-Wilson et al. (2004) revised the original IGCLC criteria for *CHD1* mutation testing (Table 23-6). Unlike the "late event" loss of E-cadherin expression expected from a somatic mutation, both gastric and lobular breast cancer associated with HDGC are felt to be a result of an early, potentially initiating event caused by the germline *CDH1* mutation.

The current hypothesis to explain the mechanism by which these autosomal dominant susceptibility cancers lose their *CDH1* heterozygosity, and thus their E-cadherin expression, involves a "two-hit" mutation theory. *CDH1* germline mutation carriers are assumed to have normal gastric mucosa with retention of E-cadherin expression until the second *CDH1* allele is "hit" by inactivation or downregulation. Hypermethylation of the *CDH1* promoter is a common, but not exclusive, mechanism. The result of this "second hit" is multifocal tumor clusters with loss of E-cadherin expression (Figure 23-8). Additional genetic events and changes in microenvironment most likely play a role in the progression to invasion.

The *CDH1* mutation in HDGC families is highly penetrant, and tumors present at a relatively early age. Male carriers of a germline *CDH1* mutation have a 40% to 67% lifetime risk of symptomatic gastric cancer, and female carriers have a 60% to 83% lifetime risk. Female carriers also have a 39% to 52% lifetime risk of breast cancer. Regardless of gender, the average age of diagnosis of gastric cancer is 38.

The following IGCLC guidelines were developed to support clinical management of families felt to be predisposed to gastric cancer: (1) genetic counseling and testing for the *CDH1* mutation should be offered to any family that meets the criteria of diagnosis for HDGC, and (2) those that choose to undergo E-cadherin testing must be provided pre- and post-testing genetic counseling by health care professionals experienced in cancer genetics.

HDGC surveillance is evolving; nevertheless, current options provide low sensitivity because of the insidious, multifocal growth pattern of diffuse gastric cancer within endoscopically normal gastric mucosa. Of the 40 "prophylactic gastrectomies" performed in patients known to carry the *CDH1*

TABLE 23-6

(Revised) Criteria for CDH1 Molecular Genetic Testing

1[a] Two or more cases of gastric cancer in a family, with at least one diffuse gastric cancer diagnosed before age 50

2[a] Three or more cases of gastric cancer in a family, with at least one diffuse gastric cancer, independent of age of onset

3[b] An individual diagnosed with diffuse gastric cancer before 35–45 years of age

4[c] An individual diagnosed with both diffuse gastric cancer and lobular breast cancer (no other criteria met)

5[c] One family member diagnosed with diffuse gastric cancer and another with lobular breast cancer (no other criteria met)

6[c] One family member diagnosed with diffuse gastric cancer and another with signet-ring cell colon cancer (no other criteria met)

[a] International Gastric Cancer Linkage Consortium criteria.
[b] Varies among literature.
[c] Additional revisions by Brooks-Wilson et al. (2004).

mutation reported in the literature, more than 80% have demonstrated occult intramucosal signet-ring cell adenocarcinoma despite normal endoscopic appearance and no evidence of tumor on random biopsies (Figure 23-8). These findings, combined with the currently limited screening procedures and tests for HDGC patients, make prophylactic gastrectomy a reasonable clinical option. Thus, an accurate genetic test is essential in guiding clinical decision making.

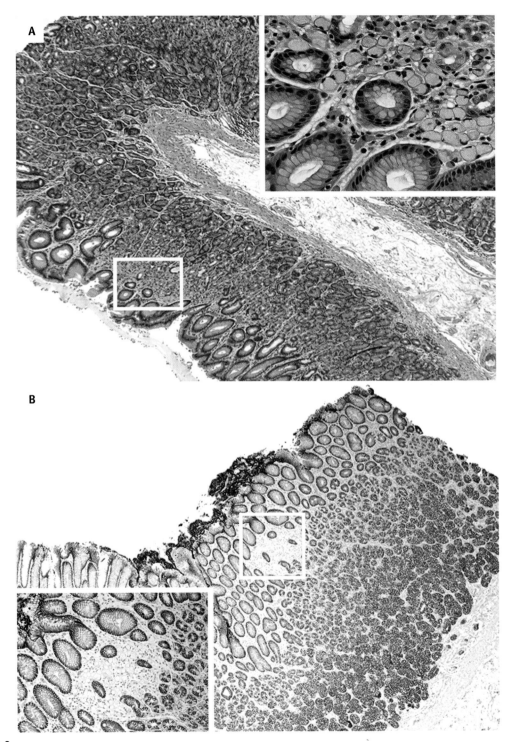

FIGURE 23-8

Multifocal intramucosal signet-ring cell adenocarcinoma in a prophylactic gastrectomy specimen from a 36-year-old male with a known *CDH1* mutation (unpublished case). **(A)** Hematoxylin and eosin section of a grossly normal-appearing stomach illustrates the insidious nature of this disease. **(B)** Focal absence of E-cadherin staining highlights the tumor cluster.

Ideally, genetic testing should begin with an index case with an established diagnosis of diffuse gastric or lobular breast cancer, although this may not be an option in all affected families. Because of the broad spectrum and distribution of *CDH1* mutations, all 16 coding exons and associated exon–intron junctions of the gene must be amplified, followed by direct DNA sequence analysis. Once the mutation is confirmed, at-risk family members can then be offered more targeted testing by DNA sequence analysis of the mutated region of the *CDH1* gene previously identified in the proband. It is important to note that this method will miss the regions of genes not analyzed (noncoding exon sequences, intron sequences other than the splice junctions, and upstream and downstream sequences, as well as large deletions or duplications).

ESOPHAGUS: BARRETT'S ESOPHAGUS

Replacement of the native esophageal squamous mucosa with a metaplastic intestinal type mucosa, Barrett's esophagus, is seen in 1.6% of the general population and 10% of patients with symptoms of gastroesophageal reflux. The diagnosis requires not only the presence of glandular epithelium with goblet cells but also the endoscopic evidence of intestinal metaplasia (although this is being challenged by some experts). Barrett's esophagus progresses through a metaplasia–dysplasia–carcinoma sequence, and patients with Barrett's esophagus have a 30- to 60-fold increased risk of developing invasive adenocarcinoma. Therefore, patients with Barrett's esophagus are enrolled in intensive endoscopic surveillance programs. Biopsy specimens are evaluated for the presence of dysplasia. When present, the degree of dysplasia must be evaluated. Dysplasia is graded according to five recognized categories: negative for dysplasia, indefinite for dysplasia, low-grade dysplasia, high-grade dysplasia, and invasive carcinoma. An accurate and reproducible diagnosis of the grade of dysplasia can be extremely challenging even for expert GI pathologists, particularly at the lower end of the spectrum. Many authors regard patients with high-grade dysplasia as having a high risk for invasive carcinoma somewhere in their esophagus; however, the natural history of low-grade dysplasia is less clear. Less is known about the molecular events that lead to esophageal dysplasia and carcinoma than in the colon. *TP53* and p16[INK4A] mutations are often found, and CpG-island methylation of tumor suppressor genes such as *APC, TERT, RUNX3,* and *TIMP3* has been described.

Numerous immunohistochemical markers such as p53, P504, MUC2, MUC1, cyclin D1, p16, and Ki-67 have been employed to aid in the diagnosis of dysplasia and to determine a patient's risk of developing progressive disease. These efforts have only met with limited success. Mutations in *TP53* typically lead to accumulation of the mutated protein, thus allowing the immunohistochemical demonstration of nuclear p53 accumulation to serve as a surrogate for a gene mutation. Indeed, immunohistologic p53 expression is usually absent in low-grade dysplasia but present in most cases of high-grade dysplasia and adenocarcinoma. In addition, increased p53 expression by immunohistochemistry was able to predict those patients with low-grade dysplasia who have a high risk of progression to high-grade dysplasia or invasive carcinoma; however, the sensitivity was relatively low (<40%). But it must be kept in mind that increased expression of p53 is not always a surrogate for a gene mutation, because false positives caused by numerous stimuli can increase p53. Indeed, some adenocarcinomas with increased p53 expression have no evidence of a mutation in *TP53*.

In a recent study, analysis of loss of heterozygosity at 8q24 *(c-Myc),* 9p21 (p16[INK4A]), 17q11.2 *(Her2/ neu),* and 20q13.2 by FISH was able to detect patients with dysplasia and adenocarcinoma. Moreover, the authors proposed that it was possible to discriminate between low- and high-grade dysplasia because low-grade dysplasia had a high percentage of loss at 9p21 but no significant chromosomal gains, whereas high-grade dysplasia and adenocarcinoma had chromosomal gains at multiple loci. Dysplastic Barrett's esophagus and adenocarcinoma are also associated with aneuploidy and an increased G2/M fraction (indicated by increased tetraploid cells) measured by flow cytometry. Moreover, 70% of patients with aneuploidy or increased G2/M fraction during initial endoscopic evaluation developed high-grade dysplasia or invasive carcinoma, whereas patients with no abnormalities did not. However, these testing methodologies are not widely available, and their adoption for routine clinical use is unlikely in the near future. Thus, endoscopic and routine histologic evaluation remains the mainstay of diagnosis.

SMALL BOWEL

Numerous inflammatory and malabsorptive disorders, both infectious and noninfectious, can be diagnosed by light microscopic examination of a duodenal mucosal biopsy obtained through endoscopy. However, for many infectious diseases, stool samples must be obtained for ova and parasite examination or cultures, and occasionally PCR or other DNA-based molecular tests are available to achieve a precise diagnosis on these specimens. These disease entities are beyond the scope of this chapter; many are discussed in other portions of this textbook.

Whipple's disease, a quite rare bacterial infection caused by *Tropheryma whipplei* that most often involves the GI tract, can be diagnosed on mucosal biopsy samples using a combination of histochemical and molecular techniques. The infection is insidious and presents with protean clinical manifestations, making diagnosis difficult. Culture of the organism from stool samples or other bodily fluids is extremely difficult and is not yet available as a diagnostic test.

Examination of a mucosal biopsy in an affected patient may reveal clusters of foamy macrophages in the lamina propria. A periodic acid Schiff stain will demonstrate clumps of the bacteria within the macrophages, or electron microscopic examination can be performed to identify the rod-shaped organisms. Unfortunately, the organisms may be sparse and patchy, and even multiple biopsies may miss the infection. Antibodies for the immunohistochemical detection of the organism in paraffin-embedded tissues are not yet widely commercially available. However, a variety of PCR-based assays targeting the 16S to 23S intergenic region of the *T. whipplei* genome have recently been developed, including a highly sensitive quantitative real-time PCR methodology. These methods can be used to assay other tissues and bodily fluids, including stool and saliva.

PANCREAS

Although the incidence of pancreatic cancer is only 10 per 100,000 people, it is the fourth leading cause of cancer deaths in the United States because most patients (80%) present with metastatic disease. Fine-needle aspiration, the preferred method of diagnosing solid pancreatic lesions, is sensitive (60% to 95%) and specific (100%) in the hands of an experienced endoscopic ultrasonographer and cytopathologist. Ancillary diagnostic techniques have been proposed based on the molecular pathogenesis of pancreatic adenocarcinoma; however, no single molecular abnormality can be used to accurately diagnose all pancreatic carcinomas, because there appear to be multiple pathways to pancreatic neoplasia. Ductal adenocarcinoma is thought to arise through preinvasive lesions termed PanIN-1A through PanIN-3. Early preinvasive lesions harbor mutations in *KRAS* and p21, whereas mutations in *TP53*, p16^{INK4A}, *DPC4/SMAD4*, and *BRCA2* are relatively late findings. An increase in telomerase activity is also common in pancreatic ductal adenocarcinomas. Telomerase is an important enzyme that adds DNA repeats to the ends of chromosomes, termed *telomeres*. Short

telomeres are indicative of replicative senescence; thus, long telomeres formed as a result of increased telomerase activity can promote tumorigenesis.

Invasive lesions arising in association with intraductal papillary mucinous tumors may arise through a different molecular pathway than ductal adenocarcinomas, because mutations in p16^{INK4A}, *SMAD4*, and *TP53* are relatively uncommon, although *KRAS* mutations and increased telomerase activity are seen in a high proportion of lesions. There is evidence that malignant transformation in intraductal papillary mucinous tumors may proceed through CpG-island methylation of tumor suppressor gene promoters. Little is known about the molecular progression in mucinous cystic neoplasms.

Hereditary forms of pancreatic cancer also exist. Patients with *BRCA2* mutations, PJS, and dysplastic nevus syndrome have an increased risk of pancreatic cancer over the general population. Recently, a mutation in a new gene, *PALLD*, which encodes palladin protein, has been described in a family with a high incidence of pancreatic cancer inherited in an autosomal dominant fashion. Palladin functions as a component of the cytoskeleton framework and is overexpressed in many pancreatic carcinoma cell lines, as well as in some sporadic carcinomas, and may represent a novel pathway to pancreatic neoplasia.

Molecular tests based on the high incidence of *KRAS* mutations and increased telomerase activity have been developed but are not routinely available in many diagnostic laboratories. Screening for codon 12 mutations in *KRAS*, along with loss of heterozygosity analysis at six tumor suppressor loci (retinoblastoma interacting zinc finger, von Hippel-Lindau, *APC*, p16^{INK4A}, *PTEN*, and *TP53*), was able to accurately separate all cases of pancreatic adenocarcinoma and cholangiocarcinoma from inflammatory conditions in a recent study. However, other researchers have found *KRAS* mutations in chronic pancreatitis, throwing its utility as a diagnostic marker into question. Two recent studies suggest that analysis of ploidy by FISH, as well as DNA content by Feulgen dye incorporation, may be helpful when the conventional cytologic analysis yields equivocal results. In these studies, trisomy 7 by FISH and a DNA content greater than 1.89 was highly suggestive of malignancy. However, chromosomal gains or losses should still be interpreted with caution, because ductal cells from chronic pancreatitis patients have been demonstrated to exhibit chromosome instability.

Increased telomerase activity is thought to be a more specific marker of invasive adenocarcinoma, because it has not been shown to be increased in inflammatory diseases. Telomerase activity can be measured using quantitative real-time reverse transcriptase–PCR or by a semiquantitative telomeric repeat amplification assay. In these molecular tests, a small amount of protein isolated from a cytology specimen is used to synthesize telomeric repeats onto a DNA substrate. The modified substrate is then amplified in a PCR reaction. Increasing amounts of PCR product correlate with the level of telomerase activity in the sampled lesion. In one study, the sensitivity for the detection of malignancy by the semiquantitative telomerase assay was 79% with a specificity of 100%. Importantly, increased telomerase activity was also found in six of seven pancreatic adenocarcinomas in which the cytology was negative. Thus, a combination of cytologic analysis, measurement of telomerase activity, and *KRAS* mutations may soon be used to increase the sensitivity of endoscopic ultrasonography.

LIVER

Most diagnostic liver biopsies are performed to evaluate hepatic medical diseases such as viral (hepatitis A, B, and C) and autoimmune hepatitis, steatohepatitis, and chronic cholestatic disorders such as primary biliary cirrhosis and primary sclerosing cholangitis. At present, these disorders do not require sophisticated molecular diagnostic testing to be performed on the liver tissue obtained. Instead, a variety of serologic and PCR tests are performed on serum samples as diagnostic and prognostic markers. These tests are beyond the scope of this chapter. Likewise, diagnostic testing for most common metabolic disorders of the liver, including α-1-antitrypsin deficiency and Wilson's disease, are performed on serum samples rather than on tissue samples. However, two inherited disorders with major hepatic manifestations, glycogen storage disease and genetic hemochromatosis, are discussed later, because testing often involves the use of liver tissue samples.

At present, the diagnosis of most primary hepatic tumors also does not require the use of molecular testing methods on tissue samples. Hepatocellular carcinoma, the most common malignant tumor of the liver, usually occurs in the setting of established cirrhosis and is most common with cirrhosis caused by chronic HBV or HCV infection, steatohepatitis, and genetic hemochromatosis. Although there is accumulating evidence that the molecular pathogenesis of hepatocellular carcinoma differs according to the cause of cirrhosis, currently none of the implicated genetic and signaling pathway defects are useful for diagnostic purposes. Instead, the diagnosis of hepatocellular carcinoma is usually based on hematoxylin and eosin examination and commonly available immunohistologic tests. Because albumin is synthesized only by hepatocytes, an in situ hybridization test for albumin messenger RNA can be used to document hepatocellular origin of a tumor.

The diagnosis of hepatoblastoma, the most common childhood malignant tumor, also is based on routine light microscopic examination and determination of the serum α-fetoprotein level.

No molecular marker of prognosis is in current use for hepatocellular carcinoma or hepatoblastoma. However, because of significant association between familial adenomatosis polyposis and hepatoblastoma, a recommendation to perform molecular testing for *APC* mutations in children with apparently sporadic hepatoblastoma has been suggested.

There has been a recent report of the use of molecular markers in the classification of hepatic adenomas to predict the likelihood of malignant degeneration to hepatocellular carcinoma. The authors reported that 46% of the adenomas they studied exhibited biallelic hepatocyte nuclear factor-1α *(HNF1α)* mutations and 14% exhibited β-catenin mutations, but none of the nearly 100 tumors analyzed had both mutations. Histologic examination revealed marked macrovesicular steatosis in the tumors with *HNF1α* mutations, and the tumors with β-catenin mutations commonly exhibited pseudoglandular formations and mild cytologic atypia. Importantly, 46% of the adenomas with β-catenin mutations contained foci of transition to hepatocellular carcinoma, compared to only 7% of the adenomas with *HNF1α* mutations. However, confirmation of these findings will be necessary before testing of adenomas for these markers is used in routine practice.

GLYCOGEN STORAGE DISEASES

The incidence of glycogen storage disease has been estimated to be 1 in 20,000 to 25,000 live births in the United States. Approximately a dozen well-defined clinical disease states are caused by genetic defects in the pathway of glycogen metabolism, but only five primarily affect the liver and produce histologic hepatic manifestations. In this subset of disorders, all but one of which are transmitted in autosomal recessive fashion, the patients generally present with hepatomegaly and are at risk for severe hypoglycemia. A liver biopsy is often performed to document abnormal glycogen deposition and to exclude other disease states. In most cases, a snap-frozen portion of the biopsy can be used for determination of the activity of the particular enzyme thought to be affected in an individual patient. Molecular diagnostic testing is possible from the biopsy sample or from DNA extracted from a skin biopsy or whole blood sample. The individual disease states are described in greater detail later (Table 23-7).

GLYCOGEN STORAGE DISEASE TYPES IA AND IB

Two severe forms of glycogen storage disease usually present in the neonatal period or in infancy with marked hepatomegaly and hypoglycemic episodes.

TABLE 23-7

Glycogen Storage Disease

Type	Gene	Clinical Features	Liver Biopsy Findings
Ia	*G6PC*, glucose-6-phosphatase	Hepatomegaly, hypoglycemic episodes, failure to thrive, growth retardation, short stature, risk of HCC	Hepatocyte swelling because of glycogen, nuclear hyperglycogenation, macrovesicular steatosis, mild portal fibrosis
Ib	*SLC374A*, glucose-6-phosphatase translocase	Same as above, neutropenia	Same as above
III	*AGL*, glycogen debrancher	15% affect liver only and 85% affect liver and muscle, fasting hypoglycemia, short stature, myopathy, cardiomyopathy	Excess glycogen, varying degrees of portal fibrosis, no steatosis
IV	Glycogen debrancher	Liver, skeletal muscle, and cardiac involvement	Fibrosis, distinctive cytoplasmic deposits (colloidal iron positive)
VI	Hepatic phosphorylase	Clinically mild, presents in adulthood	Excess glycogen, no steatosis or fibrosis
IX	*PHKB, PHKGH2,* and *PHKA2,* subunits of phosphorylase kinase	Mild hepatomegaly, fasting hyperketosis, growth retardation	Excess glycogen, no steatosis or fibrosis

HCC, hepatocellular carcinoma.

Untreated children may develop failure to thrive, growth retardation, delayed puberty, and short stature. Patients who survive into adulthood are at risk for the development of hepatic adenomas and hepatocellular carcinoma. The genetic defect responsible for glycogen storage disease type Ia occurs in the *G6PC* gene on chromosome 17q21, which codes for glucose-6-phosphatase. In glycogen storage disease type Ib, mutations of the *SLC374A* gene located on chromosome 11q23 lead to decreased activity of the glucose-6-phosphatase translocase enzyme. This defect also causes neutropenia and impairs neutrophil function, resulting in recurrent bacterial infection and GI inflammation and ulceration.

Liver biopsy specimens in both type Ia and type Ib reveal diffuse hepatocyte swelling because of excess accumulation of glycogen, nuclear hyperglycogenation, macrovesicular steatosis, and in some cases, mild portal fibrosis. Snap-frozen hepatic tissue can be assayed for glycogen content and for glucose-6-phosphatase catalytic or translocase activity. In affected individuals, the enzyme activity is reduced by more than 90%.

Targeted mutational analysis can be performed in some patient populations for which a small number of ethnic-specific mutations account for most cases. Sequence analysis of the two genes is also available in some reference laboratories. More than 75 mutations have been described for each of the two genes, most resulting in missense and nonsense sequences. Most clinical testing laboratories sequence only the exons where most (~75% to 80%) of the known mutations occur; therefore, a negative genetic test does not exclude the diagnosis. No clear genotype–phenotype correlations have been identified for glycogen storage disease type I. Heterozygotes exhibit no clinical or histologic evidence of disease, and biochemical determination of enzyme activity is unreliable in detecting carriers.

GLYCOGEN STORAGE DISEASE TYPE III

The type III form of glycogen storage disease is caused by mutation in the *AGL* gene located on chromosome 1p21, which encodes the glycogen debrancher enzyme. In about 15% of affected patients abnormal glycogen accumulation is limited to the liver, and in 85% of patients both liver and skeletal muscle (and cardiac myocytes in some) are involved. Differential transcription and alternative exon usage account for the distinct isoforms of the enzyme that are expressed in a tissue-specific fashion. The disease manifests itself during the first year of life, with fasting hypoglycemia, marked hepatomegaly, short stature, and in some patients, progressive myopathy and cardiomyopathy. Liver biopsy specimens reveal excess glycogen in hepatocytes and varying degrees of portal fibrosis but minimal steatosis (Figure 23-9). Hepatocellular carcinoma has been reported in patients with cirrhosis.

Assays for enzyme activity can be performed on snap-frozen liver tissue. Confirmation by PCR-based genetic testing on whole blood samples is available

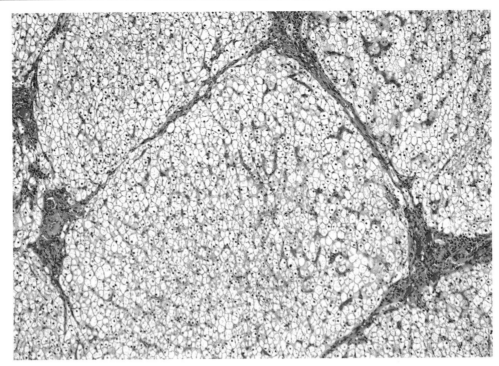

FIGURE 23-9
Glycogen storage disease type III. This native hepatectomy specimen demonstrates excess glycogen deposition in hepatocytes, as well as cirrhosis. There is no steatosis.

and is used for identifications of carriers. More than 30 mutations have been identified, most resulting in a premature stop codon. The mutations are scattered throughout the 35 exons of the gene.

Glycogen Storage Disease Type IV

The type IV disorder, which is the rarest form of glycogen storage disease involving the liver, is quite clinically heterogeneous. In many patients, skeletal or cardiac muscle involvement dominates the clinical picture, but severe hepatic involvement is also common and cirrhosis may develop in early childhood. The disease is caused by deficient branching enzyme activity. The gene is located on chromosome 3p12, but genetic testing is not available. The diagnosis rests upon assay of enzyme activity in affected tissue (liver or muscle). Confirmation on cultured skin fibroblasts is generally recommended. Liver biopsies reveal distinctive cytoplasmic deposits of amylopectin-like material, which can be highlighted by a colloidal iron stain. Progressive fibrosis may culminate in cirrhosis in some patients.

Glycogen Storage Disease Type VI

The type VI form of glycogen storage disease, which is clinically milder than the other types, usually presents in adulthood with hepatomegaly and mild to moderate hypoglycemic episodes. Confusion with hepatic glycogenosis caused by uncontrolled diabetes may occur because this disorder produces similar clinical and histologic findings. Liver biopsies demonstrate excessive hepatocellular glycogen but no steatosis or fibrosis.

A biochemical assay for hepatic phosphorylase, the defective enzyme responsible for this disorder, can be performed on snap-frozen liver tissue. Numerous splice variants and missense mutations have been described in the gene, which is located on chromosome 14q21-q22. Sequence analysis of the gene is offered by reference laboratories.

Glycogen Storage Disease Type IX

The type IX form of glycogen storage disease, which is also relatively clinically benign, develops as a result of decreased phosphorylase kinase activity caused by mutations in any of several genes that code for the subunits of the enzyme. Mutations in the *PHKB* gene on chromosome 16q12-13 or the *PHKG2* gene on chromosome 16p11-12, which encode for the α- and γ-subunits, respectively, result in a similar clinical phenotype characterized by mild hepatomegaly, fasting hyperketosis, and growth retardation, which often subside as the patient reaches adulthood. The only X-linked glycogen storage disease, caused by alteration in the α-subunit of the phosphorylase kinase protein, is caused by mutations in the *PHKA2* gene on chromosome Xp22.2-1. This disorder is phenotypically similar to the other forms of glycogen storage disease type IX.

All forms of type IX can be diagnosed by determining glycogen content and enzymatic activity in a snap-frozen sample of liver tissue. Enzymatic activity can also be determined by an assay performed on red blood cells or white blood cells from a whole blood sample. Genetic testing is not yet generally available.

HEREDITARY HEMOCHROMATOSIS

There has been a recent explosive growth in our knowledge of the molecular basis of hereditary hemochromatosis, a disease first recognized by Friedrich Daniel von Recklinghausen more than 100 years ago. In the 1970s, hereditary hemochromatosis was recognized to be an autosomal recessive disorder because of a defect in a gene located near the gene on chromosome 6 that encodes the human leukocyte antigen-A protein. Iron overload in affected patients was found to be caused by excessive absorption of iron from the small bowel, resulting in parenchymal deposition in multiple organs, particularly the liver, heart, pancreas, and joints.

Diagnosis required liver biopsy with documentation of iron deposition in hepatocytes. Iron is deposited first in the zone 1 (periportal) hepatocytes and then gradually involves the zone 2 and then zone 3 (perivenular) parenchyma. Because iron accumulates over the life of the patient, a hepatic iron index (millimoles of iron per gram of dry weight divided by the patient's age) was developed to factor in the patient's age at the time of biopsy. In the proper clinical context, a hepatic iron index of more than 1.9 was regarded as diagnostic of hereditary hemochromatosis. Quantitation of tissue iron level is performed by mass spectrophotometry performed upon a formalin-fixed, paraffin-embedded sample of liver tissue. Special handling of the tissue sample (e.g., the use of special iron-free sample containers and fixative) is no longer regarded as necessary. Although quantitative determination of hepatic iron level is becoming supplanted by the increasing use of genetic tests performed on whole blood samples, a liver biopsy is still important to stage the degree of fibrosis, document the degree of iron deposition, and guide phlebotomy treatment.

In 1996, two point mutations in the *HFE* gene, the substitutions C282Y and H63D, were identified as the basis for the most cases of hereditary hemochromatosis. Although the function of the HFE protein remained unknown, a patient who was homozygous for the C282Y substitution or the C282Y and H63D compound heterozygote was at risk for development of clinical disease. These mutations in the *HFE* gene represent the most common genetic disorder in Caucasians of northern European descent (approximately 4 per 1000).

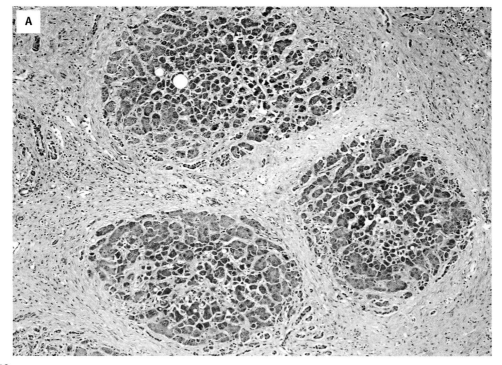

FIGURE 23-10

Juvenile hemochromatosis. **(A)** A section from an autopsy specimen from a patient with an *HJV* mutation demonstrating a micronodular pattern of cirrhosis with (trichrome stain).

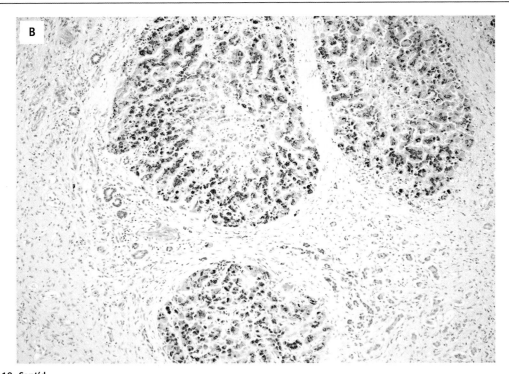

FIGURE 23-10, Cont'd.

(B) Prussian blue stain highlighting the increased deposition of iron in hepatocytes.

Soon after genetic testing became widely available, it was clear that a small proportion of patients with a clear-cut phenotype of iron overload were negative for the known *HFE* mutations. These patients tended to be significantly younger at presentation than patients with *HFE* mutations, and their disease was more severe. Over the last decade, the genetic basis for patients with so-called juvenile hemochromatosis has been elucidated. Mutation in the *HJV* gene on chromosome 1q21 is now thought to be responsible for about 90% of cases of juvenile hemochromatosis, and mutations in the *HAMP* gene on chromosome 19q13 account for the other 10% of cases. The *HAMP* gene encodes hepcidin, a protein synthesized by hepatocytes that is central to iron metabolism. Hepcidin downregulates the secretion of iron from enterocytes and macrophages by binding and degrading ferroportin, the protein responsible for iron efflux from these cells. Mutation in the *HAMP* gene causes a defective hepcidin protein, resulting in increased intestinal iron absorption and circulating iron, which in turn leads to parenchymal iron deposition and end organ damage.

The *HJV* gene encodes hemojuvelin, a protein that acts as a transcriptional regulator of hepcidin. The mutant hemojuvelin protein suppresses synthesis of hepcidin by hepatocytes, thereby causing decreased serum hepcidin levels. This results in ferroportin overactivity, which in turn produces increased intestinal iron absorption and parenchymal deposition (Figure 23-10A,B).

Mutations in either the *HAMP* or the *HJV* gene are inherited in an autosomal recessive fashion. Mutations can be detected by sequencing of the genes. No genotype phenotype correlations have been identified for the known mutations. Heterozygotes may have a subclinical abnormality in iron metabolism and may influence the phenotype of patients with *HFE* gene mutations.

Rare cases of hereditary iron overload have also been attributed to mutations in genes for transferrin receptor 2 (TFR2) and ferroportin, additional proteins important in normal iron hemostasis. Patients with mutation in the *TFR2* gene on chromosome 7q22 encoding TFR2 protein tend to present with signs and symptoms of iron overload somewhat later than patients with *HAMP* or *HJV* mutations but still at an earlier age than those with *HFE* mutations. The defective TFR2 protein results in decreased circulating hepcidin, but the mechanism is not fully understood at present. Mutations in the gene encoding ferroportin lead to an adult-onset form of hereditary hemochromatosis in which iron deposition occurs primarily in macrophages rather than parenchymal cells. Few probands have been reported in the literature for either of these two disorders, and at present diagnosis rests upon sequencing of the genes in research laboratories.

SUGGESTED READINGS

General Reading on Hereditary Colorectal Carcinoma Syndromes

Burt R, Neklason DW: Genetic testing for inherited colon cancer. Gastroenterology 2005;128(6):1696–1716.

de la Chapelle A: Genetic predisposition to colorectal cancer. Nat Rev Cancer 2004;4(10):769–780.

Kaz AM, Brentnall TA: Genetic testing for colon cancer. Nat Clin Pract Gastroenterol Hepatol 2006;3(12):670–679.

Leggett B: When is molecular genetic testing for colorectal cancer indicated? J Gastroenterol Hepatol 2002;17(4):389–393.

Hereditary Nonpolyposis Colon Cancer

Barnetson RA, Tenesa A, Farrington SM, et al: Identification and survival of carriers of mutations in DNA mismatch-repair genes in colon cancer. N Engl J Med 2006;354(26):2751–2763.

Burgart LJ: Testing for defective DNA mismatch repair in colorectal carcinoma: A practical guide. Arch Pathol Lab Med 2005;129(11):1385–1389.

Gryfe R, Kim H, Hsieh ET, et al: Tumor microsatellite instability and clinical outcome in young patients with colorectal cancer. N Engl J Med 2000;342(2):69–77.

Jass JR: Pathology of hereditary nonpolyposis colorectal cancer. Ann NY Acad Sci 2000;910:62–73; discussion 73–74.

Jass JR: Role of the pathologist in the diagnosis of hereditary nonpolyposis colorectal cancer. Dis Markers 2004;20(4–5):215–224.

Kim GP, Colangelo LH, Wieand HS, et al: Prognostic and predictive roles of high-degree microsatellite instability in colon cancer: A National Cancer Institute–National Surgical Adjuvant Breast and Bowel Project Collaborative Study. J Clin Oncol 2007;25(7):767–772.

Lagerstedt Robinson K, Liu T, Vandrocova J, et al: Lynch syndrome (hereditary nonpolyposis colorectal cancer) diagnostics. J Natl Cancer Inst 2007;99(4):291–299.

Lynch HT, Lynch JF: Lynch syndrome: History and current status. Dis Markers 2004;20(4–5):181–198.

Pawlik TM, Raut CP, Rodriguez-Bigas MA, et al: Colorectal carcinogenesis: MSI-H versus MSI-L. Dis Markers 2004;20(4–5):199–206.

Peltomaki P, Vasen H: Mutations associated with HNPCC predisposition: Update of ICG-HNPCC/INSiGHT mutation database. Dis Markers 2004;20(4–5):269–276.

Ribic CM, Sargent DJ, Moore MJ, et al: Tumor microsatellite-instability status as a predictor of benefit from fluorouracil-based adjuvant chemotherapy for colon cancer. N Engl J Med 2003;349(3):247–257.

Soreide K, Janssen EA, Söiland H, et al: Microsatellite instability in colorectal cancer. Br J Surg 2006;93(4):395–406.

Suraweera N, Duval A, Reperant M, et al: Evaluation of tumor microsatellite instability using five quasimonomorphic mononucleotide repeats and pentaplex PCR. Gastroenterology 2002;123(6):1804–1811.

Umar A, Boland CR, Terdiman JP, et al: Revised Bethesda Guidelines for hereditary nonpolyposis colorectal cancer (Lynch syndrome) and microsatellite instability. J Natl Cancer Inst 2004;96(4):261–268.

Umar A, Risinger JI, Hawk ET, Barrett JC: Testing guidelines for hereditary nonpolyposis colorectal cancer. Nat Rev Cancer 2004;4(2):153–158.

Vasen HF, Hendriks Y, de Jong AE, et al: Identification of HNPCC by molecular analysis of colorectal and endometrial tumors. Dis Markers 2004;20(4–5):207–213.

Familial Adenomatous Polyposis, Attenuated Familial Adenomatous Polyposis, and MUTYH-Associated Polyposis

Galiatsatos P, Foulkes WD: Familial adenomatous polyposis. Am J Gastroenterol 2006;101(2):385–398.

Nieuwenhuis MH, Vasen HF: Correlations between mutation site in APC and phenotype of familial adenomatous polyposis (FAP): A review of the literature. Crit Rev Oncol Hematol 2007;61(2):153–161.

Rajagopalan H, Nowak MA, Vogelstein B, Lengauer C: The significance of unstable chromosomes in colorectal cancer. Nat Rev Cancer 2003;3(9):695–701.

Rozen P, Macrae F: Familial adenomatous polyposis: The practical applications of clinical and molecular screening. Fam Cancer 2006;5(3):227–235.

Schulmann K, Pox C, Schmiegel W: The patient with multiple intestinal polyps. Best Pract Res Clin Gastroenterol 2007;21(3):409–426.

Sieber OM, Lipton L, Crabtree M, et al: Multiple colorectal adenomas, classic adenomatous polyposis, and germline mutations in MYH. N Engl J Med 2003;348(9):791–799.

Sieber OM, Segditsas S, Knudsen AL, et al: Disease severity and genetic pathways in attenuated familial adenomatous polyposis vary greatly but depend on the site of the germline mutation. Gut 2006;55(10):1440–1448.

Venesio T, Molatore S, Cattaneo F, et al: High frequency of MYH gene mutations in a subset of patients with familial adenomatous polyposis. Gastroenterology 2004;126(7):1681–1685.

Hamartomatous Polyposis Syndromes

Brosens LA, van Hattem A, Hylind LM, et al: Risk of colorectal cancer in juvenile polyposis. Gut 2007;57(5):965–967.

Chow E, Macrae F: A review of juvenile polyposis syndrome. J Gastroenterol Hepatol 2005;20(11):1634–1640.

Giardiello FM, Trimbath JD: Peutz-Jeghers syndrome and management recommendations. Clin Gastroenterol Hepatol 2006;4(4):408–415.

McGarrity TJ, Amos C: Peutz-Jeghers syndrome: Clinicopathology and molecular alterations. Cell Mol Life Sci 2006;63(18):2135–2144.

Merg A, Howe JR: Genetic conditions associated with intestinal juvenile polyps. Am J Med Genet C: Semin Med Genet 2004;129(1):44–55.

Sporadic Colorectal Carcinoma

Issa JP: CpG-island methylator phenotype in cancer. Nat Rev Cancer 2004;4(12):988–993.

Jass JR: Classification of colorectal cancer based on correlation of clinical, morphological and molecular features. Histopathology 2007;50(1):113–130.

Ogino S, Meyerhardt JA, Kawasaki T, et al: CpG-island methylation, response to combination chemotherapy, and patient survival in advanced microsatellite stable colorectal carcinoma. Virchows Arch 2007;450(5):529–537.

Ogino S, Kawasaki T, Kirkner GJ, et al: Evaluation of markers for CpG-island methylator phenotype (CIMP) in colorectal cancer by a large population-based sample. J Mol Diagn 2007;9(3):305–314.

Van Rijnsoever M, Elsaleh H, Joseph D, et al: CpG-island methylator phenotype is an independent predictor of survival benefit from 5-fluorouracil in stage III colorectal cancer. Clin Cancer Res 2003;9(8):2898–2903.

Vogelstein B, Kinzler KW: Cancer genes and the pathways they control. Nat Med 2004;10(8):789–799.

Weisenberger DJ, Siegmund KD, Campan M, et al: CpG-island methylator phenotype underlies sporadic microsatellite instability and is tightly associated with BRAF mutation in colorectal cancer. Nat Genet 2006;38(7):787–793.

Wong JJ, Hawkins NJ, Ward RL: Colorectal cancer: A model for epigenetic tumorigenesis. Gut 2007;56(1):140–148.

Inflammatory Bowel Disease–Associated Dysplasia or Carcinoma

Chen R, Rabinovitch PS, Crispin DA, et al: DNA fingerprinting abnormalities can distinguish ulcerative colitis patients with dysplasia and cancer from those who are dysplasia/cancer free. Am J Pathol 2003;162(2):665–672.

Chen R, Bronner MP, Crispin DA, et al: Characterization of genomic instability in ulcerative colitis neoplasia leads to discovery of putative tumor suppressor regions. Cancer Genet Cytogenet 2005;162:99–106.

Greten FR, Eckmann L, Greten TF, et al: IKKβ links inflammation and tumorigenesis in a mouse model of colitis-associated cancer. Cell 2004;118(3):285–296.

Itkowitz SH: Molecular biology of dysplasia and cancer in inflammatory bowel disease. Gastroenterol Clin N Am 2006;35:553–571.

Loftus EV Jr: Epidemiology and risk factors for colorectal dysplasia and cancer in ulcerative colitis. Gastroenterol Clin N Am 2006;35:517–531.

Odze RD: Pathology of dysplasia and cancer in inflammatory bowel disease. Gastroenterol Clin N Am 2006;35:533–552.

O'Sullivan JN, Bronner MP, Brentnall TA, et al: Chromosomal instability in ulcerative colitis is related to telomere shortening. Nat Genet 2002;32:280–284.

Risques R, Rabinovitch PS, Brentnall TA: Cancer surveillance in inflammatory bowel disease: New molecular approaches. Curr Opin Gastroenterol 2006;22(4):382–390.

Gastrointestinal Stromal Tumors

Connolly EM, Gaffney E, Reynolds JV: Gastrointestinal stromal tumours. Br J Surg 2003;90(10):1178–1186.

Corless CL, Schroeder A, Griffith D, et al: *PDGFR-α* mutations in gastrointestinal stromal tumors: Frequency, spectrum and in vitro sensitivity to imatinib. J Clin Oncol 2005;23(23):5357–5364.

Corless CL, Fletcher JA, Heinrich MC: Biology of gastrointestinal stromal tumors. J Clin Oncol 2004;22(18):3813–3825.

Daum O, Grossmann P, Vanecek T, et al: Diagnostic morphological features of *PDGFR-α*-mutated gastrointestinal stromal tumors: Molecular genetic and histologic analysis of 60 cases of gastric gastrointestinal stromal tumors. Ann Diagn Pathol 2007;11(1):27–33.

Druker BJ, Tamura S, Buchdunger E, et al: Effects of a selective inhibitor of the *ABL* tyrosine kinase on the growth of *BCR/ABL* positive cells. Nat Med 1996;2(5):561–566.

Emory TS, Sobin LH, Lukes L, et al: Prognosis of gastrointestinal smooth-muscle (stromal) tumors: Dependence on anatomic site. Am J Surg Pathol 1999;23(1):82–87.

Fletcher CD, Berman JJ, Corless C, et al: Diagnosis of gastrointestinal stromal tumors: A consensus approach. Int J Surg Pathol 2002;10(2):81–89.

Heinrich MC, Corless CL, Duensing A, et al: *PDGFR*-activating mutations in gastrointestinal stromal tumors. Science 2003;299(5607):708–710.

Hirota S, Isozaki K, Moriyama Y, et al: Gain-of-function mutations of c-Kit in human gastrointestinal stromal tumors. Science 1998;279(5350):577–580.

Kindblom LG, Remotti HE, Aldenborg F, Meis-Kindblom JM: Gastrointestinal pacemaker cell tumor (GIPACT): Gastrointestinal stromal tumors show phenotypic characteristics of the interstitial cells of Cajal. Am J Pathol 1998;152(5):1259–1269.

La Vecchia C, Negri E, Franceschi S, Gentile A: Family history and the risk of stomach and colorectal cancer. Cancer 1992;70(1):50–55.

Martin JF, Bazin P, Feroldi J, Cabanne F: Intramural myoid tumors of the stomach: Microscopic considerations on 6 cases. Ann Anat Pathol (Paris) 1960;5:484–497.

Mazur MT, Clark HB: Gastric stromal tumors: Reappraisal of histogenesis. Am J Surg Pathol 1983;7(6):507–519.

Miettinen M, Monihan JM, Sarlomo-Rikala M, et al: Gastrointestinal stromal tumors/smooth muscle tumors (GISTs) primary in the omentum and mesentery: Clinicopathologic and immunohistochemical study of 26 cases. Am J Surg Pathol 1999;23(9):1109–1118.

Pauls K, Merkelbach-Bruse S, Thal D, et al: *PDGFR-α*- and c-Kit-mutated gastrointestinal stromal tumours (GISTs) are characterized by distinctive histological and immunohistochemical features. Histopathology 2005;46(2):166–175.

Sakurai S, Hasegawa T, Sakuma Y, et al: Myxoid epithelioid gastrointestinal stromal tumor (GIST) with mast cell infiltrations: A subtype of GIST with mutations of platelet-derived growth factor receptor-α gene. Hum Pathol 2004;35(10):1223–1230.

Sircar K, Hewlett BR, Huizinga JD, et al: Interstitial cells of Cajal as precursors of gastrointestinal stromal tumors. Am J Surg Pathol 1999;23(4):377–389.

Stout AP: Bizarre smooth muscle tumors of the stomach. Cancer 1962;15:400–409.

Hereditary Diffuse Gastric Cancer

Berx G, Becker KF, Höfler H, van Roy F: Mutations of the human E-cadherin *(CDH1)* gene. Hum Mutat 1998;12(4):226–237.

Brooks-Wilson AR, Kaurah P, Suriano G, et al: Germline E-cadherin mutations in hereditary diffuse gastric cancer: Assessment of 42 new families and review of genetic screening criteria. J Med Genet 2004;41(7):508–517.

Caldas C, Carneiro F, Lynch HT, et al: Familial gastric cancer: Overview and guidelines for management. J Med Genet 1999;36(12):873–880.

Graziano F, Humar B, Guilford P, et al: The role of the E-cadherin gene *(CDH1)* in diffuse gastric cancer susceptibility: From the laboratory to clinical practice. Ann Oncol 2003;14(12):1705–1713.

Kaurah P, MacMillan A, Boyd N, et al: Founder and recurrent *CDH1* mutations in families with hereditary diffuse gastric cancer. JAMA 2007;297(21):2360–2372.

Oliveira C, Bordin MC, Grehan N, et al: Screening E-cadherin in gastric cancer families reveals germline mutations only in hereditary diffuse gastric cancer kindred. Hum Mutat 2002;19(5):510–517.

Pharoah PD, Guilford P, Caldas C; International Gastric Cancer Linkage Consortium: Incidence of gastric cancer and breast cancer in CDH1 (E-cadherin) mutation carriers from hereditary diffuse gastric cancer families. Gastroenterology 2001;121(6):1348–1353.

Suriano G, Yew S, Ferreira P, et al: Characterization of a recurrent germline mutation of the E-cadherin gene: Implications for genetic testing and clinical management. Clin Cancer Res 2005;11(15):5401–5409.

Barrett's Esophagus

Brankley SM, Wang KK, Harwood AR, et al: The development of a fluorescence in situ hybridization assay for the detection of dysplasia and adenocarcinoma in Barrett's esophagus. J Med Diagn 2006;8(2):260–267.

Flejou J-F, Svrcek M: Barrett's oesophagus: A pathologist's view. Histopathology 2007;50:3–14.

Keswani RN, Noffsinger A, Waxman I, Bissonnette M: Clinical use of p53 in Barrett's esophagus. Cancer Epidemiol Biomarkers Prev 2006;15(7):1243–1249.

Koppert LB, Wijnhoven BP, van Dekken H, et al: The molecular biology of esophageal adenocarcinoma. J Surg Oncol 2005;92:169–190.

Whipple's Disease

Fenollar F, Fournier PE, Raoult D, et al: R Quantitative detection of *Tropheryma whipplei* DNA by real-time PCR. J Clin Microbiol 2002;40(3):1119–1120.

Fenollar F, Fournier PE, Robert C, Raoult D: Use of genome selected repeated sequences increases the sensitivity of PCR detection of *Tropheryma whipplei*. J Clin Microbiol 2004;42(1):401–403.

Fenollar F, Puechal X, Raoult D, et al: Whipple's disease. N Engl J Med 2007;356(1):55–66.

Lepidi H, Fenollar F, Gerolami R, et al: Whipple's disease: Immunospecific and quantitative immunohistochemical study of intestinal biopsy specimens. Hum Pathol 2003;34(6):589–596.

Raoult D, Fenollar F, Birg ML, et al: Culture of *T. whipplei* from the stool of a patient with Whipple's disease. N Engl J Med 2006;355(14):1503–1505.

Rolain JM, Fenollar F, Raoult D, et al: False-positive PCR detection of *Tropheryma whipplei* in the saliva of healthy people. BMC Microbiol 2007;7:48.

Pancreatic Cancer

Cowgill SM, Muscarella P: The genetics of pancreatic cancer. Am J Surg 2003;186(3):279–286.

Hilgers W, Rosty C, Hahn SA: Molecular pathogenesis of pancreatic cancer. Hematol Oncol Clin North Am 2002;16(1):17–35, v.

Hiyama E, Kodama T, Shinbara K, et al: Telomerase activity is detected in pancreatic cancer but not in benign tumors. Cancer Res 1997;57(2):326–331.

Khalid A, Pal R, Sasatomi E, et al: Use of microsatellite marker loss of heterozygosity in accurate diagnosis of pancreaticobiliary malignancy from brush cytology samples. Gut 2004;53(12):1860–1865.

Khalid A, Finkelstein S, McGrath K, et al: Molecular diagnosis of solid and cystic lesions of the pancreas. Clin Lab Med 2005;25(1):101–116.

Kipp BR, Stadheim L, Halling SA, et al: A comparison of routine cytology and fluorescence in situ hybridization for the detection of malignant bile duct structures. Am J Gastroenterol 2004;99:1675–1681.

Mishra G, Zhao Y, Sweeney J, et al: Determination of qualitative telomerase activity as an adjunct to the diagnosis of pancreatic adenocarcinoma by EUS-guided fine-needle aspiration. Gastrointest Endosc 2006;63(4):648–654.

Moore PS, Beghelli S, Zamboni G, Scarpa A: Genetic abnormalities in pancreatic cancer. Mol Cancer 2003;2:7.

Moreno Luna LE, Kipp B, Halling KC: Advanced cytologic techniques for the detection of malignant pancreatobiliary strictures. Gastroenterology 2006;131:1064–1072.

Moskovitz AH, Linford N, Brentnall TA, et al: Chromosomal instability in pancreatic ductal cells from patients with chronic pancreatitis and pancreatic adenocarcinoma. Genes Chromosomes Cancer 2003;37: 201–206.

Niedergethmann M, Rexin M, Hildenbrand R, et al: Prognostic implications of routine, immunohistochemical, and molecular staging in resectable pancreatic adenocarcinoma. Am J Surg Pathol 2002;26(12): 1578–1587.

Pogue-Geile KL, Chen R, Bronner MP, et al: Palladin mutation causes familial pancreatic cancer and suggests a new cancer mechanism. PLoS Med 2006;3(12):2216–2228.

Sato N, Ueki T, Fukushima N, et al: Aberrant methylation of CpG islands in intraductal papillary mucinous neoplasms of the pancreas. Gastroenterology 2002;123(1):365–372.

Hepatic Tumors

Aretz S, Koch A, Uhlhaas S, et al: Should children at risk for familial adenomatous polyposis be screened for hepatoblastoma and children with apparently sporadic hepatoblastoma be screened for APC germline mutations? Pediatr Blood Cancer 2006;47(6):811–818.

Donovan A, Roy CN, Andrews NC: The ins and outs of iron homeostasis. Physiology (Bethesda) 2006;21:115–123.

Hemochromatosis

Luo JH, Ren B, Keryanov S, et al: Transcriptomic and genomic analysis of human hepatocellular carcinomas and hepatoblastomas. Hepatology 2006;44(4):1012–1024.

Pietrangelo A: Molecular insights into the pathogenesis of hereditary haemochromatosis. Gut 2006;55(4):564–568.

Swinkels DW, Janssen MC, Bergmans J, Marx JJ: Hereditary hemochromatosis: Genetic complexity and new diagnostic approaches. Clin Chem 2006;52(6):950–968.

Tiao GM, Bobey N, Allen S, et al: The current management of hepatoblastoma: A combination of chemotherapy, conventional resection, and liver transplantation. J Pediatr 2005;146(2): 204–211.

Villanueva A, Newell P, Chiang DY, et al: Genomics and signaling pathways in hepatocellular carcinoma. Semin Liver Dis 2007;27(1):55–76.

Yen AW, Fancher TL, Bowlus CL: Revisiting hereditary hemochromatosis: Current concepts and progress. Am J Med 2006;119(5):391–399.

Zucman-Rossi J, Jeannot E, Nhieu JT, et al: Genotype–phenotype correlation in hepatocellular adenoma: New classification and relationship with HCC. Hepatology 2006;43(3):515–524.

Glycogen Storage Diseases

Chou JY, Matern D, Mansfield BC, Chen YT, et al: Type I glycogen storage diseases: Disorders of the glucose-6-phosphatase complex. Curr Mol Med 2002;2(2):121–143.

Coleman RA, Winter HS, Wolf B, et al: Glycogen debranching enzyme deficiency: Long-term study of serum enzyme activities and clinical features. J Inherit Metab Dis 1992;15(6):869–881.

Demo E, Frush D, Gottfried M, et al: Glycogen storage disease type III: Hepatocellular carcinoma a long-term complication? J Hepatol 2007;46(3):492–498.

Ding JH, de Barsy T, Brown BI, et al: Immunoblot analyses of glycogen debranching enzyme in different subtypes of glycogen storage disease type III. J Pediatr 1990;116(1):95–100.

Gogus S, Kocak N, et al: Histologic features of the liver in type Ia glycogen storage disease: Comparative study between different age groups and consecutive biopsies. Pediatr Dev Pathol 2002;5(3):299–304.

McAdams AJ, Hug G, Bove KE: Glycogen storage disease, types I to X: Criteria for morphologic diagnosis. Hum Pathol 1974;5(4):463–487.

Moses SW, Parvari R: The variable presentations of glycogen storage disease type IV: A review of clinical, enzymatic and molecular studies. Curr Mol Med 2002;2(2):177–188.

Rake JP, ten Berge AM, Visser G, et al: Glycogen storage disease type Ia: Recent experience with mutation analysis, a summary of mutations reported in the literature and a newly developed diagnostic flow chart. Eur J Pediatr 2000;159(5):322–330.

Rake JP, Visser G, Labrune P, et al: Glycogen storage disease type I: Diagnosis, management, clinical course and outcome. Results of the European Study on Glycogen Storage Disease Type I (ESGSD I). Eur J Pediatr 2002;161(Suppl 1):S20–S34.

Shen JJ, Chen YT: Molecular characterization of glycogen storage disease type III. Curr Mol Med 2002;2(2):167–175.

Shin YS: Glycogen storage disease: Clinical, biochemical, and molecular heterogeneity. Semin Pediatr Neurol 2006;13(2):115–120.

Talente GM, Coleman RA, Alter C, et al: Glycogen storage disease in adults. Ann Intern Med 1994;120(3):218–226.

Wolfsdorf JI, Weinstein DA: Glycogen storage diseases. Rev Endocr Metab Disord 2003;4(1):95–102.

Molecular Endocrine Pathology

Jennifer L. Hunt

INTRODUCTION

Endocrine diseases are among the best-studied pathologic conditions in the human body at the molecular level. Significant strides have been made in our understanding of the pathogenesis of tumors, particularly in thyroid and parathyroid tumors. In other organs, such as the adrenal gland, molecular pathogenesis remains poorly understood. This chapter focuses on the best characterized molecular mutational events that have been described in three organ systems: thyroid, parathyroid, and adrenal. With a focus on understanding of the pathogenesis and potential diagnostic tools, the molecular events related to histopathologic classifications and morphologic variants of common and uncommon tumors will be discussed.

THYROID

Diseases of the thyroid gland are relatively common. The most clinical thyroid diseases are caused by abnormalities in thyroid hormone production resulting in clinical hypothyroidism or hyperthyroidism. Thyroid surgery for nodules is also common, and carcinomas of the thyroid are increasing in incidence. This section discusses the diagnostic workup and molecular alterations of neoplasms of the thyroid.

FOLLICULAR ADENOMA

The most common neoplasm of the thyroid is the benign follicular adenoma. Differentiating between follicular adenomas and hyperplastic nodules can be subjective, although some histologic criteria are used. Typical follicular adenomas are encapsulated and have a microfollicular growth pattern. Oncocytic features in follicular-derived lesions are referred to as *Hürthle cell differentiation.* The most common molecular alterations in follicular adenomas are *RAS* mutations. Few other significant mutational events

are found these benign neoplasms. Loss of heterozygosity is usually seen sporadically and only in low levels.

PAPILLARY CARCINOMA AND ITS VARIANTS

Papillary thyroid carcinoma (PTC) is the most common malignancy in the thyroid, representing up to 80% of all thyroid carcinomas. Tumors are classified by size as either less than 1 cm (microscopic PTC, often referred to as "incidental") or more than 1 cm (clinically significant PTC). There are many histologic variants of papillary carcinoma (Table 24-1).

Several distinct molecular mutational events have been identified in PTC, including translocations or intrachromosomal rearrangements between the *RET* proto-oncogene and various partner genes. The most common partner genes are *H4 (PTC1)* and *ELE1 (PTC3)* (Table 24-2). These translocations, and particularly *RET/PTC3,* are more common in radiation-induced tumors.

Another often-identified mutation is in the *BRAF* gene; this mutation occurs in between 40% and 60% of sporadic PTCs. *BRAF* mutations were originally designated as V599E, but this was corrected to V600E after discovery of a counting error in the original nucleic acid sequence. The mutation is a thymidine to adenine transition at codon 600 (nucleotide 1799) (Figure 24-1). *BRAF* mutations are most often found in conventional and tall cell variants and are uncommon in the follicular variant of papillary carcinoma. The *RET/PTC* translocations and the *BRAF* mutation are mutually exclusive and together may account for up to 70% of PTCs. The molecular mechanism behind the etiology of the remainder of conventional PTCs remains unclear.

Several variants of PTC have interesting additional molecular profiles. Follicular variant tumors, which have a low frequency of *RET/PTC* translocations and *BRAF* mutations, often harbor *RAS* gene mutations and may occasionally have a *PAX8/PPAR*γ translocation, which is usually seen in follicular carcinomas. The tall cell variant, on the other hand, has a high frequency of *BRAF* mutations. Finally, the cribriform-morular variant is associated with familial

TABLE 24-1

Variants of Papillary Carcinoma with Common Histologic Features

Morphology	Features
Conventional type	Papillary growth with nuclear features
Follicular variant	Pure follicular growth with nuclear features
Tall cell variant	Cells 2–3× as high as they are wide, distinct intracytoplasmic membranes, eosinophilic cytoplasm
Columnar cell variant	Papillary growth, stratified nuclei, nuclear features not as apparent
Warthin's-like variant	Oncocytic cells with nuclear features and prominent lymphoplasmacytic infiltrate
Cribriform-morular variant	Solid and cribriform growth with squamous morules, associated with familial adenomatosis polyposis
Diffuse sclerosis variant	Diffusely involves thyroid, abundant psammoma bodies, squamous metaplasia
Solid variant	Solid growth with nuclear features
Oncocytic variant	Oncocytic epithelial cells with nuclear features of papillary carcinoma

adenomatous polyposis syndrome, and some patients will harbor germline and somatic mutations in the adenomatous polyposis coli gene (APC).

Hyalinizing Trabecular Tumor

Hyalinizing trabecular tumor (HTT) is an unusual lesion in the thyroid that has had several different names, including "paraganglioma-like adenoma of the thyroid" and "hyalinizing trabecular adenoma."

HTTs have a characteristic morphology. The growth pattern is trabecular and should include only minimal follicular growth. There is usually deposition of an eosinophilic extracellular material that stains with collagen type IV and laminin; this can be located central to radiating trabeculae or can be deposited in the stromal compartment of the tumors. The nuclei can resemble those seen in papillary carcinoma, with intranuclear inclusions, enlargement, clearing, and grooves.

TABLE 24-2

Translocations Described in Papillary Carcinomas

Translocation	Partner Gene
RET/PTC1	H4 (10q21)
RET/PTC2	R1α (17q23)
RET/PTC3	ELE1 (10q11.2)
RET/PTC4 (or 3R2)	Ele1 (10q11.2) alternate breakpoint
RET/PTC5	RFG5 (14q22.1)
RET/PTC6	HTIF1 (7q32-34)
RET/PTC7	RFG7 (1p13.1)
RET/PTC8	RFG8 (18q21-22)
RET/KTN1	KTN1 (14q22.1)
RET/ELKS	ELKS (12p13.3)
RET/PCM1	PCM-1 (8p21-22)
TRK/T1	TPR (1q25)
TRK/T2	TPR (1q25)
TRK/TPM3	TPM3 (1q22-23)
TRK/T3	TFG (3q11-12)

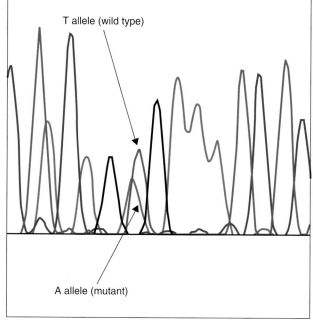

FIGURE 24-1

The sequencing results for a BRAF gene mutation at nucleotide 1799. The arrows indicate the presence of one wild-type allele (base thymidine, red) and one mutant allele (base adenine, green).

Because of histologic overlap with and possible occasional coexistence of HTT and papillary carcinoma, many investigators have studied the mutational profile of HTT for genetic similarities with papillary carcinoma. In several small series, up to 66% of HTTs have been shown to have the *RET/PTC* translocation usually characteristic of papillary carcinoma. The presence of this mutation in HTTs has been used as evidence to suggest that HTT may be a variant of papillary carcinoma. However, *BRAF* mutations have not been described in HTT. At present, controversy remains as to whether HTT is a variant of papillary carcinoma or not.

FOLLICULAR CARCINOMA (AND ONCOCYTIC VARIANT OF FOLLICULAR CARCINOMA)

Follicular-derived tumors of the thyroid gland generally have a follicular growth pattern and are composed of either typical follicular cells or Hürthle cells. The tumors are classified based on presence of invasion. Tumors are designated as minimally invasive follicular/Hürthle cell carcinoma when they show capsular invasion alone. The diagnosis of encapsulated angioinvasive follicular/Hürthle cell carcinoma is used for tumors demonstrating vascular invasion at the level of the tumor capsule. Widely invasive tumors show intra- and extrathyroidal invasion (Table 24-3). Several studies have indicated that the number of vascular invasive foci is predictive of risk of tumor recurrence.

The *RAS* genes *(KRAS, NRAS,* and *HRAS)* have long been implicated in the pathogenesis of follicular-derived tumors. In most series, *RAS* gene mutations are found in up to 50% of follicular-derived tumors. Recent evidence suggests that *RAS* gene mutations may be more common in aggressive follicular neoplasms and may be a marker for behavior.

Up to 40% of follicular carcinomas harbor a translocation between the *PAX8* gene and the *PPAR*γ gene *(PAX8/PPAR*γ). The translocation can be identified at the messenger RNA level using reverse transcription–polymerase chain reaction or at the DNA level using in situ hybridization. PPARγ protein overexpression by immunohistochemistry also correlates to some degree with the presence of the translocation. Interestingly, in microarray comparisons of tumors with and without the translocation, there are significant differences at the expression level. Tumors with Hürthle cell differentiation do not usually have *PAX8/PPAR*γ translocation or high rates of *RAS* mutations.

In studies of aneuploidy and loss of tumor suppressor genes in the follicular-derived tumors, clinically and histologically more aggressive tumors have a higher rate of loss of heterozygosity. By using a panel of tumor suppressor genes in this type of analysis, high-risk tumors can be identified by their mutational profile. Oncocytic tumors may have mutations in mitochondrial DNA, although these mutations have also been seen in other types of thyroid cancer.

POORLY DIFFERENTIATED CARCINOMAS

Papillary and follicular growth patterns are features of well-differentiated tumors. Growth patterns considered to be less well differentiated include insular, trabecular, and solid, and these have been associated with a worse prognosis. Pure insular growth in tumors is relatively uncommon, but even a minor insular growth pattern component may be significant. Other morphologic features of differentiation, such as nuclear pleomorphism, mitoses, and necrosis, have been also described in poorly differentiated tumors.

Poorly differentiated carcinomas, because of their relative rarity, have not been well studied at the molecular level. There is some indication that p53 mutations may be involved in tumorigenesis.

ANAPLASTIC (UNDIFFERENTIATED) CARCINOMAS

Undifferentiated or anaplastic thyroid carcinoma is a highly aggressive malignancy that usually presents in the elderly as a rapidly enlarging neck mass.

TABLE 24-3

Classification Scheme for Follicular-Derived Neoplasms

Criteria	Follicular Adenoma	Minimally Invasive Carcinoma	Encapsulated Angioinvasive Carcinoma	Widely Invasive Carcinoma
Capsular invasion	Absent	Mandatory	Usually present	Usually present
Vascular invasion	Absent	Absent	Mandatory	Usually present
Growth pattern	Follicular	Usually follicular	Follicular, solid, trabecular	Often solid, trabecular, or insular
Anaplasia	Minimal	Minimal	Minimal	Variable

Undifferentiated carcinomas often arise in patients who have a history of thyroid disease, including a goiter or a known well-differentiated carcinoma. Up to 50% of well-sampled anaplastic carcinomas will also have a coexisting well-differentiated thyroid carcinoma.

At the molecular level, anaplastic carcinomas have a high burden of somatic mutations, including loss of DNA in regions of common tumor suppressor genes. More than 50% will harbor point mutations in the p53 gene, and many will have loss of heterozygosity of the p53 gene (Figure 24-2). There is clear molecular evidence of a clonal connection between coexisting well-differentiated and anaplastic areas.

The V600E BRAF point mutation is found in up to half of anaplastic thyroid carcinomas, reflecting the common origin of anaplastic carcinoma from a precursor papillary carcinoma.

MEDULLARY CARCINOMA

Medullary carcinomas are derived from neoplastic C cells (or parafollicular cells). These cells are not follicular in origin but rather begin embryologically from the fourth and/or fifth branchial pouch. The C

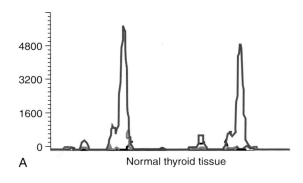

A   Normal thyroid tissue

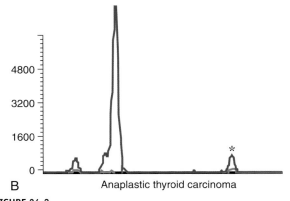

B   Anaplastic thyroid carcinoma

FIGURE 24-2

Electropherograms from normal tissue and from an anaplastic thyroid carcinoma, using primers for a polymorphism near the p53 gene. **(A)** The locus is heterozygous in the normal tissue. **(B)** The tumor has lost the second allele (*).

cells secrete calcitonin, a hormone that has a poorly understood role in calcium homeostasis. A painless thyroid nodule is the most common presentation for both hereditary and sporadic cases of medullary thyroid carcinoma. The neuroendocrine C cells in these tumors have varying morphologies, including spindled, epithelioid, or plasmacytoid cell types. In most tumors, amyloid will be detectable.

The molecular genetic understanding of medullary carcinoma is dominated by well-characterized mutations in the *RET* proto-oncogene. Germline *RET* mutations are associated with hereditary medullary carcinomas in the multiple endocrine neoplasia (MEN) syndromes. Patients with hereditary medullary carcinomas and their family members can be tested for the germline *RET* mutations genomic DNA (Table 24-4).

Multiple Endocrine Neoplasia 2A

MEN 2A syndrome patients are at high risk for medullary thyroid carcinoma, pheochromocytoma, and hyperparathyroidism. In the MEN 2A syndrome, the most common mutations are in the cysteine-coding codons 609, 611, 618, 620, and 634, which are located in exons 10 and 11. One of these six mutations is present in approximately 98% of patients with the MEN 2A clinical syndrome, with 634 being the most common ($\leq 80\%$). These mutations are missense mutations in the area encoding the extracellular domain of the RET kinase protein. The gene products from the mutated *RET* gene are constitutively dimerized through disulfide bridges.

Familial Medullary Thyroid Carcinoma

Familial medullary thyroid carcinoma (FMTC) kindreds have medullary carcinomas without the other clinical ramifications of the MEN syndrome. They have been shown to have mutations in the same cysteine-encoding codons as MEN 2A patients (609, 611, 618, 620, and 634) and rarely codons 768 and 804. However, the distribution of mutations is different, with 618 and 620 being the most common. The functional significance of the mutations appears to be different in these patients. The mutations in codons 618 and 620 appear to activate *RET* to a lesser extent than does the 634 mutation.

Multiple Endocrine Neoplasia 2B

MEN 2B syndrome patients have the clinical constellation of medullary carcinomas of the thyroid, pheochromocytoma, marfanoid habitus, and ganglioneuromatosis of the mucosal surfaces and gastrointestinal tract. In 95% of MEN 2B families, a substitution mutation of a threonine for a methionine at codon 918 in exon 16 is identified in the area encoding for the tyrosine kinase domain of the RET protein. The mutation does not appear to cause

TABLE 24-4

Mutations Associated with Medullary Carcinoma

Diagnosis	Associated Lesions	Exons	Codons
Multiple endocrine neoplasia 2A syndrome	Medullary carcinoma	Exon 10	Codon 609
	Pheochromocytoma	Exon 11	Codon 611
	Parathyroid hyperplasia		Codon 618
			Codon 620
			Codon 634
Multiple endocrine neoplasia 2B syndrome	Medullary carcinoma	Exon 16	Codon 918
	Pheochromocytoma		
	Ganglioneuromas		
Familial medullary carcinoma syndrome	Medullary carcinoma	Exon 10	Codon 609
		Exon 11	Codon 611
			Codon 618
			Codon 620
			Codon 634

dimerization of the RET protein for activation but may result in a change in substrate specificity.

SPORADIC MEDULLARY THYROID CARCINOMA

Most medullary thyroid carcinomas arise as sporadic tumors and are not the results of an inherited disorder. Somatic mutations of the *RET* proto-oncogene have been found in the tumor tissue derived from sporadic medullary thyroid carcinoma (SMTCa) in approximately 40% to 60% of cases. Some studies have suggested that tumors with mutations behave more aggressively and have a worse clinical outcome. Interestingly, when different areas of these tumors are microdissected, genotyping can reveal multiple different *RET* oncogene mutations within the same tumor.

Even in presumed sporadic disease, germline testing for *RET* mutations is often performed, because up to 6% will have an unsuspected germline mutation. In this subgroup, an overrepresentation of mutations in exons 13, 14, and 15 is often seen; thus, extending the common mutational test panel may be necessary in these patients.

RET mutations can be identified in DNA obtained from paraffin-embedded material. Testing of tumor tissues for somatic mutations may become important, given the apparent prognostic value of identifying these mutations. Testing for germline mutations in normal tissue, however, should be avoided unless appropriate informed consent is obtained, along with genetic counseling.

PARATHYROID

The major clinical manifestation of parathyroid disease is hyperparathyroidism, which is relatively common with an estimated incidence of 3 to 4 cases per 1000 people. There are primary, secondary, and tertiary forms of hyperparathyroidism (Table 24-5).

Some forms of hyperparathyroidism are associated with genetic syndromes. These include the familial disease associated with MEN syndromes and rarer forms, such hyperparathyroidism–jaw-tumor syndrome (HPT-JT). The different types of familial hyperparathyroidism are listed in Table 24-6.

CYSTS

True parathyroid cysts are rare, but cystic degeneration of a parathyroid neoplasm is much more common. Histologically, primary parathyroid cysts are lined by a bland, low, cuboidal epithelium. Parathyroid hormone immunohistochemistry stains and CK19 are positive, as are chromogranin and synaptophysin.

Parathyroid cysts and parathyroid carcinoma are key manifestations of HPT-JT; up to 15% of patients with HPT-JT will develop parathyroid carcinoma. Patients with this syndrome usually have mutations in the HRPT2 gene, a tumor suppressor gene on 1q31.1. The gene encodes for the parafibromin protein. Loss of protein expression by immunohistochemistry is also associated with parathyroid lesions in these patients.

TABLE 24-5

Causes of Hyperparathyroidism

Type	Description	Causes
Primary hyperparathyroidism	Parathyroid-related disease	Parathyroid adenoma
		Parathyroid hyperplasia (genetic)
		Parathyroid carcinoma
Secondary hyperparathyroidism	Secretion of parathyroid hormone in response to low calcium from another disease	Rickets (osteomalacia) caused by vitamin D or calcium deficiency
		Sprue
		Chronic renal failure
Tertiary hyperparathyroidism	One parathyroid gland becoming autonomous after persistent secondary hyperparathyroidism	

TABLE 24-6

Different Types of Familial Hyperparathyroidism

Syndrome Name	Pattern	Gene	Locus	Clinical Features
Multiple endocrine neoplasia type 1 (MEN1)	Dom	MEN1	11q13	Multiglandular parathyroid disease (>90%)
				Gastroenteropancreatic tumors
				Pituitary adenomas
Multiple endocrine neoplasia type 2A (MEN2A)	Dom	RET	10q21	Multiglandular parathyroid disease (20–30%)
				C cell tumors of thyroid
				Pheochromocytomas
Hyperparathyroidism–jaw-tumor syndrome (HPT-JT)	Dom	HRPT2	1q21-32	Primary hyperparathyroidism with cystic parathyroid tumors
				Parathyroid carcinoma (10–15%)
				Fibro-osseous lesions of jaws
				Kidney lesions
Familial isolated hyperparathy-roidism (FIHP)	Dom	MEN1	11q13	Benign multiglandular parathyroid disease
		CaSR	19p13.3	Carcinomas of breast, colon, endometrium, and others
Familial hypocalciuric hypercalcemic (FHH)	Dom	CaSR	3q21.1	Normal or increased calcium
			19p13.3 (type 2)	Moderate hyperphosphatemia
			19q13 (type 3)	Inappropriately low urine calcium
				Increased or normal parathyroid hormone levels
Neonatal severe hyperparathyroidism (NSHPT)	Rec	CaSR	3q21.1	Homozygous form of FHH
Autosomal dominant mild hyperparathyroidism (ADMH)	Dom	CaSR	3q21.1	

CaSR, calcium sensing receptor gene; Dom, autosomal dominant; Rec, recessive.

HYPERPLASIA

In primary hyperparathyroidism, multiglandular hyperplasia is only seen in about 10% of patients. Most multiglandular hyperplasia is secondary, often associated with renal disease. The mechanism for development of parathyroid gland hyperplasia in renal failure is the result of multiple complex pathways.

The glands in parathyroid hyperplasia are generally large, with mean weights around 1.0 g. The histologic features are nonspecific but include nodular hyperplasia, often with mixed cell types. The pathologist can rarely differentiate histologically between adenoma and hyperplasia, especially when only one parathyroid gland has been biopsied. This distinction requires the integration of clinical and laboratory data. At the molecular level, monoclonality has been reported within each gland from patients with hyperplasia in the setting of hemodialysis.

ADENOMA AND CARCINOMA

Most patients with primary hyperparathyroidism have a single glandular abnormality. Much like the distinction between hyperplasia and adenoma, adenoma and carcinoma can only be differentiated through correlation of the histology with the surgeon's intraoperative assessment of local invasion. Histologic features associated with malignancy include increased or atypical mitoses, broad bands of fibrosis, trabecular growth pattern, invasion of adjacent tissue, and perineural or angiolymphatic invasion (Table 24-7).

At the molecular level, parathyroid adenomas and carcinomas have a high rate of loss of 1p. Specific parathyroid-related genes on 1p have not yet been identified. Other genes have also been implicated in the pathogenesis of parathyroid adenomas and carcinomas, including retinoblastoma (*RB*, 13q14.3), *MEN* (11q13), and *BRCA2* (13q12.3). *HRPT2* also shows loss of heterozygosity and somatic point mutations in sporadic parathyroid carcinomas (Figure 24-3). The burden of loss of heterozygosity across a series of tumor suppressor genes correlates with the histologic evidence of malignancy.

ADRENAL GLAND

Adrenal gland tumors are most commonly derived from either the cortex (adrenal cortical adenoma and carcinoma) or the medulla (pheochromocytoma). Although diagnosing the cellular origin of these tumors is generally straightforward, diagnostic challenges arise in predicting behavior, because criteria for malignancy are not well defined. Incidental benign tumors are relatively common, whereas the malignant counterparts (adrenal cortical carcinoma and malignant pheochromocytoma) are rare. Our understanding of adrenal-derived tumors, both at the diagnostic and at the molecular levels, is limited.

TABLE 24-7

Clinical and Histologic Features of Parathyroid Carcinoma

Clinical Features	Histologic Features
High calcium level (>14 mg/dL)	Trabecular growth
Parathyroid hormone level > 5× normal	Broad intersecting fibrous bands
Palpable mass lesion	Increased mitoses
Bone symptoms	Stromal invasion
Operative findings of invasive growth (sticky, fibrotic, vascular gland)	Angiolymphatic or perineural invasion

---

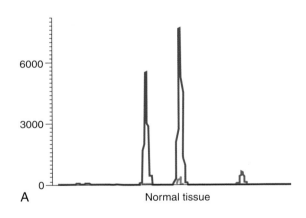

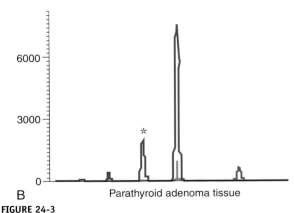

FIGURE 24-3

Electropherograms from normal tissue and from a parathyroid adenoma. The primers are specific for a short tandem repeat polymorphism on 1p. **(A)** The locus is heterozygous in the normal tissue. **(B)** Loss of heterozygosity of the first allele (*) is seen in the adenoma.

PHEOCHROMOCYTOMAS

Pheochromocytomas can be functional or non-functional. When symptoms are present, they relate to the secretion of catecholamines and include headache, perspiration, palpitations, pallor, and hypertension. Pheochromocytomas can be found in patients with several different syndromes, including MEN 2a and 2B syndromes, neurofibromatosis type I, and von Hippel-Lindau disease (Table 24-8).

Differentiating benign from malignant pheochromocytomas is difficult at the histologic level. And, unfortunately, no definitive mutational markers have been identified with either diagnostic or prognostic value.

ADRENAL CORTICAL TUMORS

In adrenal cortical tumors, the criteria used to predict malignancy are not absolute but include mitotic rate, vascular or capsular invasion, and size of the tumor. At the molecular level, these tumors are highly variable. There are reports describing loss of heterozygosity in many different genes and occasional point mutations in the oncogenes. However, no distinctive genetic alterations have been associated with malignancy, and none of these markers are currently used in the clinical setting.

CONCLUSION

The most advanced clinically applicable molecular applications in endocrine pathology relate to thyroid cancer. In thyroid tumors, there are common mutations in both tumor suppressor genes and oncogenes that have been well validated for clinical testing. Although most laboratories are not currently performing these assays, a combination of fluorescence in situ hybridization and polymerase chain reaction–based approaches for specific molecular alterations may allow diagnostic-level testing in thyroid tumors. This would be especially desirable because of the high rates of intraobserver variation that have been reported for thyroid tumors. It is anticipated that increasingly laboratories will be able to offer diagnostic molecular testing in thyroid pathology specimens, both in tissue and in fine-needle aspiration samples.

In parathyroid and adrenal tumors, the applications of molecular tests are still in the early phases. The sparse nature of data regarding malignancy and associated genetic mutational profiles, coupled with the rarity of carcinomas, makes it difficult to clinically validate new molecular tests for diagnosis. Clinically applicable diagnostic molecular testing is

---

TABLE 24-8

Genetic Syndromes Associated with Paraganglioma and Pheochromocytoma

	Gene Locus	Gene	Pheochromocytoma and Paraganglioma	Other Abnormalities
Von Hippel-Lindau	3p26	VHL	Pheochromocytoma in 10–20%	Renal cysts and renal cell carcinoma Visceral organ cysts Hemangioblastomas
Hereditary paragangliomatosis	11q23 11q13 1q21 1p36	PGL1 PGL2 PGL3 PGL4	Multiple paragangliomas (100%)	None
Neurofibromatosis type 1 (von Recklinghausen disease)	17q11.2	Neurofibroma	Pheochromocytoma in 1–5%	Neurofibromas Schwannomas Central nervous system gliomas
Multiple endocrine neoplasia type 2A	10q11.2	RET	Pheochromocytoma in 50–70%	Parathyroid hyperplasia Medullary thyroid carcinoma
Multiple endocrine neoplasia type 2B	10q11.2	RET	Pheochromocytoma in 50–70%	Medullary thyroid carcinoma Mucosal neuromas Skeletal abnormalities

(From Lester D, Thompson R: Endocrine pathology. In Hunt JL (ed): Diseases of the Paraganglia System. Philadelphia, Elsevier, 2006.)

not likely to be available for sporadic tumors for quite some time.

Endocrine tumors remain problematic at the clinical diagnostic level, both because of their heterogeneity and because of the tendency for the histology to not be entirely representative of the behavior of the tumors. As molecular diagnostics continues to develop, it would be desirable to focus development on these enigmatic tumors, where prognostication remains difficult.

SUGGESTED READINGS

Adeniran AJ, Zhu Z, Gandhi M, et al: Correlation between genetic alterations and microscopic features, clinical manifestations, and prognostic characteristics of thyroid papillary carcinomas. Am J Surg Pathol 2006;30(2):216–222.

Allolio B, Fassnacht M: Adrenocortical carcinoma: Clinical update [review]. J Clin Endocrinol Metab 2006;91(6):2027–2037.

Alsanea O, Clark OH: Familial thyroid cancer. Curr Opin Oncol 2001;13(1):44–451.

Aratake Y, Nomura H, Kotani T, et al: Coexistent anaplastic and differentiated thyroid carcinoma. Am J Clin Pathol 2006;125(3):399–406.

Baloch ZW, Puttaswamy K, Brose M, LiVolsi VA: Lack of BRAF mutations in hyalinizing trabecular neoplasm. Cytojournal 2006;3:17.

Benn DE, Robinson BG: Genetic basis of phaeochromocytoma and paraganglioma. Best Pract Res Clin Endocrinol Metab 2006;20(3):435–450.

Bertherat J, Gimenez-Roqueplo AP: New insights in the genetics of adrenocortical tumors, pheochromocytomas and paragangliomas. Horm Metab Res 2005;37(6):384–390.

Besic N, Auersperg M, Golouh R: Prognostic factors in follicular carcinoma of the thyroid—a multivariate survival analysis. Eur J Surg Oncol 1999;25(6):599–605.

Beus KS, Stack BC Jr: Parathyroid carcinoma. Otolaryngol Clin North Am 2004;37(4):845–854.

Casey MB, Sebo TJ, Carney JA: Hyalinizing trabecular adenoma of the thyroid gland: Cytologic features in 29 cases. Am J Surg Pathol 2004;28(7):859–867.

Castro P, Rebocho AP, Soares RJ, et al: PAX8/PPARγ rearrangement is frequently detected in the follicular variant of papillary thyroid carcinoma. J Clin Endocrinol Metab 2006;91(1):213–220.

Cetani F, Pardi E, Viacava P, et al: A reappraisal of the Rb1 gene abnormalities in the diagnosis of parathyroid cancer. Clin Endocrinol 2004;60(1):99–106.

Cheung CC, Boerner SL, MacMillan CM, et al: Hyalinizing trabecular tumor of the thyroid: A variant of papillary carcinoma proved by molecular genetics. Am J Surg Pathol 2000;24(12):1622–1626.

Cheung L, Messina M, Gill A, et al: Detection of the PAX8/PPARγ fusion oncogene in both follicular thyroid carcinomas and adenomas. J Clin Endocrinol Metab 2003;88(1):354–357.

Correa P, Juhlin C, Rastad J, et al: Allelic loss in clinically and screening-detected primary hyperparathyroidism. Clin Endocrinol 2002;56(1):113–117.

Cryns VL, Yi SM, Tahara H, et al: Frequent loss of chromosome arm 1p DNA in parathyroid adenomas. Genes Chromosomes Cancer 1995;13(1):9–17.

DeLellis RA: Parathyroid carcinoma: An overview. Adv Anat Pathol 2005;12(2):53–61.

French CA, Alexander EK, Cibas ES, et al: Genetic and biological subgroups of low-stage follicular thyroid cancer. Am J Pathol 2003;162(4):1053–1060.

Garcia-Rostan G, Zhao H, Camp RL, et al: Ras mutations are associated with aggressive tumor phenotypes and poor prognosis in thyroid cancer. J Clin Oncol 2003;21(17):3226–3235.

Howell VM, Haven CJ, Kahnoski K, et al: HRPT2 mutations are associated with malignancy in sporadic parathyroid tumours. J Med Genet 2003;40(9):657–663.

Kroll TG, Sarraf P, Pecciarini L, et al: PAX8/PPARγ1 fusion oncogene in human thyroid carcinoma [corrected]. Science 2000;289(5483):1357–1360.

Learoyd DL, Messina M, Zedenius J, Robinson BG: Molecular genetics of thyroid tumors and surgical decision making. World J Surg 2000;24(8):923–933.

Lombardi CP, Raffaelli M, Pani G, et al: Gene expression profiling of adrenal cortical tumors by cDNA macroarray analysis. Results of a preliminary study. Biomed Pharmacother 2006;60(4):186–190.

Lui WO, Foukakis T, Lidén J, et al: Expression profiling reveals a distinct transcription signature in follicular thyroid carcinomas with a PAX8/PPARγ fusion oncogene. Oncogene 2004;20:1–10.

Nakabashi CC, Guimaraes GS, Michaluart P, Jr., et al: The expression of PAX8/PPARγ rearrangements is not specific to follicular thyroid carcinoma. Clin Endocrinol 2004;61(2):280–282.

Nikiforov YE: Genetic alterations involved in the transition from well-differentiated to poorly differentiated and anaplastic thyroid carcinomas. Endocr Pathol 2004;15(4):319–327.

Nikiforov YE: RET/PTC rearrangement in thyroid tumors. Endocr Pathol 2002;13(1):3–16.

Nikiforova MN, Kimura ET, Gandhi M, et al: BRAF mutations in thyroid tumors are restricted to papillary carcinomas and anaplastic or poorly differentiated carcinomas arising from papillary carcinomas. J Clin Endocrinol Metab 2003;88(11):5399–5404.

Papotti M, Volante M, Giuliano A, et al: RET/PTC activation in hyalinizing trabecular tumors of the thyroid. Am J Surg Pathol 2000;24(12):1615–1621.

Quiros RM, Ding HG, Gattuso P, et al: Evidence that one subset of anaplastic thyroid carcinomas are derived from papillary carcinomas due to BRAF and p53 mutations. Cancer 2005;103(11):2261–2268.

Sakamoto A, Kasai N, Sugano H: Poorly differentiated carcinoma of the thyroid. A clinicopathologic entity for a high-risk group of papillary and follicular carcinomas. Cancer 1983;52(10):1849–1855.

Salvatore G, Chiappetta G, Nikiforov YE, et al: Molecular profile of hyalinizing trabecular tumours of the thyroid: High prevalence of RET/PTC rearrangements and absence of BRAF and NRAS point mutations. Eur J Cancer 2005;41:816–821.

Salvatore G, De Falco V, Salemo P, et al: BRAF is a therapeutic target in aggressive thyroid carcinoma. Clin Cancer Res 2006;12(5):1623–1629.

Santoro M, Melillo RM, Carlomagno F, et al: Molecular biology of the MEN2 gene. J Intern Med 1998;243(6):505–508.

Schilling T, Burck J, Sinn HP, et al: Prognostic value of codon 918 (ATG→ACG) RET proto-oncogene mutations in sporadic medullary thyroid carcinoma. Int J Cancer 2001;95(1):62–66.

Shattuck TM, Valimaki S, Obara T, et al: Somatic and germline mutations of the HRPT2 gene in sporadic parathyroid carcinoma. N Engl J Med 2003;349(18):1722–1729.

Stoler DL, Datta RV, Charles MA, et al: Genomic instability measurement in the diagnosis of thyroid neoplasms. Head Neck 2002;24(3):290–295.

Uchino S, Noguchi S, Yamashita H, et al: Mutational analysis of the APC gene in cribriform-morula variant of papillary thyroid carcinoma. World J Surg 2006;30(5):775–779.

Valimaki S, Forsberg L, Farnebo LO, Larsson C: Distinct target regions for chromosome 1p deletions in parathyroid adenomas and carcinomas. Int J Oncol 2002;21(4):727–735.

van der Harst E, de Krijger RR, Bruining HA, et al: Prognostic value of RET proto-oncogene point mutations in malignant and benign, sporadic phaeochromocytomas. Int J Cancer 1998;79(5):537–540.

Villablanca A, Farnebo F, Teh BT, et al: Genetic and clinical characterization of sporadic cystic parathyroid tumours. Clin Endocrinol 2002;56(2):261–269.

Zedenius J, Larsson C, Bergholm U, et al: Mutations of codon 918 in the RET proto-oncogene correlate to poor prognosis in sporadic medullary thyroid carcinomas. J Clin Endocrinol Metab 1995;80(10):3088–3090.

to assist in further classification of the myeloproliferative neoplasm. Correlation with the remaining clinical findings and peripheral blood and bone marrow morphology remains essential for proper classification.

Several techniques for detection of the *JAK2* V617F have been reported for testing at initial diagnosis, including allele-specific PCR or real-time PCR using fluorescence resonance energy transfer probes and melting curve analysis. Testing may be performed on either peripheral blood or bone marrow, including, in some protocols, formalin-fixed, paraffin-embedded clot preparations. An advantage of melting curve analysis is that these techniques detect and provide relative quantitative information regarding both the wild-type and the mutant alleles (Figure 25-3). However, these techniques may not be sufficiently sensitive for follow-up detection of minimal residual disease. The most appropriate technique for analysis of minimal residual disease remains to be determined.

In addition to the JAK2 exon 14 V617F mutation, two other types of mutations have also been described in Philadelphia chromosome negative myeloproliferative neoplasms. Cases of polycythemia vera lacking the JAK2 V617F have been found to have a variety of mutations located with exon 12, including point mutations and in-frame deletions. To date, the exon 12 JAK2 mutations, unlike V617F, appear to be restricted to polycythemia vera. In addition, point mutations in the thrombopoietin receptor *(MPL)* at codon 515 (W515L or W515K) have been described in approximately 5% of primary idiopathic myelofibrosis and rare cases of essential thrombocytosis. The JAK2 exon 12 mutations, JAK2 V617F, and MPL mutations all lead to disruption of the JAK-STAT signalling pathway, suggesting a common pathogenic mechanism. Exon 12

JAK2 mutations or MPL mutations may be identified by sequencing and/or allele-specific PCR.

OTHER ABNORMALITIES IN PHILADELPHIA CHROMOSOME NEGATIVE MYELOPROLIFERATIVE NEOPLASMS

Because, as described earlier, the diagnosis of non-CML myeloproliferative neoplasms can be quite challenging, other molecular techniques have been described to facilitate diagnosis. For example, overexpression of the *PRV1* gene has been described in polycythemia vera, essential thrombocytosis, and chronic idiopathic myelofibrosis. X chromosome inactivation studies have also been employed to demonstrate clonality of peripheral blood or bone marrow cells in these myeloproliferative neoplasms. However, *PRV1* studies require quantitative RT-PCR analysis of purified peripheral blood granulocytes with normalization of expression to a housekeeping gene. The complexity of this assay has limited its use in diagnostic situations. Similarly, because X chromosome inactivation studies are applicable only to female patients, this technique has not become widely used outside of a research setting.

KIT D816V IN MASTOCYTOSIS

Mast cell disease encompasses a spectrum of disorders defined by a complex set of clinicopathologic criteria. Mutations in the c-*Kit* proto-oncogene *(KIT)* have been demonstrated in many forms of mast cell disease, including urticaria pigmentosa, systemic mastocytosis, and mast cell leukemia. The most common of these abnormalities is the *KIT* D816V, which has been reported in most adult-onset mastocytosis. In the WHO classification, detection of the *KIT* D816V is

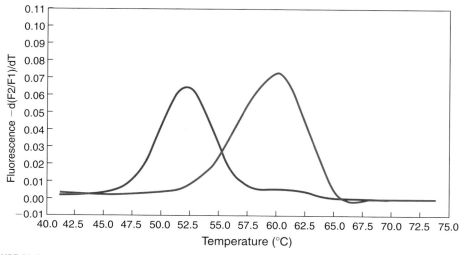

FIGURE 25-3

JAK2 V617F mutation detected by melting curve analysis. A derivative plot of the melting curve yields distinct melting peaks for the wild-type and mutant *JAK* alleles. The wild-type sequence (red curve) results in a melting point of 60°C. The mutant allele product (blue curve) with one mismatched nucleotide is less thermodynamically stable and displays a lower melting point of 52°C.

considered a minor criterion in establishing a diagnosis of systemic mastocytosis. A variety of PCR-based protocols have been reported for detection of this abnormality, including PCR restriction fragment length polymorphisms, allele-specific PCR, and real-time PCR with melting curve analysis. However, it is important to recognize that a variety of other *KIT* mutations occur in cases of mastocytosis, involving position 816 or other locations in the gene. Complete molecular analysis therefore requires employing either a panel of PCR primers or a sequencing-based approach. In many cases, however, the diagnosis of mastocytosis can be established without need for molecular studies.

MYELOID NEOPLASMS ASSOCIATED WITH EOSINOPHILIA AND ABNORMALITIES OF PDGFRA, PDGFRB OR FGFR1

The 2008 revision to the WHO Classification of Hematopoietic and Lymphoid Neoplasms recognizes category of myeloid neoplasms that are frequently associated with eosinophilia and abnormalities involving the PDGFRA, PDGFRB or FGFR1 genes. Each of these entities display distinct clinicopathologic features and correct diagnosis is essential to guide appropriate therapy.

MYELOID NEOPLASMS WITH *PDGFRA* REARRANGEMENTS

A recently described *FIP1L1/PDGFRA* fusion gene is found in a subset of patients presenting with chronic, unexplained eosinophilia. This fusion gene is

produced by an approximately 800-kilobase deletion on chromosome 4q12, with consequent fusion of the adjacent *FIP1L1* and *PDGFRA* genes. The initial reports of the *FIP1L1/PDGFRA* fusion gene identified this abnormality in cases that had previously been diagnosed as hypereosinophilic syndrome, chronic eosinophilia leukemia or systemic mastocytosis with eosinophilia. In the current WHO classification, however, these cases are categorized as a distinct myeloproliferative neoplasm with the fusion gene contained in abnormal mast cells, eosinophils, and other myeloid cells. Documentation of this abnormality is important in that it establishes the presence of a clonal, myeloid lineage neoplasm and excludes a benign reactive eosinophilia. In addition, there are important therapeutic implications, because imatinib therapy has proved efficacious in this setting.

Because the 4q12 deletion is relatively small (800 kilobases), this abnormality cannot be detected by classical cytogenetic studies, and a molecular approach is required. RT-PCR-based protocols have been described to detect the fusion transcript. However, the deletion breakpoints in the *FIP1L1* region are diverse, and it is unclear whether all occurring breakpoints can be detected by current RT-PCR-based techniques. Alternatively, a FISH-based approach has been employed that detects deletion of the *CHIC2* gene, which is normally located between the *FIP1L1* and the *PDGFRA* loci, as a surrogate marker for the fusion transcript (Figure 25-4).

MYELOID NEOPLASMS WITH *PDGFRB* REARRANGEMENTS

Uncommon myeloproliferative neoplasms, often meeting morphologic criteria for chronic myelomonocytic leukemia with accompanying eosinophilia,

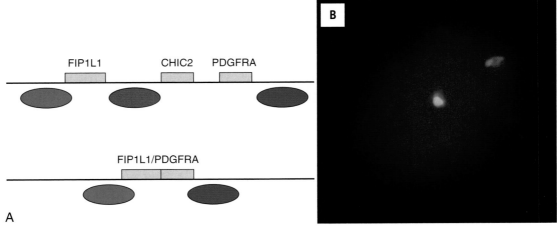

FIGURE 25-4

Fluorescence in situ hybridization (FISH) detection of *CHIC2* deletion, a surrogate marker for *PDGFR-α/FIP1L1* fusion. **(A)** FISH probes adjacent to *PDGFR-α* (aqua), *FIP1L1* (green), and *CHIC2* (red) on chromosome 4q. In the setting of a *PDGFR-α/FIP1L1* fusion, the *CHIC2* locus is deleted with loss of the red probe and retention of green and aqua signals. **(B)** Interphase FISH nucleus positive for *PDGFR-α/FIP1L1*. The normal 4q12 locus shows an intact red/green/aqua fusion, and the involved 4q12 locus displays a green/aqua fusion signal with deletion of the intervening red signal.

contain rearrangements of the *PDGFRB* locus at chromosome 5q33. More than a dozen different PDGFRB translocation partner genes have been described to date. The most frequent and best characterized of these is a t(5;12)(q33;p13) involving *TEL* at chromosome 12p13. Identification of a *PDGFRB* rearrangement is important because the majority of these abnormalities appear to respond to imatinib therapy. Translocations involving *PDGFRB* are generally detectable by metaphase cytogenetics (if informative metaphases are obtained). FISH studies using break-apart probes for *PDGFRB* rearrangements or fusion probes specific for *PDGFRB/TEL* may also be useful in diagnosis.

MYELOID NEOPLASMS WITH *FGFR1* REARRANGEMENTS

Rearrangements involving the *FGFR1* gene at 8p11 are identified in the so-called "8p11 myeloproliferative syndrome" or "stem cell leukemia/lymphoma syndrome." At least 10 different translocation partner genes have been identified, with the most frequent of these being t(8;13)(p11;q12) involving *ZNF198*. This neoplasm is characterized by eosinophilia, other myeloproliferative or myelodysplastic changes, a common progression to AML, and a high incidence of coexisting T-cell neoplasms (especially precursor T-cell lymphoblastic lymphoma). Unlike *PDGFRA* or *PDGFRB* rearrangements, myeloid neoplasms with *FGFR1* translocations do not appear to respond to imatinib therapy. Translocations of 8p11 may be detected by metaphase cytogenetics.

MYELODYSPLASTIC SYNDROMES AND MYELODYSPLASTIC–MYELOPROLIFERATIVE OVERLAP DISORDERS

The myelodysplastic syndromes and myelodysplastic–myeloproliferative overlap disorders may display a variety of cytogenetic findings. The most often found abnormalities include $-5/-5q$, $-7/-7q$, $+8$, or $-20q$. Panels of FISH probes may be employed to detect these abnormalities in interphase cells, and such panels may increase the yield of cases displaying abnormal findings compared to classical cytogenetic studies alone. However, classical cytogenetic studies are sufficient to detect these abnormalities in most cases. In addition, FISH studies provide no information regarding overall karyotype complexity, and other potentially significant abnormalities not targeted by the panel of FISH probes will not be detected. If employed for routine diagnosis, FISH panels should be used as an adjunct to and not a replacement for classical cytogenetic studies.

ACUTE MYELOID LEUKEMIA

In the WHO classification of AML, four distinct clinicopathologic entities are defined by the presence of specific recurring molecular abnormalities: *AML1/ETO, CBFβ/MYH11, PML/RARα*, and *MLL* rearrangements (Table 25-1). Other molecular abnormalities, such as mutations in the *FLT3, CBFβ*, or *NPM* genes, have been described in AML that appear to be associated with prognostic differences. Because the appropriate diagnosis and classification of AML requires correlation with the cytogenetic status, classical cytogenetic studies should be performed in all cases of suspected AML. When classical cytogenetic studies fail to identify one of the recurring cytogenetic abnormalities, FISH analysis or other molecular testing may be helpful to exclude a cryptic rearrangement or complex variant. In most laboratories, testing for these abnormalities is typically performed on peripheral blood or directly on bone marrow aspirate specimens, although, if necessary, many assays could be performed on formalin-fixed, paraffin-embedded bone marrow clot preparations.

t(8;21)(q22;q22) AML1/ETO

The t(8;21)(q22;q22), found in 5% to 12% of cases of AML, results in the *AML1/ETO* fusion transcript, which has an inhibitory effect on normal myeloid maturation. The *AML1* gene (also known as *RUNX1*) encodes the α-subunit of the core binding factor (CBF), a heterodimeric transcription factor. Because translocations involving the β subunit of the CBF also occur in AML (see discussion of *CBFβ/MYH11* later), these cases are sometimes referred to together as *CBF leukemias*. The *AML1/ETO* fusion product is believed to inhibit the normal CBF transcriptional pathways through a dominant-negative mechanism.

Morphologically, most cases of AML with *AML1/ETO* are classified as AML with maturation (FAB AML-M2), although occasional cases may lack maturation or show evidence of monocytic differentiation. Many cases display characteristic morphologic features, such as homogeneously staining, salmon-colored granules in maturing myeloid cells, abnormal large granules (pseudo-Chediak-Higashi granules), frequent Auer rods, or eosinophilia. There is often aberrant expression of CD19 and CD56 on the leukemic blasts. Clinically, these cases present at younger age and display a favorable prognosis.

At initial diagnosis, the t(8;21)(q22;q22) is readily detectable by standard cytogenetics in most cases. FISH and RT-PCR testing are useful for further evaluation of cases displaying morphologic or phenotypic

TABLE 25-1

Recurrent Cytogenetic Abnormalities in Acute Myeloid Leukemia

Abnormality	Incidence	Features	Prognosis
t(8;21)(q22;q22) *AML1/ETO*	5–12%	AML with maturation (FAB AML-M2)	Favorable
		Salmon-colored granules	
		Aberrant CD19, CD56 expression	
inv(16)(p13q22) *CBFβ/MYH11*	10–12%	Acute myelomonocytic leukemia (FAB AML-M4)	Favorable
		Abnormal eosinophils	
t(15;17)(q22;q12) *PML/RARα*	5–8%	Acute promyelocytic leukemia (FAB AML-M3)	Favorable
		Absence of CD34, HLA-DR	
11q23 *MLL*	5–6%	Acute monocytic and myelomonocytic leukemias (FAB AML-M4 and AML-M5)	Poor

AML, acute myeloid leukemia; FAB, French–American–British (classification); HLA-DR, human leukocyte antigen-DR.

findings suggesting the presence of *AML1/ETO* but for which classical cytogenetic studies failed to reveal this abnormality. In some studies, up to one third of AML with maturation and a normal karyotype are positive for *AML1/ETO* by molecular testing. For detection of minimal residual disease, a real-time quantitative RT-PCR approach has been reported, analogous to the previously discussed *BCR/ABL* minimal residual disease assays.

inv(16)(p13q22) CBFβ/MYH11

Approximately 10% to 12% of AML contain inv(16)(p13q22), producing a *CBFβ/MYH11* fusion transcript. In a few cases, the same fusion transcript is produced instead by t(16;16)(p13;q22). As with the AML1/ETO fusion protein, the *CBFβ/MYH11* is thought to function as a dominant-negative fusion protein, leading to transcriptional repression of the normal CBF pathways.

Cases of AML with *CBFβ/MYH11* usually display evidence of monocytic differentiation (acute myelomonocytic leukemia, FAB AML-M4) and characteristically contain abnormally granulated eosinophil precursors. Occasional cases, however, may lack monocytic differentiation or abnormal eosinophils. Clinically, patients with AML with *CBFβ/MYH11* tend to be younger and follow a favorable course.

Although inv(16)(p13q22) is usually detectable by standard cytogenetics at initial diagnosis, this abnormality may sometimes be subtle and may be misinterpreted as del(16)(q22) or otherwise go unrecognized. FISH or RT-PCR studies are therefore suggested when the presence of *CBFβ/MYH11* is suggested by the morphologic findings but classical cytogenetic studies have been negative or uninfor-

mative. Quantitative real-time RT-PCR approaches have been employed for monitoring of minimal residual disease.

t(15;17) and Variants

Cases of AML with *PML/RARα* translocations, which represent 5% to 8% of AML, are classified as APL. The *RARα* gene on 17q12 encodes the RARα protein that, as part of a heterodimer with retinoid-X receptors (*RXRα*), functions as a nuclear hormone receptor. The *PML* gene on 15q22 encodes a nuclear regulatory protein whose function remains incompletely understood. The PML/RARα fusion protein is thought to interfere with signaling through the normal *RARα/RXRα* pathway, resulting in transcriptional repression and lack of myeloid differentiation. Importantly, treatment with all-*trans* retinoic acid (ATRA) can alleviate the transcription repression mediated by *PML/RARα*, and combined therapy with ATRA and conventional multiagent chemotherapy has been shown to lead to a favorable prognosis compared to other forms of AML. In rare cases, variant translocations have been described in APL with translocations involving the *RARα* gene with other partner genes, including *PLZF* (11q23), *NPM* (5q35), or *NuMA* (11q13). Although cases with *PLZF/RARα* translocations are not responsive to ATRA therapy, the limited available data reported on the other variant translocations suggest they are ATRA responsive.

Patients with APL often present with easy bruising, mucosal hemorrhage, and disseminated intravascular coagulation. Morphologically, cases of APL cases display one of two patterns, consisting of either numerous atypical promyelocytes with abundant granules and many Auer rods or a microgranular variant with

B-CELL LYMPHOPROLIFERATIVE DISORDERS

In routine practice, most B-cell lymphoproliferative disorders are diagnosed on the basis of the morphologic and phenotypic findings without need for molecular analysis. However, molecular techniques can be of clinical utility in several settings. Clonality studies may be helpful in some cases, especially PCR analysis, which may be performed on paraffin-embedded tissue samples. As discussed earlier, however, a major limitation in the primers employed in most laboratories is the relatively high false-negative rate, such that a negative result cannot exclude a clonal process. In addition, several characteristic balanced translocations are associated with distinct B-cell lymphoproliferative disorders (Table 25-4). Molecular studies to detect these translocations can therefore be valuable in cases in which the morphologic and phenotypic findings are not clearly diagnostic alone. As with the Philadelphia chromosome in CML discussed earlier, multiple techniques may be employed to detect balanced translocations in non-Hodgkin's lymphomas, including classical cytogenetics, FISH analysis, or PCR-based approaches. The advantages or disadvantages of these approaches are discussed in greater detail for each entity. In general, at the time of initial diagnosis, when malignant cells are numerous, FISH studies, with or without accompanying classical cytogenetics, are the most sensitive. PCR-based techniques, on the other hand, are especially valuable for minimal residual disease studies (especially with quantitative RT-PCR protocols) or when the number of malignant cells present is quite small, such that FISH studies may give a false-negative result (<10% of the total cells).

B-CELL CHRONIC LYMPHOCYTIC LEUKEMIA

Several molecular cytogenetic abnormalities have been described in B-cell chronic lymphocytic leukemia (CLL) that are associated with differences in time to treatment and overall survival (Table 25-5). Because the malignant cells of B-cell CLL proliferate poorly in vitro, classical cytogenetic analysis is insufficiently sensitive for detection of these abnormalities in many cases. FISH studies have therefore emerged as the technique of choice for evaluation of B-cell CLL. It is important to remember that none of these abnormalities are specific for B-cell CLL and that their significance in other lymphoproliferative disorders may be unknown. FISH testing for prognostically significant abnormalities should therefore only be performed in cases of confirmed B-cell CLL.

Studies have also shown that the mutational status of the *IGH* locus carries prognostic significance in B-cell CLL. During normal B-cell maturation and activation, the *IGH* locus undergoes somatic hypermutation in the germinal center reaction. By sequencing portions of the clonally rearranged *IGH*, the mutational status of the neoplastic B cells may be determined. A mutated genotype (usually defined as >2% base-pair changes compared to germline) has been associated with a favorable prognosis compared to unmutated status. However, because these sequence-based studies are labor intensive, they are rarely performed in routine practice.

FOLLICULAR LYMPHOMA

Overall, approximately 80% to 90% of follicular lymphomas are associated with t(14;18)(q32;q21) involving *IGH* and *BCL2*, which leads to overexpression of the antiapoptotic BCL2 protein. The translocation is more common in cases with a grade 1 to 2 morphology

---

TABLE 25-4

Recurrent Molecular Cytogenetic Abnormalities in B-Cell Lymphoproliferative Disorders

Diagnosis	Translocation	Genes Involved	Incidence
Follicular lymphoma	t(14;18)(q32;q21)	*IGH/BCL2*	80–90%
	t(3;v)(q27;v)	*BCL6* and many partners	5–15%
Mantle cell lymphoma	t(11;14)(q13;q32)	*IGH/CCND1*	~100%
Mucosa-associated lymphoid tissue lymphoma	t(11;18)(q21;q21)	*API2/MALT1*	Variable
	t(14;18)(q32;q21)	*IGH/MALT1*	Variable
	t(1;14)(p22;q34)	*BCL10/IGH*	Uncommon
	t(3;14)(p14;q32)	*FOXP1/IGH*	Variable
Diffuse large B-cell lymphoma	t(14;18)(q32;q21)	*IGH/BCL2*	20–30%
	t(3;v)(q27;v)	*BCL6* and many partners	Up to 30%
Burkitt lymphoma	t(8;14)(q24;q32) and variants	*CMYC/IGH*	~100%

TABLE 25-5

Recurring Cytogenetic Abnormalities in B-Cell Chronic Lymphocytic Leukemia

Abnormality	Approximate Incidence	Prognosis
Del(13q)	30–50%	Good
+12	15–20%	Intermediate
Normal	20%	Intermediate
Del(11q23)	15–20%	Poor
Del(17p)	5–10%	Poor

(>90%) than in grade 3 cases (30% to 50%). Although most cases of follicular lymphoma may be diagnosed without need for molecular testing, the demonstration of *IGH/BCL2* may be useful in otherwise challenging cases to distinguish follicular lymphoma from other lymphomas of small B lymphocytes or to assist in distinguishing between follicular lymphoma and benign follicular hyperplasia. The translocation is not unique to follicular lymphoma; it is also found in approximately 30% of diffuse large B-cell lymphoma. The translocation may be detected by classical cytogenetics, FISH analysis, or PCR-based approaches. Because of variations in breakpoint locations, the most commonly employed PCR primers (targeting breakpoints in the major cluster region or minor cluster region) will not detect all forms of this translocation. At initial diagnosis, when the number of malignant cells is relatively high (>10% of total cells), FISH analysis of either whole cell preparations or paraffin sections is generally the most sensitive technique for detection of this translocation. PCR-based approaches have also been employed for detection of minimal residual disease.

Translocations involving the *BCL6* gene are identified in approximately 15% of follicular lymphoma, with *BCL6* abnormalities being most prevalent in cases displaying grade 3B morphology and in those lacking a t(14;18)(q32;q21). More than 30 partner genes have been identified in translocations with *BCL6* to date. *BCL6* translocations are less specific for follicular lymphoma than the *IGH/BCL2* translocation because *BCL6* translocations may be found as a secondary abnormality in many forms of B-cell lymphoma, including diffuse large B-cell lymphoma, mantle cell lymphoma, and some marginal zone lymphomas. Despite the nonspecific nature of *BCL6* translocations, identification of this abnormality may assist in selected differential diagnoses, such as between follicular hyperplasia and follicular lymphoma. Because of the large number of potential *BCL6* translocation partner genes, FISH studies using a break-apart probe flanking the *BCL6* gene are the most appropriate technique to screen for *BCL6* translocations.

Mantle Cell Lymphoma

Using WHO criteria, essentially all cases of mantle cell lymphoma contain the t(11;14)(q13;q32) involving *IGH* and *CCND1,* which leads to aberrant expression of the cell cycle protein cyclin D1. In routine practice, most cases of mantle cell lymphoma may be diagnosed by immunohistochemical detection of the cyclin D1 protein. However, many of the currently employed cyclin D1 antibodies are suboptimal and may sometimes be difficult to interpret because of weak staining. When the morphologic features or phenotype are suggestive of mantle cell lymphoma, and cyclin D1 immunohistochemistry is either unavailable (e.g., as with peripheral blood samples) or equivocal, molecular studies are helpful in further evaluation. The *IGH/CCND1* translocation may be detected by classical cytogenetics, PCR-based strategies, or FISH analysis. Because of widely scattered translocation breakpoints, PCR studies may not detect more than half of all *IGH/CCND1* translocations. Among these techniques, FISH studies have been shown to have the highest sensitivity and have emerged as the gold standard for detection of this abnormality.

In addition to mantle cell lymphoma, the t(11;14) (q13;q32) also occurs in approximately 20% of plasma cell myeloma and in a subset of cases previously reported as B-cell prolymphocytic leukemia. It is currently unclear, however, how many of the latter group of cases actually represent a leukemic presentation of mantle cell lymphoma. Cyclin D1 protein expression also occurs in the absence of t(11;14)(q13;q32) in a subset of cases of hairy cell leukemia. Recent gene expression profiling studies have suggested that cases of cyclin D1 protein–negative, *IGH/CCND1*-negative mantle cell lymphoma may exist. However, such cases are controversial and the most appropriate designation for such cases remains unclear.

Marginal Zone Lymphomas

In the WHO classification, three forms of marginal zone lymphoma are recognized: extranodal marginal zone B-cell lymphomas of the mucosa-associated lymphoid tissue (MALT) type, primary nodal marginal zone lymphoma, and splenic marginal zone lymphoma. The molecular cytogenetic findings in these three forms of marginal zone lymphoma partially overlap. For example, trisomy 3 and trisomy 18 are the most common numeric abnormalities in each category. However, because these abnormalities are not specific for this form of lymphoma, assays for these trisomies are rarely performed in routine practice.

Several translocations have been described that appear to be specific for marginal zone lymphomas of the MALT type, including t(11;18)(q21;q21) involving *API2* and *MALT1,* t(14;18)(q32;q21) involving *IGH* and *MALT1*, t(1;14)(p22;q34) involving *BCL10* and *IGH*, and t(3;14)(p14;q32) involving *FOXP1* and *IGH*. The frequency of each of these abnormalities varies dramatically based on the anatomic site at which the MALT lymphoma arises. For example, the *API2/MALT1* translocation occurs often in pulmonary and gastric MALT lymphoma but only rarely in cutaneous and salivary cases. The clinical significance of MALT lymphoma–associated abnormalities has been best established in the case of the t(11;18)(q21;q21) in gastric MALT lymphoma. In this setting, the translocation is associated with advanced disease and unresponsiveness to antibiotic therapy directed against *Helicobacter pylori*. The clinical significance of these abnormalities in other forms of MALT lymphoma remains a topic of ongoing study. Because tissue biopsies of extranodal MALT lymphomas tend to be of limited size, classical cytogenetic studies are rarely performed in such cases. FISH studies, which can be performed on touch preparations or on paraffin-embedded tissue, are particularly valuable in these cases. Dual-color, break-apart probes spanning the *MALT1* locus are commercially available and are useful to screen for the presence of a *MALT1* translocation. If testing with the break-apart probe is positive, follow-up analysis with probes specific for the *API2/MALT1* and *IGH/MALT1* translocations may be used to confirm the identify of the translocation partner. RT-PCR studies for the *API2/MALT1* translocation may also be performed on fresh or paraffin-embedded tissue. It must also be noted that because the *BCL2* and *MALT1* genes are both located at chromosome 18q21, classical cytogenetic analysis cannot distinguish between *IGH/BCL2* and *IGH/MALT1* translocations. Molecular techniques, such as

FISH studies, are therefore required to definitively distinguish these abnormalities.

Splenic marginal zone lymphomas display deletions of chromosome 7q21-32 in up to 40% of cases. This abnormality can be detected by either classical cytogenetics or FISH analysis. However, del(7q) is a relatively nonspecific finding that may also be found in other forms of B-cell lymphoma. Testing for this abnormality is therefore currently of limited utility. There are no known specific molecular abnormalities in primary nodal marginal zone lymphoma.

LYMPHOPLASMACYTIC LYMPHOMA

Lymphoplasmacytic lymphoma is a neoplasm of lymphocytes, plasmacytoid lymphocytes, and plasma cells that, in some cases, may be difficult to distinguish from other small B-cell lymphomas with plasmacytic differentiation. In the past, it was reported that up to half of cases diagnosed as lymphoplasmacytic lymphoma contained t(9;14)(p13;q32) involving *PAX5* and *IGH*. However, more recent studies employing WHO criteria have demonstrated no association with this abnormality. Currently, there are no diagnostically useful molecular markers of lymphoplasmacytic lymphoma.

DIFFUSE LARGE B-CELL LYMPHOMA

Gene expression profiling studies have identified two major subtypes of diffuse large B-cell lymphoma: one that recapitulates a normal germinal center B-cell genotype (GC type) and one that corresponds to an activated B-cell genotype (ABC type) (Figure 25-6).

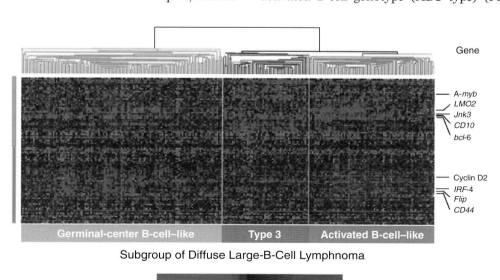

FIGURE 25-6

Gene expression profiling in diffuse large B-cell lymphoma. Two distinct subsets of diffuse large B-cell lymphoma have been identified by gene expression profiling studies: one with a genotypic profile resembling germinal center B cells and one with a profile resembling activated B cells. Cases not classifiable into either category are illustrated as type 3. (From Rosenwald, et al: The use of molecular profiling to predict survival after chemotherapy for diffuse large B-cell lymphoma. New Engl J Med 2002;346:1937–1947.)

These two forms of diffuse large B-cell lymphoma have been shown to have clinical significance, with a better prognosis identified in the GC type than in the ABC type. Because of the time-consuming and costly nature of gene expression profiling studies, such assays are not employed in routine clinical practice. However, it has been shown that immunohistochemistry for the germinal center–associated markers CD10 and BCL6 and the postgerminal center marker MUM1 can be used as a surrogate to distinguish GC and non-GC cases.

Numerous recurring cytogenetic abnormalities have been described in diffuse large B-cell lymphoma, including t(14;18)(q32;q21) *IGH/BCL2* and rearrangements of *BCL6* at 3q27, both of which are present in up to a third of cases. *MYC* abnormalities have been described in 5% to 10% of cases. However, testing for these abnormalities is not typically performed in straightforward cases of diffuse large B-cell lymphoma.

Primary mediastinal large B-cell lymphoma *(PMLBCL)* is a subtype of diffuse large B-cell lymphoma that displays distinct clinicopathologic features. Gene expression profiling studies have demonstrated that PMLBCL displays a unique expression signature that is distinct from the GC or ABC types of diffuse large B-cell lymphoma. Recurring molecular abnormalities in PMLBCL include gains on chromosome 9p or amplification of the *REL* locus on chromosome 2p. However, neither of these abnormalities is specific for PMLBCL. Currently, there is no specific molecular marker for PMLBCL suitable for routine clinical use.

Burkitt Lymphoma

As defined in the WHO classification, all cases of Burkitt lymphoma contain a translocation involving *MYC* at 8q24. This typically takes the form of t(8;14)(q24;q32) involving *MYC* and *IGH*. In 10% to 15% of cases, however, the translocation involves the immunoglobulin κ- or λ-light chain loci: t(2;8)(p12;q24) or t(8;22)(q24;q11.2), respectively. Dysregulation of *MYC* leads to marked proliferation, with Burkitt lymphoma characteristically displaying a proliferative fraction of more than 95% by Ki-67 (MIB-1) immunohistochemistry. *MYC* translocations may also be identified as secondary abnormalities in other forms of lymphoma, including diffuse large B-cell lymphoma, follicular lymphoma, and mantle cell lymphoma. The diagnosis of Burkitt lymphoma therefore requires correlation of the *MYC* status with the morphologic and phenotypic findings. Translocations involving *MYC* may be detected by classical cytogenetic studies or by FISH analysis. Dual-color, break-apart probes for the *MYC* locus are particularly useful to screen for *MYC* translocations. In the case of a positive break-apart study, subsequent analysis with a probe set specific for t(8;14)(q24;q32) may be employed to distinguish between classical *MYC/IGH*

translocation and other variant translocations. There are wide variations in translocation breakpoints in Burkitt lymphoma. For example, endemic cases typically contain breakpoints 5′ to the MYC locus, and the sporadic form displays breakpoints between the first and the second exons. In light of these widespread breakpoints, PCR studies are not suitable for detection of *MYC* rearrangements in clinical practice. In the past, Southern blot studies were often performed to assess for *MYC* translocations, but these have been largely supplanted by FISH analysis.

Recent studies have also characterized cases that may morphologically resemble Burkitt lymphoma (or "Burkitt-like" lymphoma in former classification schemes) but contain both a *MYC* translocation and a t(14;18)(q32;q21) *IGH/BCL2*. The presence of BCL2 protein expression or the *IGH/BCL2* translocation excludes a diagnosis of Burkitt lymphoma according to WHO criteria. Cases displaying both translocations are reported to be highly resistant to chemotherapy with an aggressive clinical course. Although precise classification of such dual-translocation cases is controversial, they are generally categorized as diffuse large B-cell lymphoma.

PLASMA CELL NEOPLASMS

Cytogenetic abnormalities are present in essentially all cases of plasma cell myeloma, and a subset of abnormalities has been associated with prognostic differences (Table 25-6). Classical cytogenetic studies demonstrate an abnormal karyotype in only one third of cases because of the low proliferative rate of plasma cells in vitro. The demonstration of any

TABLE 25-6

Prognostically Significant Molecular Abnormalities in Plasma Cell Myeloma

Abnormality	Genes Involved	Frequency*	Prognosis
−13/−13q	Unknown	~50%	Unfavorable
−17p	*TP53*	10%	Unfavorable
t(11;14)(q13;q32)	*CCND1/IGH*	15–20%	Neutral to favorable
t(4;14)(p16;q32)	*MMSET/IGH*	15–20%	Unfavorable
t(14;16)(q32;q23)	*CMAF/IGH*	5–10%	Unfavorable

*Frequency defined by fluorescence in situ hybridization analysis.

karyotypic abnormality by metaphase cytogenetics is a surrogate marker of a relatively high proliferative rate and is associated with an adverse prognosis, irrespective of the specific abnormalities present. In recent years, FISH studies have emerged as the favored technique for cytogenetic analysis of plasma cell myeloma. Indeed, the t(4;14)(p16;q32), which is associated with a poor prognosis, is cryptic by standard cytogenetics and is detected only by molecular diagnostic techniques. With some abnormalities, the prognostic impact varies with the detection technique employed. For example, chromosome 13 or 13q abnormalities have a greater prognostic significance when detected by metaphase cytogenetics than when detected by FISH. Therefore, FISH analysis is best interpreted with metaphase cytogenetics, and FISH panels, although valuable in the prognostic assessment of myeloma, are not an adequate substitute for classical cytogenetic analysis.

T-CELL LYMPHOPROLIFERATIVE DISORDERS

T-cell lymphoproliferative disorders are less common than their B-cell counterparts, and specific molecular abnormalities have not yet been identified in many T-cell disorders. However, molecular studies may be important in many cases. By far the most employed molecular assay in suspected T-cell disorders is clonality assessment by PCR analysis or Southern blot. The available, commonly employed PCR primers for T-cell receptor γ-chain rearrangement display a much lower false-negative rate than the commonly used primers for *IGH* rearrangements. Details of clonality assays are discussed in Chapter 13. In addition, several recurrent cytogenetic abnormalities have been described in specific types of T-cell lymphoproliferative disorders that may offer additional assistance in diagnosis or assessment of prognosis (Table 25-7), as described further later.

AUTOIMMUNE LYMPHOPROLIFERATIVE SYNDROME

Autoimmune lymphoproliferative syndrome (ALPS) is a rare, inherited disorder with onset in early childhood that is characterized by lymphadenopathy, autoimmune phenomenon, and increased risk of malignancy. The lymphadenopathy is caused by an increased number of αβ T cells that lack expression of both CD4 and CD8 (double-negative T cells). Double-negative T cells normally represent no more than approximately 1% of the total circulating lymphocytes. In ALPS, there is a deficiency in the programmed cell death pathways that normally regulate the double-negative T-cell population. Studies have identified several mutations in ALPS patients, leading to a molecular classification of ALPS (Table 25-8). In most cases, the defect is a mutation in the FAS gene, *TNFRSF6* (type 1a). In rare cases, mutations have been described in Fas ligand (type 1b) or in the caspase 8 or caspase 10 genes that function downstream in the Fas signaling pathway (type 2). In still other cases, the genetic loci involved have yet to be identified (type 3). The diagnosis of ALPS may be strongly suspected on the basis of the clinical findings and the demonstration of an increased double-negative T-cell population. Molecular studies may also be helpful. Clonality studies will demonstrate a polyclonal T-cell expansion. Sequence-based testing for *TNFRSF6* mutations in type 1a ALPS is clinically available from reference laboratories for definitive diagnosis. Genetic testing for the other types of mutations is currently performed only in research laboratories.

T-CELL PROLYMPHOCYTIC LEUKEMIA

In most cases, a diagnosis of T-cell prolymphocytic leukemia can be rendered on the basis of the morphologic and phenotypic findings. Clonality studies may also be useful to confirm the presence of a monoclonal T-cell population. Other molecular studies, however, may be of assistance in some cases. Approximately 80% of cases contain inv(14)(q11q32)

TABLE 25-7

Recurrent Molecular Cytogenetic Abnormalities in T-Cell Lymphoproliferative Disorders

Diagnosis	Translocation	Genes	Incidence
Anaplastic large-cell lymphoma	t(2;5)(p23;q35) and variants	*ALK/NPM* and other variant *ALK* translocations	60–80%
T-cell prolymphocytic leukemia	inv(14)(q11q32) or t(14;14)(q11;q32)	*TCRAD/TCL1A, TCRAD/TCL1B*	80–90%
Hepatosplenic γδ T-cell lymphoma	iso(7q)	Unknown	>80%

TABLE 25-8

Mutations Identified in Autoimmune Lymphoproliferative Syndrome

Subtype	Mutation	Frequency
Type 1a	Fas (TNFRSF6)	75%
Type 1b	Fas ligand (TNFSF6)	Rare
Type 2	Caspase 8 or caspase 10	~2%
Type 3	Undefined	20–25%

involving the *TCL1* or *TCL1β* genes at 14q32 and the T-cell receptor-αδ (TCR-αδ) locus at 14q11. In an additional 10% of cases, a similar abnormality is produced by t(14;14)(q11;q32) rather than an inversion. The *TCL1* gene, an activator of the AKT signaling pathway, has been implicated in the development of both B-cell and T-cell lymphoproliferative disorders. In rare cases of T-cell prolymphocytic leukemia, a t(X;14)(q28;q11) involves the TCR-αδ locus and the *MTCP1* gene, which is homologous to *TCL1*. These abnormalities may be detected by classical cytogenetic analysis. Break-apart FISH probes spanning the *TCL1* locus and the TCR-αδ locus are also available and may be particularly useful when classical cytogenetics are unavailable or noninformative.

ANAPLASTIC LARGE-CELL LYMPHOMA

Approximately 60% to 80% of cases of anaplastic large-cell lymphoma contain a translocation involving the *ALK* gene at 2p23, with the frequency of *ALK* rearrangements being highest in pediatric patients. Roughly 75% of the time, the *ALK* translocation is t(2;5)(p23;q35) involving the *ALK* and *NPM* genes. The ALK tyrosine kinase protein is not normally expressed in lymphoid cells. In the presence of an *ALK/NPM* translocation, however, a fusion protein is produced including the N-terminal region of *NPM* and the intracytoplasmic domain of *ALK*. The fusion protein is localized to both the nucleus and the cytoplasm, leading to dysregulated *ALK* kinase activity. In the remaining 25% of translocations, a variety of translocation partner genes have been identified, including *TPM3* (1q25), *TFG* (3q35), *ATIC* (2q35), and *CLTC* (17q23). In routine practice, *ALK* dysregulation can typically be demonstrated by immunohistochemistry. Molecular studies may be employed to confirm the presence of an *ALK* rearrangement or to further evaluate cases with equivocal staining. RT-PCR may be employed to detect the presence of

an *ALK/NPM* rearrangement. However, RT-PCR studies will not detect the presence of the less common variant translocations. FISH analysis using break-apart probes spanning the *ALK* locus are therefore the most sensitive molecular methodology to detect the presence of an *ALK* translocation at initial diagnosis. Classical cytogenetic analysis may also be helpful in identifying the translocation partner locus involved. Importantly, *ALK* translocations are not pathognomonic of anaplastic large-cell lymphoma. Rare cases of diffuse large B-cell lymphoma (especially those with plasmacytic features) have been shown to contain *ALK* translocations. *ALK* translocations also often occur in inflammatory myofibroblastic tumors and appear to occur in other mesenchymal tumors with low frequency. The detection of an *ALK* rearrangement in anaplastic large-cell lymphoma is associated with a favorable prognosis, and *ALK*-negative anaplastic large-cell lymphomas display a prognosis more similar to peripheral T-cell lymphoma, unspecified.

HEPATOSPLENIC γδ T-CELL LYMPHOMA

Hepatosplenic γδ T-cell lymphoma is an unusual neoplasm of cytotoxic γδ T cells that may be difficult to classify with certainty. Clonality studies are helpful to confirm the presence of a monoclonal T-cell population. Most cases are associated with an isochromosome 7q, and this may be a consistent finding. Abnormalities of chromosome 8 are also often found. Classical cytogenetic studies are typically used to assess for these abnormalities. FISH probes for isochromosome 7q have also been devised that may offer an increased sensitivity.

HODGKIN'S LYMPHOMA

Molecular studies are typically not performed in the routine diagnosis of Hodgkin's lymphoma except to assist in excluding other non-Hodgkin lymphomas that may be in the differential diagnosis. Using combined immunofluorescence and FISH analysis, it has recently been shown that many cases of nodular lymphocyte-predominant Hodgkin's disease contain *BCL6* translocations in the malignant cells. However, this abnormality is of limited clinical utility because of the nonspecific nature of *BCL6* translocations. In addition, because the malignant cells are few, it is difficult to evaluate for molecular abnormalities by either typical FISH protocols or classical cytogenetics. No diagnostically useful recurrent molecular abnormalities have been described in classical Hodgkin's lymphoma to date.

CONCLUSION

Already an integral part of routine hematopathology practice in many cases, the role of molecular diagnostic techniques can only be expected to grow. Ongoing studies are continuing to define molecular cytogenetic abnormalities of diagnostic and prognostic significance in lymphoid and myeloid disorders, and there is growing interest in the potential clinical significance of point mutations, especially in the myeloid disorders, analogous to the *JAK2* mutations in polycythemia vera and other myeloproliferative neoplasms. Ongoing expression microarray studies will likely continue to further define molecularly based subtypes of myeloid and lymphoid disorders, which may be tested for by microarray, multiplex RT-PCR, or some other platform that would offer diagnostic or prognostic information in routine clinical practice. Gene expression profiling studies, at least for the foreseeable future, may augment but are unlikely to replace traditional morphologic and phenotypic studies in hematopathology. It therefore remains important that pathologists evaluating peripheral blood, bone marrow, and lymphoid tissue samples continue to be familiar with the spectrum of available molecular diagnostic techniques and be able to integrate their results with the findings of other ancillary studies.

SUGGESTED READINGS

Chronic Myeloid Leukemia

Faderl S, Hochhaus A, Hughes T: Monitoring of minimal residual disease in chronic myeloid leukemia. Hematol Oncol Clin North Am 2004;18: 657–670.

Hughes TP, Deininger MW, Hochhaus A, et al: Monitoring CML patients responding to treatment with tyrosine kinase inhibitors: Review and recommendations for "harmonizing" current methodology for detecting *BCR/ABL* transcripts and kinase domain mutations and for expressing results. Blood 2006. 108(1):28–37.

Hughes TP, Kaeda J, Branford S, et al: Frequency of major molecular responses to imatinib or interferon alfa plus cytarabine in newly diagnosed chronic myeloid leukemia. N Engl J Med 2003;349:1423–1432.

Olavarria E, Kanfer E, Szydlo R, et al: Early detection of *BCR/ABL* transcripts by quantitative reverse transcriptase–polymerase chain reaction predicts outcome after allogeneic stem cell transplantation for chronic myeloid leukemia. Blood 2001;97:1560–1565.

Radich JP, Gehly G, Gooley T, et al: Polymerase chain reaction detection of the *BCR/ABL* fusion transcript after allogeneic marrow transplantation for chronic myeloid leukemia: Results and implications in 346 patients. Blood 1995;85:2632–2638.

Radich JP, Gooley T, Bryant E, et al: The significance of *BCR/ABL* molecular detection in chronic myeloid leukemia patients "late," 18 months or more after transplantation. Blood 2001;98:1701–1707.

Tefferi A, Dewald GW, Litzow ML, et al: Chronic myeloid leukemia: Current application of cytogenetics and molecular testing for diagnosis and treatment. Mayo Clin Proc 2005;80:390–402.

Nonchronic Myeloid Leukemia Myeloproliferative Disorders and Mast Cell Disease

Baxter EJ, Scott LM, Campbell PJ, et al: Acquired mutation of the tyrosine kinase *JAK2* in human myeloproliferative disorders. Lancet 2005;365: 1054–1061.

Cools J, DeAngelo DJ, Gotlib J, et al: A tyrosine kinase created by fusion of the *PDGFR*-α and *FIP1L1* genes as a therapeutic target of imatinib in idiopathic hypereosinophilic syndrome. N Engl J Med 2003;348: 1201–1214.

James C, Ugo V, Le Couedic JP, et al: A unique clonal *JAK2* mutation leading to constitutive signaling causes polycythaemia vera. Nature 2005;434:1144–1148.

Jones AV, Kreil S, Zoi K, et al: Widespread occurrence of the *JAK2* V617F mutation in chronic myeloproliferative disorders. Blood 2005;106: 2162–2168.

Kralovics R, Passamonti F, Buser AS, et al: A gain-of-function mutation of *JAK2* in myeloproliferative disorders. N Engl J Med 2005;352:1779–1790.

Levine RL, Wadleigh M, Cools J, et al: Activating mutation in the tyrosine kinase *JAK2* in polycythemia vera, essential thrombocythemia, and myeloid metaplasia with myelofibrosis. Cancer Cell 2005;7:387–397.

Longley BJ, Tyrrell L, Lu SZ, et al: Somatic *c-Kit* activating mutation in urticaria pigmentosa and aggressive mastocytosis: Establishment of clonality in a human mast cell neoplasm. Nat Genet 1996;12: 312–314.

Nagata H, Worobec AS, Oh CK, et al: Identification of a point mutation in the catalytic domain of the protooncogene c-kit in peripheral blood mononuclear cells of patients who have mastocytosis with an associated hematologic disorder. Proc Natl Acad Sci USA 1995;92: 10560–10564.

Pardanani A, Ketterling RP, Li CY, et al: *FIP1L1/PDGFR*-α in eosinophilic disorders: Prevalence in routine clinical practice, long-term experience with imatinib therapy, and a critical review of the literature. Leuk Res 2006;30(8):965–970.

Tefferi A, Elliott MA, Pardanani A: Atypical myeloproliferative disorders: Diagnosis and management. Mayo Clin Proc 2006;81:553–563.

Valent P, Horny HP, Escribano L, et al: Diagnostic criteria and classification of mastocytosis: A consensus proposal. Leuk Res 2001;25: 603–625.

Myelodysplastic Syndromes and Acute Myeloid Leukemia

Boissel N, Renneville A, Biggio V, et al: Prevalence, clinical profile, and prognosis of NPM mutations in AML with normal karyotype. Blood 2005;106:3618–3620.

Dash A, Gilliland DG: Molecular genetics of acute myeloid leukaemia. Best Pract Res Clin Haematol 2001;14:49–64.

Ferrara F, Del Vecchio L: Acute myeloid leukemia with t(8;21)/*AML1/ETO*: A distinct biological and clinical entity. Haematologica 2002;87:306–319.

Frohling S, Scholl C, Gilliland DG, et al: Genetics of myeloid malignancies: Pathogenetic and clinical implications. J Clin Oncol 2005;23:6285–6295.

Gilliland DG, Griffin JD: The roles of *FLT3* in hematopoiesis and leukemia. Blood 2002;100:1532–1542.

Jaffe E, Harris N, Stein H, Vardiman JW: Tumours of Haematopoietic and Lymphoid Tissues. Lyon, IARC Press, 2001.

Nishino HT, Chang CC: Myelodysplastic syndromes: Clinicopathologic features, pathobiology, and molecular pathogenesis. Arch Pathol Lab Med 2005;129:1299–1310.

Schoch C, Schnittger S, Klaus M, et al: AML with 11q23/*MLL* abnormalities as defined by the WHO classification: Incidence, partner chromosomes, FAB subtype, age distribution, and prognostic impact in an unselected series of 1897 cytogenetically analyzed AML cases. Blood 2003;102:2395–2402.

Steensma DP, List AF: Genetic testing in the myelodysplastic syndromes: Molecular insights into hematologic diversity. Mayo Clin Proc 2005;80: 681–698.

Yanada M, Matsuo K, Suzuki T, et al: Prognostic significance of FLT3 internal tandem duplication and tyrosine kinase domain mutations for acute myeloid leukemia: A meta-analysis. Leukemia 2005;19:1345–1349.

Precursor B-Cell and Precursor T-Cell Acute Lymphoblastic Leukemia or Lymphoma

Armstrong SA, Look AT: Molecular genetics of acute lymphoblastic leukemia. J Clin Oncol 2006;23:6306–6314.

Douet-Guilbert N, Morel F, Le Bris MJ, et al: Cytogenetic studies in T-cell acute lymphoblastic leukemia (1981–2002). Leuk Lymphoma 2004;45:287–290.

Harrison CJ: The detection and significance of chromosomal abnormalities in childhood acute lymphoblastic leukaemia. Blood Rev 2001;15: 49–59.

Silverman LB, Sallan SE: Newly diagnosed childhood acute lymphoblastic leukemia: Update on prognostic factors and treatment. Curr Opin Hematol 2003;10:290–296.

Yeoh EJ, Ross ME, Shurtleff SA, et al: Classification, subtype discovery, and prediction of outcome in pediatric acute lymphoblastic leukemia by gene expression profiling. Cancer Cell 2002;1:133–143.

B-Cell Lymphoproliferative Disorders

Bagg A: Molecular diagnosis in lymphoma. Curr Hematol Rep 2005;4:313–323.

Bosga-Bouwer AG, van Imhoff GW, Boonstra R, et al: Follicular lymphoma grade 3B includes 3 cytogenetically defined subgroups with primary t(14;18), 3q27, or other translocations: t(14;18) and 3q27 are mutually exclusive. Blood 2003;101:1149–1154.

Cook JR, Aguilera NI, Reshmi-Skarja S, et al: Lack of *PAX5* rearrangements in lymphoplasmacytic lymphomas: Reassessing the reported association with t(9;14). Hum Pathol 2004;35:447–454.

Cook JR: Paraffin section interphase fluorescence in situ hybridization in the diagnosis and classification of non-Hodgkin lymphomas. Diagn Mol Pathol 2004;13:197–206.

Dave SS, Fu K, Wright GW, et al: Molecular diagnosis of Burkitt lymphoma. N Engl J Med 2006;354:2431–42.

Dewald GW, Brockman SR, Paternoster SF, et al: Chromosome anomalies detected by interphase fluorescence in situ hybridization: Correlation with significant biological features of B-cell chronic lymphocytic leukaemia. Br J Haematol 2003;121:287–295.

Farinha P, Gascoyne RD: Molecular pathogenesis of mucosa-associated lymphoid tissue lymphoma. J Clin Oncol 2005;23:6370–6378.

Guo Y, Karube K, Kawano R, et al: Low-grade follicular lymphoma with t(14;18) presents a homogeneous disease entity otherwise the rest comprises minor groups of heterogeneous disease entities with *BCL2* amplification, *BCL6* translocation or other gene aberrances. Leukemia 2005;19:1058–1063.

Kanungo A, Medeiros LJ, Abruzzo LV, et al: Lymphoid neoplasms associated with concurrent t(14;18) and 8q24/c-Myc translocation generally have a poor prognosis. Mod Pathol 2006;19:25–33.

Krober A, Seiler T, Benner A, et al: V(H) mutation status, CD38 expression level, genomic aberrations, and survival in chronic lymphocytic leukemia. Blood 2002;100:1410–1416.

Oscier DG, Gardiner AC, Mould SJ, et al: Multivariate analysis of prognostic factors in CLL: Clinical stage, *IGVH* gene mutational status, and loss or mutation of the p53 gene are independent prognostic factors. Blood 2002;100:1177–1184.

Ott G, Katzenberger T, Lohr A, et al: Cytomorphologic, immunohistochemical, and cytogenetic profiles of follicular lymphoma: 2 types of follicular lymphoma grade 3. Blood 2002;99:3806–3812.

Remstein ED, Kurtin PJ, Buno I, et al: Diagnostic utility of fluorescence in situ hybridization in mantle-cell lymphoma. Br J Haematol 2000;110:856–862.

Savage KJ, Monti S, Kutok JL, et al: The molecular signature of mediastinal large B-cell lymphoma differs from that of other diffuse large B-cell lymphomas and shares features with classical Hodgkin lymphoma. Blood 2003;102:3871–3879.

Shipp MA, Ross KN, Tamayo P, et al: Diffuse large B-cell lymphoma outcome prediction by gene expression profiling and supervised machine learning. Nat Med 2002;8:68–74.

Streubel B, Simonitsch-Klupp I, Mullauer L, et al: Variable frequencies of MALT lymphoma–associated genetic aberrations in MALT lymphomas of different sites. Leukemia 2004;18:1722–1726.

Wotherspoon AC, Dogan A, Du MQ: Mucosa-associated lymphoid tissue lymphoma. Curr Opin Hematol 2002;9:50–55.

Wright G, Tan B, Rosenwald A, et al: A gene expression–based method to diagnose clinically distinct subgroups of diffuse large B-cell lymphoma. Proc Natl Acad Sci USA 2003;100:9991–9996.

Plasma Cell Neoplasms

Bergsagel PL, Kuehl WM, Zhan F, et al: Cyclin D dysregulation: An early and unifying pathogenic event in multiple myeloma. Blood 2005;106:296–303.

Bergsagel PL, Kuehl WM: Molecular pathogenesis and a consequent classification of multiple myeloma. J Clin Oncol 2005;23:6333–6338.

Fonseca R, Barlogie B, Bataille R, et al: Genetics and cytogenetics of multiple myeloma: A workshop report. Cancer Res 2004;64: 1546–1558.

Fonseca R, Blood EA, Oken MM, et al: Myeloma and the t(11;14)(q13;q32): Evidence for a biologically defined unique subset of patients. Blood 2002;99:3735–3741.

Gertz MA, Lacy MQ, Dispenzieri A, et al: Clinical implications of t(11;14)(q13;q32), t(4;14)(p16.3;q32), and –17p13 in myeloma patients treated with high-dose therapy. Blood 2005;106:2837–2840.

Mattioli M, Agnelli L, Fabris S, et al: Gene expression profiling of plasma cell dyscrasias reveals molecular patterns associated with distinct *IGH* translocations in multiple myeloma. Oncogene 2005;24:2461–2473.

Moreau P, Facon T, Leleu X, et al: Recurrent 14q32 translocations determine the prognosis of multiple myeloma, especially in patients receiving intensive chemotherapy. Blood 2002;100:1579–1583.

Stewart AK, Fonseca R: Prognostic and therapeutic significance of myeloma genetics and gene expression profiling. J Clin Oncol 2005;23:6339–6344.

T-Cell Lymphoproliferative Disorders

Ballester B, Ramuz O, Gisselbrecht C, et al: Gene expression profiling identifies molecular subgroups among nodal peripheral T-cell lymphomas. Oncogene 2006;25:1560–1570.

Belhadj K, Reyes F, Farcet JP, et al: Hepatosplenic γδ T-cell lymphoma is a rare clinicopathologic entity with poor outcome: Report on a series of 21 patients. Blood 2003;102:4261–4269.

Kadin ME, Carpenter C: Systemic and primary cutaneous anaplastic large-cell lymphomas. Semin Hematol 2003;40:244–256.

Pekarsky Y, Zanesi N, Aqeilan R, et al: Tcl1 as a model for lymphomagenesis. Hematol Oncol Clin North Am 2004;18:863–879, ix.

Ravandi F, Kantarjian H, Jones D, et al: Mature T-cell leukemias. Cancer 2005;104:1808–1818.

Renedo M, Martinez-Delgado B, Arranz E, et al: Chromosomal changes pattern and gene amplification in T-cell non-Hodgkin's lymphomas. Leukemia 2001;15:1627–1632.

Rizvi MA, Evens AM, Tallman MS, et al: T-cell non-Hodgkin lymphoma. Blood 2006;107:1255–1264.

ten Berge RL, Oudejans JJ, Ossenkoppele GJ, et al: *ALK*-negative systemic anaplastic large-cell lymphoma: Differential diagnostic and prognostic aspects—a review. J Pathol 2003;200:4–15.

Wlodarska I, Martin-Garcia N, Achten R, et al: Fluorescence in situ hybridization study of chromosome 7 aberrations in hepatosplenic T-cell lymphoma: Isochromosome 7q as a common abnormality accumulating in forms with features of cytologic progression. Genes Chromosomes Cancer 2002;33:243–251.

Worth A, Thrasher AJ, Gaspar HB: Autoimmune lymphoproliferative syndrome: Molecular basis of disease and clinical phenotype. Br J Haematol 2006;133:124–140.

Zettl A, Rudiger T, Konrad MA, et al: Genomic profiling of peripheral T-cell lymphoma, unspecified, and anaplastic large T-cell lymphoma delineates novel recurrent chromosomal alterations. Am J Pathol 2004;164:1837–1848.

26 Molecular Pathology of Bone and Soft Tissue Tumors

Brian P. Rubin • Alexander J.F. Lazar • Andre M. Oliveira

INTRODUCTION

Molecular pathology is an essential component of the pathology of bone and soft tissue tumors. Although the diagnosis is largely based on clinical, histologic, and immunohistochemical features, molecular diagnosis is useful and sometimes necessary as an adjunct for diagnosis and prognostication, especially in morphologically or clinically unusual lesions. Bone and soft tissue tumors can be classified broadly into those neoplasms with complex and nonspecific cytogenetic and molecular genetic features and those harboring relatively simple cytogenetic profiles with consistent and recurrent genetic aberrations (Table 26-1). In this chapter, we highlight the molecular features of various bone and soft tissue tumors, with special emphasis on molecular diagnosis. With well over 100 different neoplasms, it is beyond the scope of this chapter to comment on every entity. Instead, we focus on those neoplasms with diagnostic aberrations that are useful clinically or that provide interesting insights into pathogenesis. The 2002 World Health Organization Classification of Tumors of Bone and Soft Tissue is used.

BONE AND SOFT TISSUE TUMORS WITH COMPLEX CYTOGENETIC FEATURES

Neoplasms in this category have complex karyotypes and lack known consistent chromosomal translocations that are useful for diagnosis. It is still useful to karyotype these lesions; the presence of a complex karyotype can be useful in supporting a difficult diagnosis, because more complex karyotypes usually imply greater malignant potential. Furthermore, much has been learned about the tumors in this category as summarized in the sections that follow. Unless explicitly stated, molecular tests do not play a role in the diagnosis or prognosis of bone and soft tissue tumors with complex cytogenetic features.

ANGIOSARCOMA

Angiosarcomas are malignant neoplasms showing varying degrees of vascular differentiation. These tumors arise in several general settings: cutaneous angiosarcomas arising in sun-exposed skin; cutaneous angiosarcoma arising in a prior radiation field (such as treatment for breast carcinoma); angiosarcomas arising deep soft tissue; and angiosarcoma arising in the setting of chronic lymphedema (Stewart-Treves syndrome). Although they can be quite solid histologically, they usually exhibit focal vascular cleft formation or endothelial vacuolization. Angiosarcomas are infiltrative malignancies with a predilection for aggressive local behavior and the ability to metastasize. The diagnosis can be confirmed by immunoexpression of vascular markers, such as CD34, CD31, and FLI1; use of multiple vascular markers is often helpful, because none of them is completely specific and antigens are sometimes lost in the course of malignant transformation.

Minimal cytogenetic data is available for angiosarcoma. Nevertheless, those cases that have been karyotyped reveal complex cytogenetic changes. Some recurrent changes have been observed in several cases, including gains of 5pter-p11, 8p12-qter, and 20pter-q12; losses of 4p, 7p15-pter, and -Y; and aberrations involving 22q.

In contrast to Kaposi's sarcoma, which is characterized by involvement by human herpes virus 8 (HHV-8), angiosarcoma does not contain HHV-8 sequences. Thorium and vinyl chloride exposures are known risk factors for angiosarcoma. Genetic analysis reveals *KRAS2* and *TP53* mutations in angiosarcomas from patients with exposure to thorium and vinyl chloride, as well as sporadic angiosarcoma.

The authors would like to thank Kim Vu for artistic assistance with the figures in this chapter.

TABLE 26-1

Characteristic Cytogenetic and Molecular Alterations in Bone and Soft Tissue Tumors

Complex Molecular and Cytogenetic Profile	Cytogenetic Alterations	Molecular Alterations
Angiosarcoma	Complex	??
Chondrosarcoma	Complex	??
Leiomyosarcoma	Complex with frequent deletion/ rearrangement of 1p	??
Malignant peripheral nerve sheath tumor	Complex	??
Osteosarcoma	Complex	??
Pleomorphic liposarcoma	Complex	??
Pleomorphic rhabdomyosarcoma	Complex	??
Pleomorphic sarcoma, NOS (MFH)	Complex	??
Simple Molecular and Cytogenetic Profile		
Alveolar soft part sarcoma	t(X;17)(p11;q25)	*TFE3/ASPL* fusion
Aneurysmal bone cyst	t(16;17)(q22;p13)	*CDH11/USP6* fusion
	t(1;17)(p34;p13)	*TRAP150/USP6* fusion
	t(3;17)(q13;p13)	*ZNF9/USP6* fusion
	t(17;17)(q21;p13)	*COL1A/USP6* fusion
	t(9;17)(q22;p13)	*OMD/USP6* fusion
Angiomatoid fibrous histiocytoma	t(12;16)(q13;p11)	*FUS/ATF1* fusion
	t(12;22)(q13;q12)	*EWSR1/ATF1* fusion
	t(2;22)(q33;q12)	*EWSR1/CREB1* fusion
Bizarre parosteal osteochondromatous proliferation	t(1;17)(q32;q21)	Unknown fusion
Clear cell sarcoma	t(12;22)(q13;q12)	*EWSR1/ATF1 fusion*
Chondromyxoid fibroma	Rearrangements of 6q13 and 6q25	??
	t(2;22)(q33;q12)	*EWSR1/CREB1* fusion
Dermatofibrosarcoma protuberans	Ring form of chromosomes 17 and 22	*COL1A1/PDGF*-B fusion
	t(17;22)(q21;q13)	*COL1A1/PDGF*-B fusion
Desmoid fibromatosis	Trisomies 8 and 20 and loss of 5q21	*CTNNB1* or *APC* mutation
Desmoplastic small round cell tumor	t(11;22)(p13;q12)	*EWSR1/WT1* fusion
Endometrial stromal sarcoma	t(7;17)(p15;q21)	*JAZF1/JJAZ1* fusion
	t(6;7)(p21;p15)	*JAZF1/PHF1* fusion
	t(6;10)(p21;p11)	*EPC1/PHF1* fusion
Epithelioid hemangioendothelioma	t(1;3)(p36;q25)	Unknown fusion
Ewing sarcoma or PNET	t(11;22)(q24;q12)	*EWSR1/FLI1* fusion
	t(21;22)(q12;q12)	*EWSR1/ERG* fusion
	t(2;22)(q33;q12)	*EWSR1/FEV* fusion
	t(7;22)(p22;q12)	*EWSR1/ETV1* fusion
	t(17;22)(q12;q12)	*EWSR1/E1AF* fusion
	inv(22)(q12q;12)	*EWSR1/ZSG* fusion
	t(16;21)(p11;q22)	*FUS/ERG* fusion
Extraskeletal myxoid chondrosarcoma	t(9;22)(q22;q12)	*EWSR1/NR4A3* fusion
	t(9;17)(q22;q11)	*TAF2N/NR4A3* fusion
	t(9;15)(q22;q21)	*TCF12/NR4A3* fusion
	t(3;9)(q11;q22)	*TFG/NR4A3* fusion
Fibrous dysplasia		*GNAS1* mutation
Gastrointestinal stromal tumor	Monosomies 14 and 22	*KIT* mutation
	Deletion of 1p	??

TABLE 26-1

Characteristic Cytogenetic and Molecular Alterations in Bone and Soft Tissue Tumors—cont'd

Simple Molecular and Cytogenetic Profile	Cytogenetic Alterations	Molecular Alterations
Hibernoma	11q13 rearrangements	??
Infantile fibrosarcoma	t(12;15)(p13;q26)	*ETV6/NTRK3* fusion
	Trisomies 8, 11, 17, and 20	??
Inflammatory myofibroblastic tumor	t(1;2)(q22;p23)	*TPM3/ALK* fusion
	t(2;19)(p23;p13)	*TPM4/ALK* fusion
	t(2;17)(p23;q23)	*CLTC/ALK* fusion
	t(2;2)(p23;q13)	*RANB2/ALK* fusion
Kaposi sarcoma	Normal	*HHV8* infection
Leiomyoma	12q15 and 6p21 rearrangements	*HMEAL* and *HMGA* overexpression
Lipoblastoma	8q11-13 rearrangements	*HAS2/PLAG1* fusion
		COL1A2/PLAG1 fusion
Lipoma, chondroid subtype	t(11;16)(q13;p12-p13)	Unknown fusion
Lipoma, spindle cell or pleomorphic subtype	13q or 16q rearrangements	??
Low-grade fibromyxoid sarcoma	t(7;16)(q33;p11)	*FUS/CREB3L2* fusion
	t(11;16)(p11;p11)	*FUS/CREB3L1* fusion
Myxoid or round cell liposarcoma	t(12;16)(q13;p11)	*FUS/DDIT3* fusion
	t(12;22)(q13;q12)	*EWSR1/DDIT3* fusion
Myxoma	Normal	*PRKAR1α* and *GNAS*
Neurofibroma	Normal	*NF1* mutation
Osteochondroma	Rearrangements of 8q24 and 11p11 or p13	*EXT1* or *EXT2* mutation
Pericytoma	t(7;12)(p21-22;q13-15)	*ACTB/GLI* fusion
Rhabdomyosarcoma, alveolar	t(2;13)(q35;q14)	*PAX3/FOXO1A* fusion
	t(1;13)(p36;q14), double minutes	*PAX7/FOXO1A* fusion
	t(2;2)(q35;p23)	*PAX3/NCOA1* fusion
	t(X;2)(q35;q13)	*PAX3/AFX* fusion
Rhabdomyosarcoma, embryonal	Trisomies 2q, 8, and 20	Loss of heterozygosity at 11p15
		EWSR1/ATF1 fusion
Schwannoma	Monosomy 22	*NF2* mutation
Subungual exostosis	t(X;6)(q24-q26;q15-21)	Unknown fusion
Synovial chondromatosis	Rearrangement of 6p	??
Synovial sarcoma, biphasic	t(X;18)(p11;q11)	Predominantly *SS18/SSX1* fusion
Synovial sarcoma, monophasic	t(X;18)(p11;q11)	*SS18/SSX1, SS18/SSX2,* or *SS18/SSX4* fusion
Tenosynovial giant cell tumor	Rearrangement of 1p11-13	*CSF1* overexpression
Well-differentiated liposarcoma	Ring form of chromosome 12	Amplification of *MDM2, CDK4,* and others

MFH, malignant fibrous histiocytoma; NOS, not otherwise specified; PNET, primitive neuroectodermal tumor.

CHONDROSARCOMA

Conventional chondrosarcomas are malignant neoplasms with cartilaginous differentiation. The lesions have a permeative growth pattern and often destroy bone and invade the surrounding soft tissues. Although most chondrosarcomas arise within bone (central chondrosarcomas), some periosteal variants arise on the surface of bone and some known as secondary or peripheral chondrosarcomas are associated with osteochondromas. Overall, chondrosarcomas have complex cytogenetic findings. However, chromosomal losses and gains more commonly involve 1p36, 1p13-22, 4, 5q13-31, 6q22-ter, 9p22-ter, 10p, 10q24-ter, 11p13-ter, 11q25, 13q21-ter, 14q24-ter, 18p, 18q22-ter, and 22q13 (loss) and 7p13-ter, 12q15-ter, 19, 20pter-q11, and 21q (gain). Increasing aneuploidy, TP53 mutations, loss of CDKN2A (9p21), and loss of 13q are associated with a worse prognosis. The enchondromatosis syndromes—Ollier disease and Maffucci syndrome—may lead to an increased incidence of chondrosarcoma formation.

Despite the molecular complexity, identifiable molecular pathways appear to be present in central and peripheral chondrosarcomas. Although initiating events differ, both chondrosarcomas are characterized by abnormal parathyroid hormone–like hormone pathway signaling, which is important in cartilage development. Activation of the parathyroid hormone–like hormone pathway suggests a therapeutic strategy whereby proteins in this pathway could be targeted pharmacologically.

LEIOMYOSARCOMA

Leiomyosarcomas are malignant tumors that show varying degrees of smooth muscle differentiation. They tend to arise in older individuals and can occur in skin, deep soft tissue, the uterus, other parenchymal organs, and large blood vessels such as the inferior vena cava. Generally, they are composed of spindle-shaped cells with eosinophilic cytoplasm and tapering or "cigar-shaped" nuclei. Rare cases of leiomyosarcoma have an epithelioid cytomorphology, and some cases are extraordinarily pleomorphic. In difficult cases, immunoreactivity for smooth muscle actin, desmin, and h-caldesmon is helpful.

Cytogenetic studies have been reported on more than 100 leiomyosarcomas. The karyotypes are complex, and no two identical karyotypes have been published. Differences among subtypes have not been seen. Most leiomyosarcomas have structural aberrations of chromosomes 1, 7, 10, 13, and 14. Common gains or losses of chromosomal material are losses on 1p, 3p21-23, 8p21-pter, 13q12-13, and 13q32-qter and gain of 1q12-31.

Leiomyosarcoma often shows loss of RB1 and is the most common soft tissue sarcoma seen in hereditary retinoblastoma patients. Abnormalities in other retinoblastoma pathway proteins, including CDKN2A, CCND1, and CCND3, are also seen in sporadic leiomyosarcoma. Mutation in TP53 is seen in leiomyosarcoma and has been correlated with adverse prognostic factors.

Pediatric leiomyosarcoma is rare. However, there is an association with HIV-positive or post-transplant patients, and in either of these settings Epstein-Barr virus (EBV) infection is also seen. Therefore, it is important to assay for EBV by immunohistochemistry for EBV-latent membrane protein or by fluorescence in situ hybridization (FISH) for EBV RNA.

MALIGNANT PERIPHERAL NERVE SHEATH TUMOR

Malignant peripheral nerve sheath tumors (MPNSTs) are malignant neoplasms with schwannian or, rarely, perineurial differentiation. They are generally cellular and mitotically active and consist of fascicles of monomorphic spindle cells with fine chromatin and scant cytoplasm. Rare cases of MPNSTs have epithelioid cytomorphology. Most MPNSTs are negative or only focally positive for S100. However, epithelioid MPNSTs are diffusely and strongly positive for S100. Most MPNSTs are thought to arise from neurofibromas, and occasionally, neurofibroma is associated histologically with MPNSTs. There is a greatly increased risk of MPNSTs in type 1 neurofibromatosis (NF1).

Cytogenetic studies reveal MPNSTs to have complex karyotypes, often with a near-triploid chromosomal complement. In one large study, chromosomal rearrangements were seen in 1p11, 11q21, 14q24, 5p15, 5q13, 6q21, 8q10, 11q13, 17q21, 17q25, and 20q13. Frequent losses were seen in 1p12-13, 1p21-36, 9p13-24, 10p11-15, 11p, 11q21-25, 15p, 16q24, 17p, 17q11-12, 17q21-25, 22p, and 22q11-13, and gains were seen in 1q25-44, 5q13-15, 7p21, q36, 7p22, and 8q11-23. There are no differences between sporadic and NF1-associated MPNSTs.

Biallelic loss of NF1 is common in both sporadic and NF1-associated MPNSTs, but loss of NF1 function is thought to be an initiating event that is more important in the development of precursor neurofibromas than in progression to MPNSTs (Figure 26-1). Mutation of TP53 and p53 pathway members, including INK4A (CKDN2A), are found in MPNSTs but not neurofibromas, thus implicating loss of the p53 pathway in progression from neurofibroma to MPNST.

MPNST is usually a diagnosis of exclusion. The histomorphology of MPNST often closely mimics synovial sarcoma; thus, the absence of an SYT/SSX fusion can be helpful in supporting the diagnosis of MPNST.

OSTEOSARCOMA

Osteosarcomas are malignant neoplasms with at least focal osteoid formation. There are three major subtypes—fibroblastic, osteoblastic, and chondroblastic—but others have been described. Osteosarcomas arise most often within the medullary cavity but can occur on the surface of the bone. Extraskeletal osteosarcoma is a rare soft tissue tumor that tends to affect older individuals and should not be mistaken for metaplastic (sarcomatoid) carcinoma with heterologous bone formation. Cytogenetic studies of osteosarcoma reveal a

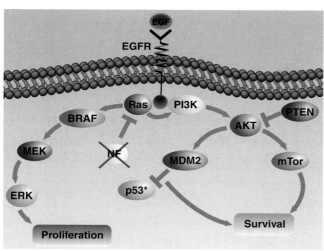

FIGURE 26-1

Major signal transduction pathways involved in neurofibroma and malignant peripheral nerve sheath tumor (MPNST). The Ras/ERK and phosphatidylinositol 3'-kinase (PI3K)/AKT pathways generally promote proliferation and survival, respectively. Neurofibromin (NF) inactivates Ras from its active guanine triphosphate (GTP)–bound state. One inactive NF1 allele is in the germline in neurofibromatosis, and there is additional loss of the remaining functional allele, which leads to increased activation of Ras-responsive pathways and neurofibroma formation. Additional mutations in the p53 pathway are often noted in MPNSTs.

variety of findings, including rearrangements of 1p11-13, 1q10-12, 1q21-22, 11p15, 12p13, 17p12-13, 19q13, and 22q11-13, as well as losses or gains of 6q, 9, 10, 13, and 17 (loss) or 1 (gain). More refined techniques have shown consistent amplification of 6p12-p21 (28%) and 17p11.2 (32%), as well as a variety of other less common findings. Osteosarcoma is associated with several genetic disorders, most notably hereditary retinoblastoma, Li-Fraumeni syndrome, Rothmund-Thomson syndrome, Werner syndrome, and familial Paget disease. Association of osteosarcoma with sporadic Paget disease of the bone is rare. Patients with hereditary retinoblastoma have germline mutations of the *RB1* gene, which encodes a tumor suppressor important in cell cycle control. Alterations in the retinoblastoma pathway, including loss of *RB1* and *CDKN2A* and amplification of *CDK4* and cyclin D1 (*CCND1*) are found in most sporadic osteosarcomas. Patients with Li-Fraumeni syndrome have germline loss-of-function mutations of TP53, which encodes a complex protein with important function in cell cycle regulation and cell survival. Loss-of-function mutations of *TP53* occur in approximately 50% of sporadic osteosarcomas. *MDM2* amplification, which leads to TP53 degradation, is seen in 7% to 15% of sporadic osteosarcoma; deletion of p14 *(ARF)*, which inhibits MDM2, is seen in 10%. Rothmund-Thomson syndrome and Werner syndrome are characterized by loss-of-function mutations in genes that encode RECQ helicases, which are important in DNA repair. However, the role of RECQ

helicases in sporadic oteosarcoma is not clear. Although there is often chromosomal gain of the *RECQL4* locus at 8q24.3, which is often mutated in Rothmund-Thomson syndrome, gene sequencing of 74 osteosarcomas failed to identify any meaningful mutations. About 30% of patients with familial Paget's disease carry mutations in *SQSTM1* on chromosome 5q35, which encodes sequesosome 1 (also known as p62) associated with several pathways involved in osteoclastogenesis. It is not known whether mutation in *SQSTM1* plays an important role in sporadic osteosarcoma.

Both *MYC* and *FOS* have been shown to be overexpressed in osteosarcomas. However, it is not known whether they are important in the pathogenesis of these tumors. Compelling mouse data indicates a role for *FOS* in osteosarcoma formation. HER2 amplification or overexpression has also been evaluated by several groups, but the results have differed dramatically. Further studies need to be performed to evaluate the role of *HER2* overexpression in osteosarcoma. Ezrin, a member of the ezrin–radixin–moesin group of proteins involved in cell migration and metastasis, has been shown to correlate with a shorter disease-free interval and higher risk of metastatic relapse when expressed at high levels.

PLEOMORPHIC SARCOMAS: PLEOMORPHIC SARCOMA NOS (MALIGNANT FIBROUS HISTIOCYTOMA), PLEOMORPHIC RHABDOMYOSARCOMA, PLEOMORPHIC LIPOSARCOMA

Sarcomas in this category exhibit pleomorphic histology. They range from unclassifiable sarcomas (also known as malignant fibrous histiocytoma) to those with either focal or diffuse rhabdomyoblasts (pleomorphic rhabdomyosarcoma) or focal or diffuse lipoblasts (pleomorphic liposarcoma). They are usually high grade with numerous atypical mitotic figures and frequent necrosis.

Most show complex cytogenetic rearrangements with intratumoral heterogeneity in the form of clonal and nonclonal cytogenetic aberrations. Many show marker chromosomes that cannot be assessed without sophisticated methods, such as spectral karyotyping. More aggressive lesions tend to have more complex karyotypes (Figure 26-2).

BONE AND SOFT TISSUE TUMORS WITH SIMPLE CYTOGENETIC FEATURES

ALVEOLAR SOFT PART SARCOMA

Alveolar soft part sarcoma (ASPS) is a rare mesenchymal neoplasm, representing less than 1% of soft tissue sarcomas. It usually occurs in the lower

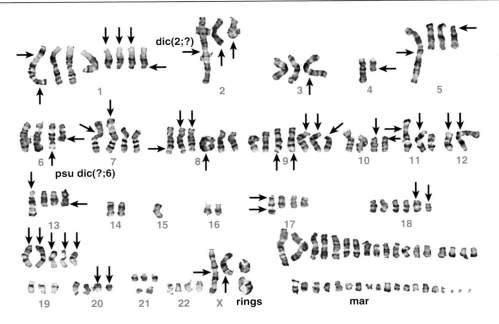

FIGURE 26-2

Complex karyotype from a high-grade unclassified sarcoma. This pleomorphic sarcoma shows extensive aneuploidy, many structural and numeric abnormalities, and a broad array of marker chromosomes that cannot be definitively categorized.

extremities of adolescents and young adults. In children, the head and neck area is preferentially involved. Histologically, ASPS is characterized by a pseudoalveolar pattern composed of richly vascularized fibrous septa lined by polygonal cells. Periodic acid Schiff–positive intracytoplasmic inclusions are common and have a characteristic crystalline rhomboid shape on ultrastructural analysis. These inclusions were recently shown to contain monocarboxylate transporter 1 and its partner CD147. Metastases to lungs, brain, and bone are common. Despite the often-multiple metastases present in more than 70% of patients, ASPS is associated with prolonged intermediate survival, although most patients with metastases ultimately succumb to the disease.

Cytogenetic and molecular studies have shown that the nonbalanced translocation der(17)t(X;17) (p11;q25) is characteristic of ASPS and results in fusion of the novel gene *ASPSCR1* (formerly *ASPL*) to the transcription factor *TFE3*. The fusion product retains the DNA-binding domains of *TFE3* and appears to work as an aberrant transcription factor. Two types of *ASPSCR1/TFE3* fusion transcripts have been described: type 1 and type 2 (Figure 26-3) that occur in similar proportion. Interestingly, type 2 is a longer transcript that retains the activation domain of *TFE3*. *ASPSCR1/TFE3* is also seen in pediatric renal cell carcinomas with unique histologic features. However, in these cases, the fusion gene results from a balanced rearrangement between chromosomes X and 17 (Figure 26-3). Other *TFE3*

fusion genes have been described in pediatric renal cell carcinomas with Xp11.2 rearrangements.

Either FISH or reverse transcriptase–polymerase chain reaction (RT-PCR) can be used for the molecular diagnosis of ASPS. The advantage of FISH for *TFE3* rearrangements is that the same probe can be used not only for the diagnosis of ASPS but also for the identification of renal cell carcinomas with *TFE3* rearrangements in the appropriate clinicopathologic context. However, immunohistochemistry for *TFE3* is an attractive alternative to molecular approaches because the identification of TFE3 protein overexpression is highly specific and sensitive for tumors with *TFE3* rearrangements.

ANEURYSMAL BONE CYST

Aneurysmal bone cyst (ABC) is a locally recurrent bone tumor that was initially described in 1942 by Jaffe and Lichtenstein. The tumor affects mainly young patients and has a predilection for the metaphyses of long bones and the posterior elements of the vertebral bodies. Histologically, ABC is mainly characterized by a loose spindle cell proliferation associated with multiple bloody cystic spaces, multinucleated giant cells, and a peculiar type of basophilic metaplastic bone formation ("blue bone"). ABC has a benign clinical course, but local recurrences can be observed in up to 70% of cases.

Initially, ABC was regarded as a reactive process, and many theories were proposed for its pathogenesis. The reactive nature of ABC was supported by the

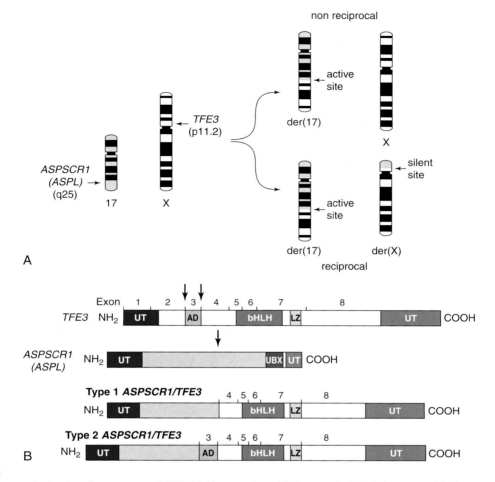

FIGURE 26-3

Translocation events in alveolar soft part sarcoma (ASPS). **(A)** The nonreciprocal fusion event in ASPS is demonstrated in the upper portion of the panel. Of interest, the translocation is reciprocal when encountered in pediatric kidney tumors, as seen in the lower right. **(B)** As seen in these exonic gene diagrams, the *TFE3* gene contributes either exons 3 to 8 or 4 to 8. The breakpoint in *ASPSCR1* (previously termed *ASPL*) is constant. This results in fusion transcripts termed type 1 and type 2. Type 2 transcripts contain the activation domain of *TFE3*, whereas type 1 does not, but both form novel transcription factors incorporating the DNA-binding domain of *TFE3* with the activation domain of *ASPSCR1*. Differences in function of the protein or clinical outcomes are not described; type 1 fusion events may be more common than type 2 events, but only a limited number of cases have been characterized. UT, untranslated region; AD, activation domain; bHLH, basic helix–loop–helix domain; UBX, UBX homology domain; LZ, leucine zipper domain.

presence of the ABC-like areas in a variety of bone neoplasms, especially giant cell tumor of bone, chondroblastoma, and osteoblastoma. For these cases, the terminology *secondary ABC* was coined.

The reactive nature of ABC was initially challenged by the work of Panoutsakopoulos et al., who demonstrated that some primary ABCs exhibited the chromosomal t(16;17)(q22;p13) as a recurrent cytogenetic abnormality (Figure 26-4). These initial observations were later confirmed by others. Recent cloning of this chromosomal translocation revealed fusion of the promoter region of the osteoblast cadherin 11 gene *(CDH11)* on chromosome 16q22 to the entire coding sequence of the ubiquitin protease *USP6* gene (also known as *TRE2* or *TRE17*) on chromosome 17p13, suggesting that the pathogenesis of most primary ABCs involves upregulation of *USP6* transcription

driven by the highly active *CDH11* promoter. In a subsequent study of 52 primary ABCs, rearrangements of *CDH11, USP6,* or both were identified in almost 70% of the cases. Rearrangements of these genes were restricted to the spindle cells in the walls of ABC and were not found in multinucleated giant cells, inflammatory cells, endothelial cells, or osteoblasts. *CDH11* and *USP6* rearrangements were also investigated in 17 secondary ABCs but with negative results, suggesting that the so-called secondary ABC represents a nonspecific morphologic pattern associated with a diverse group of neoplasms. Furthermore, the presence of *CDH11* and *USP6* rearrangements was not associated with any clinicopathologic variable, including recurrence-free survival.

Recently, four novel *USP6* fusion genes were cloned in ABC. All partner genes seem highly expressed in

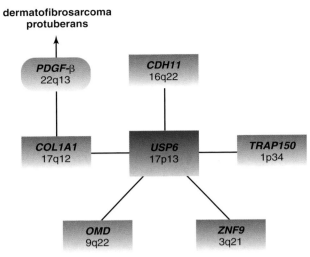

FIGURE 26-4

Gene fusion network for aneurysmal bone cyst (ABC). *USP6* (17p13) is noted to be fused with five genes (purple boxes) in ABC. One of these, *COL1A1*, is also a fusion partner with *PDGF-β* (red box) in dermatofibrosarcoma protuberans (see the relevant section in Chapter 22).

the mesenchymal or osteoblast context, including *TRAP150, ZNF9,* osteomodulin, and *COL1A1*. It is still uncertain how *USP6* transcriptional upregulation drives ABC pathogenesis, but recent work reveals that the *USP6* gene product regulates actin remodeling and vesicular trafficking and may thus regulate cell motility and invasiveness. The mechanism of a strong relatively tissue-specific promoter driving overexpression of a gene that promotes tumorigenesis is similar to the mechanism in dermatofibrosarcoma protuberans, where the *COL1A1* promoter drives overexpression of platelet-derived growth factor-β (PDGF-B). (See dermatofibrosarcoma protuberans in Chapter 22.)

Currently, few laboratories perform molecular tests for the diagnosis of ABC. Classic cytogenetics is able to detect 17p13 rearrangements with a variety of partner chromosomes. FISH can also detect *USP6* rearrangements and seems to be the most appropriate molecular diagnostic methodology for ABC because of its reasonable sensitivity (70%) and high specificity (100%). The large number of alternate *USP6* fusion genes and splicing variants observed in ABC make other methodologic approaches less attractive, especially for paraffin-embedded tissues.

ANGIOMATOID FIBROUS HISTIOCYTOMA

Angiomatoid fibrous histiocytoma (AFH), previously known as *angiomatoid malignant fibrous histiocytoma,* is a rare subcutaneous tumor that arises predominantly in the extremities of young patients. AFH is characterized by low rates of local recurrence (10% to 20%) and limited metastatic potential (<2%).

Surgical excision is considered the treatment of choice. Histologically, AFH is characterized by a nodular proliferation of oval to spindle cells associated with pseudovascular spaces. A rich lymphoplasmacytic infiltrate often surrounds the lesion, simulating a lymph node. Immunohistochemical studies suggest a possible myoid phenotype similar to the fibroblastic reticulum cells found in the connective tissue of lymph nodes. Initially, two structurally similar fusion genes were identified in AFH: *FUS/ATF1* and *EWSR1/ATF1,* resulting from the chromosomal t(12;16)(q13;p11) and t(12;22)(q13;q12), respectively. However, more recently, it was realized that most AFHs harbor the fusion gene *EWSR1/CREB1* because of the chromosomal t(2;22)(q33;q12). Both *ATF1* and *CREB1*—as well a related paralog, *CREM*—belong to the cyclic adenosine monophosphate response element–binding protein (CREB) family of transcription factors (see Figure 26-5 in the next section). These genes are involved in several processes, including cellular metabolism and growth factor–dependent cell survival (see Figure 26-15 in the section of fibrous dysplasia). Interestingly, *EWSR1/CREB1* is also seen in a subset of clear cell sarcomas that occur in the gastrointestinal tract (see the next section). As is seen with *ETV6/NTRK3* and anaplastic lymphoma kinase *(ALK)* fusion genes, this represents another instance in which identical fusion transcripts can be seen in two tumors with widely distinct histology and natural history (see Figure 26-12 in the section on Ewing sarcoma). AFH is often diagnosed by its distinct morphology, but unusual histologic features, such as nuclear pleomorphism or myxoid changes, may occasionally be seen. In these cases, molecular confirmation may be useful. Given the number of fusion partners, FISH for *EWSR1* or *FUS* may be used, although RT-PCR approaches are also possible. RT-PCR is complicated by the presence of at least three fusion transcripts, although the *EWSR1/CREB1* event appears to be the most common.

CLEAR CELL SARCOMA

Clear cell sarcoma, also known as *melanoma of soft parts,* is a rare soft tissue neoplasm that predominantly occurs in the distal extremities of adolescents and young adults. Histologically, it is characterized by a nested proliferation of clear or eosinophilic polygonal cells separated by fibrous septa and sometimes associated with multinucleated giant cells. The tumor expresses several melanocytic markers, and premelanosomes can be observed in approximately 50% of cases at the ultrastructural level. Clinically, clear cell sarcoma is characterized by the development of metastasis in 50% of patients, most commonly to lungs and lymph nodes. The overall 5-year survival rate is of 47% to 67%.

Cytogenetically, clear cell sarcoma is characterized by a t(12;22)(q13;q12) in almost all cases, which results in fusion of *EWSR1* to the CREB family transcription factor *ATF1*. The fusion protein EWSR1/ATF1 was shown to bind to the promoter of the microphthalmia-associated transcriptor factor and stimulate the activity of the melanocyte-stimulating hormone, an amplified oncogene observed in melanomas and an important regulator of melanocytic differentiation. At least four major *EWSR1/ATF1* splicing variants have been described (Figure 26-5). Type 1 is the most common and results in fusion of *EWSR1* exon 8 to *ATF1* exon 4 (85% of cases). In all splicing variants, the transcriptional activation domain of *EWSR1* and the *ATF1* bZIP DNA domain are preserved. In the descriptions of the major types of fusion transcripts, two groups use opposite designations for the types 2 and 3 transcripts, which this can cause confusion. In Figure 26-5, we chose to use the nomenclature in which types 1 and 2 represent the most commonly encountered fusion transcripts. Few type 4 fusion transcripts have been described. Quantification of percentages is complicated because some reports indicate that, apparently because of alternative splicing, up to two-thirds of cases may contain a mixture of type 1 and type 2 transcripts. This phenomenon has not been reported universally. The type of fusion transcript or transcripts present does not appear to effect clinical outcome.

Both RT-PCR and FISH may be used for molecular diagnosis of clear cell sarcoma. RT-PCR is specific and sensitive but can be challenging on paraffin-embedded tissues. FISH for *EWSR1* lacks specificity, given the involvement of this locus in multiple neoplasms (Figure 26-12); however, in a tumor showing immunohistochemical evidence of melanocytic differentiation, clear cell sarcoma can be readily distinguished from melanoma because *EWSR1* rearrangements have not been described in melanoma.

Recently, a unique type of clear cell sarcoma that occurs in the gastrointestinal tract was described. Two fusion genes have been described for this variant: the classic *EWSR1/ATF1* and a novel *EWSR1/CREB1* characterized at the chromosomal level by t(2;22)(q32;q12). *EWSR1/CREB1* has also been recently described in AFH.

Chondromyxoid Fibroma

Chondromyxoid fibroma is a rare, benign bone tumor with a predilection for males in the second and third decades of life. The lesions occur most commonly in the distal femur and proximal tibia but can arise in virtually any bone. Histologically, chondromyxoid fibroma is characterized by lobules of distinctive stellate-shaped fibroblasts set in a myxoid matrix. The lobules tend to be more hypercellular at the periphery. Despite

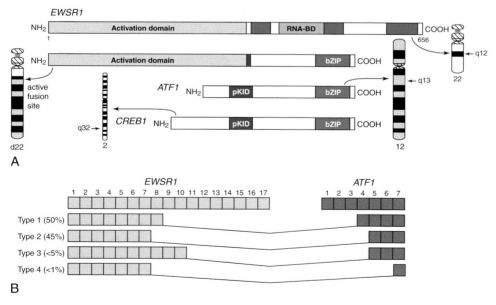

FIGURE 26-5

Clear cell sarcoma gene fusion. (A) *EWSR1* (22q12) provides the transactivation domain, and *ATF1* (12q13) provides the DNA-binding domain for the fusion gene in clear cell sarcoma produced on the derivative chromosome 22. *CREB1* (2q32), a cyclic adenosine monophosphate (cAMP)–responsive transcription factor homolog of *ATF1,* can form a similar fusion transcript in some clear cell sarcomas of the gastrointestinal tract. Similar fusion events are encountered in angiomatoid fibrous histiocytoma. **(B)** The fusion transcripts produced are of two major types, with two less common forms also encountered. Different authors have numbered these transcripts in different manners; the nomenclature employed in panel B is adapted from Panagopoulos et al. (2002). The prevalence of the fusion transcripts is complicated because some groups report the presence of both types 1 and 2 in a significant proportion of their cases, presumably because of alternative splicing, although this is not a universal finding. The percentages here include all reports of the presence of the transcripts, whether present singly or combined, and are normalized to sum to 100%. RNA-BD, RNA-binding domain.

its suggestive name, the presence of hyaline cartilage is uncommon. The immunophenotype is rather non-specific and generally not useful other than to exclude neoplasms that might mimic this tumor.

Only a few cases have been characterized cytogenetically and recurrent rearrangements of chromosome bands 6q13 and 6q25 have been observed. However, the involved genes have not been elucidated.

DESMOID FIBROMATOSIS

Desmoids are fibroblastic or myofibroblastic neoplastic proliferations that present on the extremities, trunk, or intraabdominal locations, with head and neck being a less commonly involved region. Based on clinical considerations, the deep fibromatoses are generally considered to fall into two broad classes—intraabdominal and extraabdominal. The tumors arise in young patients, often in their 30s. Primarily intraabdominal, but also extremity, desmoids can be seen in the context of familial adenomatous polyposis or Gardner syndrome, where a variant of the tumor is termed *Gardner fibroma.* Although these tumors do not metastasize, they have a strong propensity to recur locally (20% to 50%). It is important to note that these deep fibromatoses are clinically and pathogenically distinct from the superficial fibromatoses such as Dupuytren (palmar), Ledderhose (plantar), and Peyronie (penile) disease.

Approximately half of desmoid (deep fibromatosis) cases show evidence of clonal chromosomal aberrations, more often trisomies of 8 and 20 and loss or rearrangements of 5q21. These cytogenetic findings are generally absent in superficial fibromatoses.

The most common known genetic event in desmoid tumors is activating mutation of exon 3 of *CTNNB1,* the gene encoding β-catenin (Figure 26-6) This protein directly interacts with the tumor suppressor protein APC (discussed later) and is a key effector in Wnt signaling (Figure 26-7). Its role is highly variable and dependent on cellular context, but it is generally involved in proliferation, migration, and cell division. Mutations in exon 3 of *CTNNB1* are seen in many tumor types, both benign and malignant. Mutations in β-catenin block the phosphorylation necessary for degradation; thus, it accumulates in the nucleus, resulting in constitutive signaling. Interestingly, the mutations are present almost exclusively at codons 41 (Thr41Ala) and 45 (Ser45Phe and Ser45Pro). More than 80% of sporadic desmoids have these mutations. In desmoids associated with familial adenomatous polyposis or Gardner syndrome, loss of heterozygosity at the *APC* locus (5q) is present and leads to inability to form a phosphorylation complex with β-catenin, which targets the complex for destruction in the proteasome. Interestingly, certain types of germline mutations in *APC* are associated with more severe forms of

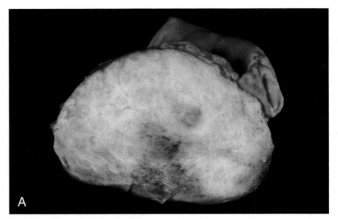

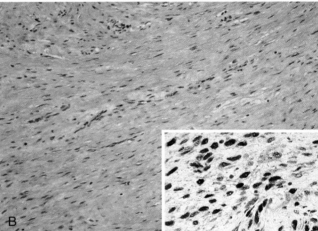

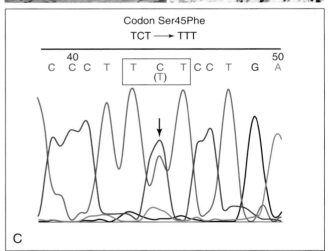

FIGURE 26-6

Desmoid tumor. A gross image of a bisected desmoid associated with the small bowel mesentery **(A)** shows a relatively bland spindle cell proliferation of fibroblastic-type cells **(B),** with intense nuclear staining for β-catenin on immunohistochemistry (inset). **(C)** Sequencing of exon 3 of *CTNNB1* revealed a missense mutation encoding a critical serine required for proteolytic degradation.

fibromatosis. These genetic features are generally absent in superficial fibromatoses.

Clinical and histologic features are usually sufficient for making the diagnosis of desmoid tumor. Immunohistochemistry for nuclear β-catenin can

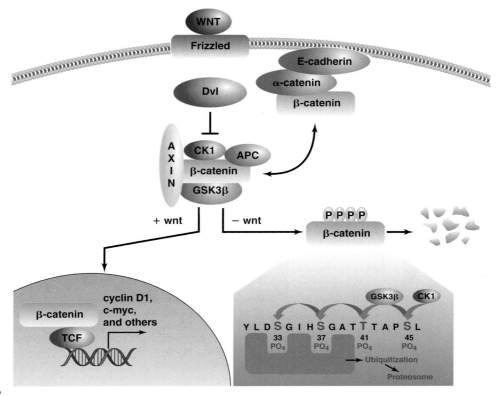

FIGURE 26-7

β-Catenin signaling pathway. β-Catenin is sequestered in adhesion junctions in the membrane with E-cadherin but can also translocate into the nucleus when the Wnt signaling pathway is activated. Thus, this protein is involved in both intracellular signaling and adhesion; the relationship between these two protein pools is unclear. A complex of proteins, including axin and APC, phosphorylates β-catenin at four critical serine and threonine residues as depicted in the lower right, marking the protein for immediate degradation in the proteasome. Active signaling through the Wnt pathway, inactivating mutations in *APC*, and mutation in exon 3 of *CTNNB1*, the gene encoding β-catenin that prevent phosphorylation, all lead to accumulation of β-catenin in the nucleus and activation of target genes such as cyclin D1, *MYC*, and others. Mutation in *CTNNB1* is the predominant change in sporadic desmoids, and germline-inactivating mutation in *APC* with subsequent loss of heterozygosity is seen in familial syndromes, such as Gardner, that are associated with desmoid fibromatosis.

sometimes be useful, especially in small biopsies (Figure 26-6). Examination for mutations in *CTNNB1* is generally not performed but could be potentially useful in small biopsies or for consideration of scar versus recurrent disease.

Desmoplastic Small Round Cell Tumor

Desmoplastic small round cell tumor (DSRCT) is a rare and highly malignant soft tissue tumor that tends to occur in adolescents or young adults and shows a striking male predominance. These tumors have a characteristic appearance of a small round cell neoplasm associated with desmoplastic stroma. The proportions of small cell and desmoplastic components can vary greatly. The tumors cells display an unusual polyphenotypic immunophenotype consisting of positivity for desmin (often dot-like), cytokeratin, neuron-specific enolase, and Wilms' tumor gene 1 (WT1).

The cytogenetic profiles in this disease may be complex, as seen in Figure 26-8, but a diagnostic reciprocal translocation involving chromosomes 11p13 and 22q12 is present in most cases.

The characteristic fusion transcript for DSRCT fuses the activation domain from *EWSR1* (22q12) to the DNA-binding domain of *WT1* (11p13), resulting in an aberrant transcription factor (Figure 26-8). Although *WT1* is a classic tumor suppressor gene, the fusion protein behaves as an oncogene. As with most *EWSR1*-related fusion transcripts, multiple microsubtypes occur between different exons of the *EWSR1* gene.

Cytogenetics can readily identify the t(11;22) (p13;q12). The diagnosis of DSRCT can also be supported by FISH for rearrangement of the *EWSR1* locus in the context of a supportive immunohistochemical profile. RT-PCR-based detection of the fusion transcript can also be performed and may be particularly helpful if Ewing sarcoma enters the differential diagnosis.

Endometrial Stromal Sarcoma

Endometrial stromal sarcoma (ESS) is a low-grade sarcoma that tends to arise from myometrium and is characterized by nodules of uniform, spindle-shaped cells arranged in vague fascicles. The lesional cells

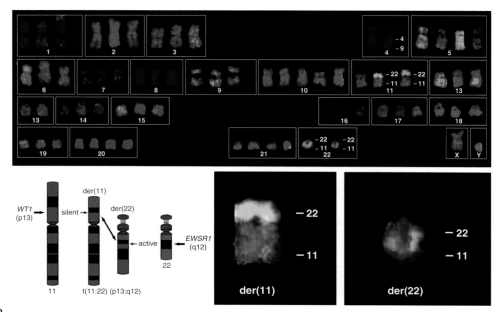

FIGURE 26-8

Desmoplastic small round cell tumor karyotype. This complex, predominantly triploid karyotype was demonstrated to have a t(11;22)(p13;q12) translocation using spectral karyotyping, and the *EWSR1/WT1* fusion transcript was confirmed by reverse transcriptase–polymerase chain reaction. The derivative chromosomes are enlarged in the two lower right panels. The active fusion site is on derivative chromosome 22, as depicted in the idiotype in the lower left.

are reminiscent of endometrial stroma and tend to invade the wall of lymphatics in a characteristic "endolymphatic" distribution.

Cytogenetically, ESS is characterized by t(7;17) (p15;q21), which results in *JAZF1/JJAZ1* fusion. This fusion gene is found in most endometrial stromal nodules and in at least 50% of low-grade ESS. Less commonly, *JAZF1* is fused to *PHF1,* which is characterized by t(6;17)(p21;p15). There is also a single example with the fusion of *EPC1* to *PHF1.* All of these gene fusions appear to encode chimeric transcription factors.

Although not commercially available, break-apart FISH for *JAZF1* would detect most cases of ESS. RT-PCR could also be performed to confirm the diagnosis.

EPITHELIOID HEMANGIOENDOTHELIOMA

Epithelioid hemangioendothelioma (EHE) is a relatively rare malignant neoplasm showing vascular differentiation. EHE can occur in bone, soft tissue, or parenchymal organs, especially lungs and liver. It has a tendency for multicentricity. Histologically, it is a poorly circumscribed proliferation of epithelioid cells arranged in cords and strands in a myxohyaline matrix. The lesional cells frequently have vacuolated cytoplasm, often containing red blood cells.

There is minimal cytogenetic information for EHE. However, two of four cases that have been reported in the literature contain an identical t(1;3)(p36.3;q25). Both the prevalence and the significance of this rearrangement remain to be defined.

EWING SARCOMA OR PRIMITIVE NEUROECTODERMAL TUMOR

Ewing sarcoma or primitive neuroectodermal tumor (PNET) was the first sarcoma to be associated with a recurrent chromosomal translocation and as such represents the archetype for translocation-associated sarcomas. It is also a prototypic "small round cell tumor" with a broad histologic differential diagnosis that includes leukemia, lymphoma, some melanomas and carcinomas, and other mesenchymal tumors, such as rhabdomyosarcoma and neuroblastoma. Although this tumor usually involves the long bones of children and young adults, extraskeletal Ewing sarcoma usually involves the trunk and lower extremities. PNET is best viewed as a subtype of Ewing sarcoma showing histological, ultrastructural, or immunohistochemical evidence of neuroectodermal differentiation such as Homer-Wright and Flexner-Wintersteiner rosettes or pseudorosettes. There appears to be a continuous spectrum between Ewing sarcoma and PNET. Ewing sarcoma is essentially undifferentiated, but PNET shows neural differentiation. Immunohistochemical evidence of distinct, crisp membranous expression of CD99/mic-2 is helpful in making the diagnosis but it is not specific.

The most common translocation in Ewing sarcoma and PNET is t(11;22)(q24;q12). The chromosome 22 breakpoint is within the *EWSR1* gene, and the chromosome 11 breakpoint falls within the *FLI1* gene (Figure 26-9). The *EWSR1* gene consists of 17 exons and encodes a protein with a transactivation domain (exons 1 to 7), a domain homologous to the putative RNA-binding site of RNA polymerase II (exons 11 to

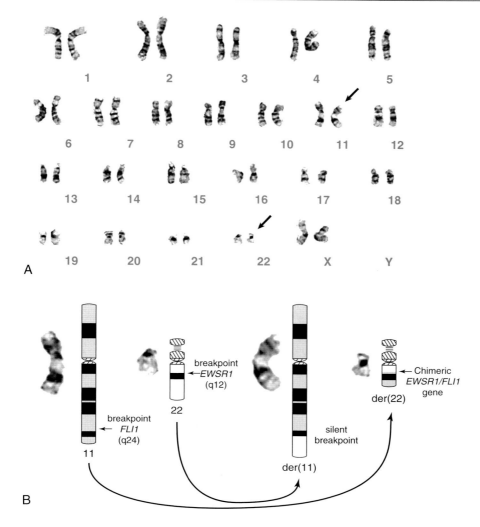

FIGURE 26-9

Karyotype of Ewing sarcoma and primitive neuroectodermal tumor (PNET). **(A)** The karyotype shows the translocation between chromosomes 11 and 22 characteristic for Ewing sarcoma and PNET as the single identifiable genetic event. The t(11;22)(q24;q12) is illustrated with karyotype and idiotype chromosomes, which demonstrates exchange of material between the long arms and creation of the active chimeric or fusion *EWSR1/FLI1* gene on the derivative chromosome 22. The fusion event on the derivative chromosome 11 does not produce a functional chimeric gene.

13), and a zinc-binding finger domain (exon 15). The precise function of this protein is not known yet. Most breakpoints are in introns 7 or 8, between exons 7 and 8, or between exons 8 and 9. If present, exon 8 is spliced out during RNA processing; thus, only exons 1 to 7 encoding the transactivation domain are present in the chimeric fusion transcript. Fusion transcripts have been categorized broadly into either type 1 (*EWSR1/FLI1*) or non-type 1 (all others). However, consensus is lacking as to whether the precise fusion transcript (either fusion partner or structural type) affects prognosis, with several conflicting small retrospective studies being reported.

FLI1 encodes a DNA-binding protein that seems to function as a transcription factor of uncertain function (Figure 26-10). The FLI1 protein has homology to the protein encoded by *ETS1,* which is developmentally regulated during cranial neural crest migration and may be involved in vasculogenesis. Thus, the fusion

transcript in its many forms, presented in Figure 26-11, fuses the transactivation domain encoded by *EWSR1* to the DNA-binding domain encoded by *FLI1.* This produces a transcription factor with aberrant activity that promotes tumorigenesis by transcriptional dysregulation in a fashion not completely understood at this time. As indicated in Figure 26-12, multiple members of the ETS family of genes form fusion transcripts with *EWSR1,* although *FLI1* (>90%) and *ERG* (≤5%) are by far the most common.

EWSR1 plays a role in the fusion transcripts of multiple soft tissue lesions. *EWSR1* can be substituted by a homologous gene, *TLS/FUS,* in some fusion transcripts for several tumors, including myxoid liposarcoma, angiomatoid fibrous histiocytoma, and rare cases of Ewing sarcoma/PNET, as indicated in Figure 26-13.

Given the broad differential diagnosis of this tumor, there is accumulating consensus that genetic

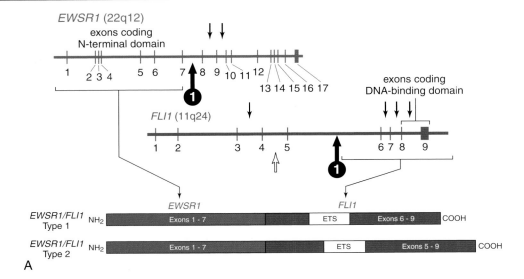

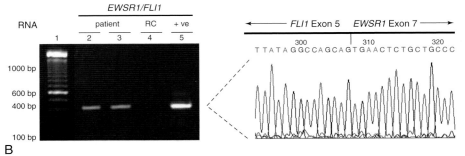

FIGURE 26-10

Gene structures of *EWSR1* and *FLI1*. **(A)** The *EWSR1* gene is composed of 17 exons separated by variably sized introns, and the *FLI1* gene is composed of 9 exons. The major breakpoints in the various introns are depicted by black-and-white arrows below the gene diagrams, with minor breakpoints marked by the small black arrows above the genes. **(B)** The two major fusion transcripts are below. The fusion transcripts can be detected from reverse-transcribed messenger RNA using polymerase chain reaction with confirmation by sequencing, as seen for the type 2 transcript. The fusion events are most readily detected from reverse-transcribed RNA, because the breakpoints with the large introns are quite variable and complicate amplification schemes.

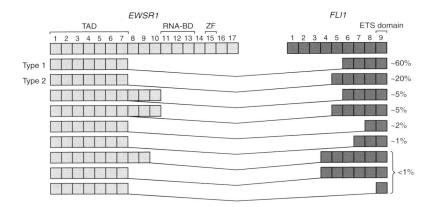

FIGURE 26-11

EWSR1/FLI1 fusion transcripts. A variety of fusion transcripts are encountered resulting from the *EWSR1/FLI1* gene fusion. Because of post-transcriptional splicing, *EWSR1* exons 1 to 7 or 1 to 10 (or rarely, 1 to 9) are always present, regardless of the breakpoint. The *FLI1* gene can contribute a variety of exons, but these always include exon 9 containing the ETS DNA-binding domain. Thus, all fusions retain the transcriptional activation domain of *EWSR1* and the DNA-binding domain of *FLI1*. Types 1 and 2 are the most common fusion transcripts, and as a whole, the *EWSR1/FLI1* types constitute 90% to 95% of all fusion events seen in Ewing sarcoma. TAD, transactivation domain; RNA-BD, RNA-binding domain; ZF, zinc finger domain.

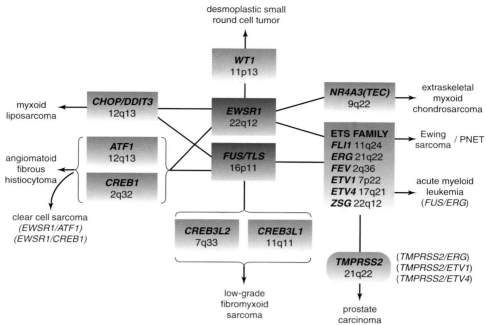

FIGURE 26-12

Depiction of *EWSR1* and *FUS* interacting fusion partners. Several genes are found in sarcomas that form fusion genes with multiple partners. *EWSR1* is the most promiscuous in this regard and can be substituted by *FUS* in some instances. The multiple interacting partners and resulting tumors involving these two genes are depicted here.

confirmation of this diagnosis is important. The tests are particularly useful for unusual morphologic variants or uncommon clinical presentations. Classic cytogenetics is a reasonable approach but is labor intensive and requires fresh tumor material (Figure 26-9). In addition to the cytogenetic translocations already described, a second common characteristic cytogenetic abnormality is the der(16)t(1;16), which has not been characterized to date. FISH using break-apart probes at the *EWSR1* locus at 22q12 is an excellent diagnostic option, because most of the currently described fusion transcripts employ the *EWSR1* locus (Figure 26-13), with the possible exception of the rare cases with *FUS/ERG* fusion because of t(16;21) and others.

It is important to remember that multiple other soft tissue tumors are associated with fusion transcripts involving the *EWSR1* locus. Because FISH using break-apart probes for the *EWSR1* locus only gives evidence of rearrangement at this locus, it is important to correlate the molecular cytogenetic results with the other pathologic and clinical data to rule out other entities that involve this locus. RT-PCR can be used to directly demonstrate the *EWSR1/FLI1* fusion transcript, although the structure of the fusion transcript can vary and usually more than one primer set is required for full coverage (Figure 26-10). Confirmation of a viable fusion transcript by direct DNA sequencing is important. Different primer sets are required to detect each of the six members of the ETS family that can fuse with *EWSR1,* but fortunately *FLI1* (11q24) and *ERG* (21q22) represent more than 97% of cases. Thus, only

these two are routinely tested. RT-PCR has the advantage of being able to detect small amounts of tumor in a background of normal tissue, but FISH is usually a more robust test that is amenable to samples such as older paraffin blocks, where it is difficult to extract quality RNA. It is important to remember that neither of these tests should ever be interpreted outside of a sensible clinical and pathologic evaluation and should only be employed when Ewing sarcoma or PNET is a reasonable diagnostic consideration. Interpretation of molecular results outside of this context can lead to diagnostic confusion.

Preliminary studies of RT-PCR using peripheral blood have shown some association with disease recurrence after treatment and thus poor outcome. Additional studies are needed to determine whether such avenues truly provide clinical utility.

EXTRASKELETAL MYXOID CHONDROSARCOMA

Although these rare soft tissue tumor neoplasms were originally thought to show primitive cartilaginous differentiation, the name is a misnomer because, with more sophisticated, modern techniques, there is no evidence of chondroid differentiation. This tumor is encountered in older adults with a male predominance. The tumor usually involves the deep soft tissues of the lower extremities. Immunohistochemical features are relatively non-specific and show that, in contrast to conventional chondrosarcomas, most extraskeletal myxoid chondrosarcomas are negative or

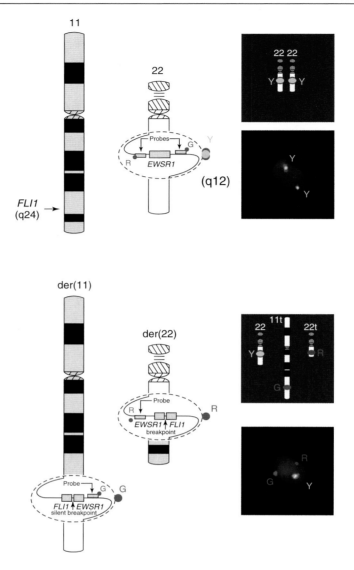

FIGURE 26-13

Detection of *EWSR1* rearrangement by fluorescence in situ hybridization (FISH). Using a break-apart strategy, the centromeric (red) and telomeric (green) flanking regions of the *EWSR1* genes are hybridized with fluorescently labeled probes. In cells in which the two loci are together, the overlapping emission spectrum of the two probes produces two yellow-appearing signals, as diagrammed in the upper panels and demonstrated in a 4'-6-diamidino-2-phenylindole (DAPI)–stained nucleus. In the lower panels, translocation between chromosomes 11 and 22 results in a derivative chromosome 22 that retains the centromeric (red) probe, and the telomeric (green) probe is transferred to the derivative chromosome 11. These two chromosomes then segregate independently in the nucleus, resulting in three signals per nucleus: the separated green and red probes and the combined (yellow) probes at the remaining intact *EWSR1* locus. The advantage of FISH with break-apart probes is that it will detect virtually all rearrangements at the *EWSR1* locus, although it cannot provide insight into the identity of the fusion partner.

focally positive only for S100, epithelial membrane antigen, or cytokeratin. Interestingly, neuroendocrine differentiation has been observed in cases of extraskeletal myxoid chondrosarcoma.

The cytogenetics of this tumor involves reciprocal translocations of the 9q22 locus with chromosomes 3q11, 15q21, 17q11, and 22q12. Other cytogenetic events can be seen but are not characteristic. The most common translocation involves the *EWSR1* locus at 22q12 and the *NR4A3* (also known as *CHN* and *TEC*) locus at 9q22. As often seen in chimeric transcripts involving *EWSR1,* the transactivation

domain of *EWSR1* is fused to the DNA-binding domain of *NR4A3*. Several types of fusion products can be seen, depending on which exons are involved. *NR4A3* is an orphan nuclear receptor that can activate the *FOS* promoter and plays a poorly understood role in the regulation of hematopoietic growth and differentiation. Unlike Ewing sarcoma or PNET, where the transactivation domain of *EWSR1* is constant and DNA targeting domains from a variety of proteins are employed, in extraskeletal myxoid chondrosarcomas the DNA-binding domain is constant and the transactivation domains of several genes are

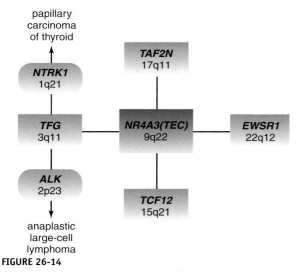

FIGURE 26-14

Gene fusion network for extraskeletal myxoid chondrosarcoma. *NR4A3(TEC)/CHN* (9q22) can combine with any of the four genes diagrammed in extraskeletal myxoid chondrosarcoma. Interestingly, *TFG* can also combine with *NTRK1* or *ALK* to form other tumors as indicated.

involved (Figure 26-14). These genes include *TAF2N* (17q11) encoding an RNA-binding protein that is a subunit of RNA polymerase II, *TCF12* (15q21) encoding a transcription factor in the basic helix–loop–helix family, and *TFG* (3q11) encoding a regulator of the nuclear factor-κB (NF-κB) pathway with homology to *FUS* and *EWSR1* in its N-terminal region. *TFG* is also seen as a fusion transcript with *ALK* (2p23) in anaplastic large-cell lymphoma and with *NTRK1* (1q21) in some thyroid papillary carcinomas. Interestingly, recent evidence indicates that tumors with these various translocations have similar gene expression profiles.

Cytogenetics is useful in revealing the various translocations diagnostic of extraskeletal myxoid chondrosarcoma. Because most translocations in this entity involve the *EWSR1* locus, FISH with break-apart, commercially available probes for this locus is a solid diagnostic option in the appropriate histologic context. Even better is the use of an *NR4A3* break-apart probe, which should be more sensitive and specific for extraskeletal myxoid chondrosarcoma. RT-PCR is a less attractive option because of the large number of fusion partners.

FIBROUS DYSPLASIA

Fibrous dysplasia is an osteofibrous neoplastic disease of bone characterized by a proliferation of spindle cells intermixed with disorganized lamellae of woven bone. Weakening of the involved bone can occur, leading to pathologic fracture. The disease can be either monostotic (involving a single bone) or polyostotic (involving multiple bones). Commonly

involved sites include the jaw bones, femur, tibia, ribs, and skull. The distal extremities are rarely involved. Rarely, osteosarcoma has been described to arise in the context of fibrous dysplasia. This condition is encountered as part of the spectrum of McCune-Albright syndrome, which also features endocrine organ and skin pigmentation disorders. Mazabraud syndrome is the rare combination of soft tissue myxomas and fibrous dysplasia.

Cytogenetic aberrations in fibrous dysplasia are seen, but no widely recurrent defect has been found in the limited cases described. The presence of cytogenetic aberrations in multiple cases supports the neoplastic nature of this disease.

Fibrous dysplasia is associated with activating point mutations in *GNAS1*, which encodes the α-stimulatory subunit of heterotrimeric G proteins (Gα$_s$). Patients with McCune-Albright syndrome have germline mosaicism (post zygotic) for a mutation in the *GNAS1* gene. Mutation affects the ability of the protein to undergo inactivation by hydrolyzing bound guanine triphosphatase; thus, increased signaling flux occurs, leading to increased activation of adenylyl cyclase and sustained increases in cellular levels of cyclic adenosine monophosphate. Ultimately, this leads to increased activation of protein kinase A (PKA) and increased activation of CREB1, which drives transcription of genes under the control of cyclic adenosine monophosphate response elements, as illustrated in Figure 26-15.

Mutations in *GNAS1* are seen in most sporadic fibrous dysplasia cases. Although most cases can be diagnosed in the absence of molecular confirmation, direct polymerase chain reaction (PCR) of tumor-derived DNA can be used to demonstrate the mutation in difficult cases, especially in the discrimination from low-grade osteosarcomas. This test is simplified because the mutations are described at but two sites, leading to Arg201His or Arg201Cys (95%), and Gln227Leu (5%). This allows for primer design leading to a short amplicon easily derived from formalin-fixed tissue. Excessive acidic decalcification methods sometimes employed in these specimens can preclude extraction of quality DNA. However, because the assay involves the detection of point mutations in a relatively short stretch of tumor genomic DNA, the assay is reasonably robust.

GASTROINTESTINAL STROMAL TUMOR

Gastrointestinal stromal tumors (GISTs) are the most common mesenchymal tumors of the gut. They have a predilection for the stomach and small bowel but occur along the entire length of the gastrointestinal tract and rarely occur in the omentum, retroperitoneum, and pelvis. They range in clinical behavior from low-grade to high-grade or clinically aggressive

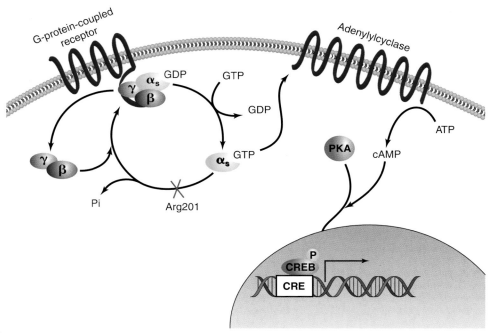

FIGURE 26-15

G-protein cyclic adenosine monophosphate (cAMP) regulatory network in fibrous dysplasia. In the presence of ligand for the G-protein-coupled receptor, guanosine diphosphate (GDP) is displaced from the G protein α-subunit, which then binds guanine triphosphatase (GTP). As a result, the Gα subunit is dissociated from the βγ-subunit complex, and can activate adenylyl cyclase to produce cAMP from adenosine triphosphate (ATP). The α-subunit is a guanosine triphosphatase that eventually hydrolases its bound GTP to GDP, thus inactivating itself. It then returns to form the initial receptor G-protein-αβγ-heterotrimeric complex. Protein kinase A (PKA) is activated by cAMP, leading to phosphorylation of *CREB*, which then binds to the cAMP response element (CRE) to activate gene transcription. In fibrous dysplasia, *GNAS*, the encoding Gα$_s$, is mutated, often at Arg201, preventing the intrinsic hydrolysis of GTP and causing constitutive activation of the cAMP pathway with subsequent tumorigenesis.

lesions. Histologically, they are composed of spindle cells, epithelioid cells, or both, and there is great heterogeneity in histologic appearance. Immunohistochemistry is helpful in difficult cases because approximately 95% of GISTs are strongly positive for *KIT, DOG1,* and phosphokinase C-θ. Most GISTs are also positive for CD34.

GISTs have a relatively simple karyotype without structural rearrangements but frequent loss of 1p, 9p, 14q, and 22q and gain of 8p and 17q. Loss of 9p corresponds to loss of *CDKN2A* (p16^{INK4a} and AKF) and is associated with aggressive clinical behavior. Approximately 85% to 90% of GISTs have activating mutations in *KIT,* a receptor tyrosine kinase (RTK) important in the development and maintenance of interstitial cells of Cajal, which likely share a common precursor with GIST. The mutations include in-frame deletions, insertions (duplications), and point mutations, but all encode virtually full-length KIT protein. Mutations are most common in exon 11 (encoding the so-called juxtamembrane domain) but occur less commonly within exon 9 (encoding part of the extracellular domain), in exons 13 and 17 (encoding the tyrosine kinase catalytic domains), and rarely in other exons. About 5% of GISTs have activating mutations within *PDGFR-α,* an RTK related to *KIT.* These mutations occur in exons 12, 14, and 18,

which are analogous to exons 11, 13, and 17 in *KIT* (Figure 26-16). About 5% to 10% of GISTs are negative for *KIT* or *PDGFR-α* mutations.

Imatinib mesylate (Gleevec™, Novartis), an orally administered small molecule compound that inhibits *KIT,* has been successful in the treatment of unresectable, recurrent/metastatic GIST. Interestingly, different mutations show variations in response to imatinib. Exon 11 mutants tend to respond well, and exon 9 mutants have an intermediate response. Recent studies have shown that exon 9 mutants respond better to increased doses of imatinib. *KIT* exon 17 mutants and the most common *PDGFR-α* mutants tend to respond poorly, but some *KIT* exon 17 mutants, *PDGFR-α* mutants, and even *KIT/PDGFR-α* wild-type GISTs respond to imatinib. Therefore, all patients with unresectable GISTs receive imatinib as first-line therapy. Some GISTs develop resistance to imatinib after prolonged treatment through the occurrence of additional mutations, which interfere with imatinib binding. Many patients who develop resistance benefit from treatment with sunitinib maleate (Sutent™, Pfizer), another orally administered small molecule inhibitor that inhibits KIT and has antivascular endothelial growth factor receptor activity. Many other targeted therapeutics are in GIST clinical trials.

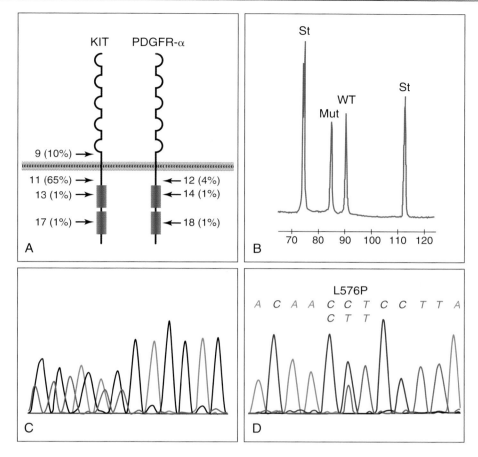

FIGURE 26-16

KIT mutation in gastrointestinal stromal tumors. The approximate mutational frequencies of various exons in *KIT* and *PDGFR*-α are noted **(A)**. With mutations or deletions, size fractionation chromatography of the polymerase chain reaction amplicon can give rapid indication of the mutation type. An in-frame 6-base-pair deletion is shown **(B)** with DNA sequencing of the reverse strand **(C)**. Point mutations are not readily detected by chromatography but are easily detected by sequencing **(D)**. Mut, mutant test DNA; St, size standard; WT, wild-type control DNA.

Determining the mutation status of GIST has not been universally recommended. However, because of differences in response to the available GIST therapies, it is likely that determination of *KIT/PDGFR*-α mutation status will become mandatory for proper clinical care.

HIBERNOMA

Hibernoma is a benign adipose tissue tumor showing brown fat differentiation. This tumor occurs mainly in the thigh of young adults. Cytogenetic analysis has shown that chromosome band 11q13 is recurrently rearranged. More recent molecular cytogenetic studies show that these rearrangements often lead to large submicroscopic chromosomal deletions that include *MEN1* and other genes. The clinical application of these findings remains to be determined. More importantly, these tumors lack the cytogenetic features of well-differentiated liposarcoma or the complex karyotype of pleomorphic liposarcoma, tumors with which hibernomas are sometimes confused.

INFANTILE FIBROSARCOMA

Infantile fibrosarcoma (IFS) (also known as congenital fibrosarcoma) is a rare neoplasm of infancy with a predilection for the distal extremities and a favorable prognosis. It is composed of a monomorphic cellular proliferation of spindle cells with fine chromatin and minimal cytoplasm. Mitotic figures are usually numerous, and necrosis is often observed. The neoplasm usually infiltrates into the surrounding soft tissues. In contrast to its aggressive appearance, IFS usually has a good prognosis.

IFS is characterized by the chromosomal t(12;15) (p13;q26), which can be difficult to recognize at the cytogenetic level because it involves the tips of chromosomes 12p and 15q. This rearrangement leads to fusion of *ETV6* (also known as *TEL*) to *NTRK3* (also known as *TRKC*). *ETV6* is a nuclear transcription factor and *NTRK3* is an RTK. The fusion gene encodes a chimeric constitutively activated RTK composed of the N-terminal oligomerization domain of *ETV6* and the kinase domain of *NTRK3*. Trisomies of chromosomes 8, 11, 17, and 20 are also characteristic of IFS and represent secondary changes involved in tumor progression subsequent to initiation by *ETV6/NTRK3* gene fusion. Trisomy 11 in particular is a characteristic finding and may be diagnostically useful in selected contexts. Cellular and mixed cellularity mesoblastic nephroma, a renal neoplasm of infancy with histology identical to that of IFS, also has the *ETV6/NTRK3* gene fusion and thus represents IFS of the kidney. This gene fusion has also been demonstrated in a case of adult acute myeloid leukemia and in most cases of secretory breast carcinoma.

Cytogenetics is helpful in confirming the diagnosis of IFS but may be challenging because of the nature of the rearrangement (described earlier). Interestingly, the identification of trisomy 11 may be a red flag for the presence of an apparently unrecognized t(12;15). FISH and RT-PCR are useful in making the diagnosis when cytogenetics is not available or in cytogenetically ambiguous cases.

INFLAMMATORY MYOFIBROBLASTIC TUMOR

Inflammatory myofibroblastic tumor was first described in the lung but is now recognized to occur in virtually any anatomic location. This diagnostic term is somewhat confusing because some have applied it to what they describe as reactive pseudotumors of the bladder and other sites. Here we employ the term for a mesenchymal neoplasm with potential for local recurrence and minimal propensity to metastasize; morbidity and mortality are primarily caused by destructive local involvement.

The major recurrent chromosomal aberrations are balanced translocations involving the *ALK* locus at 2p23. This cytogenetic feature is more commonly encountered in younger patients and may portend a more favorable course of disease. Approximately a third to half of cases diagnosed in patients younger than 30 are associated with translocations involving *ALK*.

ALK encodes a membrane-bound RTK (Figure 26-17) that is normally expressed in certain areas of the brain. The various translocation events direct the catalytic domain of this receptor to the cytoplasm or the nucleus, where it presumably signals in an unregulated fashion and promotes tumorigenesis. Proteins described as chimeric partners for *ALK* include tropomyosins (*TPM3* on 1q21 and *TPM4* on 19p13), clathrin heavy chain polypeptide (*CLTC;* 17q11), *CARS* (11p15), *ATIC* (2q35), *SEC31A* (4q21), and *RANBP2* (2q13) (Figure 26-18). In each case, the C-terminal cytoplasmic portion of ALK with its kinase domain is bound to the N-terminus of the partner protein that results in improper compartmentalization. The fusion partner with ALK appears to provide an oligomerization domain that leads to constitutive activation of ALK. In the first four fusion partners, the chimeric protein is present

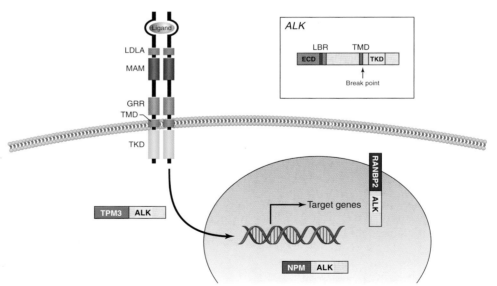

FIGURE 26-17

Anaplastic lymphoma kinase (ALK) pathway in inflammatory myofibroblastic tumor (IMT). *ALK* (2p23; CD246) encodes a receptor tyrosine kinase consisting of an extracellular domain (ECD) composed of a low-density lipoprotein–like domain (LDLA), MAM domain, glycine-rich region (GRR), transmembrane domain (TMD), and cytoplasmic tyrosine kinase domain (TKD). The extracellular and transmembrane portions of *ALK* are lost in the fusion event, and the dimerization and cellular compartment targeting are provided by the fusion partner. *TPM3* targets to the cytoplasm, *RANBP2* to the nuclear membrane, and *NPM* (seen anaplastic large-cell lymphoma but not in IMT) to the nucleus. Although not clearly understood, downstream effectors seem to modify gene expression as a result of activation. Among the downstream effector molecules that have been implicated is phospholipase C-γ. The protein encoded by ALK is shown in the membrane, and the gene diagram and breakpoint are depicted in the inset at the upper right.

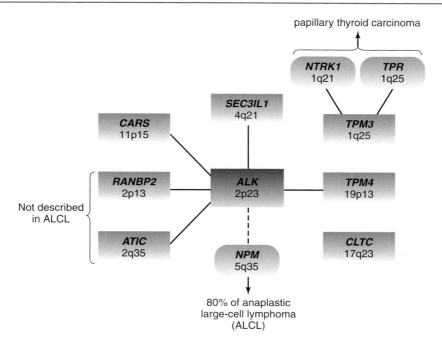

FIGURE 26-18

Anaplastic lymphoma kinase *(ALK)* gene fusion network in inflammatory myofibroblastic tumor (IMT). *ALK* (2p23) can form fusion genes with multiple partners (green boxes). All but two of these are also seen in anaplastic large-cell lymphoma (ALCL). Interestingly, *NPM,* the most common fusion partner, seen in 80% of ALCL cases, has not been described in IMT. *TPM3* fusion with *ALK* is seen in both IMT and ALCL and is fused with other genes (*NTRK1* and *TPR,* red boxes) in papillary carcinoma of the thyroid.

in the cytosol whereas with the last, RANBP2, the fusion protein is targeted to the nuclear membrane. Similar translocations are present in anaplastic large-cell lymphoma, and more than 10 fusion partners are described. In contradistinction, anaplastic large-cell lymphoma employs *NPM* (5q35) in approximately 80% of cases with distinct nuclear localization.

Immunohistochemistry can be helpful to demonstrate nuclear or cytoplasmic distribution of ALK. Immunoreactivity usually indicates translocation of ALK because expression of this protein is usually quite restricted to neural and some lymphoid cells and may even suggest the type of fusion gene present because cytoplasmic or nuclear localization can be characteristic of certain fusion events (Figure 26-17). However, the presence of ALK reactivity in a variety of sarcomas lacking ALK rearrangements has been reported; thus, molecular cytogenetic confirmation is often helpful. Break-apart FISH strategies at the *ALK* 2p23 locus are also commonly employed, given the broad array of potential binding partners.

Kaposi's Sarcoma

Although the name implies that this condition is a sarcoma, most data seem to indicate that this lesion, although sometimes clonal in nature and aggressive in certain clinical settings, is best considered a neoplasm

driven by infectious etiology. Infection with HHV-8 is seen in virtually all cases of Kaposi's sarcoma, regardless of the clinical subtype. Furthermore, Kaposi's sarcoma tends to regress when the underlying immune deficiency is treated (particularly in the aggressive cases associated with HIV or AIDS), indicating that the lesion lacks the ability to grow independently in immune-competent individuals, although there may be exceptions to this general finding. Despite differences of opinion on the nature of this endothelial proliferation, immunohistochemistry demonstrating nuclear HHV-8-associated antigens and histologic features are usually sufficient for diagnosis. This lesion is further discussed in Chapter 22.

Leiomyoma

Leiomyomas are benign smooth muscle tumors that can be seen in three distinct clinical contexts: uterine leiomyoma, superficial or cutaneous leiomyoma, and leiomyoma of deep soft tissue. Morphologic and immunohistochemical features are usually sufficient for the diagnosis of these neoplasms, and the main difficulty is in distinguishing benign from malignant forms in a small subset of cases. Criteria for malignancy vary based on the site of the tumor. In general, deep (nonuterine) smooth muscle tumors are best considered malignant until proven otherwise, given the prevalence of leiomyosarcoma at deep sites. Genetic syndromes of multiple leiomyomata are also known—most importantly, hereditary leiomyomatosis and renal cell carcinoma (HLRCC) syndrome. Leiomyomatosis associated with EBV infection is rarely encountered but well described.

Most cytogenetic findings are based on uterine leiomyomas. Recurrent cytogenetic features are encountered in up to 40% of leiomyomas; the most common finding is t(12;14)(q15;q24). Other chromosomes, including 1, 5, 8, and 10, have also been reported to fuse with 12q15. Deletions of 7q are also noted. Extrauterine leiomyomas can show deletions of 1p that can also be seen in leiomyosarcomas. In contrast, however, leiomyosarcomas show 1p deletions in the context of aneuploid, highly complex karyotypes resulting from widespread genomic instability. Cutaneous leiomyomas are less well studied. A curious entity known as benign metastasizing leiomyoma has recently been shown to demonstrate terminal deletions in 19q and 22q, a feature seen in only about 3% of benign uterine leiomyomas.

Although fusion transcripts between *HMGA2* (12q15) and *RAD51L1* (14q24) can be detected, these are not seen in most cases, and the precise significance of this translocation remains obscure. HLRCC syndrome (sometimes termed Reed syndrome) is inherited through a defective fumarate hydratase allele (1q42) in an autosomal dominant fashion. It is unclear how a mitochondrial enzyme involved in the Krebs cycle leads to uterine and cutaneous leiomyomata and renal cancer, but it is suspected that increased dependence on glycolysis is required. The gene contains 10 exons that encode a 5′ DNA-binding domain and a 3′ substrate-binding or catalytic domain. Inherited mutations are usually deletions, and missense mutations cause frameshifts and loss of the ability to produce functional protein; about 90 HLRCC families have such mutations. Loss of heterozygosity at this locus appears to drive tumorigenesis. Interestingly, an autosomal recessive disorder of fumarate hydratase deficiency is associated with severe encephalopathy.

At this point, the only relevant clinical testing would be for germline-inactivating mutations in the fumarate hydratase *(FH)* gene, because these patients are at risk for papillary renal cell carcinoma and confirmation of the diagnosis may be helpful for risk assessment and planning of clinical follow-up. Although not done routinely, evidence of a highly complex karyotype would be concerning for leiomyosarcoma.

LIPOBLASTOMA

Lipoblastoma is a benign adipocytic tumor that predominantly occurs in the extremities of young patients. Histologically, it is characterized by a lobulated proliferation of lipoblasts at various stages of differentiation, often set in a myxoid matrix with a typical plexiform vascular pattern. The clinical course is usually uneventful, but local recurrences may occur in up to 20% of cases.

Cytogenetic analyses of lipoblastoma often show rearrangements of chromosome 8q11~q13 with different chromosome partners. Gains of chromosome 8 are also commonly seen and may occur with or without rearrangements of 8q. Two fusion genes have been described in lipoblastoma—*HAS2/PLAG1* and *COL1A2/PLAG1*—and it seems that the major oncogenic mechanism is pleomorphic adenoma gene 1 *(PLAG1)* transcriptional upregulation by promoter swapping with *HAS2* or *COL1A2*. *PLAG1* encodes for a zinc finger transcription factor that was initially identified as a fusion partner with β-catenin *(CTNNB1)* in a promoter-swapping mechanism in pleomorphic adenomas with t(3;8)(p21;q12). Interestingly, another collagen gene with a strong promoter—*COL1A1*—also contributes to the transcriptional upregulation of *PDGF*-β and *USP6* in dermatofibrosarcoma protuberans and ABC, respectively (see Figure 26-4 in the section on aneurysmal bone cyst).

At present, the diagnosis of lipoblastoma is primarily histologic, although cytogenetics could serve a confirmatory role in morphologically unusual cases.

LIPOMA AND VARIANTS

Lipoma is a benign adipose tissue tumor that can occur in any age group but is more commonly found in the adult population. Lipomas typically occur in the subcutaneous tissues but can be seen in deeper locations. Lipomas are classified into many subtypes, primarily based on specific histologic features. The most important subtypes are conventional lipoma, angiolipoma, chondroid lipoma, and spindle cell or pleomorphic lipoma.

Conventional Lipoma

Conventional or ordinary lipoma is the most common mesenchymal neoplasm in humans, particularly in obese individuals. Histologically, lipomas are characterized by a lobular proliferation of mature adipocytes, similar in appearance to normal adipose tissue. Cytogenetically, lipomas exhibit abnormal but simple karyotypes in up to 80% of cases. The most common cytogenetic abnormality is rearrangement of chromosome 12q13~q15 with involvement of the chromatin remodeling gene *HMGA2* (previously known as *HMGIC*). This gene has been shown to be rearranged not only in lipomas but also in many other benign and malignant neoplasms, including pulmonary chondroid hamartoma, leiomyoma, pleomorphic adenoma, endometrial stromal polyp, aggressive angiomyxoma, fibroadenoma of breast, enchondroma, chondrosarcoma, osteosarcoma, and liposarcoma (see Figure 26-17 in the section on inflammatory myofibroblastic tumor). A few *HMGA2* fusion genes have been described in lipomas, including *HMGA2/LPP*, *HMGA2/LHFP*, and *HMGA2/RDC1*. The first is the most common and results from the chromosomal t(3;12)(q37;q15). However, in many cases of lipoma with *HMGA2* rearrangements, no partner gene has been identified. The *HMGA2* rearrangements observed in malignant neoplasms, in contrast to benign tumors, are usually accompanied by amplification.

The role of *HMGA2* in the pathogenesis of lipoma remains poorly understood despite extensive investigation, including the development of mouse models. Nevertheless, it became evident that transcriptional upregulation of this gene (or its upstream DNA-binding domains) seems to play an important role in the pathogenesis of these tumors. Recently, it has been suggested that loss of microRNA *let7* consensus sequences at the 3′ untranslated region of *HMGA2*, which normally function as repressor transcriptional units, plays a critical role for upregulation of *HMGA2* transcription.

Other cytogenetic abnormalities have been observed in ordinary lipomas. Approximately 5% to 10% of these tumors also show structural abnormalities of chromosome 6p21 with rearrangements of the *HMGA2* homolog *HMGA*.

Identification of *HMGA2* or *HMGA1* rearrangements can be readily seen by FISH, which may be used as a molecular diagnostic tool in specific situations. However, this approach has not been fully explored in clinical applications. Real-time RT-PCR or semiquantitative RT-PCR may be used to identify *HMGA2* transcriptional upregulation, which can be of clinical relevance in specific settings.

Angiolipoma

Angiolipoma is one of the most common variants of lipoma and often occurs as multiple painful tumors. Histologically, it is characterized by a proliferation of mature adipose tissue intermixed with clusters of capillary-sized vessels, often displaying intraluminal microthrombi. Cytogenetically, except for a single case, the few cases karyotyped have all shown normal karyotypes. No specific genetic abnormality has been found in angiolipoma.

Chondroid Lipoma

Chondroid lipoma is a rare variant of lipoma more commonly observed in the proximal extremities of females. Histologically, it is characterized by a mixture of mature adipocytes and chondrocyte-like lipoblasts immersed in a myxoid matrix. Only two examples have been karyotyped, and both showed the same chromosomal t(11;16)(q13;p12~p13). The genes involved remain unknown.

Spindle Cell and Pleomorphic Lipoma

Spindle cell lipoma and pleomorphic lipoma represent ends of a histologic continuum of the same clinicopathologic entity. These tumors often occur in the head and neck region and upper trunk of older male patients. Histologically, spindle cell lipoma is characterized by bland spindle cells intermixed with ropey collagen bundles and mature adipose tissue in varying proportions. Also characteristic is the presence of scattered mast cells and the strong expression of CD34 by the spindle cell component. Pleomorphic lipoma is characterized by the presence of hyperchromatic cells and multinucleated "floret-type" giant cells, in addition to the spindle cell component. Both tumors are well circumscribed and rarely recur locally.

Cytogenetically, spindle cell or pleomorphic lipoma is characterized by relatively simple karyotypes, often hypodiploid and often exhibiting deletions of unbalanced rearrangements of chromosomes 13q or 16q. These abnormalities may have diagnostic utility in specific situations, especially in the discrimination between pleomorphic lipoma and well-differentiated liposarcoma, although depth, location, and size are usually sufficient for definitive classification. Until now, no specific molecular abnormality has been found in spindle cell or pleomorphic lipoma.

LOW-GRADE FIBROMYXOID SARCOMA

Low-grade fibromyxoid sarcoma is characterized by a low-grade-appearing spindle cell proliferation with a fascicular growth pattern. The tumor typically exhibits alternating hypo- and hypercellular areas. Although the former tends to show a more fibrous stroma, the later is more myxoid. Delicate, arcading vessels are also typical, and occasional giant, fibroblastic rosettes can be seen. The tumor is cytogenetically characterized by the chromosomal translocation t(7;16)(q33;p11), which leads to the formation of the fusion gene *FUS/CREB3L1* (see Figure 26-12 in the section on Ewing sarcoma). Recently, a second fusion gene—*FUS/CREB3L2*—was described at the molecular level in a single case, likely because of the t(11;16)(p11;p11). It seems that the transcriptional upregulation of both fusion genes is driven by the strong *FUS* promoter, which provides a transcriptional activation domain to the DNA-binding domain of *CREB3L1*. The fusion breakpoints occur within exons 6 to 7 of *FUS* and exon 5 of *CREB3L1*. The fusion genes seem to be specific for low-grade fibromyxoid sarcoma and have not been detected in other tumors. A recent study showed that the fusion gene *FUS/CREB3L1* can be successfully amplified by RT-PCR from paraffin-embedded tissues for diagnostic confirmation. Another approach uses FISH to identify *FUS* in histologically suspicious cases. Although

FISH is less specific than RT-PCR (other sarcomas contain *FUS* rearrangements; see Figure 26-12 in the section on Ewing sarcoma), the most common differential diagnoses of low-grade fibromyxoid sarcoma—myxofibrosarcoma and perineurioma—do not harbor *FUS* rearrangements.

Myxoid/Round Cell Liposarcoma

Myxoid liposarcoma is the second most common type of liposarcoma and occurs mainly during the fourth to fifth decades of life; it typically arises in the lower extremities, and this tumor shows a strong propensity to metastasize. Histologically, myxoid liposarcoma is composed of spindle and stellate cells immersed in a myxoid matrix, with a characteristic branching capillary vascular pattern. Round cell liposarcoma is the cellular and poorly differentiated or high-grade form of myxoid liposarcoma. Myxoid liposarcoma has been associated with a relatively good prognosis, with a 5-year overall survival rate of 75%, but the presence of round cell differentiation is an important adverse prognostic factor.

Cytogenetic and molecular studies have shown that myxoid and round cell liposarcomas share the same genetic abnormalities. They exhibit the chromosomal translocation t(12;16)(q13;p11) in up to 90% to 95% of cases, which results in fusion of *FUS* to *DDIT3* (also known as *FUS/CHOP*) (see Figure 26-12 in the section on Ewing sarcoma). Several *FUS/DDIT3*-splicing variants have been described in myxoid or round cell liposarcoma. The most common are types 1 (30%) and 2 (60%), but their discrimination has been shown to have no prognostic relevance. FUS (previously termed TLS) encodes for a RNA-binding protein similar to the EWSR1 protein. *DDIT3* encodes for a DNA-damage-inducible negative transcription regulator involved in adipocyte differentiation. The second most common chromosomal translocation—t(12;22)(q13;q12)—results in the fusion gene *EWSR1/DDIT3*. Both FUS/DDIT3 and EWSR1/DDIT3 chimeric proteins can transform NIH3T3 fibroblasts, and recent work has shown that a myxoid liposarcoma–like phenotype is induced by transfecting *FUS/DDIT3* in mesenchymal progenitor cells or HT1080 sarcoma cells.

Three major approaches are useful for the diagnosis of myxoid liposarcoma: traditional cytogenetics (Figure 26-19), FISH, and RT-PCR. FISH for *DDIT3* rearrangements is more feasible at the clinical level, and specifically for paraffin-embedded tissues, because rearrangements of this gene have been seen only in myxoid or round cell liposarcoma. RT-PCR-based assays can also be employed but are less attractive because of the presence of at least two fusion genes and many splicing variants.

Myxoma

Myxoma is a relatively hypocellular spindle cell neoplasm with extensive myxoid stroma. Myxomas tend to occur in large muscles and are benign. Interestingly, myxomas can be seen in the context of several heritable syndromes, including Carney complex and Mazabraud syndrome. Carney complex classically consists of primary pigmented nodular adrenocortical disease, leading to primary hypercortisolism; pigmented lesions of the skin including ephelides, lentigines, and blue nevi that are often cellular (these lesions can also be present at mucosal sites); and a variety of endocrine and nonendocrine tumors, including myxomas that affect sites such as cardiac atria, skin, and breast. Other unusual tumors described include melanotic psammomatous schwannoma and large-cell calcifying Sertoli cell tumor. Mazabraud syndrome is an extremely rare syndrome in which patients have

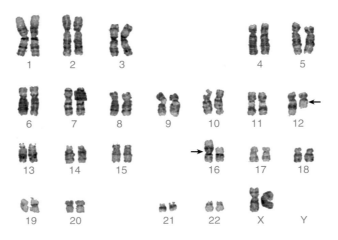

FIGURE 26-19

Karyotype of myxoid liposarcoma. This simple karyotype of myxoid liposarcoma demonstrates the characteristic chromosomal t(12;16)(q13;p11) as the only detectable cytogenetic aberration.

both fibrous dysplasia and multiple intramuscular myxomas.

Cytogenetic aberrations, including translocations, have been described in cardiac myxomas, but none of these are clearly recurrent. Deep soft tissue myxomas are less well studied.

Carney complex is associated with inactivating mutations in *PRKAR1α*, a regulatory subunit of PKA in up to 65% of cases (Figure 26-20). Rare mutations in *MYH8* have also been seen in this syndrome. Mazabraud syndrome is associated with activating mutations in *GNAS1,* a heterotrimeric G-protein-activating subunit (see Figure 26-15 in the section on fibrous dysplasia). It appears that sporadic cardiac myxomas are rarely associated with inactivating *PRKAR1α* or *GNAS1* mutations. The presence of these mutations in sporadic soft tissue myxomas is not clearly documented.

The clinical utility of examining for *PRKAR1α* or *GNAS1* mutations in myxomas is not established but may not be particularly insightful outside of evaluation for establishing the rare Carney complex patient or the even less common Mazabraud syndrome patient.

NEUROFIBROMA

Conventional neurofibromas are common neoplasms that occur most often in skin but also in subcutaneous and deep soft tissue. They are usually circumscribed but unencapsulated and composed of a combination of Schwann cells, perineurial-like cells, and fibroblasts with a variably prominent collagenous component. They are variably positive for S100, CD34, and neurofilaments.

Patients with NF1 tend to develop multiple cutaneous and deep-seated neurofibromas. These patients are born with loss-of-function germline mutations in the *NF1* gene. Interestingly, although NF1 is often familial, many cases arise sporadically in the absence of a family history. This is likely because of propensity toward mutagenesis at the *NF1* locus; the large size of the *NF1* gene may be a contributing factor. *NF1* encodes the protein neurofibromin, which has a guanosine triphosphatase activity that inactivates RAS (see Figure 26-1 in the section on MPNST). Neurofibroma formation results with loss of the other *NF1* allele. Patients with neurofibromatosis have a greatly increased risk of developing MPNSTs in neurofibromas, especially deep-seated neurofibromas that often have a plexiform growth pattern. Biallelic loss of *NF1* is also likely the pathogenetic mechanism in sporadic neurofibromas.

OSTEOCHONDROMA

Osteochondroma is a benign neoplasm characterized by an osteocartilaginous outgrowth at the bone surface, usually seen at the metaphyseal regions of

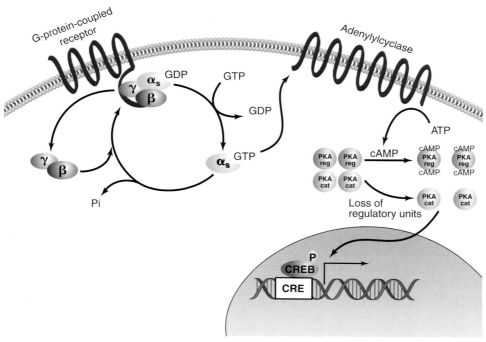

FIGURE 26-20

Protein kinase A in Carney complex. Mutations in the regulatory subunit of protein kinase A (PKA reg) allow the catalytic subunits (PKA cat) to overstimulate the cyclic adenosine monophosphate (cAMP) response pathway leading to increased activation of genes controlled by cAMP response elements. The precise mechanism of this dysfunction is still being clarified, but it appears to lead to the various endocrine tumors associated with the Carney complex, as well as the characteristic myxomas. ATP, adenosine triphosphate; CRE, cAMP response element; CREB, cAMP response element–binding protein; GDP, guanosine diphosphate; GTP, guanine triphosphatase.

the distal femur, upper tibia, and proximal humerus. Osteochondromas predominate in the first three decades of life, and most are found incidentally. They can be solitary or multiple. Multiple osteochondromas may occur in the setting of a few genetic disorders, including hereditary multiple exostosis syndrome, Langer-Giedion syndrome, and Potocki-Shaffer syndrome. Multiple hereditary exostosis is an autosomal dominant disorder characterized by short stature, multiple osteochondromas, and increased risk for the development of chondrosarcoma. It is mainly caused by mutations of the exostosin genes *EXT1* on chromosome 8 (type 1) or *EXT2* on chromosome 11 (type 2). A third locus (type 3) has been linked to chromosome 19. Langer-Giedion syndrome (trichorhinophalangeal syndrome type 2) is an autosomal dominant contiguous gene syndrome characterized by mental retardation, dysmorphic features, and multiple exostosis, and it results from loss of functional copies of the *TRPS1* and *EXT1* genes on 8q24. Potocki-Shaffer syndrome is another contiguous gene syndrome involving *EXT2* and other genes on chromosome 11p11-p13. It is characterized by cranial dysostosis and multiple exostosis.

EXT1 and *EXT2* genes encode for transmembrane glycoproteins involved in heparin sulfate polymerization, and their inactivation leads to altered Indian hedgehog, parathyroid hormone–related peptide and fibroblast growth factor signaling, which may underlie the pathogenesis of osteochondromas. Interestingly, cytogenetic clonal abnormalities are common in sporadic enchondromas, and they often involve chromosomes 8q22~q24 and 11p11~p13, where the *EXT1* and *EXT2* genes, respectively, are located.

Osteochondromas are primarily diagnosed at the histologic and radiologic levels. Cytogenetic and molecular genetic tests are usually not necessary for the diagnosis, but molecular testing can play a role in clinical management and genetic counseling for patients with the genetic syndromes above discussed.

PERICYTOMA WITH t (7;12)

A group of hemangiopericytic tumors exhibiting the chromosomal t(7;12)(p21-22;q13~15) was recently identified. Three of the five cases reported occurred in the tongue with an apparently benign clinical course. Histologically, the tumor is characterized by a lobular perivascular proliferation of ovoid to spindle-shaped cells and a hemagiopericytoma-like vasculature. Smooth muscle actin expression is universal. The chromosomal translocation results in the fusion of the 5′ end of the actin gene *ACTB* on chromosome 7 to the 3′ end of oncogene *GLI* on chromosome 12 (see Figure 26-20 in the section on myxoma). The structure of the fusion gene shows that the DNA-binding zinc finger domains of *GLI* are retained

and indicates that *GLI* transcriptional upregulation is likely mediated through the strong ectopic *ACTB* promoter.

RHABDOMYOSARCOMA

Rhabdomyosarcomas are divided into alveolar, embryonal, and pleomorphic subtypes. Botryoid and spindle cell rhabdomyosarcomas are generally considered embryonal in type. Embryonal rhabdomyosarcoma is usually encountered in children to young adults, whereas alveolar rhabdomysarcoma has a wider age distribution. Pleomorphic rhabdomyosarcoma is usually encountered in elderly patients. Histopathologic features such as eosinophilic cytoplasm with cross-striations can be helpful in establishing the diagnosis. Immunohistochemistry showing nuclear reactivity for the master myogenic regulatory transcription factors MyoD1 and myogenin is extremely helpful in confirming skeletal muscle differentiation. Distinction of the alveolar and the embryonal subtypes can often be achieved by noting the smaller, more primitive cells in the embryonal type and the large cells with more abundant cytoplasm and alveolar architecture in the alveolar type. This distinction can be complicated by the occurrence of the solid form of the alveolar subtype, which may be indistinguishable at the histologic level from other small round cell tumors. Pleomorphic rhabdomyosarcoma is discussed in the Pleomorphic Sarcomas section of this chapter and is associated with a highly complex cytogenetic profile.

Cytogenetic analysis of embryonal rhabdomyosarcoma often shows trisomies of chromosomes 2, 8, and 20, and loss of heterozygosity at 11p15 is present in most instances. Microcell hybridization transfer experiments have indicated at least two tumor suppressor loci in this chromosome band. Recent work in mice suggests that synergistic loss of *INK4A/ARF* and *MET* signaling disruption, as well as concomitant inactivation of *TP53* and *FOS,* may be important for the pathogenesis of rhabdomyosarcoma.

Two major chromosomal translocations are noted in alveolar rhabdomyosarcoma: t(2;13)(q35;q14) and t(1;13)(p36;q14). Both the translocations in alveolar rhabdomyosarcoma involve *FOXO1A* (also known as *FKHR*) at 13q14. The t(2;13)(q35;q14) and t(1;13)(p36;q14) translocations fuse the paired box transcription factors *PAX3* and *PAX7,* respectively, to *FOXO1A.* PAX3/FOXO1A is the most common fusion gene and occurs in approximately 60% to 75% of the cases; *PAX7/FOXO1A* occurs in 10% (Figure 26-21). The fusion proteins stimulate transcription on PAX-binding sites with higher potency than the corresponding wild-type PAX proteins. In addition, *PAX7/FOXO1A* is often amplified in the form of double minutes. *PAX3* and *PAX7* are specifically expressed during the development of the dorsal

from chromosome 12q13~q15, which includes *MDM2, SAS, HMGA2,* and *CDK4,* among other genes. Amplification of these genes is not specific for well-differentiated or dedifferentiated liposarcoma because they can be seen in many other sarcomas, including leiomyosarcomas, pleomorphic sarcomas, and non-mesenchymal tumors (Figure 26-24A). Recently, assays that can detect amplification of these genes on clinical specimens have raised interest because the discrimination between well-differentiated liposarcoma with minimal cytologic atypia and lipoma may be histologically challenging. Amplification of at least one of these genes, especially *MDM2,* is seen in almost all cases of well-differentiated liposarcoma but not in lipoma (Figure 26-24B). Several diagnostic methodologies have been used in this regard, including immunohistochemistry for the detection of MDM2 protein overexpression, PCR and real-time PCR, and FISH. The latter seems the most specific and sensitive because even cells devoid of cytologic atypia exhibit high levels of *MDM2* amplification. Furthermore, it is predicted that new bright-field in situ hybridization approaches may replace FISH because of lower costs and easy applicability on paraffin-embedded tissues.

SUGGESTED READINGS

Bone and Soft Tissue Tumors with Complex Cytogenetic Features

Fletcher CDM, Unni KK, Mertens F (eds): World Health Organization Classification of Tumours: Pathology and Genetics of Tumours of Soft Tissue and Bone. Lyon, IARC Press, 2002.
Naka N, Tomita Y, Nakanishi H, et al: Mutations of p53 tumor suppressor gene in angiosarcoma. Int J Cancer 1997;71:952–955.
Przygodzki RM, Finkelstein SD, Keohavong P, et al: Sporadic and thorotrast-induced angiosarcomas of the liver manifest frequent and multiple point mutations in *KRAS*-2. Lab Invest 1997;76:153–159.
Zietz C, Rossie M, Haas C, et al: *MDM2* oncoprotein overexpression, p53 gene mutation, and VEGF upregulation in angiosarcomas. Am J Pathol 1998;153:1425–1433.

Chondrosarcoma

Bovee JVMG, Cleton-Jansen AM, Taminiau HM, Hogendoorn CW: Emerging pathways in the development of chondrosarcoma of bone and implications for targeted treatment. Lancet Oncol 2005;6: 599–607.
Mandahl N, Gustafson P, Mertens F, et al: Cytogenetic aberrations and their prognostic impact in chondrosarcoma. Genes Chromosomes Cancer 2002;33:188–200.
Sandberg AA: Genetics of chondrosarcoma and related tumors. Curr Opin Oncol 2004;16:342–54.
Tallini G, Dorfman H, Brys P, et al: Correlation between clinicopathological features and karyotype in 100 cartilaginous and choroids tumours: A report from the Chromosomes and Morphology (CHAMP) Collaborative Study Group. J Pathol 2002;196:194–203.

Leiomyosarcoma

Chadwick EG, Connor EJ, Hanson IC, et al: Tumors of smooth-muscle origin in HIV-infected children. JAMA 1990;263:3182–3184.
Dei Tos AP, Maestro R, Doglioni C, et al: Tumor suppressor genes and related molecules in leiomyosarcoma. Am J Pathol 1996;148:1037–1045.
Fletcher CDM, Unni KK, Mertens F (eds): World Health Organization Classification of Tumours: Pathology and Genetics of Tumours of Soft Tissue and Bone. Lyon, IARC Press, 2002.

Sandberg AA: Updates on the cytogenetics and molecular genetics of bone and soft tissue tumors: Leiomyosarcoma. Cancer Genet Cytogenet 2005;161:1–19.

Malignant Peripheral Nerve Sheath Tumor

Kleihues P, Cavenee WK (eds): World Health Organization Classification of Tumours: Pathology and Genetics of Tumours of the Nervous System. Lyon, IARC Press, 2000.
Mertens F, Dal Cin P, De Wever I, et al: Cytogenetic characterization of peripheral nerve sheath tumours: A report of the CHAMP study group. J Pathol 2000;190:31–38.
Mertens F, Rydhom A, Bauer HF, et al: Cytogenetic findings in malignant peripheral nerve sheath tumors. Int J Cancer 1995;61:793–798.

Osteosarcoma

Boehm AK, Neff JR, Squire JA, et al: Cytogenetic findings in 36 osteosarcoma specimens and a review of the literature. Ped Pathol Mol Med 2000;19:359–376.
Bridge JA, Nelson M, McComb E: Cytogenetic findings in 73 osteosarcoma specimens and a review of the literatures. Cancer Genet Cytogenet 1997;95:74–87.
LauCC, Harris CP, Lu XY, et al: Frequent amplification and rearrangement of chromosomal bands 6p12-p21 and 17p11.2 in osteosarcoma. Genes Chromosomes Cancer 2004;39:11–21.
Wang LL: Biology of osteogenic sarcoma. Cancer J 2005;11:294–305.

Pleomorphic Sarcomas Pleomorphic Sarcoma, Nos (Malignant Fibrous Histiocytoma), Pleomorphic Rhabdomyosarcoma, Pleomorphic Liposarcoma

Fletcher CDM, Unni KK, Mertens F (eds): World Health Organization Classification of Tumours: Pathology and Genetics of Tumours of Soft Tissue and Bone. Lyon, IARC Press, 2002.
Mertens F, Fletcher CDM, Dal Cin P, et al: Cytogenetic analysis of 46 pleomorphic soft tissue sarcomas and correlation with morphologic and clinical features: A report of the CHAMP study group. Genes Chromosomes Cancer 1998;22:16–25.

Bone and Soft Tissue Tumors with Simple Cytogenetic Features

Alveolar Soft Part Sarcoma

Argani P, Ladanyi M: Translocation carcinomas of the kidney. Clin Lab Med 2005;25:363–378.
Argani P, Lal P, Hutchinson B, et al: Aberrant nuclear immunoreactivity for *TFE3* in neoplasms with *TFE3* gene fusions: A sensitive and specific immunohistochemical assay. Am J Surg Pathol 2003;27:750–761.
Argani P, Antonescu CR, Illei PB, et al: Primary renal neoplasms with the *ASPL/TFE3* gene fusion of alveolar soft part sarcoma: A distinctive tumor entity previously included among renal cell carcinomas of children and adolescents. Am J Pathol 2001;159:179–192.
Ladanyi M, Lui MY, Antonescu CR, et al: The der(17)t(X;17)(p11;q25) of human alveolar soft part sarcoma fuses the *TFE3* transcription factor gene to *ASPL,* a novel gene at 17q25. Oncogene 2001;20:48–57.
Ladanyi M, Antonescu CR, Drobnjak M, et al: The precrystalline cytoplasmic granules of alveolar soft part sarcoma contain monocarboxylate transporter 1 and CD147. Am J Pathol 2002;160:1215–1221.
Lazar AJ, Das P, Tuvin D, et al. Angiogenesis-promoting gene patterns in alveolar soft part sarcoma. Clin Cancer Res. 2007;15;13(24):7314-7321.
Lieberman PH, Brennan MF, Kimmel M, et al: Alveolar soft-part sarcoma: A clinicopathologic study of half a century. Cancer 1989;63:1–13.
Ordonez N, Ladanyi M, et al: Alveolar soft part sarcoma. In Fletcher CD, Unni KK, Mertens F (eds): World Health Organization Classification of Tumours: Pathology and Genetics of Tumours of Soft Tissue and Bone. Lyon, IARC Press, 2002, pp. 208–210.

Aneurysmal Bone Cyst

Dal Cin P, Kozakewich HP, Goumnerova L, et al: Variant translocations involving 16q22 and 17p13 in solid variant and extraosseous forms of aneurysmal bone cyst. Genes Chromosomes Cancer 2000;28:233–234.

Jaffe H, Lichtenstein L: Solitary unicameral bone cyst, with emphasis on the roentgen picture, the pathologic appearance and the pathogenesis. Arch Surg 1942;44:1004–1025.

Martinu L, Masuda-Robens JM, Robertson SE, et al: The TBC (Tre-2/Bub2/Cdc16) domain protein TRE17 regulates plasma membrane–endosomal trafficking through activation of Arf6. Mol Cell Biol 2004;24:9752–9762.

Masuda-Robens JM, Kutney SN, Qi H, Chou MM: The TRE17 oncogene encodes a component of a novel effector pathway for Rho GTPases Cdc42 and Rac1 and stimulates actin remodeling. Mol Cell Biol 2003;23:2151–2161.

Oliveira AM, Perez-Atayde AR, Dal Cin P, Gebhardt MC, et al: Aneurysmal bone cyst variant translocations upregulate USP6 transcription by promoter swapping with the ZNF9, COL1A1, TRAP150, and OMD genes. Oncogene 2005;24:3419–3426.

Oliveira AM, Hsi BL, Weremowicz S, Rosenberg AE, et al: USP6 (Tre2) fusion oncogenes in aneurysmal bone cyst. Cancer Res 2004;64:1920–1923.

Oliveira AM, Perez-Atayde AR, Inwards CY, Medeiros F, et al: USP6 and CDH11 oncogenes identify the neoplastic cell in primary aneurysmal bone cysts and are absent in so-called secondary aneurysmal bone cysts. Am J Pathol 2004;165:1773–1780.

Panoutsakopoulos G, Pandis N, Kyriazoglou I, Gustafson P, et al: Recurrent t(16;17)(q22;p13) in aneurysmal bone cysts. Genes Chromosomes Cancer 1999;26:265–266.

Rosenberg A, Nielsen G, Fletcher J: Aneurysmal bone cyst. In Fletcher CD, Unni KK, Mertens F (eds): World Health Organization Classification of Tumours: Pathology and Genetics of Tumours of Soft Tissue and Bone. Lyon, IARC Press, 2002, pp.338–339.

Angiomatoid Fibrous Histiocytoma

Antonescu CR, Dal Cin P, Nafa K, Teot LA, et al: EWS/CREB1 is the predominant gene fusion in angiomatoid fibrous histiocytoma Genes Chromosomes Cancer 2007;46:1051–1060.

Antonescu CR, Nafa K, Segal NH, et al: EWS/CREB1: A recurrent variant fusion in clear cell sarcoma—association with gastrointestinal location and absence of melanocytic differentiation. Clin Cancer Res 2006;12:5356–5362.

Costa MJ, Weiss SW: Angiomatoid malignant fibrous histiocytoma. A follow-up study of 108 cases with evaluation of possible histologic predictors of outcome. Am J Surg Pathol 1990;14:1126–1132.

Enzinger FM: Angiomatoid malignant fibrous histiocytoma: A distinct fibrohistiocytic tumor of children and young adults simulating a vascular neoplasm. Cancer 1979;44:2147–2157.

Hallor KH, Micci F, Meis-Kindblom JM, et al: Fusion genes in angiomatoid fibrous histiocytoma. Cancer Lett 2006;25:158–163.

Hallor KH, Mertens F, Jin Y, et al: Fusion of the EWSR1 and ATF1 genes without expression of the MITF-M transcript in angiomatoid fibrous histiocytoma. Genes Chromosomes Cancer 2005;44:97–102.

Waters BL, Panagopoulos I, Allen EF: Genetic characterization of angiomatoid fibrous histiocytoma identifies fusion of the FUS and ATF1 genes induced by a chromosomal translocation involving bands 12q13 and 16p11. Cancer Genet Cytogenet 2000;121:109–116.

Clear Cell Sarcoma

Antonescu CR, Nafa K, Segal NH, et al: EWS/CREB1: A recurrent variant fusion in clear cell sarcoma: Association with gastrointestinal location and absence of melanocytic differentiation. Clin Cancer Res 2006;12:5356–5362.

Chung EB, Enzinger FM: Malignant melanoma of soft parts: A reassessment of clear cell sarcoma. Am J Surg Pathol 1983;7:405–413.

Coindre JM, Hostein I, Terrier P, et al: Diagnosis of clear cell sarcoma by real-time reverse transcriptase–polymerase chain reaction analysis of paraffin embedded tissues: Clinicopathologic and molecular analysis of 44 patients from the French sarcoma group. Cancer 2006;107:1055–1064.

Davis IJ, Kim JJ, Ozsolak F, et al: Oncogenic MITF dysregulation in clear cell sarcoma: Defining the MiTF family of human cancers. Cancer Cell 2006;9:473–484.

Kawai A, Hosono A, Nakayama R, et al: Clear cell sarcoma of tendons and aponeuroses: A study of 75 patients. Cancer 2007;109:109–116.

Panagopoulos I, Mertens F, Isaksson M, et al: Molecular genetic characterization of the EWS/ATF1 fusion gene in clear cell sarcoma of tendons and aponeuroses. Int J Cancer 2002;99:560–567.

Patel RM, Downs-Kelly E, Weiss SW, et al: Dual-color, break-apart fluorescence in situ hybridization for EWS gene rearrangement distinguishes

clear cell sarcoma of soft tissue from malignant melanoma. Mod Pathol 2005;18:1585–1590.

Sandberg AA, Bridge JA: Updates on the cytogenetics and molecular genetics of bone and soft tissue tumors: Clear cell sarcoma (malignant melanoma of soft parts). Cancer Genet Cytogenet 2001;130:1–7.

Sciot R, Speleman F: Clear cell sarcoma of soft tissue. In Fletcher CD, Unni KK, Mertens F (eds): World Health Organization Classification of Tumours: Pathology and Genetics of Tumours of Soft Tissue and Bone. Lyon, IARC Press, 2002, pp.211–212.

Zucman J, Delattre O, Desmaze C, et al: EWS and ATF1 gene fusion induced by t(12;22) translocation in malignant melanoma of soft parts. Nat Genet 1993;4:341–345.

Chondromyxoid Fibroma

Granter SR, Renshaw AA, Kozakewich HP, Fletcher JA. The pericentromeric inversion, inv (6)(p25q13), is a novel diagnostic marker in chondromyxoid fibroma. Mod Pathol 1998;11:1071–1074.

Safar A, Nelson M, Neff JR et al. Recurrent anomalies of 6q25 in chondromyxoid fibroma. Hum Pathol 2000;31:306–311.

Tallini G, Dorfman H, Brys P, et al. Correlation between clinicopathological features and karyotype in 100 cartilaginous and chordoid tumours. A report from the chromosomes and morphology (CHAMP) collaborative study group. J Pathol. 2002;196:194–203.

Ostrowski JM, Spjut HJ, Bridge JA. Chondromyxoid Fibroma In Fletcher CD, Unni KK, Mertens F (eds): World Health Organization Classification of Tumours: Pathology and Genetics of Tumours of Soft Tissue and Bone. Lyon, IARC Press, 2002 pp. 243-245.

Desmoid Fibromatosis

Bhattacharya B, Dilworth HP, Iacobuzio-Donahue C, et al: Nuclear β-catenin expression distinguishes deep fibromatosis from other benign and malignant fibroblastic and myofibroblastic lesions. Am J Surg Pathol 2005;29:653–659.

Latchford A, Volikos E, Johnson V, et al: APC mutations in FAP-associated desmoid tumours are nonrandom but not "just right." Hum Mol Genet 2007;16:78–82.

Lev D, Kotilingam D, Wei C, et al: Optimizing treatment of desmoid tumors. J Clin Oncol 2007;25:1785–1791.

Tejpar S, Nollet F, Li C, et al: Predominance of β-catenin mutations and β-catenin dysregulation in sporadic aggressive fibromatosis (desmoid tumor). Oncogene 1999;18:6615–6620.

Desmoplastic Small Round Cell Tumor

Antonescu CR, Gerald WL, Magid MS, Ladanyi M: Molecular variants of the EWS/WT1 gene fusion in desmoplastic small round cell tumor. Diagn Mol Pathol 1998;7:24–28.

Fletcher CDM, Unni KK, Mertens F (eds): World Health Organization Classification of Tumours: Pathology and Genetics of Tumours of Soft Tissue and Bone. Lyon, IARC Press, 2002.

Sandberg AA, Bridge JA: Updates on the cytogenetics and molecular genetics of bone and soft tissue tumors. desmoplastic small round-cell tumors. Cancer Genet Cytogenet 2002;138:1–10.

Endometrial Stromal Sarcoma

Koontz JI, Soreng AL, Nucci M, et al: Frequent fusion of the JAZF1 and JJAZ1 genes in endometrial stromal tumors. Proc Natl Acad Sci USA 2001;98:6348–6353.

Micci F, Panagopoulos I, Bjerkehagen B, Heim S: Consistent rearrangement of chromosomal band 6p21 with generation of fusion genes JAZF1/PHF1 and EPC1/PHF1 in endometrial stromal sarcoma. Cancer Res 2006;66:107–112.

Epithelioid Hemangioendothelioma

Boudousquie AC, Lawce HJ, Sherman R, et al: Complex translocation (7;22) identified in an epithelioid hemangioendothelioma. Cancer Genet Cytogenet 1996;92:116–121.

He M, Das K, Blacksin M, et al: A translocation involving the placental growth factor gene is identified in an epithelioid hemangioendothelioma. Cancer Genet Cytogenet 2006;168:150–154.

Mendlick MR, Nelson M, Pickering D, et al: Translocation t(1;3)(p36.3;q25) is a nonrandom aberration in epithelioid hemangioendothelioma. Am J Surg Pathol 2001;25:684–687.

Ewing Sarcoma or Primitive Neuroectodermal Tumor

Avigad S, Cohen IJ, Zilberstein J, et al: The predictive potential of molecular detection in the nonmetastatic Ewing family of tumors. Cancer 2004;100:1053–1058.

Bridge RS, Rajaram V, Dehner LP, et al: Molecular diagnosis of Ewing sarcoma/primitive neuroectodermal tumor in routinely processed tissue: A comparison of two FISH strategies and RT-PCR in malignant round cell tumors. Mod Pathol 2006;19:1–8.

Fletcher CDM, Unni KK, Mertens F (eds): World Health Organization Classification of Tumours: Pathology and Genetics of Tumours of Soft Tissue and Bone. Lyon, IARC Press, 2002.

Folpe AL, Goldblum JR, Rubin BP, et al: Morphologic and immunophenotypic diversity in Ewing family tumors: A study of 66 genetically confirmed cases. Am J Surg Pathol 2005;29:1025–1033.

Khoury JD: Ewing sarcoma family of tumors. Adv Anat Pathol 2005;12: 212–220.

Sandberg AA, Bridge JA: Updates on cytogenetics and molecular genetics of bone and soft tissue tumors: Ewing sarcoma and peripheral primitive neuroectodermal tumors. Cancer Genet Cytogenet 2000;123:1–26.

Extraskeletal Myxoid Chondrosarcoma

Fletcher CDM, Unni KK, Mertens F (eds): World Health Organization Classification of Tumours: Pathology and Genetics of Tumours of Soft Tissue and Bone. Lyon, IARC Press, 2002.

Sjogren H, Meis-Kindblom JM, Orndal C, et al: Studies on the molecular pathogenesis of extraskeletal myxoid chondrosarcoma: Cytogenetic, molecular genetic, and cDNA microarray analyses. Am J Pathol 2003;162:781–792.

Fibrous Dysplasia

Cohen MM Jr: The new bone biology: Pathologic, molecular and clinical correlates. Am J Med Genet A 2006;40:2646–2706.

de Sanctis L, Delmastro L, Russo MC, et al: Genetics of McCune-Albright syndrome. J Pediatr Endocrinol Metab 2006;19(Suppl 2):577–582.

Idowu BD, Al-Adnani M, O'Donnell P, et al: A sensitive mutation-specific screening technique for GNAS1 mutations in cases of fibrous dysplasia: The first report of a codon 227 mutation in bone. Histopathology 2007;50:691–704.

Gastrointestinal Stromal Tumor

Rubin BP, Duensing A: Mechanisms of resistance to small molecule kinase inhibition in the treatment of solid tumors. Lab Invest 2006;86: 981–986.

Rubin BP, Heinrich MC, Corless CL: Gastrointestinal stromal tumour. Lancet 2007;369:1731–1741.

Rubin BP: Gastrointestinal stromal tumors: An update. Histopathology 2006;48:83–96.

Hibernoma

Gisselsson D, Hoglund M, Mertens F, et al: Hibernomas are characterized by homozygous deletions in the multiple endocrine neoplasia type I region. Metaphase fluorescence in situ hybridization reveals complex rearrangements not detected by conventional cytogenetics. Am J Pathol 1999;155:61–66.

Maire G, Forus A, Foa C, et al: 11q13 alterations in two cases of hibernoma: Large heterozygous deletions and rearrangement breakpoints near GARP in 11q13.5. Genes Chromosomes Cancer 2003;37:389–395.

Mrozek K, Karakousis CP, Bloomfield CD: Band 11q13 is nonrandomly rearranged in hibernomas. Genes Chromosomes Cancer 1994;9:145–147.

Infantile Fibrosarcoma

Bourgeois JM, Knezevich SR, Mathers JA, Sorensen PH: Molecular detection of the ETV6/NTRK3 gene fusion differentiates congenital fibrosarcoma from other childhood spindle cell tumors. Am J Surg Pathol 2000;24:937–946.

Fletcher CDM, Unni KK, Mertens F (eds): World Health Organization Classification of Tumours: Pathology and Genetics of Tumours of Soft Tissue and Bone. Lyon, IARC Press, 2002.

Knezevich SR, McFadden DE, Tao W, et al: A novel ETV6/NTRK3 gene fusion in congenital fibrosarcoma. Nat Genet 1998;18:184–187.

Lannon CL, Sorensen PH: ETV6/NTRK3: A chimeric protein kinase with transformation activity in multiple cell lineages. Semin Cancer Biol 2005;15:215–223.

Inflammatory Myofibroblastic Tumor

Coffin CM, Hornick JL, Fletcher CD: Inflammatory myofibroblastic tumor: Comparison of clinicopathologic, histologic, and immunohistochemical features including ALK expression in atypical and aggressive cases. Am J Surg Pathol 2007;31:509–520.

Lawrence B, Perez-Atayde A, Hibbard MK, et al: TPM3/ALK and TPM4/ALK oncogenes in inflammatory myofibroblastic tumors. Am J Pathol 2000;157:377–384.

Ma Z, Hill DA, Collins MH, et al: Fusion of ALK to the Ran-binding protein 2 (RANBP2) gene in inflammatory myofibroblastic tumor. Genes Chromosomes Cancer 2003;37:98–105.

Leiomyoma

Alam NA, Rowan AJ, Wortham NC, et al: Genetic and functional analyses of FH mutations in multiple cutaneous and uterine leiomyomatosis, hereditary leiomyomatosis and renal cancer, and fumarate hydratase deficiency. Hum Mol Genet 2003;12:1241–1252.

Hornick JL, Fletcher CD: Criteria for malignancy in nonvisceral smooth muscle tumors. Ann Diagn Pathol 2003;7:60–66.

Nucci MR, Drapkin R, Cin PD, et al: Distinctive cytogenetic profile in benign metastasizing leiomyoma: Pathogenetic implications. Am J Surg Pathol 2007;31:737–743.

Quade BJ, Weremowicz S, Neskey DM, et al: Fusion transcripts involving HMGA2 are not a common molecular mechanism in uterine leiomyomata with rearrangements in 12q15. Cancer Res 2003;63:1351–1358.

Tomlinson IP, Alam NA, Rowan AJ, et al: Germline mutations in FH predispose to dominantly inherited uterine fibroids, skin leiomyomata and papillary renal cell cancer. Nat Genet 2002:30:406–410.

Lipoblastoma

Gisselsson D, Hibbard MK, Dal Cin P, et al: PLAG1 alterations in lipoblastoma: Involvement in varied mesenchymal cell types and evidence for alternative oncogenic mechanisms. Am J Pathol 2001;159:955–962.

Hibbard MK, Kozakewich HP, Dal Cin P, et al: PLAG1 fusion oncogenes in lipoblastoma. Cancer Res 2000;60:4869–4872.

Kas K, Voz ML, Röijer E, et al: Promoter swapping between the genes for a novel zinc finger protein and β-catenin in pleiomorphic adenomas with t(3;8)(p21;q12) translocations. Nat Genet 1997;15:170–174.

Lawrence B, Perez-Atayde A, Hibbard MK, et al: TPM3/ALK and TPM4/ALK oncogenes in inflammatory myofibroblastic tumors. Am J Pathol 2000;157:377–384.

Sciot R, Mandahl N: Lipoblastoma. In Fletcher CD, Unni KK, Mertens F (eds): World Health Organization Classification of Tumours: Pathology and Genetics of Tumours of Soft Tissue and Bone. Lyon, IARC Press, 2002, pp.26–27.

Lipoma and Variants

Bartuma H, Hallor KH, Panagopoulos I, et al: Assessment of the clinical and molecular impact of different cytogenetic subgroups in a series of 272 lipomas with abnormal karyotype. Genes Chromosomes Cancer 2007;46(6):594–606.

Dal CP, Sciot R, Polito P, et al: Lesions of 13q may occur independently of deletion of 16q in spindle cell/pleomorphic lipomas. Histopathology 1997;31:222–225.

Fedele M, Battista S, Manfioletti G, et al: Role of the high mobility group A proteins in human lipomas. Carcinogenesis 2001;22:1583–1591.

Mayr C, Hemann MT, Bartel DP: Disrupting the pairing between let-7 and HMGA2 enhances oncogenic transformation. Science 2007;315:1576–1579.

Mietinnen MM, Mandahl N: Spindle cell lipoma / pleomorphiclipoma. In Fletcher CD, Unni KK, Mertens F (eds): WorldHealth Organization Classification of Tumours: Pathology and Genetics of Tumours of Soft Tissue and Bone. Lyon, IARC Press, 2002, pp. 31-32.

Nielsen GP, Mandahl N: Lipoma. In Fletcher CD, Unni KK, Mertens F (eds): World Health Organization Classification of Tumours: Pathology and Genetics of Tumours of Soft Tissue and Bone. Lyon, IARC Press, 2002, pp. 20–22, 31–32.

Pedeutour F, Forus A, Coindre JM, et al: Structure of the supernumerary ring and giant rod chromosomes in adipose tissue tumors. Genes Chromosomes Cancer 1999;24:30–41.

Petit MM, Mols R, Schoenmakers EF, et al: V LPP, the preferred fusion partner gene of HMGIC in lipomas, is a novel member of the LIM protein gene family. Genomics 1996;36:118–129.

Sandberg AA: Updates on the cytogenetics and molecular genetics of bone and soft tissue tumors: Lipoma. Cancer Genet Cytogenet 2004;150:93–115.

Willen H, Akerman M, Dal Cin P, et al: Comparison of chromosomal patterns with clinical features in 165 lipomas: A report of the CHAMP study group. Cancer Genet Cytogenet 1998;102:46–49.

Low-Grade Fibromyxoid Sarcoma

Matsuyama A, Hisaoka M, Shimajiri S, et al: Molecular detection of FUS/CREB3L2 fusion transcripts in low-grade fibromyxoid sarcoma using formalin-fixed, paraffin-embedded tissue specimens. Am J Surg Pathol 2006;30(9):1077–1084.

Mertens F, Fletcher CD, Antonescu CR, et al: Clinicopathologic and molecular genetic characterization of low-grade fibromyxoid sarcoma, and cloning of a novel FUS/CREB3L1 fusion gene. Lab Invest 2005;85(3):408–415.

Panagopoulos I, Moller E, Dahlen A, et al: Characterization of the native CREB3L2 transcription factor and the FUS/CREB3L2 chimera. Genes Chromosomes Cancer 2007;46(2):181–191.

Panagopoulos I, Storlazzi CT, Fletcher CD, et al: The chimeric FUS/CREB3l2 gene is specific for low-grade fibromyxoid sarcoma. Genes Chromosomes Cancer 2004;40(3):218–228.

Storlazzi CT, Mertens F, Nascimento A, et al: Fusion of the FUS and BBF2H7 genes in low grade fibromyxoid sarcoma. Hum Mol Genet 2003;12(18):2349–2358.

Myxoid or Round Cell Liposarcoma

Antonescu CR, Tschernyavsky SJ, Decuseara R, et al: Prognostic impact of p53 status, TLS/CHOP fusion transcript structure, and histological grade in myxoid liposarcoma: A molecular and clinicopathologic study of 82 cases. Clin Cancer Res 2001;7:3977–3987.

Crozat A, Aman P, Mandahl N, Ron D: Fusion of CHOP to a novel RNA-binding protein in human myxoid liposarcoma. Nature 1993;363:640–644.

Engstrom K, Willén H, Kåbjörn-Gustafsson C, et al: The myxoid/round cell liposarcoma fusion oncogene FUS/DDIT3 and the normal DDIT3 induce a liposarcoma phenotype in transfected human fibrosarcoma cells. Am J Pathol 2006;168:1642–1653.

Kilpatrick SE, Doyon J, Choong PF, et al: The clinicopathologic spectrum of myxoid and round cell liposarcoma. A study of 95 cases. Cancer 1996;77:1450–1458.

Panagopoulos I, Höglund M, Mertens F, et al: Fusion of the EWS and CHOP genes in myxoid liposarcoma. Oncogene 1996;12:489–494.

Panagopoulos I, Mertens F, Isaksson M, Mandahl N: A novel FUS/CHOP chimera in myxoid liposarcoma. Biochem Biophys Res Commun 2000;279:838–845.

Rabbitts TH, Forster A, Larson R, Nathan P: Fusion of the dominant-negative transcription regulator CHOP with a novel gene FUS by translocation t(12;16) in malignant liposarcoma. Nat Genet 1993;4:175–180.

Riggi N, Cironi L, Provero P, et al: Expression of the FUS/CHOP fusion protein in primary mesenchymal progenitor cells gives rise to a model of myxoid liposarcoma. Cancer Res 2006;66:7016–7023.

Myxoma or Cellular Myxoma

Boikos SA, Stratakis CA: Carney complex: The first 20 years. Curr Opin Oncol 2007;19:24–29.

Faivre L, Nivelon-Chevallier A, Kottler ML, et al: Mazabraud syndrome in two patients: Clinical overlap with McCune-Albright syndrome. Am J Med Genet 2001;99:132–136.

Fletcher CDM, Unni KK, Mertens F (eds): World Health Organization Classification of Tumours: Pathology and Genetics of Tumours of Soft Tissue and Bone. Lyon, IARC Press, 2002.

Kirschner LS, Carney JA, Pack SD, et al: Mutations of the gene encoding the protein kinase A type I-α regulatory subunit in patients with the Carney complex. Nat Genet 2000;26:89–92.

Stratakis CA, Kirschner LS, Carney JA: Clinical and molecular features of the Carney complex: Diagnostic criteria and recommendations for patient evaluation. J Clin Endocrinol Metab 2001;86:4041–4046.

Neurofibroma

Kleihues P, Cavenee WK (eds): World Health Organization Classification of Tumours: Pathology and Genetics of Tumours of the Nervous System. Lyon, IARC Press, 2000.

Maertens O, Brems H, Vandesompele J, et al: Comprehensive NF1 screening on cultured Schwann cells from neurofibromas. Hum Mutat 2006;27:1030–1040.

Osteochondroma

Bridge JA, Nelson M, Orndal C, et al: Clonal karyotypic abnormalities of the hereditary multiple exostoses chromosomal loci 8q24.1 (EXT1) and 11p11-12 (EXT2) in patients with sporadic and hereditary osteochondromas. Cancer 1998;82:1657–1663.

Duncan G, McCormick C, Tufaro F: The link between heparan sulfate and hereditary bone disease: Finding a function for the EXT family of putative tumor suppressor proteins. J Clin Invest 2001;108:511–516.

Tallini G, Dorfman H, Brys P, et al: Correlation between clinicopathological features and karyotype in 100 cartilaginous and choroids tumours: A report from the Chromosomes and Morphology (CHAMP) Collaborative Study Group. J Pathol 2002;196:194–203.

Tiet TD, Alman BA: Developmental pathways in musculoskeletal neoplasia: Involvement of the Indian Hedgehog–parathyroid hormone–related protein pathway. Pediatr Res 2003;53:539–543.

Unni K, Inwards C, Bridge J, et al: Tumors of the bones and joints. Washington, DC, Armed Forces Institute of Pathology, 2005.

Wuyts W, Van HW: Molecular basis of multiple exostoses: Mutations in the EXT1 and EXT2 genes. Hum Mutat 2000;15:220–227.

Zak BM, Crawford BE, Esko JD: Hereditary multiple exostoses and heparan sulfate polymerization. Biochim Biophys Acta 2002;19;1573:346–355.

Pericytoma with t(7;12)

Dahlen A, Fletcher CD, Mertens F, et al: Activation of the GLI oncogene through fusion with the β-actin gene (ACTB) in a group of distinctive pericytic neoplasms: Pericytoma with t(7;12). Am J Pathol 2004;164:1645–1653.

Dahlen A, Mertens F, Mandahl N, Panagopoulos I: Molecular genetic characterization of the genomic ACTB/GLI fusion in pericytoma with t(7;12). Biochem Biophys Res Commun 2004;325:1318–1323.

Rhabdomyosarcoma

Barr FG, Qualman SJ, Macris MH, et al: Genetic herterogeneity in the alveolar rhabdomyosarcoma subset without typical gene fusions. Cancer Res 2002;62:4704–4710.

Fletcher CDM, Unni KK, Mertens F (eds): World Health Organization Classification of Tumours: Pathology and Genetics of Tumours of Soft Tissue and Bone. Lyon, IARC Press, 2002.

Fritsch MK, Bridge JA, Schuster AE, et al: Performance characteristics of a reverse transcriptase–polymerase chain reaction assay for the detection of tumor-specific fusion transcripts from archival tissue. Pediatr Dev Pathol 2003;6:43–53.

Nishio J, Althof PA, Bailey JM, et al: Use of a novel FISH assay on paraffin-embedded tissues as an adjunct to diagnosis of alveolar rhabdomyosarcoma. Lab Invest 2006;86:547–556.

Sorensen PH, Lynch JC, Qualman SJ, et al: PAX3/FKHR and PAX7/FKHR gene fusions are prognostic indicators in alveolar rhabdomyosarcoma: A report from the children's oncology group. J Clin Oncol 2002;20:2672–2679.

Schwannoma

Baser ME: Contributors to the international NF2 mutation database. Hum Mutat 2006;27:297–306.

Brooks DG: The neurofibromatosis: Hereditary predisposition to multiple peripheral nerve tumors. Neurosurg Clin N Am 2004;15:145–155.

Kleihues P, Cavenee WK (eds): World Health Organization Classification of Tumours: Pathology and Genetics of Tumours of the Nervous System. Lyon, IARC Press, 2000.

Subungual Exostosis and Bizarre Parosteal Osteochondromatous Proliferation

Endo M, Hasegawa T, Tashiro T, et al: Bizarre parosteal osteochondromatous proliferation with a t(1;17) translocation. Virchows Arch 2005;447:99–102.

Nilsson M, Domanski HA, Mertens F, Mandahl N: Molecular cytogenetic characterization of recurrent translocation breakpoints in bizarre parosteal osteochondromatous proliferation (Nora's lesion). Hum Pathol 2004;35:1063–1069.

Storlazzi CT, Wozniak A, Panagopoulos I, et al: Rearrangement of the COL12A1 and COL4A5 genes in subungual exostosis: Molecular cytogenetic delineation of the tumor-specific translocation t(X;6)(q13-14;q22). Int J Cancer 2006;118:1972–1976.

Zambrano E, Nosé V, Perez-Atayde AR, et al: Distinct chromosomal rearrangements in subungual (Dupuytren) exostosis and bizarre parosteal osteochondromatous proliferation (Nora lesion). Am J Surg Pathol 2004;28:1033–1039.

Synovial Chondromatosis

Buddingh EP, Krallman P, Neff JR, et al: Chromosome 6 abnormalities are recurrent in synovial chondromatosis. Cancer Genet Cytogenet 2003;140:18–22.

Sandberg AA: Genetics of chondrosarcoma and related tumors. Curr Opin Oncol 2004;16:342–354.

Unni K, Inwards C, Bridge J, et al: Tumors of the bones and joints. Washington, DC, Armed Forces Institute of Pathology, 2005.

Synovial Sarcoma

Amary MF, Berisha F, Bernardi Fdel C, et al: Detection of SS18/SSX fusion transcripts in formalin-fixed paraffin-embedded neoplasms: Analysis of conventional RT-PCR, qRT-PCR and dual color FISH as diagnostic tools for synovial sarcoma. Mod Pathol 2007;20:482–496.

Clark J, Rocques PJ, Crew AJ, et al: Identification of novel genes, SYT and SSX, involved in the t(X;18)(p11.2;q11.2) translocation found in human synovial sarcoma. Nat Genet 1994;7:502–508.

Guillou L, Benhattar J, Bonichon F, et al: Histologic grade, but not SYT/SSX fusion type, is an important prognostic factor in patients with synovial sarcoma: A multicenter, retrospective analysis. J Clin Oncol 2004;22:4040–4050.

Haldar M, Hancock JD, Coffin CM, et al: A conditional mouse model of synovial sarcoma: Insights into a myogenic origin. Cancer Cell 2007;11:375–388.

Jin L, Majerus J, Oliveira A, et al: Detection of fusion gene transcripts in fresh-frozen and formalin-fixed paraffin-embedded tissue sections of soft-tissue sarcomas after laser capture microdissection and rt-PCR. Diagn Mol Pathol 2003;12:224–230.

Kawai A, Woodruff J, Healey JH, et al: SYT/SSX gene fusion as a determinant of morphology and prognosis in synovial sarcoma. N Engl J Med 1998;338:153–160.

Ladanyi M: Fusions of the SYT and SSX genes in synovial sarcoma. Oncogene 2001;20:5755–5762.

Lim FL, Soulez M, Koczan D, et al: A KRAB-related domain and a novel transcription repression domain in proteins encoded by SSX genes that are disrupted in human sarcomas. Oncogene 1998;17:2013–2018.

Oliveira AM, Fletcher CD: Molecular prognostication for soft tissue sarcomas: Are we ready yet? J Clin Oncol 2004;22:4031–4034.

Sandberg AA, Bridge JA: Updates on the cytogenetics and molecular genetics of bone and soft tissue tumors: Synovial sarcoma. Cancer Genet Cytogenet 2002;133:1–23.

Weiss SW, Goldblum JR: Enzinger and Weiss Soft Tissue Tumors. St Louis, Mosby, 2001.

Tenosynovial Giant Cell Tumor

Fletcher CDM, Unni KK, Mertens F (eds): World Health Organization Classification of Tumours: Pathology and Genetics of Tumours of Soft Tissue and Bone. Lyon, IARC Press, 2002.

West RB, Rubin BP, Miller MA, et al: A landscape effect in tenosynovial giant-cell tumor from activation of CSF1 expression by a translocation in a minority of tumor cells. Proc Natl Acad Sci USA 2006;103:690–695.

Well-Differentiated and Dedifferentiated Liposarcoma

Binh MB, Sastre-Garau X, Guillou L, et al: MDM2 and CDK4 immunostainings are useful adjuncts in diagnosing well-differentiated and dedifferentiated liposarcoma subtypes: A comparative analysis of 559 soft tissue neoplasms with genetic data. Am J Surg Pathol 2005;29:1340–1347.

Cordon-Cardo C, Latres E, Drobnjak M, et al: Molecular abnormalities of MDM2 and p53 genes in adult soft tissue sarcomas. Cancer Res 1994;54:794–799.

Dei Tos A, Pedeutour F: Dedifferentiated lipsarcoma. In Fletcher CD, Unni KK, Mertens F (eds): WorldHealth Organization Classification of Tumours: Pathology and Genetics of Tumours of Soft Tissue and Bone. Lyon, IARC Press, 2002, pp. 38-39.

Dei Tos A, Pedeutour F: Atypical lipomatous tumour/well differentiated liposarcoma. In Fletcher CD, Unni KK, Mertens F (eds): World Health Organization Classification of Tumours: Pathology and Genetics of Tumours of Soft Tissue and Bone. Lyon, IARC Press, 2002, pp.35–37.

Hostein I, Pelmus M, Aurias A, et al: Evaluation of MDM2 and CDK4 amplification by real-time PCR on paraffin wax–embedded material: A potential tool for the diagnosis of atypical lipomatous tumours/well-differentiated liposarcomas. J Pathol 2004;202:95–102.

Jacob E, Erickson-Johnson M, Wang X, et al: Assessment of MDM2 amplification using fluorescence in situ hybridization on paraffin-embedded tissues discriminates atypical lipomatous tumors from lipomas. Lab Invest 2006;86(13A 45 Suppl):13a.

Liquori CL, Ricker K, Moseley ML, et al: Myotonic dystrophy type 2 caused by a CCTG expansion in intron 1 of ZNF9. Science 2001;293:864–867.

Lucas DR, Nascimento AG, Sanjay BK, Rock MG: Well-differentiated liposarcoma. The Mayo Clinic experience with 58 cases. Am J Clin Pathol 1994;102:677–683.

Oliveira AM, Dei Tos AP, Fletcher CD, Nascimento AG: Primary giant cell tumor of soft tissues: A study of 22 cases. Am J Surg Pathol 2000;24:248–256.

Pedeutour F, Suijkerbuijk RF, Forus A, et al: Complex composition and coamplification of SAS and MDM2 in ring and giant rod marker chromosomes in well-differentiated liposarcoma. Genes Chromosomes Cancer 1994;10:85–94.

Pedeutour F, Forus A, Coindre JM, et al: Structure of the supernumerary ring and giant rod chromosomes in adipose tissue tumors. Genes Chromosomes Cancer 1999;24:30–41.

Sandberg AA: Updates on the cytogenetics and molecular genetics of bone and soft tissue tumors: Liposarcoma. Cancer Genet Cytogenet 2004;155:1–24.

Weaver J, et al: Fluorescence in situ hybridization (FISH) for MDM2 gene amplification in formalin-fixed paraffin-embedded tissue (FFPET) as a diagnostic tool in lipomatous neoplasms. Mod Pathol 2007;20(21A–22A 78 Suppl 2):.

Weiss SW, Goldblum JR: Liposarcoma. In Weiss SW, Goldblum JR (eds): Enzinger and Weiss's soft tissue tumors. St Louis, Mosby, 2001, p. 641.

Weiss SW, Rao VK: Well-differentiated liposarcoma (atypical lipoma) of deep soft tissue of the extremities, retroperitoneum, and miscellaneous sites. A follow-up study of 92 cases with analysis of the incidence of "dedifferentiation." Am J Surg Pathol 1992;16:1051–1058.

27 Molecular Pathology of Breast Cancer

David G. Hicks

INTRODUCTION

Adenocarcinoma of the breast is one of the leading causes of cancer morbidity and mortality among women worldwide. In the United States alone, there are more than 200,000 newly diagnosed cases of invasive breast cancer and in excess of 40,000 cancer-related deaths each year. When a new diagnosis of breast cancer is made, the most immediate issues for each patient involve what the diagnosis means for her future, whether or not she will survive, and whether therapies beyond primary surgery might be of additional benefit. There has been an encouraging decline in mortality from breast cancer over the past years, which can be attributed to several factors, likely largely related to public education and screening programs that lead to the discovery of the disease at an earlier and more treatable stage. In addition, there have been several significant and important treatment advances, with improvements in hormonal therapies, the development of more effective combination chemotherapy regimens, and the development of biologic therapeutics such as the targeted therapy against the human epidermal growth factor receptor 2 (HER2) receptor tyrosine kinase. This evolution of therapeutic modalities for breast cancer has yielded an increasingly complex array of treatment options, both local and systemic, necessitating the development of some rational way of stratifying patients as to the most appropriate treatment regimen based on an assessment of the likelihood for disease recurrence after completion of local–regional therapy.

ASSESSMENT OF BREAST CANCER

TRADITIONAL MORPHOLOGIC PROGNOSTIC FACTORS

A major challenge in the treatment of breast cancer is to identify those patients more likely to develop recurrence so that the most appropriate therapy can be provided. Useful prognostic information is routinely obtained from the careful assessment of the clinical resection specimen from the newly diagnosed breast cancer patient. The validated pathologic metrics that have been demonstrated to provide clinically useful prognostic information in breast cancer include tumor size, histologic type, tumor grade, lymph node staging, and evidence of vascular or lymphatic invasion. This information has been deemed helpful in determining the probability of local and/or distant recurrence and the likelihood that the patient will benefit from the addition of hormonal therapy, chemotherapy, or both to the treatment regimen. Despite the validated clinical utility of these pathologic prognostic factors, this traditional assessment does not provide sufficient information to allow accurate individual risk assessment. This is particularly true for the newly diagnosed early-stage breast cancer patient. These clinical realities, along with the significant cost and potential toxicities associated with systemic adjuvant and targeted therapies, have necessitated an intense search for molecular factors that, in addition to the "tried and true" traditional clinicopathologic metrics, can help better predict the likelihood of recurrence, as well as the potential benefit from adjuvant therapies for patients with breast cancer.

HORMONE RECEPTORS

The first of the prognostic and predictive biomarkers in breast cancer to enter routine clinical use, the steroid hormone receptors are in fact not new. It has been known for more than a century that oophorectomy increases the survival for some patients with advanced breast cancer. In addition, it has been known for some time that around 60% to 70% of breast carcinomas express estrogen receptors (ERs) and progesterone receptors (PRs) (Figure 27-1). Furthermore, tumors that express these receptors depend on estrogen, progesterone, or both for growth, and they preferentially concentrate radio-labeled estrogens within such breast cancer tissues. Thus, the ER

TRADITIONAL PROGNOSTIC AND PREDICTIVE MARKERS IN BREAST CANCER—FACT SHEET

AXILLARY LYMPH NODES

▶ Axillary lymph node status is the most influential traditional predictor of post-treatment recurrence and death.

▶ Absent systemic adjuvant therapy, chance of recurrence within 10 years is 24% for patients with negative axillary lymph nodes.

▶ A direct relationship exists between number of involved lymph nodes and risk for distant recurrence. (The 5-year survival rate for 1 to 3 positive lymph nodes is 73%, 4 to 12 lymph nodes is 45%, and more than 12 lymph nodes is 28%.)

Tumor Size

▶ Tumor size is prognostic regardless of the method used for measurement, including clinical estimates, imaging (mammogram, MRI), and gross and histologic measure.

▶ Size is directly correlated with increased probability of involved axillary lymph nodes, as well as increasing distant recurrence rates with larger tumor size.

▶ The 20-year recurrence-free survival rate is 88% for tumors less than 1 cm, 72% for tumors 1.1 to 3 cm, and 59% for tumors 3.1 to 5 cm.

▶ For node-negative patients, size is the most important prognostic factor and is routinely used to make decisions about adjuvant treatment. (Tumors >1 to 2 cm warrant consideration of adjuvant therapy because the distant recurrence rate may be >20%.)

Tumor Grade and Histologic Type

▶ Microscopic tumor characteristics have prognostic significance.

▶ Several special subtypes, including tubular, mucinous, and medullary, have a more favorable prognosis than carcinoma of no special type.

▶ The most accepted standard grading in use is the Nottingham Combined Histologic Grade or Elston-Ellis/modified Scarff-Bloom-Richardson, which are based on a semiquantitative assessment of the degree of tubular formation, nuclear pleomorphism, and mitotic activity.

▶ Some studies have shown poor reproducibility, however, when performed by experienced pathologists; histologic grade has been demonstrated to correlate with clinical outcome.

Lymphatic and Vascular Invasion

▶ Peritumoral lymphatic vessel and vascular invasion have been demonstrated to have prognostic significance for the risk of local and distant recurrence.

▶ Recurrence for stage I disease with lymphatic invasion was 38%, compared with 22% for lymphatic invasion–negative disease.

▶ Lymphatic invasion is useful in therapeutic decision making for node-negative patients with borderline tumor size.

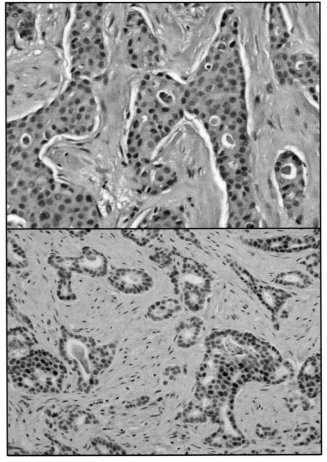

FIGURE 27-1

Immunohistochemistry for the evaluation of estrogen receptor (ER). This case shows a moderately differentiated infiltrating ductal carcinoma (Scarff-Bloom-Richardson grade 2), which shows strong ER reactivity in the nuclei of approximately 60% of tumor cells (mouse monoclonal antibody 1D5).

MOLECULAR PROGNOSTIC AND PREDICTIVE FACTORS

HER2

became the first target for either treatment by therapeutic hormonal manipulations with ER antagonists such as tamoxifen or treatment with aromatase inhibitors, which will decrease the local concentrations of estrogen within the tumor microenvironment of mammary tissue or within metastatic deposits. The presence of ERs in breast cancer is a weak prognostic factor; however, it is optimally useful as a predictive factor for the benefit of adjuvant tamoxifen or aromatase inhibitor therapy.

The next major advance in the evolving role of prognostic and predictive markers in the diagnosis and therapeutic decision making for breast cancer came with the discovery of the importance of the *HER2* receptor tyrosine kinase in the biology and the clinical course of disease in breast cancer. Normal cells have one copy of the *HER2* gene on each chromosome 17 (CHR17), and when this gene is expressed in normal breast epithelial cells, it is translated into a 185-kDa transmembrane growth factor receptor with cytoplasmic tyrosine kinase activity, which transmits signals regulating cell growth and survival. In approximately 15% to 25% of breast cancers, the *HER2* gene is found to be amplified 2-fold to greater than 20-fold in each tumor cell nucleus relative to CHR17, and this amplification drives gene expression, generating up to

ESTROGEN AND PROGESTERONE RECEPTORS—FACT SHEET

Estrogen is the main hormone that controls breast cancer proliferation, interacting with breast epithelial cells through ER.

▶ Two isoforms of ER are known, ER-α and ER-β. ER-α is the dominant mediator of estrogen signaling in breast cancer pathogenesis.

▶ ER-α expression has been shown to be a strong predictive factor for benefit from adjuvant hormonal therapy.

▶ Recent studies suggest that a shift in expression to ER-β receptors may occur in endocrine-resistant breast tumors.

▶ Validated methods for the assessment of ER in breast tissue include measurement of the ER content of the tumor using biochemical ligand-binding assays such as the dextran-coated charcoal assay, which has been replaced by immunohistochemistry (IHC) performed on formalin-fixed, paraffin-embedded tissues; the IHC correlates well with results from biochemical assays.

▶ An emerging method to assess ER is by quantitative reverse transcriptase–polymerase chain reaction (RT-PCR) to measure messenger RNA levels.

PR is a surrogate marker of ER activity in breast cancer.

▶ ER and PR are codependent variables, and PR is a weaker predictor of response to endocrine therapy than ER when both are included in multivariate analysis.

▶ An ER-positive, PR-negative breast cancer phenotype may represent a distinct subset of ER-positive breast cancer, with a more aggressive clinical course and increased resistance to antiendocrine therapy.

▶ The PR status of the tumor may reflect activated HER1/HER growth factor signaling in these tumors.

▶ Loss of PR in ER-positive tumors may represent a surrogate marker for increased growth factor signaling and tamoxifen resistance.

100 times the normal number of *HER2* receptor proteins at the cell surface.

HER2, also known as *ERBB2,* is a member of a family of transmembrane growth factor receptors, all of which are involved in regulating normal cell proliferation and survival. Like *HER2,* other members of this receptor family have been implicated in cancer. Several high-affinity ligands bind to several of the *HER* family members, which leads to receptor dimerization, activation of the cytoplasmic tyrosine kinase, and initiation of downstream signaling. It is now believed that *HER2* functions as the preferred dimerization partner for other *HER* members, leading to increased stability and prolonged activation of signal transduction. This, in turn, results in a proliferative drive, increased cell migration, and survival of those tumor cells that aberrantly overexpress this protein. Therefore, for those tumors with the *HER2* molecular alteration, the overexpression of the receptor plays a direct pivotal role in mediating the tumor's biologic and clinical behavior. As a result, *HER2*-positive breast cancers tend to be more aggressive, resulting in a significantly shortened disease-free survival rate and overall survival rate regardless of other prognostic factors. Furthermore,

HER2-positive breast cancer is significantly correlated with several unfavorable pathologic tumor characteristics, including larger tumor size, positive axillary nodes, higher nuclear grade, and higher proliferative index. In addition to the prognostic significance, retrospective studies have suggested that *HER2* overexpression may have a predictive role for response to adjuvant chemotherapy and endocrine therapy.

The location of the HER2 protein on the surface of the tumor cell, along with its pivotal role in determining the clinical course of disease for these patients, makes this molecule an ideal target for therapy. Trastuzumab (Herceptin®, Genetech), a humanized antibody that combined the mouse recognition sequence of a monoclonal antibody with the framework of a human IgG1, was developed as a biologic targeted therapeutic against an extracellular epitope of the HER2 receptor. The Herceptin molecule has been shown to demonstrate a high specificity and affinity for the HER2 protein and in preclinical studies was shown to be most effective against tumor cells with *HER2* overexpression. The therapeutic efficacy and tolerability of Herceptin therapy has been investigated in several clinical trials, and this drug has proved to be a remarkably effective therapeutic agent in both the metastatic and, more recently, the adjuvant setting, particularly in combination with cytotoxic chemotherapy. What is clear from these trials is that a positive *HER2* status, as assessed by either IHC (Figure 27-2) for protein overexpression or fluorescence in situ hybridization (FISH) (Figures 27-3 through 27-6) for gene amplification, is predictive for a clinical response from Herceptin treatment, thus providing a rationale for testing all newly diagnosed breast cancer patients. In contrast, patients who test negative for *HER2* have been shown to receive no additional benefit from the inclusion of Herceptin to their therapeutic regimen. Given the increasingly important role of this testing for patient selection and therapeutic decision making, the performance of *HER2* assays on clinical samples has become a priority for laboratory quality control and pathologic standardization. As an alternative to FISH for genotyping breast cancer, bright-field in situ hybridization methodologies (CISH™ and SISH™) have been developed, which allow detection of gene copy status using conventional bright-field microscopy (Figures 27-7 through 27-12). Such assays allow direct light microscopic evaluation and better correlation with morphology, and their results have been shown to correlate well with FISH assays, as well as demonstrate the potential to predict clinical outcomes in breast cancer.

Unlike most tests performed by diagnostic surgical pathologists, the results of a *HER2* assay does not serve as an adjunct to rendering a diagnosis but, rather, stands alone in determining which

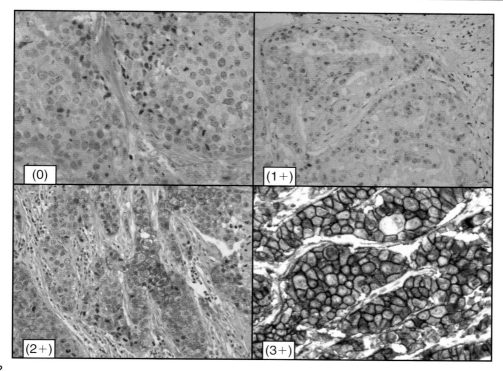

FIGURE 27-2

Immunohistochemistry (IHC) for the assessment of the level of HER2 protein expression at the tumor cell membrane. The assessment of HER2 by IHC needs to be evaluated critically and semiquantitatively to be clinically relevant. HER2-negative cases either show an absence of membrane staining, and are scored as 0 (upper left panel), or demonstrate partial weak membrane staining of tumor cells with no complete circumferential staining, and are scored as 1+ (upper right panel). Equivocal cases, scored as 2+, demonstrate circumferential membrane staining of tumor cells, but the staining ring is thin (lower left panel). HER2-positive cases demonstrate circumferential membrane staining of at least 30% of the tumor cells, but the staining ring is thick, has a retractile quality, and is scored as 3+ (lower right panel). Only cases with strong circumferential membrane staining (3+) show a good concordance with HER2 gene amplification by fluorescence in situ hybridization, and it is these patients who should be considered candidates for targeted treatment and who are the most likely to benefit from Herceptin therapy.

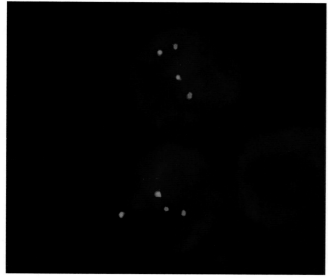

FIGURE 27-3

Fluorescence in situ hybridization image, invasive ductal carcinoma, demonstrating the absence of *HER2* gene amplification (red signals) and two chromosome 17 signals (green) (×1000). (From Tubbs RR, Hicks DG, Downs-Kelly E, et al: Fluorescence in situ hybridization (FISH) as primary methodology for the assessment of *HER2* status in adenocarcinoma of the breast: A single institution experience. Diagn Mol Pathol 2007;16:207–210.)

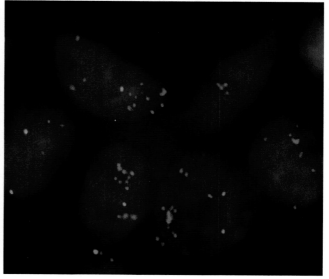

FIGURE 27-4

Fluorescence in situ hybridization image, invasive ductal carcinoma, demonstrating the presence of *HER2* gene amplification (red signals) and two chromosome 17 green signals (×1000). (From Tubbs RR, Hicks DG, Downs-Kelly E, et al: Fluorescence in situ hybridization (FISH) as primary methodology for the assessment of *HER2* status in adenocarcinoma of the breast: A single institution experience. Diagn Mol Pathol 2007;16:207–210.)

FIGURE 27-5

Fluorescence in situ hybridization image, invasive ductal carcinoma, demonstrating chromosome 17 polysomy/aneusomy (green signals) and deletion of the *HER2* locus (red signals). The signal enumeration results for this case were as follows: *HER2* = 2.8, CEP17 = 4.5, *HER2*/CEP17 ratio = 0.6 (×1000).

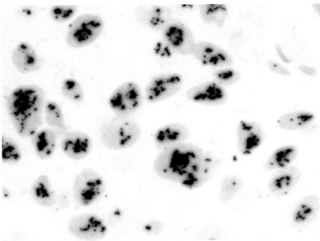

FIGURE 27-7

Silver in situ hybridization image, invasive ductal carcinoma, demonstrating the presence of *HER2* gene amplification (metallic silver, black). Note the presence of an endogenous *HER2* signal in a stromal cell (upper right).

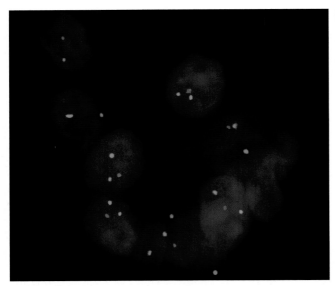

FIGURE 27-6

Fluorescence in situ hybridization image, invasive ductal carcinoma, demonstrating monoallelic *HER2* deletion. Only one *HER2* red signal in nuclei with two chromosome 17 signals (green) is identified. The *HER2*/CEP17 ratio for this case was 0.5 (×1000).

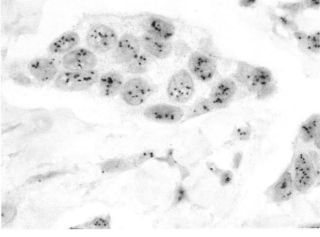

FIGURE 27-8

Dual-color silver in situ hybridization (SISH) image, invasive ductal carcinoma, demonstrating genomic heterogeneity and the presence of low-level *HER2* gene amplification in a subpopulation of tumor cells (upper left) (metallic silver, black). Some tumor cells are eusomic for chromosome 17 (red CHR17 centromeric signals); others tumor cells are aneusomic/polysomic for CHR17. Note the presence of endogenous *HER2* and CHR17 signals in stromal cells. The dual-color SISH staining was performed by Dr. Hiro Nitta and is gratefully acknowledged.

breast cancer patients are the most likely to benefit from Herceptin treatment. As such, this testing needs to be accurate, precise, and reproducible to help ensure that only the most appropriate patients will be selected for therapy. Given concerns about cost, potential side effects, and toxicities, it is criti-

cally important that Herceptin only be used in selected patients whose tumors have been evaluated by a validated *HER2* assay. Data from clinical trials with Herceptin in both the adjuvant and the metastatic settings have demonstrated that the incidence of cardiac dysfunction was higher in patients who

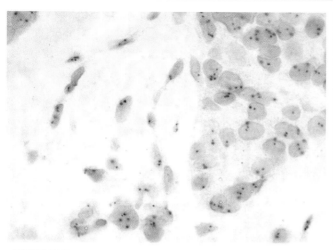

FIGURE 27-9

Dual-color silver in situ hybridization (SISH) image, invasive ductal carcinoma, demonstrating absence of *HER2* gene amplification (metallic silver, black). Tumor cells are eusomic for chromosome 17 (red CHR17 centromeric signals). Note the presence of endogenous *HER2* and CHR17 signals in stromal cells. The dual-color SISH staining was performed by Dr. Hiro Nitta and is gratefully acknowledged.

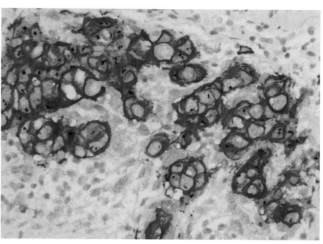

FIGURE 27-11

Dual-color silver in situ hybridization Pro (SISHPro) image, invasive ductal carcinoma, simultaneously demonstrating *HER2* gene amplification (metallic silver, SISH component, black) and overexpression of HER2-encoded protein (fast red/naphthol phosphate, immunohistochemistry component, red). Note the presence of endogenous *HER2* signals in stromal cells. The dual-color SISHPro combined in situ hybridization and immunohistochemistry staining was performed by Dr. Hiro Nitta and is gratefully acknowledged.

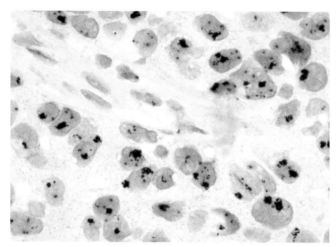

FIGURE 27-10

Dual-color silver in situ hybridization (SISH) image, invasive ductal carcinoma, demonstrating the presence of overt *HER2* gene amplification as large clusters of *HER2* signals in tumor cells (metallic silver, black). Some tumor cells are eusomic for chromosome 17 (red CHR17 centromeric signals); others tumor cells are aneusomic/polysomic for CHR17. Note the presence of endogenous *HER2* and CHR17 signals in stromal cells. The dual-color SISH staining was performed by Dr. Hiro Nitta and is gratefully acknowledged.

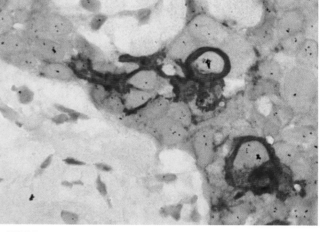

FIGURE 27-12

Dual-color silver in situ hybridization Pro (SISHPro) image, invasive ductal carcinoma, simultaneously demonstrating phenotypic and genotypic heterogeneity; *HER2* gene amplification (metallic silver, SISH component, black) and overexpression of HER2-encoded protein (fast red/naphthol phosphate, immunohistochemistry component, red) are identified in a subset of tumor cells, but other contiguous tumor cells do not demonstrate *HER2* gene amplification or overexpression. Note the presence of endogenous *HER2* signals in stromal cells. The dual-color SISHPro combined in situ hybridization and immunohistochemistry staining was performed by Dr. Hiro Nitta and is gratefully acknowledged.

received Herceptin in addition to chemotherapy compared with those receiving chemotherapy alone. In the metastatic setting, the incidence and severity of cardiac dysfunction was particularly high in patients who received Herceptin concurrently with an anthracycline.

Among the most important lessons learned from our experience with *HER2* testing is the need for standardization of all aspects of the handling of clinical biopsies or resection samples, which will require some form of testing for a predictive biomarker like *HER2*. This standardization includes all aspects of preanalytic tissue sample acquisition and handling, the type and duration of fixation, tissue processing, assay performance, interpretation, and reporting. Regardless of the laboratory methodology employed, specific guidelines and training to gain proficiency in *HER2* testing are needed to ensure accuracy, specificity, and reproducibility of the test results. National guidelines (see fact sheets) recommend that *HER2* overexpression or amplification be evaluated for every newly diagnosed breast cancer patient. Per these guidelines, both IHC and FISH (Boxes 27-1 and 27-2) are appropriate testing methodologies for clinical laboratories, provided that high concordance rates are established and appropriate quality control procedures are in place. As articulated by the guidelines developed by the American Society of Clinical Oncology and the College of American Pathologists (ASCO/CAP) (see fact sheets), a rigorous quality control program, experience, and proper training for accurate interpretation and proficiency testing is now mandatory for all laboratories engaged in *HER2* testing. The goal should be to achieve a greater than 95% concordance between IHC negative/FISH negative (gene nonamplified) and IHC positive (3+)/FISH positive (gene amplified) within a given

laboratory and across laboratories; this concordance should be established for each laboratory engaged in testing by rigorous test validation.

21st-Century Molecular Prognostic and Predictive Factors

The expansion of our knowledge of human DNA sequences brought about by the completion of the Human Genome Project, along with an explosion of genomic technologies, has brought us to a new crossroad in diagnostic prognostic and predictive markers that hold great promise to improve the care of patients with breast cancer. Technology has been the primary driving force in many of these efforts, and methodologies including quantitative real-time PCR, gene expression microarrays, and array-based comparative genomic hybridization, as outlined in earlier chapters, have all been applied to clinical samples from breast cancer patients with surprising results. What has emerged from these studies (summarized later) is a rapidly evolving understanding of the molecular alterations and cellular pathways underlying the clinical

BOX 27-1   ASCO/CAP GUIDELINE RECOMMENDATIONS FOR THE OPTIMAL ALGORITHM FOR HER2 TESTING BY IHC

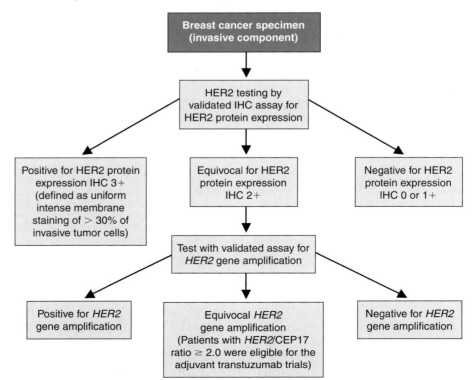

(Modified from Arch Pathol Lab Med 2007;131:18–43.)

BOX 27-2   ASCO/CAP GUIDELINE RECOMMENDATIONS FOR THE OPTIMAL ALGORITHM FOR HER2 TESTING BY FISH OR SISH

(Modified from Arch Pathol Lab Med 2007;131:18–43.)

GENOMIC ALTERATIONS AND THEIR ASSOCIATION WITH TUMOR GRADE

heterogeneity and driving the clinical course of the disease, as well as new insights into predictive markers for response to specific therapies. The ensuing discussion examines some of these new molecular methodologies and their evolving role in helping better define breast cancer biology and taxonomy, as well as in helping identify potential new and improved prognostic and predictive biomarkers that can be used to guide therapeutic decision making.

The application of conventional cytogenetics, loss of heterozygosity, FISH, and more recently, comparative genomic hybridization has begun to define the complex genomic aberrations and recurrent genomic imbalances that characterize mammary carcinomas. Among the most common recurrent genomic changes identified are gains in regions of chromosomes 1q, 8q, 11q, 17q, and 20q and losses in regions of chromosomes 8p, 11q, 13q, 16q, and 18q. It is noteworthy that many of these recurrent chromosomal changes occur in regions that harbor known proto-oncogenes, as well as tumor suppressor genes. Interestingly,

when these genomic patterns or signatures were compared with traditional clinicopathologic metrics, what was found was that both the number and the pattern of genomic aberrations differed most significantly in breast cancer when stratified by tumor grade. The prototype would be the amplification of the HER2 gene on the long arm of CHR17 (17q12), a genomic change that is significantly correlated with high-grade tumors.

What these finding suggest is that the pathogenesis and pathways leading to the development of low-grade and high-grade breast cancers differ and that tumorigenesis is associated with unique patterns of genomic alterations for low- and high-grade breast carcinomas. Further support for this notion comes from the finding that these differential changes found in low- and high-grade infiltrating tumors are also shared with low- and high-grade ductal carcinoma in situ, suggesting that these changes occur early in the course of the disease and play a role in pathogenesis. In addition, recent gene expression profiling studies have shown that both low- and high-grade tumors have distinctive gene signatures, adding further support to the view that low- and high-grade breast cancers represent independent pathobiologic entities.

HER2 RECEPTOR TYROSINE KINASE STATUS—FACT SHEET

HER2 Proto-oncogene on the Long Arm of Chromosome 17 (17q12)

▶ The official gene name is *ERBB2,* but *HER2* is used most commonly.

▶ *HER2* encodes a 185-kDa transmembrane protein growth factor receptor with cytoplasmic tyrosine kinase activity, which transmits signals regulating cell growth.

▶ In 20% to 30% of breast cancers, the *HER2* gene is amplified 2-fold to greater than 20-fold, driving gene expression and generating up to 100 times the normal number of HER2 receptor proteins on the cell surface.

▶ *HER2* is a member of a family of transmembrane growth factor receptors involved in regulating normal cell proliferation and survival.

▶ No high-affinity ligand has been described for the *HER2* receptor, and it is now believed that *HER2* functions as the preferred dimerization partner for other HER family members, leading to increased stability and prolonged activation of signaling.

▶ *HER2*-positive breast cancers tend to be more aggressive than *HER2*-negative disease, resulting in significantly shorter disease-free survival and overall survival rates.

▶ *HER2*-positive breast cancer significantly correlates with several other poor prognostic factors and unfavorable pathologic tumor characteristics, including large tumor size, positive lymph nodes, higher proliferative index, and high nuclear grade.

▶ The *HER2* oncoprotein is a therapeutic target for the drug Herceptin, a humanized monoclonal antibody against an extracellular portion of the receptor.

▶ Patients whose tumor cells overexpress the *HER2* protein by IHC or demonstrate amplification of the *HER2* gene by FISH are candidates for Herceptin-targeted therapy.

Herceptin: Potential Mechanisms of Action

▶ The *HER2* receptor tyrosine kinase, when activated, initiates multiple cellular signaling pathways, including mitogen-activated protein kinase and phosphatidylinositol 3-kinase signaling cascades.

▶ The binding of Herceptin to the juxtamembrane region of *HER2* leads to reduced signaling in these pathways, along with increased expression of p27^{Kip1} levels, which promotes cell cycle arrest and apoptosis.

▶ The efficacy of Herceptin could be partly related to induction of an immune response through antibody-dependent cellular cytotoxicity.

FDA-APPROVED HER2 TESTING METHODOLOGIES—FACT SHEET

Immunohistochemistry Assays

▶ HercepTest™ (Dako) IHC assay, polyclonal antibody

▶ Pathway® (Ventana Medical Systems) IHC assay–rabbit monoclonal antibody 4B5

▶ Intended use, semiquantitative determination of HER2 protein overexpression

▶ Uses formalin-fixed, paraffin-embedded tissue section of invasive breast cancer

▶ Indicated as an aid in the assessment of patients for whom Herceptin treatment is being considered

▶ Uses ASCO/CAP criteria rather than historical scoring criteria for HER2 IHC, as follows:

IHC Level of Expression (Score)	Tumor Cell Membrane Staining Pattern
Negative (0)	Absence of staining
Negative (1+)	Faint incomplete membrane staining, >10% of cells
Equivocal (2+)	Weak complete membrane staining, >10% of cells
Positive (3+)	Strong complete membrane staining, >30% of cells

Fluorescence In Situ Hybridization Assays

▶ PathVysion® (Abbot Molecular) FISH assay, *HER2*/CEP17

▶ *HER2* FISH PharmDx™ assay (Dako)

▶ Intended use, detect amplification of the *HER2* gene relative to chromosome 17

▶ Calculated ratio, average number of *HER2* gene copies/CEP17 copies (*HER2*/CEP17 ratio > 2.2 considered *HER2* gene amplification using ASCO/CAP guidelines)

Scoring Principles Using a Fluorescence Microscope with Appropriate Filter Set

▶ Count *HER2* and CEP17 signals in invasive tumor cells

▶ Count 30 to 40 nonoverlapping tumor nuclei of uniform size in at least two areas of invasive tumor using 100X oil immersion objective

▶ Calculate average number of *HER2* gene signals and CEP17 signals per tumor nuclei, then calculate *HER2*/CEP17 ratio

Silver In Situ Hybridization Assay

▶ Inform® *HER2* (Ventana Medical Systems)

▶ Intended use, detect amplification of the *HER2* gene relative to CHR17

▶ Calculate the ratio from semiquantitative and pattern recognition analysis of two separate slides in current U.S. Food and Drug Administration (FDA)–approved format

▶ *HER2*/CHR17 ratio more than 2.2 considered *HER2* gene amplification using ASCO/CAP guidelines

▶ Uses formalin-fixed, paraffin-embedded tissue section of invasive breast cancer

▶ Indicated as an aid in the assessment of patients for whom Herceptin treatment is being considered

(Modified from Arch Pathol Lab Med 2007;131:18–43.)

SUMMARY OF ASCO/CAP GUIDELINE RECOMMENDATIONS FOR THE OPTIMAL ALGORITHM FOR HER2 TESTING—FACT SHEET

Optimal Algorithm for HER2 Testing

▶ Positive for *HER2* is either IHC HER2 3+ (defined as uniform intense membrane staining of >30% of invasive tumor cells) or FISH, silver in situ hybridization (SISH), or chromogenic in situ hybridization (CISH) amplified (*HER2*/CHR17 ratio > 2.2 or average *HER2* gene copy number of >6 signals/nucleus for those test systems without an internal control probe).

▶ Equivocal for *HER2* is defined as either the IHC 2+ or in situ hybridization ratio of 1.8 to 2.2 or the average *HER2* gene copy number of 4 to 6 signals/nucleus for test systems without an internal control probe.

▶ Negative for *HER2* is defined as either the IHC 0 to 1+ or in situ hybridization ratio of less than 1.8 or the average *HER2* gene copy number of less than four signals/nucleus for test systems without an internal control probe.

These definitions depend on laboratory documentation of the following:

  ▶ Proof of initial testing validation in which positive and negative *HER2* categories are 95% concordant with an alternative validated method or the same validated method for HER2; reference validation materials should not include equivocal cases

  ▶ Ongoing internal quality assurance (QA) procedures

  ▶ Participation in external proficiency testing

  ▶ Current accreditation by a valid accrediting agency

(Modified from Arch Pathol Lab Med 2007;131:18–43.)

SUMMARY OF ASCO/CAP GUIDELINE RECOMMENDATIONS FOR THE OPTIMAL TISSUE HANDLING, ASSAY VALIDATION, QA/QC, AND ACCREDITATION FOR HER2 TESTING—FACT SHEET

Optimal Tissue Handling Requirements

▶ Time from tissue acquisition to fixation should be as short as possible; samples for HER2 testing are fixed in formalin for 6 to 48 hours; samples should be sliced at 5- to 10-mm intervals after appropriate gross inspection and margins designation and should be placed in sufficient volume of formalin.

▶ Sections should ideally not be used for HER2 testing if cut more than 6 weeks earlier; this may vary with primary fixation or storage conditions.

▶ Time to fixation and duration of fixation if available should be recorded for each sample.

Optimal Internal Validation Procedure

▶ Validation of a test must be done before the test is offered. The validation set should not include reference cases with equivocal results.

▶ Initial test validation requires 25 to 100 samples tested by an alternative validated method in the same laboratory or by a validated method in another laboratory.

▶ Proof is required of initial testing validation in which positive and negative HER2 categories are 95% concordant with an alternative validated method or the same validated method for HER2.

▶ Ongoing validation should be done biannually.

Optimal Internal Quality Assurance

▶ Initial test validation procedures

▶ Ongoing quality control and equipment maintenance

▶ Initial and ongoing laboratory personnel training and competency assessment

▶ Use of standardized operating procedures, including routine use of control materials

▶ Revalidation of procedure if changed

▶ Ongoing competency assessment and education of pathologists

Optimal External Proficiency Assessment

▶ Participation is required in an external proficiency testing program with at least two testing events (mailings)/year.

▶ Satisfactory performance requires at least 90% correct responses on graded challenges for either test.

▶ Unsatisfactory performance will require the laboratory to respond according to accreditation agency program requirements.

Optimal Laboratory Accreditation

▶ Onsite inspection is required every other year, with an annual requirement for self-inspection.

▶ Reviews of laboratory validation, procedures, QA results and processes, results, and reports are necessary.

▶ Unsatisfactory performance results in suspension of laboratory testing for HER2 for that method.

SUMMARY OF ASCO/CAP GUIDELINE RECOMMENDATIONS FOR THE OPTIMAL FISH AND IHC TESTING FOR HER2—FACT SHEET

Optimal Fluorescence In Situ Hybridization Testing Requirements

▶ Fixation for fewer than 6 hours or longer than 48 hours is not recommended.
▶ The test is rejected and repeated if
  ▶ Controls are not as expected.
  ▶ The observer cannot find and count at least two areas of invasive tumor.
  ▶ More than 25% of signals are unscorable because of weak signals.
  ▶ More than 10% of signals occur over cytoplasm.
  ▶ Nuclear resolution is poor.
  ▶ Autofluorescence is strong and masks signals.
▶ Interpretation is done by counting at least 20 cells; a pathologist must confirm that counting involved the invasive tumor.
▶ The sample is subjected to increased counting, repeated counting if equivocal, or both; the report must include guideline-detailed elements (lower right).

Optimal Immunohistochemistry Testing Requirements

▶ Fixation for fewer than 6 hours or longer than 48 hours is not recommended.
▶ The test is rejected and repeated or tested by FISH if
  ▶ Controls are not as expected.
  ▶ Artifacts involve most of the sample.
  ▶ The sample has strong membrane staining of normal breast ducts (internal controls).
▶ Interpretation follows guideline recommendation.
▶ A positive HER2 result requires a homogeneous, dark circumferential (chicken wire) pattern in more than 30% of the invasive tumor.
  Interpreters have a method to maintain consistency and competency.
▶ The sample is subjected to confirmatory FISH testing if it is equivocal based on initial results.
▶ The report must include guideline-detailed elements.

(Modified from Arch Pathol Lab Med 2007;131:18–43.)

SILVER IN SITU HYBRIDIZATION FOR *HER2* GENE AMPLIFICATION—FACT SHEET

Inform Silver In Situ Hybridization for HER2 and Chromosome 17

▶ The assay determines the presence or absence of *HER2* gene amplification.
▶ Semiquantitative or quantitative signal enumeration of *HER2* and CHR17 signals; two separate slides are used in the current format.
▶ The method depends upon enzyme metallography (SISH), which converts ionic silver in silver acetate to elemental (metallic) silver in the presence of peroxidase, hydroquinone, and hydrogen peroxide.
▶ There is a high level of concordance with FISH results.
▶ Interobserver interpretative reproducibility is excellent.
▶ Image analysis (VIAS™) is available for quantification.
▶ Evaluation of the internal positive control, the endogenous *HER2* and CHR17 signals in stromal cells, is essential.
▶ External xenograft controls derived from cell lines spanning the dynamic range of *HER2* gene amplification detected by SISH are also available, but identification of internal endogenous *HER2* signals in stromal cells of the test tissue is paramount.

ASCO/CAP GUIDELINES FOR IMMUNOHISTOCHEMISTRY INTERPRETATION CRITERIA—FACT SHEET

▶ Review controls; if not as expected, the test should be repeated.
▶ More than 30% of the tumor must show circumferential membrane staining for a positive result.*
▶ Membrane staining must be intense and uniform.
▶ A homogeneous, dark circumferential (chicken wire) staining pattern should be seen.
▶ Ignore incomplete or pale membrane staining.
▶ Quantitative image analysis is encouraged for cases with weak membrane staining (1 to 2+) to improve consistency of interpretation. Equivocal (2+) cases should be reflexed to an FDA-approved FISH or SISH assay.
▶ If cytoplasmic staining obscures membrane staining, repeat the assay or do FISH.
▶ Reject the sample if normal ducts and lobules show obvious staining.
▶ Reject the sample if there are obscuring artifacts.
▶ Avoid scoring ductal carcinoma in situ; score only if there is infiltrating ductal carcinoma.

*This percentage is greater than that specified in FDA-approved tests, but the value was based on expert panel consensus that this level is a more realistic threshold.
(Modified from Arch Pathol Lab Med 2007;131:18–43.)

ASCO/CAP GUIDELINES FOR FISH AND SISH INTERPRETATION CRITERIA—FACT SHEET

▶ Review the corresponding hematoxylin and eosin slide, IHC slide, or both to localize the invasive cancer; carcinoma in situ should not be scored.
▶ Review controls; if not as expected, the test should be repeated.
▶ Count at least 20 nonoverlapping cells in two separate areas of invasive cancer.
▶ Reject if signals are nonuniform (>25%).
▶ Reject if autofluorescence is high or nuclear resolution is poor.
▶ Reject if background obscures signal resolution (>10% over cytoplasm).
▶ If the *HER2*/CHR17 ratio is between 1.8 and 2.2, have an additional person recount. If the final ratio is 1.8 to 2.2, perform IHC or an alternative in situ hybridization assay (FISH or SISH if not previously performed) using an FDA-approved method.
▶ If there is heterogeneous expression, have an additional person recount.
▶ Counting can be done by a trained technologist, but a pathologist must confirm that result (count) is correct and that the invasive tumor was counted.

Note: Tumor heterogeneity, monosomy or polysomy of CHR17, and gene deletion may influence the interpretation of the absolute ratio value and should be noted. If genomic heterogeneity is identified, an estimation of the percentage of tumor cells that are amplified should be provided in the report.

(Modified from Arch Pathol Lab Med 2007;131:18–43.)

GENOMIC PROFILES IN BREAST CANCER—FACT SHEET

The average number of chromosomal changes increases with increasing tumor grade, and the pattern of genomic alterations differs significantly when stratified by tumor grade.

Most Common Recurrent Chromosomal Genomic Gains

▶ Chromosomes 1q, 8q, 11q, 17q, 20q

Most Common Recurrent Chromosomal Genomic Losses

▶ 8p, 11q, 13q, 16q, 18q

Low-Grade Infiltrating Ductal Carcinoma

▶ Tend to be ER positive, *HER2* nonamplified, and diploid and to have a low proliferative index.
▶ Tend to have fewer chromosomal alterations compared with high-grade tumors.
▶ Most common genomic changes are losses on 16q and gains on 1q.
▶ Other reported changes include gains on 8q, 11q, 16p, and 17q and losses on 1p, 8p, 11q, 13q, and 22q.
▶ Genomic changes seen in low-grade infiltrating ductal carcinomas also present in low-grade ductal carcinoma in situ, lobular carcinoma in situ, and classic infiltrating lobular carcinoma.

High-Grade Infiltrating Ductal Carcinoma

▶ Tend to be ER negative and aneuploid; often have loss of p53 function; and tend to overexpress C-myc and *HER2* and have a high proliferative index.
▶ Tend to have more frequent, extensive, and complex chromosomal alterations.
▶ Gains are often on 8q, 17q, and 20q, and losses are on 17p, 1p, 19p, and 19q.
▶ Genomic losses are rarely seen on 16q.

GENE EXPRESSION PROFILING

The application of molecular gene expression profiling to clinical samples using new array technologies has provided significant insight into our understanding of the biologic and clinical diversity of breast cancer. This new approach allows the simultaneous examination of global changes in the patterns of gene expression within clinical samples of malignant tissue. Because these types of studies allow the simultaneous examination of thousands of genes without the need to define function, relationship between gene sets, or relevant patterns, the data has the potential to provide important insights into tumor biology and clinically meaningful tumor subtypes in an extremely rapid and unprecedented fashion. As a result, both clinical and scientific advances have proceeded in parallel, with the identification of reproducibly distinctive molecular subsets of breast cancer accompanied by differences in clinical feature, such as statistically robust differences in relapse-free survival, overall survival, and patterns of recurrence. At the same time, these studies have provided a window

of understanding into the molecular alterations and the critical pathway changes driving the biologic behavior of these distinctive breast cancer subtypes.

UNSUPERVISED MOLECULAR CLASSIFICATION OF BREAST CANCER USING EXPRESSION PROFILING

Clinicians caring for breast cancer patients have recognized for some time that all breast cancers are not the same but rather demonstrate a diversity of clinical behaviors suggesting that "breast cancers" encompass a heterogeneous group of diseases. Using complementary DNA (cDNA) microarrays and unsupervised analysis, Perou and Sorlie reported that breast cancers could be grouped into distinctive subtypes based on variations in global gene expression patterns. These molecularly defined subtypes were shown to differ in terms of the likelihood of recurrence and therapeutic responses, suggesting that the clinical heterogeneity of breast cancer can be explained, at least partly, by differences in the molecular genetic composition and global gene expression patterns of the primary tumors. These expression-based distinctive classes of breast cancer have been confirmed and validated in numerous studies. The molecularly defined subsets of breast cancer include a group of *HER2*-positive tumors, at least two categories of *HER2*-negative tumors that express hormone receptors (luminal subtypes), and a group of "basal-like" tumors that do not express hormone receptors or *HER2*. The reproducible differences in gene expression patterns among these distinct subtypes of breast cancer are likely to represent tumor phenotypes and reflect underlying differences in biology, which in turn exerts an influence on overall survival and response to therapy. One possible explanation for differences in gene expression among these tumor subsets is that they originate from different mammary epithelial cell types. This hypothesis is supported by the fact that breast tumor subtypes with patterns of gene expression similar to those of luminal epithelial cells and the patterns of at least one other subtype (basal-like) resemble the two major epithelial cell types of the normal mammary gland.

Luminal Subtypes of Breast Cancer

The luminal subtypes comprise a major group of breast cancers, distinguished by hormone receptor expression with characteristic gene expression profiles reminiscent of the luminal epithelial elements of the breast. These patterns include the expression of ER and genes associated with ER activation, as well as the epithelial cytokeratin 8/18, which are associated with luminal epithelial cells. The luminal category can be further subdivided into at least two subtypes, luminal A and luminal B, that vary in terms of gene expression and prognosis. The luminal A group in general demonstrates a higher level of expression of ER-related genes, tends to show a lower tumor histologic grade, and has a lower expression of proliferation-related genes compared with the luminal B group.

Clinical data proposes the intriguing possibility that some differences in outcome between the luminal A and the luminal B groups may be partly related to differences in response to both hormonal and conventional chemotherapy. These studies suggest that luminal A tumors may be adequately treated with hormonal therapy alone and tend to respond poorly to chemotherapy, whereas the more highly proliferative luminal B tumors may represent a subset that will benefit from chemotherapy added to endocrine treatment. Furthermore, luminal B tumors appear to have a worse outcome with tamoxifen therapy compared with luminal A, and these patients may do better if they receive an aromatase inhibitor. Although these studies show great promise to aid in guiding treatment planning, further investigation will be needed to better define and validate these observations before these factors can begin to be used in routine clinical practice and therapeutic decision making.

HER2 Subtype of Breast Cancer

The identification of a *HER2* subtype by expression profiling confirmed the clinical impression that *HER2*-overexpressing tumors represent a clinically distinct subset of breast cancer. This *HER2* subset is characterized by being hormone receptor negative and overexpressing other genes in the *HER2* amplicon, such as *GRB7*. Interestingly, the subset of *HER2*-positive tumors identified by expression profiling does not completely overlap with the group of *HER2*-positive tumors identified clinically by IHC, FISH, or both (detailed earlier). Most tumors identified as *HER2* overexpressing by clinical testing will fall into the group of *HER2*-positive tumors identified by expression profiling. However, other *HER2*-positive tumors identified by IHC or FISH also express hormone receptor and fall within the luminal subsets rather than the *HER2* subset defined by cDNA arrays. It is noteworthy that in the adjuvant clinical trials, Herceptin showed efficacy for the treatment of *HER2*-positive breast cancer identified by clinical assay, regardless of the hormone receptor status for these tumors. This strongly suggests that the most important and overriding determinant for the clinical outcome and therapeutic response for *HER2*-positive breast cancer is the *HER2* molecular alteration.

Basal-like Subtype of Breast Cancer

Among the distinctive subtypes of breast cancer identified by gene expression profiling is a group of tumors characterized by lack of hormone receptor expression; low expression of *HER2*: strong expression of the basal cytokeratins 5, 14, and 17; and high expression of proliferation-related genes. The term *basal-like tumors* has been applied to this subset of breast cancers given that the expression pattern of this subtype overlaps with that of the normal basal or myoepithelial cells of the breast by both cDNA microarrays and IHC. Morphologic studies on basal-like breast cancers initially identified by cDNA microarrays have reported several characteristic features for these tumors, including circumscription with pushing borders, high nuclear grade, high mitotic index, areas of geographic necrosis, and lymphocytic stromal reaction, all of which have also been associated with the so-called medullary or atypical medullary phenotype.

Several recent clinical reports have supported the original observations that tumors of the basal-like subtype are aggressive, more likely to be high grade with a high proliferative index, and more likely to demonstrate *TP53* mutations compared to luminal A tumors. From the clinical standpoint, this group of tumors has generated much interest given the poor prognosis, an association with hereditary breast cancer, the lack of specific biologic therapy, and the consequent dependence on chemotherapy for treatment. Gene expression profiling has also been used to study breast cancers associated with inherited *BRCA1* mutations; surprisingly, the basal-like phenotype is one of the hallmarks of these particular familial breast tumors. These studies have demonstrated that breast cancers arising in *BRCA1* mutation carriers typically have expression profiles consistent with the basal-like subtype, which suggests that basal-like sporadic cancers and familial *BRCA1* tumors could share a similar etiology. These findings might have important implications for patient management.

SUPERVISED MOLECULAR CLASSIFICATION OF BREAST CANCER USING EXPRESSION PROFILING

The goal of supervised classification of breast cancer using gene expression profiling is to detect gene expression patterns that are predictive of outcome in clinically well-defined patient cohorts. As with unsupervised expression profiling, the large amount of data generated from these sorts of studies needs to be analyzed using sophisticated statistics and mathematic models to generate genomic classifiers with prognostic and predictive value. The ultimate clinical utility of these multigene classifiers must then be rigorously validated in additional patient cohorts (other than the ones upon which the model was developed), given that the disproportion between the numbers of genes tested and the number of clinical samples used to create these models can lead to a high false-discovery rate for genes that appear to be correlated with outcome.

GENE EXPRESSION PROFILING IN BREAST CANCER—FACT SHEET

Rational for Molecular Classification of Breast Cancer Using Gene Expression Profiling

▶ Distinct subgroups of breast cancer can be identified based on reproducible differences in complex messenger RNA expression patterns.

▶ Subsets of breast cancer defined by molecular classification appear to have significantly different natural histories.

▶ Once better characterized and understood, the molecular signatures that define particular groups may lead to the discovery of therapeutic targets and treatments that are effective in particular molecular subsets.

The first studies to examine comprehensive gene expression patterns of breast cancer suggested that breast cancer can be divided into at least four molecularly defined subsets, with clinical differences in prognosis and chemotherapy sensitivity.

Luminal Subtypes

▶ These are the most common subtypes (approximately two thirds of all breast cancers).

▶ Luminal subtypes express hormone receptors and genes associated with ER activation and luminal cytokeratins (8/18).

▶ Two subtypes fall within the luminal cluster: Luminal A demonstrates a higher level of expression of ER-related genes, and luminal B shows lower levels of ER-related genes and higher expression of proliferation genes.

▶ In general, the luminal subtypes carry a good prognosis, with the luminal B group having a significantly worse prognosis than the luminal A group.

▶ Recent clinical data suggests that the luminal A group may be adequately treated with hormonal therapy alone and the luminal B group may benefit from the combination of hormonal therapy and chemotherapy.

HER2 Subtype

▶ This subset is characterized as part of the larger hormone receptor–negative group, with overexpression of HER2 and other genes on the ERBB2 amplicon, such as GRB7.

▶ These are higher-grade tumors that demonstrate higher proliferative rates, are more likely to harbor TP53 mutations, and are candidates for Herceptin therapy.

Basal-like Subtype

▶ This subset is characterized by an expression pattern reminiscent of normal breast myoepithelial cells and includes lack of expression of ER and related genes, low expression of HER2, and expression of basal cytokeratins (CK5, 6, 14, 17) and proliferation-related genes. It carries a poor prognosis.

▶ BRCA1 mutation carriers who develop breast cancer generally develop basal-like tumors, and premenopausal African American women have twice the risk of developing basal-like tumors as any other group of women.

Quantitative analysis of gene expression–based predictors for breast cancer, except for the two-gene HOXB15/ILMBR ratio, has been shown to be highly concordant and prognostic for clinical outcome. However, this exception is likely attributable to the use of a non-validated assay and the failure to confine analysis to an appropriate patient cohort.

(From Fan C, Oh D, Wessels L, et al: Concordance among gene expression–based predictors for breast cancer. N Engl J Med 2006;355(6):560–569 and Goetz MP, Ingle JN, Couch FJ. Gene expression-based predictors for breast cancer. N Engl J Med 2006;355(6):560–569.)

GENETIC TESTING FOR HEREDITARY BREAST CANCER—FACT SHEET

▶ Of women with breast cancer, 15% to 20% report a positive family history.

▶ Only 5% to 6% of all breast cancers are associated with inherited gene mutation.

▶ Two well-recognized major susceptibility genes for breast cancer are BRCA1 and BRCA2. These are among several known susceptibility genes that have been associated with breast cancer.

▶ The protein products of these genes function as a part of the mechanisms that repair double-stranded DNA breaks through recombination with undamaged, homologous DNA strands.

▶ BRCA1 and BRCA2 are inherited in an autosomal dominant fashion and are thought to account for most inherited breast cancers (also for increased risk for ovarian cancer).

▶ Lifetime risk of breast cancer for mutation carriers is between 65% and 85% by age 70.

▶ Prevalence of BRCA mutation is highest among women of Ashkenazi Jewish decent.

Genetic Testing for BRCA1 and BRCA2 Gene Mutations

▶ More than 200 mutations have been described in each gene. These mutations are distributed throughout the length of each gene, without a mutation "hotspot," necessitating full direct sequencing of both genes to exclude an obvious abnormality.

▶ Careful patient selection is important to optimize testing.

▶ Myriad Genetics Laboratories and Pharmaceuticals offers full sequencing of all exons and adjacent base pairs in the noncoding introns in the United States.

▶ Once a mutation is identified in an affected individual, analysis for the specific mutation in family members is considerably less expensive.

▶ Risk of carrying a mutation is associated with the following:
  ▶ Breast cancer onset at an early age.
  ▶ Strong family history for breast cancer, ovarian cancer, or both.
  ▶ Specific tumor characteristics such as triple negative (ER/PR/HER2) tumor, basal-like phenotype including expression of basal cytokeratins (CK5, 6, 14, 17), morphology showing pushing tumor borders, high nuclear grade, high mitotic activity, and lymphocytic host response.

▶ Several models have been developed to help predict an individual patient's risk or probability of carrying a deleterious BRCA1 or BRCA2 mutation (BRCAPRO), and the American Society of Clinical Oncology has suggested that patients whose risk of carrying a mutation exceeds 10% should be considered for testing.

Two large studies have used this supervised molecular classification approach to address broad prognostic questions involving recurrence and survival in node-negative breast cancer patients treated only with surgery. Investigators from the Netherlands Cancer Institute identified a cohort of 98 patients who were node negative and younger than 55 years of age. The patients from this cohort could be further separated into those who experienced a relapse of their disease within 5 years (34 patients) and those who were disease free at 5 years or more (44 patients). From the initial study, which looked at 25,000 genes, a system of supervised classification identified 70 genes that were independently correlated with poor prognosis, that is, different levels of gene expression that tended to be associated with the patients who developed distant metastases compared with those who did not. Subsequently, the prognostic power of the 70-gene signature was tested in a validation study in 295 patients, some of whom were lymph node positive. The patients with a good prognostic gene signature had a less than 15% risk of recurrence of 10 years, and those who demonstrated tumor genes associated with a poor prognosis had a 50% risk for distant metastases. The encouraging results from these studies have led to the development of a large clinical trial in Europe (the Microarray in Node-Negative Disease May Avoid Chemotherapy, or MINDACT, trial) (MammoPrint™, Agendia), in which more than 5000 patients will be randomized to treatment according to their 70-gene profile, as well as clinical prognostic factors. The results are awaited with great interest. Another group from Rotterdam derived a 76-gene prognostic signature from 115 node-negative breast cancer patients and validated the results on a wholly independent series of 171 samples. The results of these studies were strikingly similar to those obtained by the Amsterdam group, and again, the genomic classifier appeared to outperform all univariate tests.

Many other studies of gene expression have developed other genomic classifiers and have reported gene sets that are prognostic, predictive, or both for breast cancer patients. Interestingly, a comparison of the lists of genes derived from these apparently similar studies demonstrates little overlap in the gene sets that make up these classifiers, despite similar clinical and statistical designs. A recent study by Fan et al. compared the predictions derived from five gene expression–based models and found that these models mostly had high rates of concordance in their outcome predictions for the individual samples from 295 well-characterized breast cancer cases with follow-up, despite the different gene sets that were used for prognostication. These authors concluded that although different gene sets were being used as predictors, each appears to track a common set of biologic characteristics present in different groups and subsets of breast cancer patients, which affect clinical behavior and outcome.

Interestingly, recent studies have suggested that the application of selected antibody panels using routine IHC on formalin-fixed, paraffin-embedded breast cancer samples is also able to identify breast cancer subsets with differing outcomes and is predictive of clinical behavior. Furthermore, other studies have suggested that a limited panel of IHC markers such as ER, PR, HER2, HER1, and basal cytokeratins can be used to stratify breast cancer samples into groups remarkably similar to the subtypes defined by expression profiling. These studies have opened the door for the use of such IHC antibody panels in the routine pathologic evaluation of newly diagnosed breast cancer patients and have the potential to provide much useful information to help guide clinical decisions on adjuvant therapies. As is true for the other genomic classifiers under development, IHC panels need to be rigorously validated against multiple patient cohorts from multiple institutions to help better define their practicality and clinical utility before entering routine clinical practice.

QUANTITATIVE REVERSE TRANSCRIPTASE–POLYMERASE CHAIN REACTION–BASED PROFILING OF BREAST CANCER

A significant limitation of the expression profiling studies outlined earlier is the need for fresh or snap-frozen tissue, which contains high-quality RNA that has not degraded. IHC assays for prognosis are an appealing alternative from several practical perspectives, including the ability to use formalin-fixed tissue samples, the broad availability of IHC technology, the morphologic confirmation of the tissue tested, a lower cost, and a more rapid turnaround time. However, significant concerns over the limitations of IHC for such applications include the influence of preanalytic variables such as the effects of fixation on antigenicity, the subjectivity and interobserver variability of manual scoring, and the current lack of the ability for practical and meaningful quantitative assay results.

A more recent, alternative approach to the molecular profiling of clinical specimens by cDNA microarrays has been to apply quantitative real-time RT-PCR to formalin-fixed, paraffin-embedded clinical samples to quantify the expression of potentially clinically important, tumor-related gene transcripts in a multigene approach. Using a multistep developmental method, a validated 21-gene assay (Oncotype DX®) has been developed for use in formalin-fixed, paraffin-embedded breast cancer samples through collaborations between Genomic Health and the National Surgical Adjuvant Breast and Bowel Project (NSABP). The assay quantifies the expression of 21 tumor-related genes using TaqMan® quantitative PCR (Applied Biosystems). The development of the assay used a candidate gene approach, in which 250 genes were selected for RT-PCR assays based on the published literature, genomic databases, and cDNA microarray analysis. These RT-PCR assays were used to study some 447 patients across three independent clinical studies. The data from all three studies were used to select a panel of 21 genes (16 cancer-related genes and 5 reference genes used for normalization of gene expression) that consistently showed a strong correlation with the likelihood of distant disease recurrence. An algorithm, based on the levels of expression of these genes, was developed and used to calculate a recurrence score (RS) for each breast cancer sample. The calculated RS ranges from 0 to 100 and is divided into three risk groups: low (<18), intermediate (18 to 31), and high (>31).

The difference in the risk of distant recurrence between patients with a low RS and those with a high RS has been consistently found to be large and highly statistically significant across several studies. Taking advantage of the NSABP paraffin archive of tissue blocks from patients treated on numerous clinical trials, several studies have been performed to evaluate the performance of the RS in predicting distant recurrence-free survival in node-negative, ER-positive breast cancers. One such study looked at material from NSABP B-14, a landmark clinical trial that established the value of tamoxifen in the treatment of hormone receptor–positive breast cancer. The paraffin blocks from 668 ER-positive patients from the tamoxifen-treated arm of B-14 were used for a validation study of the 21-gene RT-PCR assay. The technical success rate of the assay was 99%, and the study met its prospectively defined end points, demonstrating that the RSs were independent and highly significant predictors of recurrence-free survival. Risk of distant recurrence at 10 years for patients with a low RS was 6.8%; for those with an intermediate RS, the risk was 14.3%; and for patients with a high RS, the risk for distant recurrence was 30.5%. In further studies, the RS has also been shown to be prognostic in untreated patients, predictive for tamoxifen efficacy (patient with low RS appear to receive greatest benefit from tamoxifen), and predictive for response to chemotherapy (patients with high RS appear to receive greatest benefit from chemotherapy). Approximately 50% of patients fall within the low RS category in the published series, and the data suggests that these patients are likely to be adequately treated with hormonal therapy alone and unlikely to receive additional benefit from the addition of chemotherapy to their adjuvant treatment regimen.

Based on these encouraging results, a large National Cancer Institute–sponsored clinical trial involving the Oncotype DX breast cancer assay (PACCT-1 or TAILORx: Trial Assigning Individualized Options for Treatment) has recently been launched in the United States and is being coordinated by the Eastern Cooperative Oncology Group. The results of the Oncotype DX assay will be used to molecularly triage patients into treatment groups. Patients with a low RS will be assigned to hormonal therapy alone, patients with a high RS will be assigned to receive hormonal and chemotherapy, and patients with an intermediate RS will be randomized to receive either chemohormonal therapy or hormonal therapy alone. As is true for the European MINDACT trial, TAILORx represents a

new direction for clinical trial design. The results of these two trials are eagerly awaited.

Interestingly, 8 of the 16 genes included in the calculation of the RS consisting of ER-related genes and proliferation-related genes are also a component of the gene sets used to distinguish the luminal A from

---

GENE EXPRESSION PROFILING IN BREAST CANCER USING QUANTITATIVE RT-PCR—FACT SHEET

Oncotype DX

▶ The assay quantifies the expression of 21 tumor-related genes, using TaqMan quantitative PCR, from formalin-fixed, paraffin-embedded tissue blocks.

▶ The assay is validated to assess the risk of 10-year distant recurrence for women with node-negative, ER-positive breast cancer who will receive hormonal therapy.

▶ Additional data suggests that the assay is valuable to help predict the likelihood of patient survival within 10 years of diagnosis and the magnitude of chemotherapy.

▶ The measured level of expression of 16 tumor-related genes and 5 reference genes is used to calculate an RS using a mathematic algorithm.

▶ The RS score is used to predict patient prognosis. It ranges from 0 to 100 and is divided into three risk groups: low (<18), intermediate (18 to 31), and high (>31).

Final Gene Sets Used to Calculate Recurrence Score

▶ Proliferation gene set
  ▶ Ki-67
  ▶ STK15
  ▶ Survivin
  ▶ CCNB1 (cyclin B1)
  ▶ MYBL2
▶ Estrogen-related gene set
  ▶ ER
  ▶ PGR
  ▶ *BCL2*
  ▶ SCUBE2
▶ HER2 gene set
  ▶ *GRB7*
  ▶ *HER2*
▶ Invasion gene set
  ▶ MMP11 (stromelysin 3)
  ▶ CTSL2 (cathepsin L2)
▶ Unrelated gene set
  ▶ GSTM1
  ▶ CD68
  ▶ BAG1
▶ Reference gene set
  ▶ β-Actin
  ▶ GAPDH
  ▶ RPLPO
  ▶ GUS
  ▶ TFRC

Results of Clinical Studies of the Recurrence Score

▶ RS is prognostic in untreated patients.
▶ RS is predictive of lack of efficacy of tamoxifen.
▶ RS is predictive of response to chemotherapy.

MOLECULAR GRADE INDEX (MGI) AND *HOXB13:IL17BR* INDEX (HI INDEX) IN BREAST CANCER UTILIZING QRT-PCR—FACT SHEET

► MGI Assay quantifies the expression of five cell cycle, tumor-related genes using quantitative real time RT-PCR, from formalin fixed paraffin embedded tissue blocks

► MGI has been shown to be a robust strong prognostic factor comparable to a more complex 97-gene genomic grade index in multiple data sets

► MGI and the HI Index are complementary prognostic tests in early stage breast cancer: MGI has been associated with significantly worse outcome only in the context of a high HI Index, and a high HI Index is associated with significantly worse outcome only in the context of high level MGI

► The combination of MGI and HII molecular signatures selects a group of ER positive breast cancer patients treated with anti-hormonal therapy with significantly worse clinical outcome

---

the luminal B subtypes of breast cancer by expression profiling. The data now seems to indicate that tumors with a low RS are of the luminal A subtype whereas tumors with a high RS are of the luminal B subtype, again supporting the notion that these markedly different approaches to the molecular classification of breast cancer appear to have narrowed to a common set of biologic features that influence tumor biology and clinical outcomes and may affect the response to specific adjuvant therapies. The possibility that existing slide-based tools—IHC, FISH, CISH, SISH, and/or QDot detection—with quantification by image analysis and weighed integration of quantified data, can be modified to provide a result equivalent to the Oncotype DX RS has not been fully investigated.

CONCLUSION

The most clinically relevant, practical, affordable, and broadly available ancillary testing to help determine the prognosis for breast cancer patients, as well as testing to help guide the selection of the most beneficial treatment regimens, will continue to be an area of active research. The current clinical reality is that our ability to accurately determine which breast cancer patients are likely to develop metastatic disease on an individual basis, based on established prognostic and predictive factors, is limited. As a result, we still treat with toxic therapeutic regimens far too many patients who would have been destined to do well without therapy beyond local–regional treatment of their cancer. In contrast, many other patients, despite

receiving established standard adjuvant therapy, subsequently develop recurrent metastatic disease. If robust prognostic markers were available and could be used at initial diagnosis to help accurately stratify an individual patient's risk, this information would be invaluable clinically in helping improve and optimize treatment decisions. For those patients who were at a high risk for recurrence, appropriate systemic adjuvant therapy could be initiated with confidence; others with an excellent prognosis would receive local and hormonal therapies and avoid unnecessary and likely toxic treatment regimens that may be of little or no additional benefit.

Breast cancer diagnosis and progress in treatment will continue to rapidly evolve from our growing understanding of the molecular basis for a tumor's biologic and clinical behavior. The explosion of new molecular and cellular technologies has led to an overwhelming amount of new data that encompasses myriad information on cellular alterations, all the way from the genome to the transcriptome and the proteome in tumor samples. All of this new information is confusing and in some cases contradictory. Clinicians are in a quandary about what to make of and how to begin to apply this information to the care of their patients. To make matters worse, much of this new molecular information has ignored most existing validated clinical data used by clinicians and instead has clustered patients together for the purposes of these studies. In addition, many of the reported studies thus far are limited by small sample sizes (another reason for clustering patients), varying assay methodologies, varying treatment regimens, and retrospective analysis.

The task at hand is to begin to sort through the mountain of new molecular data that exists and to start separating the golden nuggets of clinically useful information from the sediment. The pathology community has an unprecedented opportunity to play a critically important role in these efforts and must join with general scientists and clinicians to help translate molecular differences among tumors within a clinical and morphologic context. The natural progression of these sorts of multidisciplinary studies will almost certainly lead to the development of validated diagnostic assay procedures and the identification of novel targeted therapeutic strategies for dealing with malignant disease. Moving forward, it will also be necessary to evaluate prospectively new, potentially useful prognostic assays in uniformly treated patient populations using standardized assay procedures and state-of-the-art statistical methods. The fruits of all these efforts will be to one day achieve the goal of tailoring individual treatment regimens for breast cancer patients to maximize the benefit from therapy for every newly diagnosed patient.

SUGGESTED READINGS

General References and Traditional Prognostic and Predictive Factors

Arpino G, Weiss H, Lee AV, et al: Estrogen receptor–positive, progesterone receptor–negative breast cancer: Association with growth factor receptor expression and tamoxifen resistance. J Natl Cancer Inst 2005;97:1254–1261.

Early Breast Cancer Trialists' Collaborative Group: Tamoxifen for early breast cancer: An overview of the randomized trials. Lancet 1998;351:1451–1467.

Greenlee RT, Murray T, Bolden S, Wingo PA: Cancer statistics 2000. CA Cancer J Clin 2000;50:7–34.

Hayes DF: Prognostic and predictive factors revisited. Breast 2005;14: 493–499.

Rosen PP, Groshen S, Kinne DW, et al: Factors influencing prognosis in node-negative breast carcinoma: Analysis of 767 T1N0M0/T2N0M0 patients with long-term follow-up. J Clin Oncol 1993;11:2090–2100.

Rosen PP, Groshen S, Saigo PE, et al: Pathological prognostic factors in stage I (T1N0M0) and stage II (T1N1M0) breast carcinoma: A study of 644 patients with median follow-up of 18 years. J Clin Oncol 1989; 1239–1251.

Singletary SE, Allred C, Ashley P, et al: Staging system for breast cancer: Revision for the 6th edition of the AJCC Cancer Staging Manual. Surg Clin North Am 2003;83:803–819.

Molecular Prognostic and Predictive Factors: HER2

Cobleigh MA, Vogel CL, Tripathy D, et al: Multinational study of the efficacy and safety of humanized anti-HER2 monoclonal antibody in women who have HER2-overexpressing metastatic breast cancer that has progressed after chemotherapy for metastatic disease. J Clin Oncol 1999;17:2639–2648.

Dietel M, Ellis IO, Höfler H, et al: Comparison of automated silver enhanced in situ hybridization (SISH) and fluorescence ISH (FISH) for the validation of HER2 gene status in breast carcinoma according to the guidelines of the American Society of Clinical Oncology and the College of American Pathologists. Virchows Arch 2007;45:19–25.

Downs-Kelly E, Pettay J, Hicks D, et al: Analytical validation and interobserver reproducibility of EnzMet GenePro: A second-generation brightfield metallography assay for concomitant detection of HER2 gene status and protein expression in invasive carcinoma of the breast. Am J Surg Pathol 2005;29:1505–1511.

Downs-Kelly E, Stoler M, Tubbs RR, et al: The Influence of polysomy 17 (CEP17+) on HER2 gene and protein expression in adenocarcinoma of the breast: A fluorescent in situ hybridization (FISH), immunohistochemical (IHC) and isotopic mRNA in situ hybridization (ISH) study. Am J Surg Pathol 2005;29:1221–1227.

Fitzgibbons PL, Murphy DA, Dorfman DM, et al, for the Immunohistochemistry Committee, College of American Pathologists: Interlaboratory comparison of immunohistochemical testing for HER2: Results of the 2004 and 2005 College of American Pathologists HER2 Immunohistochemistry Tissue Microarray Survey. Arch Pathol Lab Med 2006;130:1440–1445.

Hicks DG, Pettay J, Swain E, et al: The incidence of topoisomerase II-α (TOP2A) genomic alterations in adenocarcinoma of the breast, and their relationship to HER2 gene amplification: A fluorescence in situ hybridization (FISH) study. Hum Pathol 2005;36:348–356.

Hicks DG, Tubbs RR: Assessment of the HER2 status in breast cancer by fluorescence in situ hybridization (FISH): A technical review with interpretative guidelines. Hum Pathol 2005;36:250–261.

Laudadio J, Quigley DI, Tubbs R, Wolff DJ: HER2 testing: A review of detection methodologies and their clinical performance. Expert Rev Mol Diagn 2007;7:53–64.

Paik S, Bryant J, Tan-Chiu E, et al: Real-world performance of HER2 testing: National Surgical Adjuvant Breast and Bowel Project experience. J Natl Cancer Inst 2002;94:852–854.

Pauletti G, Dandekar S, Rong H, et al: Assessment of methods for tissuebased detection of the HER-2/neu alteration in human breast cancer: A direct comparison of fluorescence in situ hybridization and immunohistochemistry. J Clin Oncol 2000;18:3651–3664.

Perez EA, Suman VJ, Davidson NE, et al: HER2 testing by local, central, and reference laboratories in specimens from the north central cancer treatment group N9831 intergroup adjuvant trial. J Clin Oncol 2006;24: 3032–3038.

Persons DL, Tubbs RR, Cooley LD, et al: HER2 fluorescence in situ hybridization (FISH): Results from the survey program of the College of American Pathologists (CAP). Arch Path Lab Med Arch Pathol Lab Med 2006;130:325–331.

Press M, Bernstein L, Thomas P, et al: HER-2/neu gene amplification by fluorescence in situ hybridization: Evaluation of archival specimens and utility as a marker of poor prognosis in node-negative invasive breast carcinomas. J Clin Oncol 1997;15:2894–2904.

Press MF, Slamon DJ, Flom KJ, et al: Evaluation of HER2 gene amplification and overexpression: Comparison of frequently used assay methods in a molecularly characterized cohort of breast cancer specimens. J Clin Oncol 2002;20:3095–3105.

Roche PC, Suman VJ, Jenkins RB, et al: Concordance between local and central laboratory HER2 testing in the breast intergroup trial N9831. J Natl Cancer Inst 2002;94:855–857.

Romond EH, Perez EA, Bryant J, et al: Trastuzumab plus adjuvant chemotherapy for operable HER2-positive breast cancer. N Engl J Med 2005;353:1673–1684.

Slamon DJ, Clark GM, Wong SG, et al: Human breast cancer: Correlation of relapse and survival with amplification of the HER-2/neu oncogene. Science 235:177–182, 1987.

Slamon DJ, Godolphin W, Jones L, et al: Studies of the HER-2/neu proto-oncogene in human breast and ovarian cancer. Science 244:707–712, 1989.

Slamon DJ, Leyland-Jones B, Shak S, et al: Use of chemotherapy plus a monoclonal antibody against HER2 for metastatic breast cancer that overexpresses HER2. N Engl J Med 2001;344:783–792.

Tan-Chiu E, Yothers G, Romond E, et al: Assessment of cardiac dysfunction in a randomized trial comparing doxorubicin and cyclophosphamide followed by paclitaxel, with or without trastuzumab as adjuvant therapy in node-positive, human epidermal growth factor receptor 2–overexpressing breast cancer: NSABP B-31. J Clin Oncol 2005;23: 7811–7819.

Tubbs RR, Hicks DG, Downs-Kelly E, et al: Fluorescence in situ hybridization (FISH) as primary methodology for the assessment of HER2 status in adenocarcinoma of the breast: A single institution experience. Diagn Mol Pathol 2007;16:207–210.

Tubbs RR, Pettay J, Hicks D, et al: Novel bright field molecular morphology methods for detection of HER2 gene amplification. J Mol Histol 2004;35:589–594.

Wolff AC, Hammond MEH, Schwartz JN, et al: American Society of Clinical Oncology/College of American Pathologists: Guideline recommendations for HER2 testing in breast cancer. J Clin Oncol 2007;25:118–145.

Yarden Y, Sliwkowski MX: Untangling the ErbB signaling network. Nat Rev/Mol Cell Biol 2001;2:127–137.

Yaziji H, Goldstein LC, Barry TS, et al: HER-2 testing in breast cancer using parallel tissue-based methods. JAMA 2004;291:1972–1977.

Molecular Prognostic and Predictive Factors: Genomic Alterations

Buerger H, Simon R, Schafer KL, et al: Genetic relation of lobular carcinoma in situ, ductal carcinoma in situ, and associated invasive carcinoma of the breast. Mol Pathol 2000;53:118–121.

Cingoz S, Altungoz O, Canda T, et al: DNA copy number changes detected by comparative genomic hybridization and their association with clinicopathologic parameters in breast tumors. Cancer Genet Cytogenet 2003;145:108–114.

Jain AN, Chin K, Borresen-Dale A-L, et al: Quantitative analysis of chromosomal CGH in human breast tumors associates copy number abnormalities with p53 status and patient survival. Proc Natl Acad Sci USA 2001;98:7952–7957.

Jones C, Ford E, Gillett C, et al: Molecular cytogenetic identification of subgroups of grade III invasive ductal breast carcinomas with different clinical outcomes. Clin Cancer Res 2004;10:5988–5997.

Loveday RL, Greenman J, Simcox DL, et al: Genetic changes in breast cancer detected by comparative genomic hybridization. Int J Cancer 2000;86:494–500.

Robanus-Maandag EC, Bosch CA, Kristel PM, et al: Association of C-MYC amplification with progression from the in situ to the invasive stage in C-MYC–amplified breast carcinomas. J Pathol 2003;201:75–82.

Roylance R, Gorman P, Harris W, et al: Comparative genomic hybridization of breast tumors stratified by histologic grade reveals new insights into the biological progression of breast cancer. Cancer Res 1999;59: 1433–1436.

Stange DE, Radlwimmer B, Schubert F, et al: High-resolution genomic profiling reveals association of chromosomal aberration on 1q and 16p with histologic and genetic subgroups of invasive breast cancer. Clin Cancer Res 2006;12:345–352.

Tsuda H, Fukutomi T, Hirohashi S: Pattern of gene alteration in intraductal breast neoplasms associated with histological type and grade. Clin Cancer Res 1995;1:261–267.

Molecular Prognostic and Predictive Factors: Gene Expression Profiling

Ahr A, Karn T, Solbach C, et al: Identification of high-risk breast cancer patients by gene expression profiling. Lancet 2002;359:131–132.

Bogaerts J, Cardoso F, Buyse M, et al: Gene signature evaluation as a prognostic tool: Challenges in the design of the MINDACT trial. Nat Clin Prac 2006;3(10):540–551.

Chang HY, Nuyten DS, Sneddon JB, et al: Robustness, scalability, and integration of a wound-response gene expression signature in predicting breast cancer survival. Proc Natl Acad Sci USA 2005;102:3738–3743.

Fan C, Oh D, Wessels L, et al: Concordance among gene expression–based predictors for breast cancer. N Engl J Med 2006;355(6):560–569.

Hu Z, Fan C, Oh DS, et al: The molecular portraits of breast tumors are conserved across microarray platforms. BMC Genomics 2006;7:96.

Huang E, Cheng SH, Dressman H, et al: Gene expression predictors of breast cancer outcomes. Lancet 2003;361:1590–1596.

Ivshina AV, George J, Senko O, et al: Genetic reclassification of histologic grade delineates new clinical subtypes of breast cancer. Cancer Res 2006;66:10292–10301.

Ma XJ, Wang Z, Ryan PD, et al: A two-gene expression ratio predicts clinical outcome in breast cancer patients treated with tamoxifen. Cancer Cell 2004;5:607–616.

Perou CM, Sorlie T, Eisen MB, et al: Molecular portraits of human breast tumours. Nature 2000;406:747–752.

Rouzier R, Perou CM, Symmans WF, et al: Breast cancer molecular subtypes respond differently to preoperative chemotherapy. Clin Cancer Res 2005;11:5678–5685.

Sargent DJ, Conley BA, Allegra C, et al: Clinical trial designs for predictive marker validation in cancer treatment trials. J Clin Oncol 2005;23:2020–2027.

Sorlie T, Perou CM, Fan C, et al: Gene expression profiles do not consistently predict the clinical treatment response in locally advanced breast cancer. Mol Cancer Ther 2006;5:2914–2918.

Sorlie T, Perou CM, Tibshirani R, et al: Gene expression patterns of breast carcinomas distinguish tumor subclasses with clinical implications. Proc Natl Acad Sci USA 2001;98:10869–10874.

Sorlie T, Tibshirani R, Parker J, et al: Repeated observation of breast tumor subtypes in independent gene expression data sets. Proc Natl Acad Sci USA 2003;100:8418–8423.

van de Vijver MJ, He YD, van't Veer LJ, et al: A gene expression signature as a predictor of survival in breast cancer. N Engl J Med 2002;347:1999–2009.

van't Veer LJ, Dai H, van de Vijver MJ, et al: Gene expression profiling predicts clinical outcome of breast cancer. Nature 2002;415:530–536.

Wang Y, Klijn JG, Zhang Y, et al: Gene expression profiles to predict distant metastasis of lymph node–negative primary breast cancer. Lancet 2005;365:671–679.

Molecular Prognostic and Predictive Factors: Gene Expression by RT-PCR

Gianni L, Zambetti M, Clark K, et al: Gene expression profiles in paraffin-embedded core biopsy tissue predict response to chemotherapy in women with locally advanced breast cancer. J Clin Onc 2005;23:7265–7277.

Goetz MP, Ingle JN, Couch FJ: Gene-expression-based predictors for breast cancer. M Engl J Med. 2007;356(7):752.

Ma XJ, Salunga R, Dahiya S, Wang W, et al. A five-gene molecular grade index and HOXB13:IL17BR are complementary prognostic factors in early stage breast cancer. Clin Cancer Res 2008;14(9):2601–2608.

Paik S, Shak S, Tang G, et al: A multigene assay to predict recurrence of tamoxifen-treated, node-negative breast cancer. N Engl J Med 2004;351:2817–2826.

Paik S, Tang G, Shak S, et al: Gene expression and benefit of chemotherapy in women with node-negative, estrogen receptor–positive breast cancer. J Clin Onc 2006;24:3726–3734.

Perreard L, Fan C, Quackenbush JF, et al: Classification and risk stratification of invasive breast carcinomas using a real-time quantitative RT-PCR assay. Breast Cancer Res 2006;8:R23.

Molecular Prognostic and Predictive Factors: IHC Marker Profiling

Abd El-Rehim DM, Ball G, Pinder SE, et al: High-throughput protein expression analysis using tissue microarray technology of a large well-characterized series identifies biologically distinct classes of breast cancer confirming recent cDNA expression analyses. Int J Cancer 2005;116:340–350.

Abd El-Rehim DM, Pinder SE, Paish CE, et al: Expression of luminal and basal cytokeratins in human breast carcinoma. J Pathol 2004;203:661–671.

Dolled-Filhart M, Ryden L, Cregger M, et al: Classification of breast cancer using genetic algorithms and tissue microarrays. Clin Cancer Res 2006;12:6459–6468.

Farshid G, Balleine RL, Cummings M, et al: Morphology of breast cancer as a means of triage of patients for BRCA1 genetic testing. Am J Surg Pathol 2006;30:1357–1366.

Hicks DG, Short SM, Prescott NL, et al: Breast cancers with brain metastases are more likely to be estrogen receptor negative, express the basal cytokeratin CK5/6, and overexpress HER2 or EGFR. Am J Surg Pathol 2006;30:1097–1104.

Jacquemier J, Ginestier C, Rougemont J, et al: Protein expression profiling identifies subclasses of breast cancer and predicts prognosis. Cancer Res 2005;65:767–779.

Livasy C, Karaca G, Nanda R, et al: Phenotypic evaluation of the basal-like subtype of invasive breast carcinoma. Mod Pathol 2006;19:264–271.

Nielsen TO, Hsu FD, Jensen K, et al: Immunohistochemical and clinical characterization of the basal-like subtype of invasive breast carcinoma. Clin Cancer Res 2004;10:5367–5374.

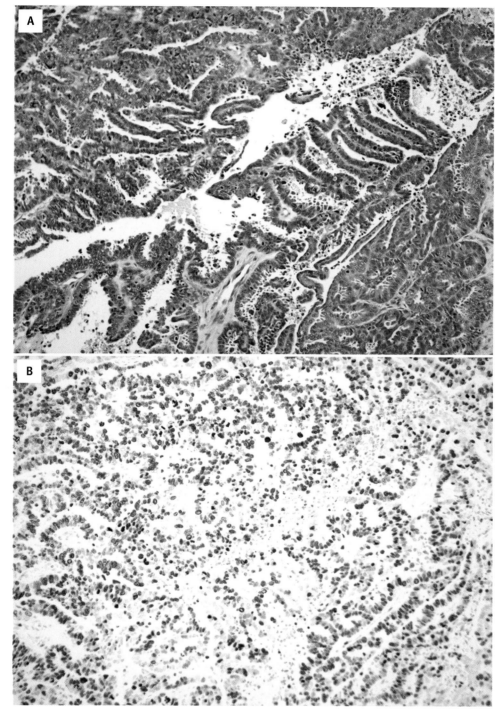

FIGURE 29-5

Immunohistochemistry of uterine serous carcinoma. **(A)** Hematoxylin and eosin stain of a serous tumor. **(B)** Ki-67 stain of the serous tumor, showing diffuse, intense staining.

EPITHELIAL OVARIAN AND FALLOPIAN TUBE CARCINOMA

The four main histologic subtypes of epithelial ovarian cancer are papillary serous, endometrioid, clear cell, and mucinous adenocarcinomas. Oligonucleotide microarray studies support the idea that these four types are distinct from one another and likely arise from different pathogenetic processes. This section discusses all four, with particular focus on the most common papillary serous subtype. Ovarian cancer is the fourth most common malignancy diagnosed in women in the United States and the most lethal

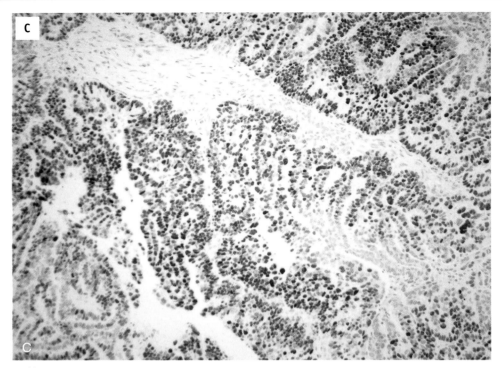

FIGURE 29-5, cont'd.
(C) P53 stain with the diffuse, intense staining often seen with p53 missense mutations.

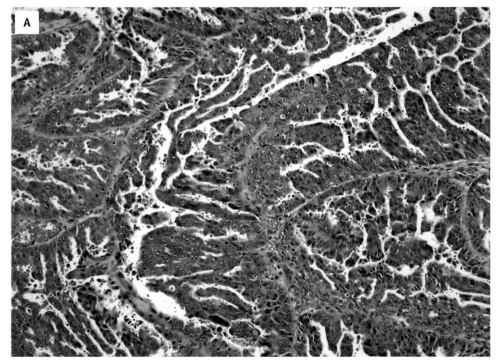

FIGURE 29-6
Immunohistochemistry of uterine serous carcinoma. **(A)** Hematoxylin and eosin stain of a serous tumor.

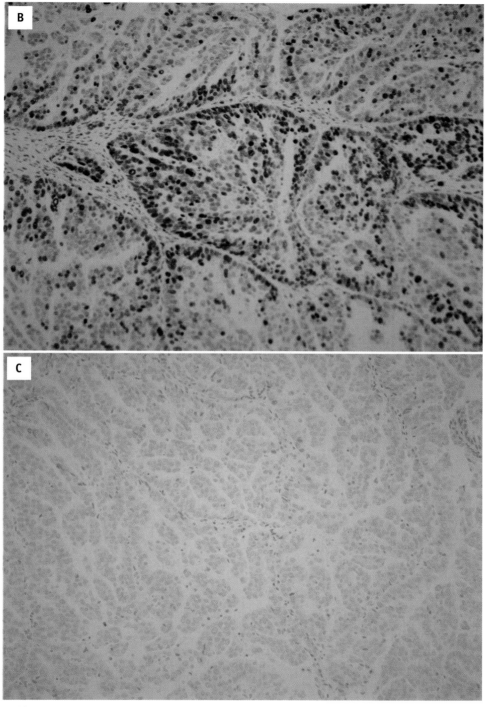

FIGURE 29-6, cont'd.

(B) Ki-67 stain of the serous tumor, showing diffuse, intense staining. **(C)** P53 stain with the negative staining often seen with frameshift and nonsense mutations.

gynecologic malignancy, with more than 21,650 newly diagnosed cases and 15,520 deaths due to ovarian cancer expected in 2008. Symptoms of ovarian cancer may be subtle and include increasing abdominal girth, bloating, abdominal or pelvic pain, early satiety, and difficulty eating. No effective screening programs exist for the early diagnosis of ovarian cancer, and more than two-thirds of cases are diagnosed at an advanced stage. Approximately 10% of ovarian cancers are thought to be caused by hereditary genetic alterations, and 90% are sporadic. The ovarian surface and the fallopian tube epithelium are derived from the same coelomic epithelium. Histologically, ovarian and fallopian tube carcinomas are identical, and recent data suggest that many serous ovarian tumors arise from the fallopian tube. Thus, this section pertains to both entities.

OVARIAN SEROUS CARCINOMA

Ovarian serous carcinoma accounts for most ovarian cancers that are diagnosed. The molecular alterations most commonly found in serous carcinoma are mutations of *TP53,* which produce an abnormal expression of the p53 protein. It has been shown to be the most common molecular genetic alteration in epithelial ovarian carcinoma. Although p53 overexpression is rare in benign ovarian epithelium and tumors of low malignant potential, *TP53* is mutated in approximately 45% of invasive epithelial ovarian carcinomas, with the highest percentage seen in serous carcinomas. In addition, the frequency of *TP53* mutations increases with increasing stage and tumor grade. It is known to be an independent indicator of poor prognosis. Recently, it was also shown that 67% of stage 1 and 2 ovarian serous cancers harbor a *TP53* mutation, compared to only 10% to 20% of early-stage clear cell, endometrioid, and mucinous ovarian cancers. This finding suggests that *TP53* mutations are early events in the pathogenesis of ovarian serous carcinomas and supports the hypothesis that distinct molecular pathways are involved in the pathogenesis of different histologic subtypes.

Clinically, p53 protein expression is often used to identify aberrations in *TP53.* Missense mutations that result in altered amino acid sequences lead to accumulation in the nucleus detected by immunohistochemical analysis, whereas frameshift and nonsense mutations that result in truncated protein products often manifest as a complete absence of staining.

Recently, studies have identified *WT1* as a specific marker for ovarian, fallopian tube, and primary peritoneal serous carcinoma (Figure 29-7). *WT1* is a gene encoded on 11p13 that translates into four protein isoforms and is involved in the development of the urogenital tissues. Because *WT1* is expressed in a limited number of human tissues—i.e., ovarian, fallopian tube, testis, kidney, and mesothelium—it is a useful marker for tumors of urogenital or mesothelial origin. *WT1* expression has been used to distinguish ovarian adenocarcinoma from breast and pancreatic carcinomas. In addition, because *WT1* is not expressed in endometrial epithelium, it has been shown to distinguish uterine papillary serous carcinoma from ovarian and primary peritoneal serous carcinomas, even in the presence of metastatic peritoneal disease. These findings suggest that serous carcinoma

may have a different pathogenesis based on site of origin, where USC arises via a different pathway from ovarian, fallopian tube, and primary peritoneal carcinomas. Thus, *WT1* is a marker with significant clinical utility and likely one that will be studied in greater detail.

Ovarian Serous Tumors of Low Malignant Potential

Although high-grade serous carcinomas harbor *TP53* mutations in most cases, even in early-stage disease, molecular studies provide evidence for a second pathway of tumorigenesis from atypical proliferating tumors, otherwise known as *serous borderline tumors* or *tumors of low malignant potential,* to invasive low-grade serous carcinomas. More than 88% of serous borderline tumors and low-grade invasive serous carcinomas harbor mutations of *KRAS* and *BRAF;* however, mutations of *TP53* are rare in this group. Thus, an alternative pathway of tumorigenesis is suggested and has been further supported by the presence of identical mutations in benign serous cystadenomas adjacent to serous borderline tumors harboring a *KRAS* or *BRAF* mutation. These findings suggest that the mutation occurs early in tumorigenesis, before the identification of morphologic changes that can be found by light microscopy.

OVARIAN ENDOMETRIOID CARCINOMA

The Wnt signaling pathway appears to have a prominent role in the development of endometrioid ovarian carcinomas, with up to 40% of these tumors exhibiting deregulation of β-catenin, which results in nuclear accumulation of β-catenin and can be seen by immunohistochemical analysis. Most ovarian endometrioid carcinomas that have nuclear accumulation of β-catenin will have mutations in exon 3 of *CTNNB1,* the gene that encodes for β-catenin. A smaller percentage will exhibit inactivation of the *APC* gene, also in the Wnt signaling pathway, which is the gene inactivated in a large percentage of colorectal carcinomas. Tumors with β-catenin nuclear accumulation will often present with squamous differentiation morphologically, and this has been shown both in ovarian carcinoma and in UEC. In the ovary, the presence of β-catenin mutation is often associated with low-grade histology and has an overall favorable prognosis compared to the high-grade serous and clear cell carcinomas.

OVARIAN CLEAR CELL CARCINOMA

Clear cell ovarian cancer is associated with poor prognosis compared to other histologic subtypes of epithelial ovarian cancer, including ovarian serous

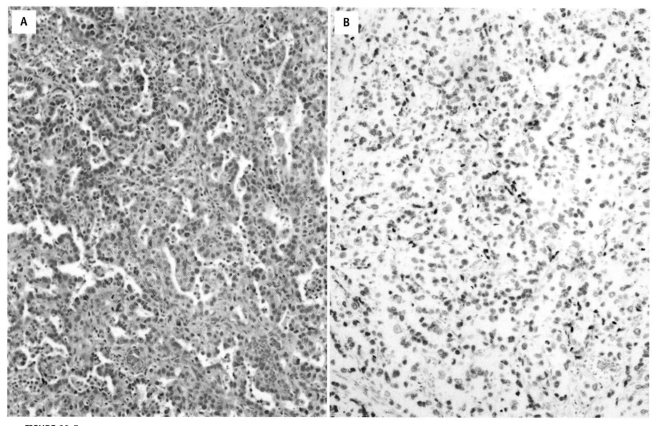

FIGURE 29-7

Immunohistochemistry of ovarian serous carcinoma. **(A)** Hematoxylin and eosin stain of ovarian serous carcinoma. **(B)** Wilms' tumor gene 1 immunohistochemical stain, with strong, homogeneous staining. (Courtesy of Dr. Mark H. Stoler.)

carcinoma. In addition, response rates with conventional chemotherapy for ovarian cancer are lower for patients with clear cell histology; thus, a lower overall survival rate is seen in these patients. Oligonucleotide microarrays used to evaluate the gene expression profiles of the different histologic subtypes have shown a distinct molecular profile for clear cell ovarian cancer when compared to serous and endometrioid ovarian cancers. In addition, a recent microarray study evaluated clear cell ovarian, endometrial, and renal cell carcinomas and found that the expression patterns of these tumors were similar regardless of the organ of origin, in distinct contrast to the gene expression patterns of serous and endometrioid ovarian and endometrial cancers, which segregated by organ rather than histologic subtype. Morphologically, clear cell carcinomas can be confused with endometrioid carcinomas with secretory features. Thus, although currently no markers specifically identify clear cell carcinoma by immunohistochemistry, as the microarray technology becomes more available as a clinical tool it may be useful to identify clear cell ovarian and endometrial cancers that arise in a mixed

background and cannot be identified definitively by light microscopy.

OVARIAN MUCINOUS TUMORS

Activating mutations of the *KRAS* oncogene are seen in approximately 50% of invasive mucinous ovarian cancers, but they are relatively rare in high-grade serous, clear cell, and endometrioid ovarian cancers. Missense mutations are commonly seen in codons 12, 13, and 61. In addition, most mucinous tumors of low malignant potential also harbor *KRAS* mutations, suggesting a possible common pathway of tumorigenesis.

Diagnostically, it is often difficult to differentiate mucinous ovarian carcinomas from metastatic tumors that have spread to the ovary such as gastrointestinal, pancreatic, and biliary tract carcinomas. Immunohistochemical markers such as cytokeratin 7 and 20 (CK7 and CK20) have been somewhat useful in distinguishing these entities. CK7-positive and CK20-negative profiles are seen commonly in primary ovarian mucinous tumors, whereas lower intestinal tract carcinomas (i.e., colorectal and appendiceal cancers) have a CK7-negative and CK20-positive staining pattern. The primary carcinoma is often difficult to determine when the staining pattern is CK7 positive and CK20 positive, because it may be seen in more than 74% of primary mucinous ovarian tumors, 78% of upper gastrointestinal tract carcinomas, 88% of endocervical adenocarcinomas, 11% of colorectal cancers, and 35% of appendiceal carcinomas metastatic to the ovary, according to a recent comprehensive study. When this combination is observed, it may be beneficial to characterize the staining pattern. With the primary mucinous ovarian cancers, there will typically be diffuse staining with CK7 and focal expression of CK20 (Figure 29-8). In contrast, when a lower intestinal tract tumor displays positivity for both CK7 and CK20, it will often have focal CK7 and diffuse CK20 expression.

Given that the staining pattern of CK7 and CK20 is similar for primary mucinous ovarian tumors and upper gastrointestinal tract carcinomas, such as gastric, pancreatic, and biliary, it becomes necessary to identify other markers that may be used with these two. For endocervical cancers, which also are largely positive for both CK7 and CK20, p16 has been useful in distinguishing these tumors when metastatic to the ovary. Recently, a nuclear transcription factor involved in intestinal differentiation, CDX2, has been shown to differentiate primary ovarian mucinous tumors from upper

gastrointestinal tract carcinomas when used with CK7 and CK20. As a single marker, CDX2 has a significantly lower expression rate of 40% in primary mucinous ovarian tumors versus the rate in metastatic mucinous carcinomas of both the upper (74%) and the lower (90%) gastrointestinal tract. When CDX2 is combined with CK7 and CK20 expression, the CK7-positive and CDX2-negative profile pattern is significantly more common than the CK7-positive and CK20-negative pattern in primary mucinous ovarian tumors (60% versus 17%), suggesting that the combination of CK7 and CDX2 may be better at discriminating between primary ovarian and metastatic lower intestinal tract carcinomas. In addition, the combination may be used to distinguish metastases from primary upper gastrointestinal tract tumors, because more than 60% of the primary mucinous ovarian tumors will be CK7 positive and CDX2 negative but only 26% of the upper gastrointestinal tract tumors will display the same pattern. Thus, the coordinate expression of all three markers may be beneficial in the determination of the primary source of mucinous ovarian carcinomas.

Importantly, recent studies using these immunohistochemical markers have suggested that primary mucinous carcinomas are quite rare and that most mucinous carcinomas involving the ovary are metastases from other sites (gastrointestinal and endocervical).

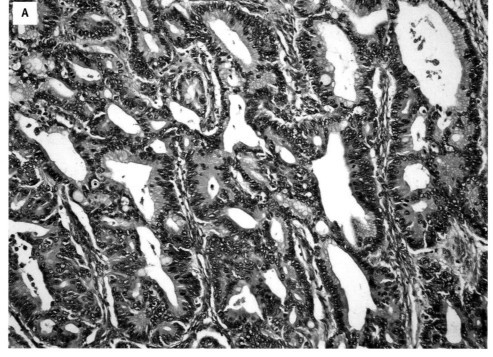

FIGURE 29-8

Immunohistochemical staining of mucinous carcinoma involving the ovary. **(A)** Hematoxylin and eosin (H&E) stain of ovarian mucinous carcinoma.

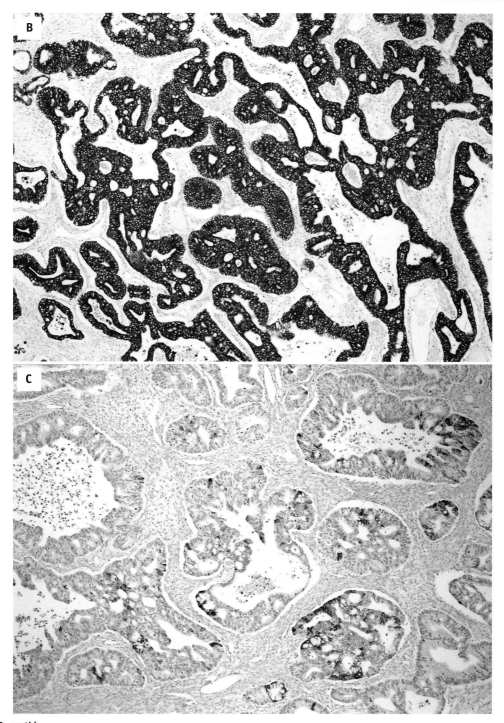

FIGURE 29-8, cont'd.
(B) Cytokeratin 7 (CK7) stain of the ovarian carcinoma. **(C)** Cytokeratin 20 (CK20) stain of the ovarian carcinoma.

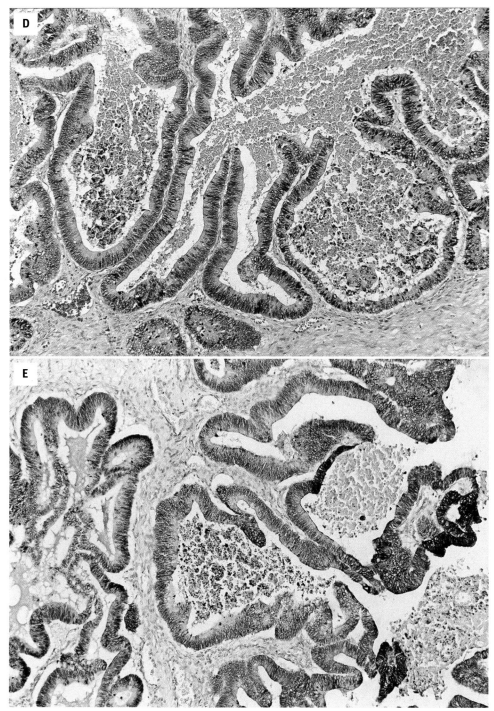

FIGURE 29-8, cont'd.
(D) H&E stain of colon cancer metastatic to the ovary. **(E)** CK7 stain of the colon carcinoma.

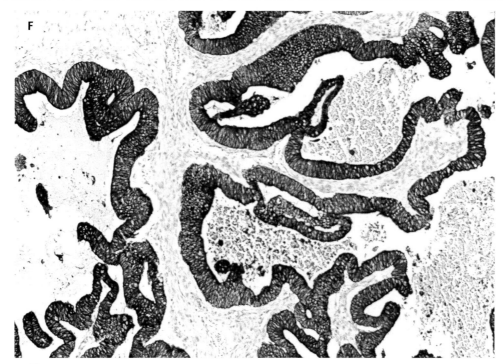

FIGURE 29-8, cont'd.

(F) CK20 stain of the colon carcinoma. (Courtesy of Dr. Brigitte M. Ronnett.)

CONCLUSION

In clinical practice, we are steadily moving toward a more molecular approach in the diagnosis of gynecologic malignancies. In addition to recently identified protein markers that have clinical utility by immunohistochemical analysis, such as WT1 and CDX2, molecular analysis has become possible in the clinical setting with the advent of high-throughput technology such as PCR, automated sequencing, and messenger RNA oligonucleotide microarray analysis. In the next decade, we are likely to have these techniques routinely incorporated into clinical practice. The molecular genetic differences in the various subtypes provide clues in the clinical setting as to why all cancers from one organ site do not behave uniformly and some are more aggressive than others. As this chapter highlights, the histologic variants of gynecologic malignancies arise from different pathogenetic pathways, and molecular studies have aided in our understanding of these diverse pathways.

SUGGESTED READINGS

Cervical Carcinoma

Keating JT, Cviko A, Riethdorf S, et al: Ki-67, cyclin E, and p16INK4 are complementary surrogate biomarkers for human papilloma virus–related cervical neoplasia. Am J Surg Pathol 2001;25(7):884–891.

Kong CS, Balzer BL, Troxell ML, et al: p16INK4A Immunohistochemistry is superior to HPV in situ hybridization for the detection of high-risk HPV in atypical squamous metaplasia. Am J Surg Pathol 2007;31(1): 33–43.

Liotta LA. Tumor invasion and metastases: role of the basement membrane. Am J Pathol 1984;117:339-348.

Pirog EC, Baergen RN, Soslow RA, et al: Diagnostic accuracy of cervical low grade squamous intraepithelial lesions is improved with MIB-1 immunostaining. Am J Surg Pathol 2001;26:70–75.

Pirog EC, Isacson C, Szabolcs MJ, et al: Proliferative activity of benign and neoplastic endocervical epithelium and correlation with HPV DNA detection. Int J Gynecol Pathol 2002;21(1): 22–26.

Rush D, Hyjek E, Baergen RN, et al: Detection of microinvasion in vulvar and cervical intraepithelial neoplasia using double immunostaining for cytokeratin and basement membrane components. Arch Pathol Lab Med 2005;129(6):747–753.

Endometrial Carcinoma

An HJ, Logani S, Isacson C, Ellenson LH: Molecular characterization of uterine clear cell carcinoma. Mod Pathol 2004;17: 530–537.

Bokhman JV. Two pathogenetic types of endometrial carcinoma. Gynecol Oncol 1983;15(1):10-17.

Hayes MP, Wang H, Espinal-Witter R, et al: *PIK3CA* and *PTEN* mutations in uterine endometrioid carcinoma and complex atypical hyperplasia. Clin Cancer Res 2006;12:5932–5935.

Lax SF, Kendall B, Tashiro H, et al: The frequency of p53, *KRAS* mutations, and microsatellite instability differs in uterine endometrioid and serous carcinoma: Evidence of distinct molecular genetic pathways. Cancer 2000;88:814–824.

Oda K, Stokoe D, Taketani Y, McCormick F: High frequency of coexistent mutations of PIK3CA and PTEN genes in endometrial carcinoma. Cancer Res 2005;65:10669–10673.

Risinger JI, Hayes AK, Berchuck A, Barrett JC: *PTEN/MMAC1* mutations in endometrial cancers. Cancer Res 1997;57:4736–4738.

Santin AD, Bellone S, Van Stedum S, et al: Determination of *Her2/neu* status in uterine serous papillary carcinoma: Comparative analysis of immunohistochemistry and fluorescence in situ hybridization. Gynecol Oncol 2005;98:24–30.

Tashiro H, Blazes MS, Wu R, et al: Mutations in *PTEN* are frequent in endometrial carcinoma but rare in other common gynecological malignancies. Cancer Res 1997;57:3935–3940.

Taylor NP, Zighelboim I, Huettner PC, et al: DNA mismatch repair and *TP53* defects are early events in uterine carcinosarcoma tumorigenesis. Mod Pathol 2006;19:1333–1338.

Epithelial Ovarian and Fallopian Tube Carcinoma

Euscher ED, Malpica A, Deavers MT, Silva EG: Differential expression of WT1 in serous carcinomas in the peritoneum with or without associated serous carcinoma in endometrial polyps. Am J Surg Pathol 2005;29:1074–1078.

Ho CL, Kurman RJ, Dehari R, et al: Mutations of *BRAF* and *KRAS* precede the development of ovarian serous borderline tumors. Cancer Res 2004;64:6915–6918.

Leitao MM, Soslow RA, Baergen RN, et al: Mutation and expression of the *TP53* gene in early stage epithelial ovarian carcinoma. Gynecol Oncol 2004;93:301–306.

Schwartz DR, Kardia SL, Shedden KA, et al: Gene expression in ovarian cancer reflects both morphology and biological behavior, distinguishing clear cell from other poor-prognosis ovarian carcinomas. Cancer Res 2002;62:4722–4729.

Vang R, Gown AM, Wu LS, et al: Immunohistochemical expression of CDX2 in primary ovarian mucinous tumors and metastatic mucinous carcinomas involving the ovary: Comparison with CK20 and correlation with coordinate expression of CK7. Mod Pathol 2006;19:1421–1428.

Wu R, Zhai Y, Fearon ER, Cho KR: Diverse mechanisms of β-catenin deregulation in ovarian endometrioid adenocarcinomas. Cancer Res 2001;61:8247–8255.

Zorn KK, Bonome T, Gangi L, et al: Gene expression profiles of serous, endometrioid, and clear cell subtypes of ovarian and endometrial cancer. Clin Cancer Res 2005;11:6422–6430.

30 Pediatric Molecular Pathology

Robin LeGallo

INTRODUCTION

The use of molecular and cytogenetic testing has become the standard of care in the diagnosis and treatment of childhood solid tumors. The molecular events underlying childhood cancer include the inactivation of tumor suppressor genes and activation of proto-oncogenes, as well as the creation of novel fusion genes, and each is a target for molecular detection (Table 30-1). The classification of a small round blue cell tumor can typically be made by light microscopy with immunohistochemistry or electron microscopy, but morphologic and immunophenotypic overlap or aberrant antigen expression may result in diagnostic challenges. For example, both the Ewing family of tumors (EFT) and poorly differentiated synovial sarcoma show membranous CD99 staining and variable reactivity with epithelial markers. The identification of an *EWS* or *SYT* rearrangement can confirm a diagnosis.

Molecular prognostic or predictive markers are increasingly being incorporated into therapy protocols. This is perhaps best exemplified by *MYCN* amplification status in neuroblastoma (NB), which, combined with clinical and pathologic features, identifies those patients in need of the most aggressive therapy. Likewise, the absence of specific genetic alterations may allow decreased therapy to minimize toxicity during vulnerable stages of development. Because current mainstream therapy is nonspecifically targeted against proliferating cells, its potential detrimental effects to rapidly growing normal tissue should not be underestimated.

Much of what is known about the biology of pediatric solid tumors has been generated from cooperative group studies. In the United States, more than 70% of children with cancer are enrolled in a clinical trial sometime during their treatment course. Many of these studies incorporate tumor biology into risk stratification or are prospectively investigating the prognostic significance of molecular events. Appropriate tissue procurement is essential and is increasingly difficult with smaller biopsies and even cytologic samples. Communication among the pathologist,

surgeon, and oncologist is vital to establish a plan to obtain an adequate sample for tissue diagnosis, ancillary studies, and cooperative study protocol enrollment. Biology protocol requirements differ for individual tumors, and these should be reviewed preoperatively. Touch preparations with or without frozen sections should be performed to determine appropriate triage of tissue. General guidelines for tissue procurement (Table 30-2) should be followed for undifferentiated small blue cell tumors for which a diagnosis is unknown. However, adequate tissue for light microscopy continues to take precedence and should not be compromised in attempts to obtain tissue for other studies.

NEUROBLASTOMA

NB is the most common pediatric solid tumor outside the central nervous system, with 500 to 700 cases diagnosed annually in the United States. NB is a tumor of young children; it is the most often detected congenital malignancy, and more than 95% of tumors are diagnosed before the age of 5. NB usually arises within the region of the adrenal gland and paraspinal tissue but can occur in all sites of sympathetic ganglia or paraganglia. The morphologic diagnosis is based on the identification of the neuroblast with evidence of ganglion cell differentiation, variable amounts of neuropil, or both (Figure 30-1). In undifferentiated tumors, immunohistochemistry, electron microscopy, or both are necessary to make the diagnosis. NB is variably immunoreactive for markers of neuronal differentiation, which can also be expressed in EFT. NB should not be positive for CD99 or FLI1. Neuroblastic tumors are categorized as having or favorable or unfavorable histology using the International Neuroblastoma Pathology Classification (INPC) system based on the amount of schwannian stroma, ganglion cell differentiation, and mitotic karyorrhexis index, combined with patient age. NB perhaps has the widest spectrum of biologic behavior of any malignancy; it ranges from spontaneous regression to widespread

411

TABLE 30-1

Molecular Pathogenesis of Pediatric Solid Tumors

Tumor	Mechanism	Locus	Gene	Percentage
Neuroblastoma	Oncogene amplification	2p24	*MYCN*	15–25%
	Tumor suppressor	1p36	*Unknown*	25–35%
	Tumor suppressor	11q23	*Unknown*	30–35%
	Oncogene amplification	17q	*Unknown*	50–60%
Wilms tumor	Tumor suppressor	11p13	*WT1*	30–40%
	Tumor suppressor	11p15	*WT2*	30%
Congenital mesoblastic nephroma	Fusion gene	t(12;15)(p13;q26)	*ETV6/NTRK*	90%
Malignant rhabdoid tumor	Tumor suppressor	22q11.2	*INI1*	95%
Alveolar rhabdomyosarcoma	Fusion gene	t(2;13)(q35;q14)	*PAX3/FKHR*	50–60%
		t(1;13)(p36;q14)	*PAX7/FKHR*	15–25%
Ewing family of tumors	Fusion gene	t(11;22)(q24;q12)	*EWS/FLI1*	80–85%
		t(21;22)(q22;q12)	*EWS/ERG*	10–15%
		t(7;22)(p22;q12)	*EWS/ETV1*	Rare
		t(17;22)(q21;q12)	*EWS/ETV4*	Rare
		t(2;22)(q36;q12)	*EWS/FEV*	Rare
		t(6;21)(p11;q22)	*FUS/ERG*	Rare
Desmoplastic small round cell tumor	Fusion gene	t(11;22)(p13;q12)	*EWS/WT1*	90–95%
Hepatoblastoma	Activation mutation	3p22-p21.3	*β-Catenin*	50%
Infantile fibrosarcoma	Fusion gene	t(12;15)(q13;q26)	*ETV6/NTRK*	90%
Retinoblastoma	Tumor suppressor	13q14	*RB*	95–100%

TABLE 30-2

Tissue Procurement for Pediatric Small Blue Cell Tumors

Snap-frozen tumor: ≥0.5 g but up to 10 g

OCT-embedded frozen tumor: ≥0.5 g

Fresh tumor in tissue transport media: >0.2 g

Touch preparations from tumor: 8–95% alcohol fixed and unstained

Fresh tumor in 2% glutaraldehyde: 1-mm pieces

Formalin-fixed tumor: Additional block

Snap-frozen normal tissue: ≥0.5 g but up to 10 g

Snap-frozen metastatic tumor: ≥0.5 g

OCT, optimal cutting temperature

metastases, and therapy spans observation alone to radiotherapy and multimodality chemotherapy with stem cell rescue. The current risk stratification system combines stage (International Neuroblastoma Staging System), patient age, MYCN status, INPC histology, and in select cases DNA ploidy to assign a patient to a low-, intermediate-, or high-risk group. Additional genomic aberrations and gene expression patterns have been shown to be of significance and will likely be implemented in future risk assessment protocols.

DIAGNOSTIC FACTORS

Clonal karyotypic abnormalities can be identified in 80% to 90% of primary NBs by conventional cytogenetics, and a complex karyotype is often present, particularly in advanced-stage tumors. Although none of these abnormalities are entirely specific for NB, many are nonrandom and are present in a significant subset of tumors. Numeric abnormalities show losses to only slightly outnumber gains, with most nonrandom losses occurring with chromosomes X, 3, 9, 10, 11, 15, and 19. Whole

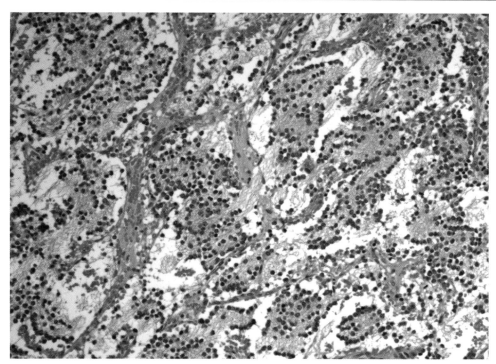

FIGURE 30-1
Neuroblastoma (NB) histologic findings. Nests of neuroblasts in a background of neuropil separated by thin fibrovascular septae is diagnostic of NB.

chromosomal loss has been documented for every chromosome except chromosome 1. Nonrandom gains are seen with chromosomes 7, 13, 17, and 20. The most common structural aberrations involve 17q, 1p, 11q, 1q, 7q, 2p, 3p, 4p, and 6q, although a structural abnormality of every chromosome has been reported. *MYCN* amplification can often be seen in metaphases as double minutes. *MYCN* amplification is not specific to NB and can be seen in other pediatric solid tumors, including alveolar rhabdomyosarcoma and retinoblastoma, but it has not been reported in EFT. Finally, certain chromosomal abnormalities tend to act in concert and correlate with defined risk groups.

PREDICTIVE AND PROGNOSTIC FACTORS

The clinical diversity of NB is underlined by its genetic heterogeneity, and through large-scale comparative genomic hybridization and loss of heterozygosity (LOH) studies, genotypic patterns have emerged that define biologic subgroups (Table 30-3). Although clinical investigation is ongoing, several genetic loci are proving to be independent predictors of outcome.

MYCN amplification is present in 15% to 25% of NBs and is a strong predictor of adverse outcome. The *MYCN* locus is 2p24, but amplification is most often expressed as extrachromosomal double-minute chromatin bodies, with a small percentage of tumors

showing linear integration of the amplified DNA as homogenously staining regions (Figure 30-2). Although most *MYCN*-amplified tumors are associated with other unfavorable factors, neither histologic nor clinical parameters can accurately predict *MYCN* status. Amplification is usually present at the time of diagnosis, and retesting the tumor at the time of relapse is not routine. Interphase fluorescence in situ hybridization (FISH) has replaced Southern blot as the method of choice and can be performed on cytogenetic cultures, direct preparations, or paraffin-embedded tissue. For clinical purposes, a tumor is considered amplified when there are more than four *MYCN* signals per chromosome 2 as defined by CEP2 signals. Low-level amplification is rare and must be distinguished from extreme hyperdiploidy. Quantitative polymerase chain reaction (PCR) is an alternative method but may lack the sensitivity of FISH in heterogeneous tumors such as nodular ganglioneuroblastoma. Several investigators have addressed the question of whether it is the genomic DNA or the messenger RNA copy number that predicts biologic behavior, with controversial results. Recent data suggest that a high level of *MYCN* expression in the absence of genomic amplification is a low-risk phenotype and is associated with high levels of TrkA expression, a favorable biologic marker.

Deletion of chromosome 1p is present in 25% to 35% of NBs. Cases of constitutional abnormalities of 1p in patients with NB make it an attractive location

TABLE 30-3

Biologic Patterns of Neuroblastoma

Factors	Group 1	Group 2	Group 3
Age	<18 months	>18 months	>18 months
Stage	Low or 4s	High	High
MYCN	Nonamplified	Nonamplified	Amplified
1p LOH	Absent	Absent	Present
17 gain	+17	+17q	+17q
11q23 LOH	Absent	Present	Absent
DNA ploidy	Triploid	Diploid/tetraploid	Diploid/tetraploid
Outcome	Favorable	Intermediate	Unfavorable

LOH, loss of heterozygosity.

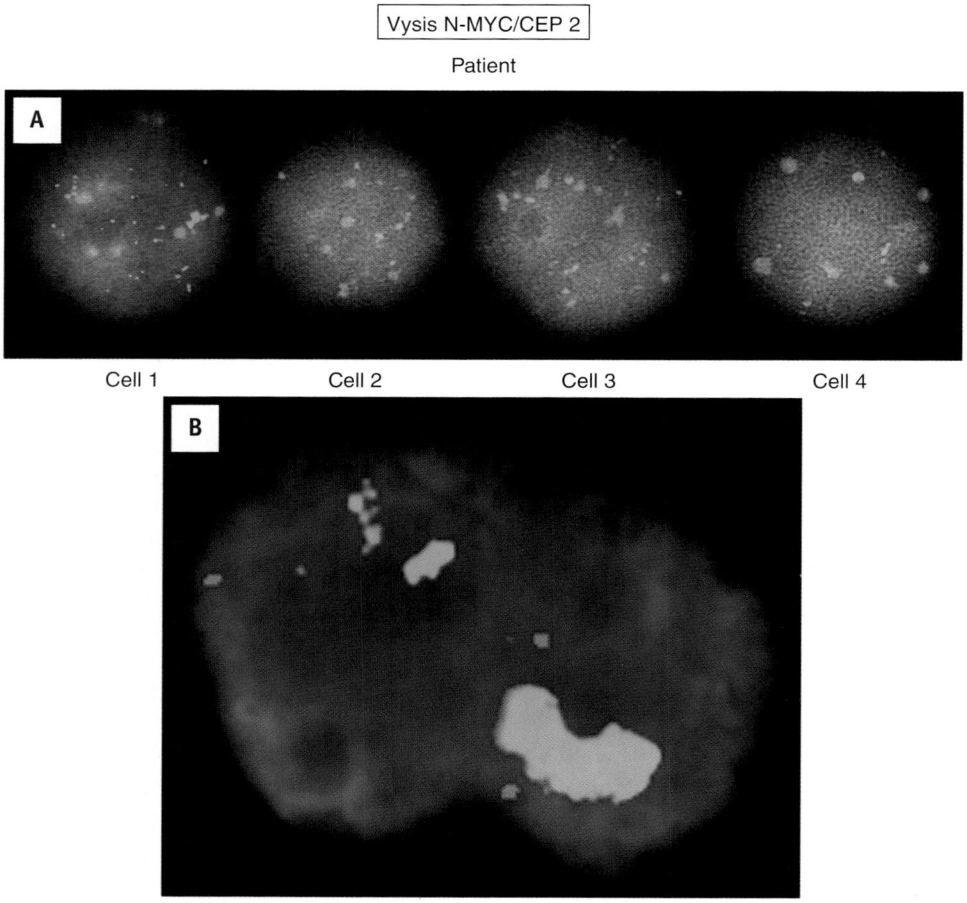

Vysis N-MYC/CEP 2

Patient

Cell 1   Cell 2   Cell 3   Cell 4

FIGURE 30-2

Neuroblastoma *MYCN* amplification. Amplification of *MYCN* is identified as double minutes **(A)** and homogenously staining regions **(B)** using interphase fluorescence in situ hybridization. *MYCN* = green probe, CEP2 = red probe. (A courtesy of Columbus Children's Hospital Cytogenetics Laboratory, B courtesy of University of Virginia Cytogenetics Laboratory.)

for one or more tumor suppressor genes. Large deletions are seen in near-diploid, *MYCN*-amplified tumors (high risk); smaller interstitial deletions are more common in nonamplified, near-triploid tumors (low risk). The difference in biologic behavior between the groups suggests the presence of more than one tumor suppressor. The smallest common region of deletion in all groups has been mapped to 1p36.3, and several candidate genes are under investigation. A promising gene is *CAMTA1,* and reduced expression has been shown to be an independent risk factor for decreased event-free survival. Deletion of 1p present in otherwise-high-risk tumors is not an independent predictor of treatment failure. In the low- and intermediate-risk groups, 1p LOH is independently associated with decreased progression-free survival but not overall survival. Most 1p deletions are large, and many are associated with a t(1;17) and thus can commonly be detected by routine cytogenetics. FISH can supplement conventional cytogenetics or be performed on direct preparations or formalin-fixed, paraffin-embedded tissues. Allelic status of 1p36 can be also be determined by Southern blot, LOH studies, and quantitative real-time PCR.

Gain of 17q is the most common genetic alteration, being present in up to 80% of NBs either as a translocation or as a whole chromosome gain. Unbalanced 17q gain, present in 50% of NBs, almost exclusively results from an unbalanced translocation, with the most common partners being 1p, 3p, and 11q. The result is gain of 17q material and loss of material from the partner chromosome. The breakpoint is highly variable but consistently involves gain of material distal to 17q22. The heterogeneity of the breakpoints makes the possibility of a fusion gene or disruption an unlikely oncogenic event. Dosage effects of one or more genes likely influence tumor progression and candidate genes are being investigated. Many studies have shown unbalanced gain of 17q to be a predictor of adverse outcome independent of other established or proposed prognostic factors, including *MYCN,* LOH of 1p, and 11q. Gain of whole chromosome 17, as seen in triploid tumors, does not carry this prognostic implication and in some studies has been shown to be a favorable prognostic marker. Most gains of 17q can be detected by conventional karyotype, but interphase FISH may pick up cases missed by routine karyotype. Quantitative PCR and LOH studies can be used and, like FISH, must take into account the 17p status to discriminate unbalanced versus whole chromosome gain.

Approximately one third of NBs show LOH for 11q23. These cases are equally distributed between those with an unbalanced loss of 11q23 with retention of 11p and those with whole chromosome loss. Both groups show an inverse correlation with *MYCN*

amplification, but only unbalanced 11q23 is an independent predictor of event-free and progression-free survival across all risk groups. Because it is usually found in the absence of *MYCN* amplification, it is potentially a valuable biologic marker for a cohort of patients with localized disease that may benefit from more intensive therapy. FISH, LOH, quantitative real-time PCR, or Southern blot can assess unbalanced 11q allelic status.

DNA ploidy can be determined by flow cytometry off of fresh, frozen, or formalin-fixed, paraffin-embedded tissue, as well as by conventional cytogenetics. Near-diploid or tetraploid tumors carry a poor prognosis, whereas hyperdiploid (near-triploid) and pentaploid tumors have a more favorable prognosis. The current risk stratification system only applies ploidy to subsets of stage 4 and 4s tumors in patients under 18 months of age.

CHILDHOOD RENAL TUMORS

WILMS TUMOR

Wilms tumor accounts for 85% of pediatric renal tumors, with approximately 500 cases diagnosed annually in the United States. The diagnosis can be made by light microscopy alone when a triphasic pattern with epithelial, blastemal, and stromal components is present. The blastemal predominant Wilms tumor must be differentiated from other undifferentiated small blue cell tumors (Figure 30-3). Stromal predominant Wilms tumor can be confused with clear cell sarcoma or other spindle cell neoplasms.

Although Wilms tumors are most often a sporadic occurrence, approximately 10% are multifocal or bilateral and a smaller subset occurs in children with a recognized malformation syndrome. These syndromes mostly can be grouped as overgrowth syndromes (i.e., Beckwith-Wiedemann, Perlman, Sotos, and Simpson-Golabi-Behmel) or those with associated genitourinary abnormalities (i.e., Denys-Drash, WAGR, and Frasier). The syndromic associations with Wilms tumor have provided clues to the pathogenesis of this tumor.

Germline mutations or deletions of Wilms tumor gene 1 *(WT1)* are present in Wilms tumor predisposition syndromes with associated genitourinary malformations and in about 2% of phenotypically normal children with Wilms tumor, which are often multiple or bilateral. *WT1* is a zinc finger transcription factor located at 11p13 and is essential for genitourinary development. Most of these germline mutations are de novo, although rare inherited mutations in *WT1* have been identified. *WT1* mutations are present in approximately 10% of sporadic Wilms

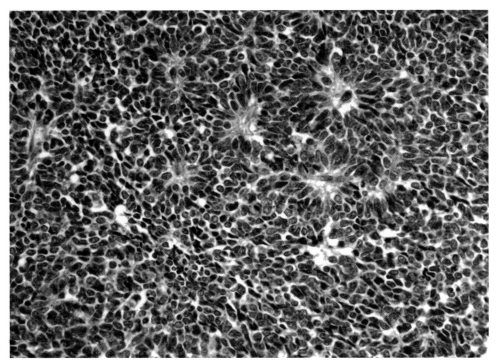

FIGURE 30-3

Blastemal Wilms tumor histology. Undifferentiated small blue cells forming Homer Wright rosettes mimics either the Ewing family of tumors or neuroblastoma.

tumors, and many of these also show β-catenin-activating mutations. Tumors with *WT1* mutations are often associated with intralobar nephrogenic rests and more often show stromal predominant histology. An additional mechanism of epigenetic silencing increases LOH at *WT1* in up to 40% of Wilms tumors. However, approximately 80% of Wilms tumors retain WT1 expression, and immunohistochemistry using antibodies against the WT1 protein is a useful marker when used in a panel to differentiate Wilms tumor from other pediatric renal and small blue cell tumors.

The increased incidence of Wilms tumor in Beckwith-Wiedemann syndrome turned attention to the 11p15 *(WT2)* locus as a possible location of a tumor suppressor. Loss of 11p15 with sparing of the *WT1* locus at 11p13 has also been reported in sporadic Wilms tumors. The imprinted genes *IGF2, H19, LIT1,* and *p57* that have been implicated in Beckwith-Wiedemann syndrome are a few of the possible tumor suppressor candidates.

Diagnostic Factors

No single chromosomal aberration is diagnostic of Wilms tumor. Approximately one third of Wilms tumors yield an apparently normal karyotype. Those with abnormal karyotypes are divided roughly equally between hyperdiploid and pseudodiploid tumors;

hypodiploidy is uncommon. The most common numeric abnormalities include gain of chromosomes 12, 8, 6, and 13 and loss of chromosomes 16 and 22 (Figure 30-4). Structural abnormalities include gain of 1q and loss of 11p, 16q, 1p, 14q, and 11q. Loss of 17p is a common finding in anaplastic Wilms tumors and corresponds to the deletion of *p53.*

Predictive and Prognostic Factors

Risk stratification has historically been based on clinical and pathologic stage and favorable versus unfavorable histology (diffuse anaplasia). Patient age and tumor size play roles in select cases, because children less than 2 years of age with favorable histology, stage 1 tumors, weighing less than 550 g may be eligible for surgery alone. Overall survival for Wilms tumor approaches 90%, but the prognosis for those with relapse or diffuse anaplasia and high-stage disease remains poor. Among the favorable histology groups, molecular markers including LOH for 1p and 16q are being used to potentially identify a group of patients at high risk for relapse.

LOH for 1p and 16q occurs in approximately 11% and 17%, respectively, of favorable histology Wilms tumors. The National Wilms Tumor Study Group investigated whether LOH of 1p and or 16q predicts an adverse outcome. In low-stage tumors

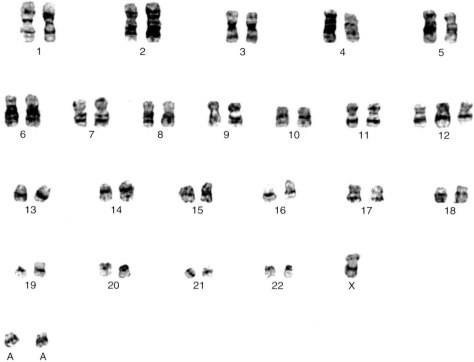

FIGURE 30-4
Wilms tumor cytogenetics. This hyperdiploid karyotype shows trisomy 12, the most common numeric abnormality found in Wilms tumor. (Courtesy of University of Virginia Cytogenetics Laboratory.)

(stage 1 or 2), LOH of either 1p or 16q is associated with increased risk of relapse. However, concurrent loss of 1p and 16q defined a subgroup with the greatest decrease in overall survival. In higher-stage tumors (stage 3 or 4), the adverse effect was limited to the group showing LOH of both 1p and 16q. Thus, loss of 1p and 16q identifies a higher-risk group, regardless of stage, that may potentially benefit from more aggressive therapy.

Congenital Mesoblastic Nephroma

Congenital mesoblastic nephroma (CMN) is a tumor of infancy, and greater than 90% of patients are diagnosed in the first year of life. CMN is subclassified into the classic and the cellular variants, which are genotypically distinct tumors. The classic variant resembles fibromatosis, with fascicles of spindle cells in a variably collagenized background extending into the adjacent renal parenchyma and soft tissue. The immunophenotype is myofibroblastic, and no consistent genetic abnormalities have been reported.

Cellular CMN is likely the renal counterpart to infantile fibrosarcoma, because both are characterized by t(12;15)(p13;q25)*(ETV6/NTRK)*. The details of this molecular alteration are present under the heading of infantile fibrosarcoma.

Clear Cell Sarcoma

Clear cell sarcoma (CCSK) makes up approximately 4% of renal childhood malignancies. Approximately half the cases are diagnosed in the second or third year of life, and males are twice as likely to be affected as females. The classic histologic pattern of CCSK is cords or nests of undifferentiated ovoid cells separated by thin fibrovascular septae, but numerous patterns have been described and often coexist within the same tumor. Patterns include myxoid, sclerosing, cellular, epithelioid, palisading, spindle, storiform, and anaplastic, sometimes making distinction from other tumors difficult. Immunohistochemical analysis shows immunoreactivity for vimentin only in most tumors. The anaplastic variant is immunoreactive to antibodies against p53. Little is known about the genetic events underlying CCSK.

Diagnostic Factors

Cytogenetics studies reveal a variety of numeric and structural abnormalities. Two cases of t(10;17)(q22;p13) have been reported. Gene expression profiling has shown a distinctive pattern with upregulation of neural markers that may be used to distinguish these tumors in large clinical trials and to further investigate the biology of CCSK.

Predictive and Prognostic Markers

CCSK continues to have a worse prognosis than favorable histology Wilms tumor, but significant improvement of survival has been achieved through cooperative group trials. Patients with CCSK had an overall survival of 83% in the fourth National Wilms Tumor Study. No molecular or biologic factors of CCSK have been reported to have prognostic significance.

RHABDOID TUMOR

Malignant rhabdoid tumor (MRT) may be renal or extrarenal or may occur in the central nervous system as an atypical teratoid or rhabdoid tumor. MRTs make up less than 2% of childhood renal tumors but are important to identify because of their distinctive therapy and poor prognosis. MRTs typically arise in children less than 2 years of age. These children are often high stage at the time of diagnosis and present with fever, hematuria, or both. The histologic hallmark is a monomorphous population of relatively discohesive cells with large, eccentric nuclei, prominent nucleoli, and eosinophilic cytoplasmic inclusions. However, a variety of patterns have been described. Immunohistochemically, the cells are polyphenotypic, with reactivity toward vimentin, keratin, epithelial membrane antigen, desmin, and neurofilament. Aberrations of chromosome 22q11.2 are present in 75% to 90% or MRTs. Cloning studies identified this as the locus of the *hSNF5/INI1,* a gene involved in chromatin remodeling and transcriptional regulation. It acts as a tumor suppressor; thus, biallelic inactivation is the rule, with deletions and point mutations being the most common mechanisms. Rare constitutional mutations have been documented that predispose to multiple tumors and are more often sporadic than inherited.

Diagnostic Factors

Despite their aggressive nature, cytogenetic studies of MRTs typically show minimal aberrations. Alterations of chromosome 22 are identified in most cases, either as deletions or as translocations involving 22q11.2 with a variety of partner chromosomes. The INI1 gene can be assessed by LOH studies, FISH, or direct sequencing. Recently, an immunohistochemical stain for the INI1 protein has become available that shows loss of staining in MRT. Small numbers of MRT cases that did not show 22q11.2 genomic aberrations have shown loss of staining, suggesting additional mechanisms for INI1 inactivation.

Predictive and Prognostic Factors

MRT is an aggressive neoplasm with an overall survival rate of 20% to 25%. Mutations in all nine exons of INI1 have been identified, and no correlation with prognosis has been attempted.

RHABDOMYOSARCOMA

Rhabdomyosarcoma (RMS) is the most common soft tissue sarcoma in the first two decades of life, accounting for about half of all soft tissue sarcomas in this age group. RMS consists of a family of tumors that demonstrate near-exclusive skeletal muscle differentiation by morphologic, immunophenotypic, or ultrastructural examination. RMS can be divided into alveolar rhabdomyosarcoma (ARMS) and embryonal rhabdomyosarcoma (ERMS), which includes the favorable botryoid and paratesticular spindle cell subtypes. ERMS tends to occur in younger patients and shows a predilection for the head and neck, genitourinary system, abdomen, and retroperitoneum. It has an embryonal appearance with hyperchromatic, spindle cells, often embedded in a myxoid stroma. Differentiation is usually in the form of strap cells. ARMS affects older patients and most commonly presents as an extremity mass. The morphology is that of a monomorphic round cell that either clings to fibrovascular cores or exhibits nested or sheet-like growth. Giant cells are common, and differentiation is usually as rhabdomyoblasts. Desmin is a highly sensitive marker for RMS but lacks the specificity of myoD1 and myogenin, transcription factors expressed early in skeletal muscle differentiation (Figure 30-5). Most cases are sporadic, but rare cases are associated with Li-Fraumeni syndrome, Beckwith-Wiedemann syndrome, neurofibromatosis type 1, and Costello syndrome and as a second malignancy in patients with inherited retinoblastoma. ARMS is characterized by t(2;13)(q35;q14) or t(1;13)(p36;q14), which juxtaposes the DNA-binding domain of either *PAX3* or *PAX7,* members of the paired box transcription factor family, to the transcriptional activation domain of *FOXO1A(FKHR),* a member of the forkhead transcription factor family. The chimeric protein acts as a more potent transcription factor than wild-type *PAX* through mechanisms of overexpression, nuclear localization, and resistance to inhibitory affects of the N-terminal PAX domain. This novel fusion has oncogenic properties, and downstream candidate target genes include *MET* and *CXCR4.* The pathogenesis of ERMS is less clear, but oncogene amplification seems to play a role in the anaplastic variant.

DIAGNOSTIC FACTORS

No cytogenetic abnormalities are diagnostic of ERMS, but LOH at 11p15 is often present. Most are hyperdiploid, with gains of chromosomes 2, 7, 8, 12, and 13 being most common. Demonstration of t(2;13) or t(1;13) is diagnostic of ARMS and is present in approximately 55% or 25% of morphologically diagnosed ARMS, respectively. The translocation can usually be

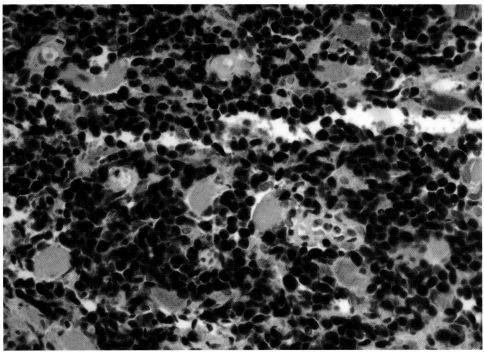

FIGURE 30-5
Alveolar rhabdomyosarcoma (ARMS). Myogenin is a transcription factor expressed early in skeletal muscle differentiation. Diffuse nuclear reactivity supports a diagnosis of ARMS, because staining is usually focal in embryonal rhabdomyosarcoma.

seen on karyotype (Figure 30-6). Common methodologies also include reverse transcriptase–polymerase chain reaction (RT-PCR) and FISH, which show equivalent sensitivity and specificity. RT-PCR requires frozen tissue, because sensitivity drops significantly with formalin-fixed, paraffin-embedded tissue with most described methods. The advantages of RT-PCR are that the fusion partner and breakpoint are identified and it can arguably be more easily run in a panel including other translocations occurring in small blue cell tumors. Furthermore, it may be more amenable for translational research including transcript quantitation and detection of micrometastatic disease in bone marrow. The benefit of FISH is that an FOX01A break-apart probe may detect variant translocations. FISH can be performed on formalin-fixed, paraffin-embedded tissue, but the interpretation can be difficult (Figure 30-7). The disadvantage of the break-apart probe is that the partner is not identified, which may have prognostic implications in the diagnosis of ARMS. Although cases of mixed ARMS and ERMS currently are classified as ARMS for treatment purposes, the translocation is infrequently demonstrated using molecular or cytogenetic techniques.

PREDICTIVE AND PROGNOSTIC FACTORS

Prognostic factors for RMS include tumor histology, stage, tumor burden, site, and patient age. Within the subgroup of ERMS, failure-free survival with localized disease exceeds 80% but drops to 40% with metastatic disease. The botryoid and paratesticular spindle cell variants are considered to have the most favorable histology; unfavorable features include focal or diffuse anaplasia. ARMS is an independent predictor of poor prognosis, with failure-free survival of approximately 65% and 20% for localized and metastatic disease, respectively. Although the *PAX3* and *PAX7* tumors show similar prognosis for localized disease, the *PAX3* tumors have a dismal prognosis when metastatic, with an overall survival of less than 10%. In addition, gene expression analysis has shown upregulation of platelet-derived growth factors and insulin-like growth factors to be associated with decreased survival for all subtypes.

THE EWING FAMILY OF TUMORS

EFT encompasses osseous and extraosseous Ewing sarcoma, peripheral primitive neuroectodermal tumor (PNET), and Askin tumor (PNET of chest wall) and is a prime example of how cytogenetic and genetic data have influenced histologic classification. EFT occurs most often in the second decade of life but may occur in both young children and adults. For extraosseous sites, chest wall, trunk, extremities,

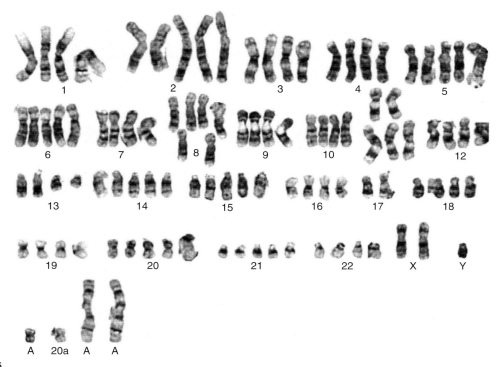

FIGURE 30-6

Alveolar rhabdomyosarcoma (ARMS) cytogenetics. This extreme hyperdiploid, complex karyotype of ARMS shows the diagnostic t(2;13). (Courtesy of University of Virginia Cytogenetics Laboratory.)

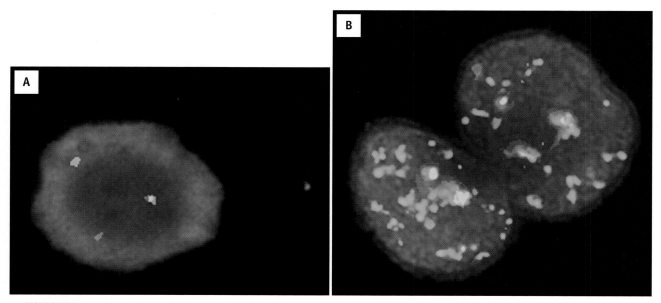

FIGURE 30-7

Alveolar rhabdomyosarcoma (ARMS). **(A)** Using break-apart fluorescence in situ hybridization on paraffin-embedded tissue, the split signal indicates a single *FOXO1A(FKHR)* rearrangement and in the correct setting is diagnostic of ARMS. **(B)** This cell shows amplification of the fusion gene, which is common with the *PAX7/FKHR* variant. (Courtesy of Columbus Children's Hospital Cytogenetics Laboratory.)

abdomen or pelvis, and head and neck are common sites, although EFT has been described just about everywhere. EFT is a small round blue cell tumor and is characterized by a monomorphic population of round cells with finely dispersed chromatin and inconspicuous nucleoli. Cytoplasm is scant and may be slightly eosinophilic, amphophilic, or cleared out. Cytoplasmic glycogen can be demonstrated with periodic acid Schiff. EFT may be difficult to differentiate from undifferentiated NB or poorly differentiated synovial sarcoma. Strong membranous immunoreactivity toward cell-surface glycoprotein CD99 has greatly aided in this diagnosis but may also be present in lymphoblastic lymphoma, RMS, and synovial sarcoma (Figure 30-8). EFT is characterized by a translocation leading to a fusion of Ewing sarcoma gene *(EWS)* on 22q12 to a member of the ETS family of transcription factors, most commonly *FLI1*. The chimeric gene juxtaposes the potent transcriptional activation domain of *EWS* to the DNA-binding domain of ETS. This creates an aberrant transcription factor that is oncogenic, although the downstream targets are not well characterized. *EWS/FLI1* tumorigenesis is likely a result of induction of genes involved in cell proliferation and survival, as well as a repression of genes involved in apoptosis and growth inhibition.

DIAGNOSTIC FACTORS

EFT usually shows a relatively simple karyotype, with few structural and numeric abnormalities. Eighty-five percent of EFT cases have the t(11;22)(q24;q12) *(EWS/FLI1)*, and this, plus variant translocations, characterizes greater than 98% of EFT cases (Table 30-4). The most common secondary abnormality in EFT is an unbalanced translocation der(16)t(1;16)(q21,q13), usually resulting in a gain of 1q and partial monosomy 16q. This aberration is not unique to EWS; it can also be seen in retinoblastomas, Wilms tumors, and RMS, among others. Among numeric chromosomal changes, trisomies 8 and 12 are most often observed.

Although *EWS/FLI1* can usually be detected by routine karyotyping, the variant translocations involving *EWS* are often complex or involve interstitial chromosomal rearrangements and are difficult to detect. FISH can be performed on direct preparations, metaphase spreads, or formalin-fixed, paraffin-embedded tissues and can use fusion gene or break-apart methodology. Although the fusion method can identify the partner, it cannot discriminate a *EWS/FLI1* type 1 variant, which may have prognostic significance. The main disadvantage of break-apart FISH is that neither the

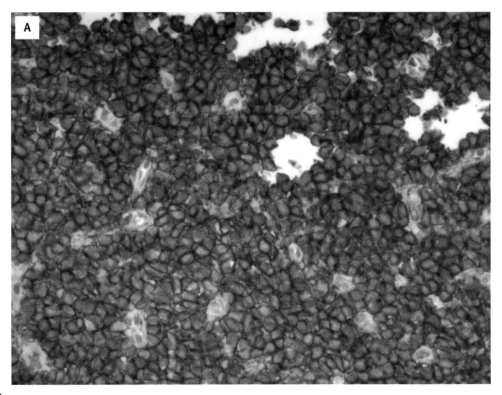

FIGURE 30-8

Immunohistochemistry of the Ewing family of tumors (EFT). **(A)** Strong and diffuse membranous staining with an antibody directed against CD99 is seen in EFT.

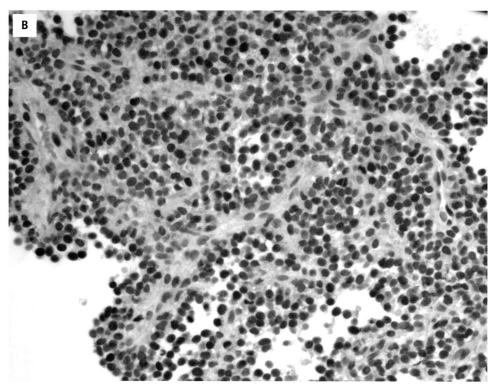

FIGURE 30-8, cont'd.

(B) Nuclear staining for FLI1 supports the diagnosis of EFT but is not specific for this tumor.

breakpoint nor the partner is identified. Thus, the EWS break-apart cannot distinguish EFT from other tumors characterized by an EWS transloca-tion (Table 30-4). RT-PCR using fresh or frozen tissue also is highly sensitive and specific, but nu-merous primers must be used to detect variant

breakpoints or partners. The sensitivity falls ap-preciably using formalin-fixed, paraffin-embedded tissues and is reported around 50% to 75%. A sec-ond potential pitfall of RT-PCR is an exquisite sensitivity for a low level of transcripts that may represent a secondary event in a tumor, but this has not been thoroughly studied. Benefits of RT-PCR are that the primers can be multiplexed and the fusion gene and breakpoint characterized. The tumor-specific fusion can be characterized, and this can be used to assay for low levels of disease in bone marrow.

PREDICTIVE AND PROGNOSTIC FACTORS

No molecular studies are routinely performed that alter the therapy of EFT, but several have po-tential prognostic significance. Studies have sug-gested that the type of *EWS/FLI1* fusion may be of prognostic value. The chromosome translocation breakpoint is restricted to introns 7 through 10 of the *EWS* gene and is variable within the partner gene. The most common rearrangements join exon 7 of *EWS* to exon 6 to 9 of *FLI1* and are designated type 1 fusion transcripts. Type 1 fusions appear to be associated with an improved overall survival over nontype 1 fusions. In general, cases with complex karyotypes with structural abnormalities

TABLE 30-4

Tumors with EWS Translocation and Partner Genes

Tumor	Gene	Breakpoint
Ewing family of tumors	*FLI1*	11q24
	ERG	21q22
	ETV1	7p22
	ETV4 (E1AF)	17q21
	FEV	2q36
Desmoplastic small round cell tumor	*WT1*	11p13
Clear cell sarcoma of soft parts	*ATF1*	12q13
Extraskeletal myxoid chondrosarcoma	*CHN (TEC)*	9q22
Myxoid liposarcoma	*CHOP*	12q13

do worse than those with simpler karyotypes. A mutation of p53 with LOH of 17p13 or a homozygous deletion of the p16/p14^{ARF} at 9p21 collectively occurs in approximately one fourth of cases, and these are highly unfavorable genotypes. Several studies also report micrometastatic disease in the bone marrow detected by RT-PCR as a predictor of poor prognosis, but this requires larger trials for confirmation.

DESMOPLASTIC SMALL ROUND CELL TUMOR

Desmoplastic small round cell tumor (DSRCT) is an aggressive malignancy with a predilection for adolescent and young adult males. An intra-abdominal mass with growth along the peritoneal surfaces is the classic presentation. Solid nests of round undifferentiated cells separated by a desmoplastic stroma are characteristic. Polyphenotypic differentiation with immunoreactivity toward vimentin, keratin, epithelial membrane antigen, desmin, and neural markers aids in the diagnosis, which can usually be made without difficulty in the typical setting. However, cases with an atypical morphology or an unusual location or patient demographic may pose a diagnostic challenge. DSRCT is characterized by a recurrent translocation. The t(11;22)(p13;q12) fuses the N-terminal activation domain of EWS to the C-terminal DNA-binding domain of *WT1*. *WT1* normally acts as a tumor suppressor, but this novel chimeric protein acts as a transcriptional activator with oncogenic properties.

DIAGNOSTIC FACTORS

Karyotyping typically reveals multiple abnormalities and is often complex. A balanced t(11;22)(p13;q12) is present in most cases, which can be visualized on conventional karyotype. Variant translocations that have been described include t(2;21;22)(p23;q22;q13) and t(11;17)(p13;q11.2). The fusion transcript messenger RNA can be detected by RT-PCR in 90% to 95% of cases. The breakpoint is most commonly in intron 7 of *EWS* and intron 7 of *WT1,* with resultant fusion of exon 7 of EWS to exon 8 of *WT1.* Variant breakpoints in intron 8 and 9 of *EWS* have been reported and seem to be associated with atypical presentations. The fusion appears to be specific for DSRCT. However, phenotypic and genotypic overlaps with EFT have been described. FISH analysis is an alternative method, although the *EWS* break-apart probe will not differentiate DSRCT from EFT. *WT1*

expression can be detected by immunohistochemistry in up to 90% of cases, with an antibody directed against the C-terminus.

PREDICTIVE AND PROGNOSTIC FACTORS

DSRCT has an overall poor prognosis, with a 5-year survival rate of 15% to 35%. Metastatic disease is present in about half the cases at the time of diagnosis. The tumor shows a poor response to chemotherapy, and aggressive surgical resection improves patient outcome. Localized tumors in an extra-abdominal location have the best prognosis, likely because of surgical resectability. No histologic or genetic markers are currently predictive of prognosis.

HEPATOBLASTOMA

Hepatoblastoma represents only 1% of pediatric cancer but is the most common malignant liver tumor in children. It almost exclusively presents within the first 5 years of life and usually grows to a large size before detection. Serum α-fetoprotein is elevated in up to 80% of tumors and is a useful marker for recurrent or metastatic disease. The histology of hepatoblastoma may be purely epithelial, which includes fetal, embryonal, macrotrabecular, and small cell undifferentiated (SCUD) variants or mixed epithelial and mesenchymal variants. The diagnostic challenges include differentiating a SCUD variant from other small round blue cell tumors and the macrotrabecular pattern from hepatocellular carcinoma. α-Fetoprotein is often not elevated in hepatoblastoma-SCUD, and the immunophenotype is polyphenotypic with coexpression of vimentin and keratin. Children at increased risk for hepatoblastoma include those with Beckwith-Wiedemann syndrome, familial adenomatous polyposis, and low birth weight. It is unclear if low birth weight is partly a consequence of prolonged medical therapy. Most hepatoblastomas have aberrant Wnt/β-catenin activation with greater than 50% of tumors carrying somatic mutations or deletions in the β-catenin gene, almost exclusively in exon 3. Inactivation of the APC gene is present in familial adenomatous polyposis–associated hepatoblastoma, as well as a subset of sporadic tumors. This results in both cytoplasmic and nuclear localization of β-catenin by immunohistochemistry, which is present in most tumors. LOH at 1p is present in approximately one third of tumors, as is LOH at 11p15. The latter is the site of maternally imprinted genes *p57, H19,* and *IGF2.*

DIAGNOSTIC FACTORS

Cytogenetic abnormalities in hepatoblastoma are divided equally between numeric and structural aberrations. Chromosome gains are more common than losses, and trisomies 20, 2, and 8 are most common (Figure 30-9). The most common translocation involves chromosome 1q, with the partner chromosome being highly varied. Normal or no karyotype generated from culture is not uncommon, and interphase FISH may pick up abnormalities in these cases.

PREDICTIVE AND PROGNOSTIC FACTORS

As of yet, no definitive molecular prognostic markers are able to predict adverse biologic behavior in hepatoblastoma. It is recognized that the hepatoblastoma-SCUD has a poor prognosis, but it is unclear how much of the tumor must show this histology to confer a more aggressive course. The macrotrabecular pattern is also considered unfavorable histology. Data suggest strong nuclear β-catenin staining by immunohistochemistry is associated with unfavorable histology. p27/KIP 1, a kinase inhibitor protein normally expressed in quiescent cells, is downregulated in embryonal and SCUD tumors, as well as tumors resected after chemotherapy, but its independent predictive value is uncertain. A pure fetal histology with low mitotic activity is the most favorable subtype,

and if at stage 1, the patient may be eligible for surgical resection alone.

INFANTILE FIBROSARCOMA

Infantile fibrosarcoma is an uncommon pediatric malignancy diagnosed predominantly within the first 2 years, and it commonly presents in the neonatal period. It has a predilection for the extremities, often distal, followed by the trunk, head, and neck. It is histologically similar to its adult counterpart, with the classic highly cellular herringbone growth and high mitotic activity. However, features such as a prominent hemangiopericytoma-like pattern and hypocellular, collagenized areas of short, intersecting bundles may raise the differential of other benign or malignant lesions, especially outside the classic presentation (Figure 30-10). Infantile fibrosarcoma has identical histology to that of cellular CMN of the kidney, and cytogenetic and molecular studies have created a nosologic link with the elucidation of a common translocation. Up to 90% of infantile fibrosarcomas have a t(12;15)(p13;q26), creating a fusion gene, *ETV6/NTRK3 (TEL/TRCKC)*. The chimeric transcript juxtaposes the dimerization domain of *ETV6* to the tyrosine kinase domain of *NTRK3*. The fusion

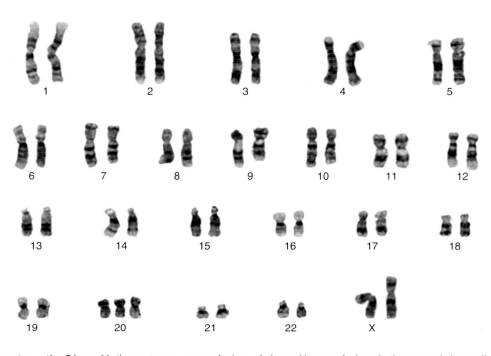

FIGURE 30-9

Hepatoblastoma cytogenetics. Trisomy 20, the most common numeric change in hepatoblastoma, is the only chromosomal abnormality identified in this case. (Courtesy of the University of Virginia Cytogenetics Laboratory.)

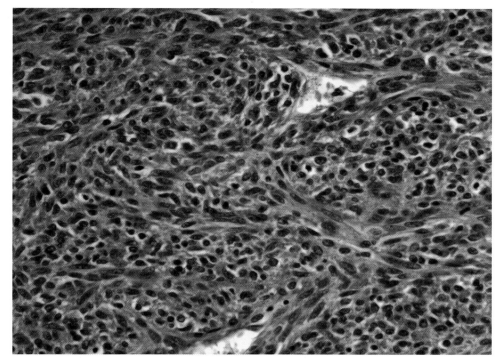

FIGURE 30-10
Infantile fibrosarcoma histology. A prominent hemangiopericytoma pattern in this case raises the differential of a cellular myofibroma or synovial sarcoma.

protein is capable of homodimerization and auto-phosphorylation with constitutive activation of the NTRK3 signal transduction pathways.

DIAGNOSTIC FACTORS

Infantile fibrosarcoma is characterized by recurrent numeric abnormalities, which are likely secondary events in tumor progression. The most consistent is trisomy 11, followed by trisomies 8, 17, and 20 (Figure 30-11). The t(12;15) is often cryptic in a conventional karyotype, and FISH or RT-PCR is indicated in cases negative by karyotype (Figure 30-12). RT-PCR is ideally performed on frozen tissue. Some studies have shown a high sensitivity using formalin-fixed, paraffin-embedded tissue, but others have suggested a much reduced sensitivity compared to frozen tissue. Interestingly, the reduced sensitivity of paraffin has not been appreciated in cellular CMN.

PREDICTIVE AND PROGNOSTIC FACTORS

Although infantile fibrosarcoma may be of an impressive size and locally destructive, metastases are rare, occurring in less than 10% of cases. Complete surgical resection is the mainstay of therapy, and chemotherapy has an established role in surgically

unresectable cases or cases in which excision would result in significant morbidity. Translocation-positive cases are reportedly chemoresponsive, although those that lack the translocation have not been thoroughly studied. The protein kinase activity of ETV6/NTRK3 makes it a potentially attractive target for pharmaceutical therapy.

RETINOBLASTOMA

Approximately 300 cases of retinoblastoma are diagnosed each year in the United States. About 40% are a result of a germline mutation, and most of these cases are bilateral. A small proportion of cases are trilateral, with the development of an intracranial neuroblastic tumor. Sporadic tumors, accounting for most cases of retinoblastoma, are unilateral, and in general the patients are older than those with the germline counterparts. Proper evaluation of the enucleated specimen is critical, because further therapy is based on pathologic staging. Usually, the globe is fixed overnight before cutting, but if the tumor is needed for genetic studies, this should only be done after the optic nerve margin has been removed. Retinoblastoma grows in an endophytic pattern from the

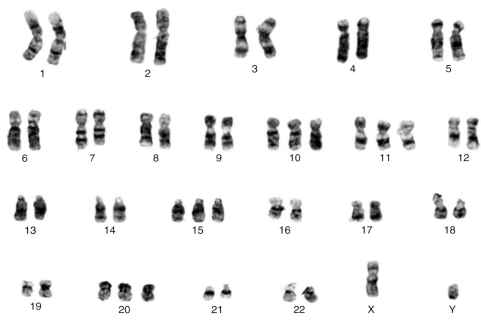

FIGURE 30-11

Infantile fibrosarcoma cytogenetics. Numeric gains of 10, 11, 15, and 20 are present in this infantile fibrosarcoma. The characteristic t(12;15) is cryptic and is not detected in this karyotype. (Courtesy of University of Virginia Cytogenetics Laboratory.)

inner retinal surface into the vitreous cavity or in an exophytic pattern from the outer retinal surface, filling the subretinal space. The histology is that of a small round blue cell tumor composed of sheets, nests, or trabeculae of cells with oval to round nuclei and scant cytoplasm. Retinal differentiation as Flexner-Wintersteiner rosettes and photoreceptor differentiation as florets may be seen, as well as Homer Wright rosettes. The diagnosis usually does

not require immunohistochemistry, but immunoreactivity for neuroendocrine or neuronal markers such as neuron-specific enolase, synaptophysin, S100, and glial fibrillary acidic protein are common. Retinoblastoma is the prototype of Alfred Knudson's two-hit hypothesis. The retinoblastoma gene at 13q14 is a tumor suppressor critical to cell cycle regulation. Biallelic inactivation is the rule, and in most inheritable forms the constitutional hit is a single base-pair

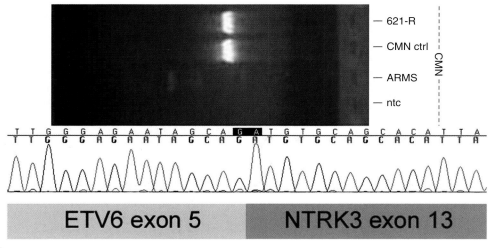

FIGURE 30-12

Infantile fibrosarcoma molecular genetics. **(A)** Reverse transcriptase–polymerase chain reaction analysis for the *ETV6/NTRK* fusion shows a band in the CMN lane. **(B)** The fusion product is confirmed by direct sequencing. 621-R, patient; ARMS, alveolar rhabdomyosarcoma; CMN, congenital mesoblastic nephroma/infantile fibrosarcoma; ntc, no tumor control. (Courtesy of Columbus Children's Hospital Molecular Genetics Laboratory.)